90 0822300 1

# Nutrition in the Clinical Management of Disease

# Nutrition in the Clinical Management of Disease

## Second Edition

Edited by
**John W T Dickerson**

Professor of Human Nutrition, University of Surrey, Guildford;
Formerly Consultant Adviser in Clinical Nutrition, South West Thames Regional Health Authority

and
**Harry A Lee**

Professor of Renal Medicine, University of Southampton;
Director of the Wessex Regional Renal and Transplant Unit

Edward Arnold
A division of Hodder & Stoughton
LONDON BALTIMORE MELBOURNE AUCKLAND

First published in Great Britain 1988

Second Edition, 1988

*British Library Cataloguing in Publication Data*

Nutrition in the clinical management of disease. — 2nd ed.
1. Diet therapy 2. Nutrition
I. Dickerson, John W.T. II. Lee, Harry A.
615.8'54 RM216

ISBN 0-7131-4514-5



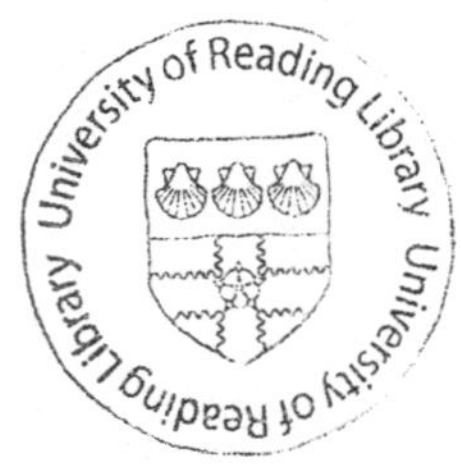


Typeset in 10/11pt California Medium by Colset, Singapore
Printed and bound in Great Britain for Edward Arnold, the educational, academic and medical publishing division of Hodder and Stoughton Limited, 41 Bedford Square, London WC1B 3DQ by Richard Clay Ltd, Bungay, Suffolk

# Contributors

---

Carol Bateman,
District Dietitian,
Hampstead Health Authority,
Royal Free Hospital, London

Israel Chanarin,
Head of Department of Haematology,
Northwick Park Hospital and Clinical Research Centre,
Harrow, Middlesex

Jennifer Coutts, District Dietitian,
Department of Dietetics,
Royal Manchester Children's Hospital,
Pendlebury

John W T Dickerson,
Professor of Human Nutrition,
Department of Biochemistry,
University of Surrey,
Guildford.
Formerly Consultant Adviser in Clinical Nutrition,
South West Thames Regional Health Authority

A. Norman Exton-Smith, CBE,
Emeritus Professor of Geriatric Medicine,
University of London,
Director, Geriatric Neurophysiology Unit,
Whittington Hospital,
London

Michael H N Golden,
Wellcome Senior Lecturer,
Tropical Metabolism Research Unit,
University of the West Indies,
Mona, Kingston,
Jamaica

Susan M Goodinson,
Lecturer in Nursing Studies,
University of Surrey,
Guildford

M A Jackson,
Consultant Physician,
Wolverhampton Health Authority

Harry Keen,
Professor of Human Metabolism.
Director, Unit for Metabolic Medicine,
United Medical and Dental Schools of Guy's and St Thomas's Hospitals,
London

Harry A Lee,
Director of the Wessex Regional Renal and Transplant Unit.
Professor of Renal Medicine,
University of Southampton

Neil McIntyre,
Professor and Chairman of The Academic Department of Medicine,
Royal Free Hospital,
London

E Bruce Mitchell,
Consultant Immunologist,
Blackrock Clinic,
Blackrock,
Dublin

Jane B Morgan,
Lecturer in Nutrition and Dietetics,
Department of Biochemistry,
University of Surrey,
Guildford

Elizabeth M E Poskitt,
Senior Lecturer in Child Health,
Institute of Child Health,
University of Liverpool,
Liverpool

Bashir Quereshi,
General Practitioner,
Hounslow, London

Trevor C B Stamp,
Consultant Physician,
Royal National Orthopaedic Hospital,
Stanmore, Middlesex

B Jacqueline Stordy,
Senior Lecturer in Nutrition,
Department of Biochemistry,
University of Surrey,
Guildford

Briony Thomas
Formerly Research Nutritionist,
Unit for Metabolic Medicine,
United Medical and Dental Schools of Guy's And St Thomas's Hospitals,
London

Celia A Williams,
Lecturer in Nutrition,
Department of Biochemistry,
University of Surrey,
Guildford

Christine M Williams,
Lecturer in Human Nutrition,
Department of Biochemistry,
University of Surrey,
Guildford

J E Wraith,
Senior Registrar,
Willink Laboratory,
Royal Manchester Children's Hospital,
Pendlebury

John Wright,
Consultant Chemical Pathologist,
Department of Biochemistry,
University of Surrey,
Guildford

# Preface to the Second Edition

The first edition of this book was published in 1978. Since then the intervening years have seen further interest in, and appreciation of the importance of nutrition in the total care of patients. For some diseases dietary modification remains the sole means of survival, whilst for others it may enhance the benefit received from other forms of treatment, or simply improve physical and mental well-being. Nutrition is a rapidly changing subject and many questions remain unanswered. However, since the publication of the first edition, advances have been made in a number of aspects of our subject and topics that were omitted have assumed an importance which cannot be ignored. The reception given to the book has persuaded us that we should proceed to a second edition in order to incorporate some of the new findings and changes of direction and opinion.

The preparation of this new edition has involved considerable revision and re-writing in order to accommodate the new material without greatly increasing the size of the book. In this revision, and in the preparation of the additional chapters, we have been careful to maintain our original approach to the subject. This was that the fundamental biochemistry and physiology have been integrated where necessary with discussions of the pathophysiology and treatment of disease. Again, we have not attempted to be exhaustive. Indeed, this would have defeated one of our initial aims which was to produce a book of handy size in which clinicians and nutritionists would find material of direct practical relevance to their patients.

This new edition starts with a discussion of the nutrition of the mother before and after conception. This is followed, as before, by chapters on nutrition during childhood, the dietary modifications necessary in the care of patients with inborn errors of metabolism and protein – energy malnutrition in children. A new chapter has been included on nutritional aspects of different dietary practices, a matter which involves both children and adults. A discussion of the problems of the elderly is followed by separate chapters on obesity, anorexia nervosa and food allergies. This latter topic has now been recognized by many as being the cause of disease in almost all systems of the body. Chapters then follow on nutrition in relation to diseases of a number of systems and on mineral metabolism. The problem of the relationship of nutrition to both the aetiology of cancer and the nutritional problems of patients with cancer is then discussed. This is followed by a discussion of nutrition in relation to disorders of the nervous system. The book concludes with five chapters on more general topics – alcohol, the inter-relationships of nutrition and drugs, the assessment of nutritional status, tube feeds and elemental diets and parenteral nutrition.

These changes have resulted in an increase in the number of chapters to 23 and in the number of pages to about 500.

We are grateful to our colleagues for their willing co-operation in the revision of their chapters and to our new Authors for entering into the spirit of the venture as well as providing what we hope will prove to be a useful addition to the book. This new edition owes much to those who provided us with helpful criticisms of the first edition. Their interest and comments were very much appreciated and we hope that this second edition will consequently be a better and more useful book.

Guildford, 1988

JWTD
HAL

# Contents

# Nutrition for and during pregnancy

Jane B. Morgan



## Introduction

Pregnancy represents only a part of the reproductive cycle of a woman. In a biological sense the cycle can be extended for a further 9 months when the breast takes the place of the placenta (Jelliffe *et al.*, 1975). Indeed, a woman's ability to lactate is nutritionally far more demanding than that of bearing a fetus *in utero* (Thomson and Hytten, 1973).

However, there is no doubt that pregnancy represents a time of physiological stress to the mother primarily because of increases in metabolism associated with the production of new tissue in the placenta, fetal membranes, fetus and mammary gland. Her ability to support and sustain these physiological demands depends not entirely on her nutritional status during pregnancy – her diet prior to conception, indeed from her own conception, has an important influence on the efficiency of human reproduction. The evidence for this is far more convincing than the evidence relating to her diet during pregnancy (Thomson and Hytten, 1973). For example, maternal size has a dominating influence on birthweight. Forty years ago Baird (1945) reported that short mothers giving birth to their first infant had lighter, shorter babies than tall primigravidae. International studies confirm this trend for different ethnic groups, i.e. that mean birthweight increases with maternal height. Thus, the quality of the mother's diet prior to conception is of paramount importance in her ability to bear children successfully.

Pregnancy has been described as a parasitic state – that of the fetus on the mother. However, the mother does have remarkable powers of physiological adaptation. In pregnancy the concentration of many nutrients in the maternal blood circulation is reduced (albeit that the pattern of these changes varies depending on the substance) compared with levels occurring in the non-pregnant state. Hytten and Chamberlain (1980) have suggested that these changes favour the transfer of substances across the placental barrier to the fetus.

Therefore it may be closer to the truth to describe the relationship between healthy well-nourished women and their fetus as a state of symbiosis, and the full benefits become apparent to both the mother and her offspring only when breast feeding is fully established.

This chapter will consider our knowledge concerning the impact of nutrition on the reproductive performance of normal healthy women. It will also be concerned with the effects that various specific disorders (obesity, hypertension) have on the outcome of pregnancy, and the occurrence of primary nutritional deficiencies seen more commonly in pregnancy than in the non-pregnant state. A section on disadvantaged women within the community, e.g. women who exist on very low incomes or in extreme poverty or deprived conditions, and the pregnant adolescent will complete the chapter.

## Nutrition and pregnancy in the normal state

For a woman to support a fetus successfully throughout pregnancy she must be healthy and free from infection, both prior to conception and through the 9 months gestational period.

Figures of perinatal and infant mortality rates and birthweight are statistics used frequently to measure the success or otherwise of pregnancy since there is an inverse relationship between infant mortality and birthweight. (It is of interest to note that data are rarely collected on the woman herself to estimate or evaluate the physiological consequences of pregnancy to her.) Nutritional status at the time of conception is a culmination of a woman's lifetime nutritional experience and is an important determinant of reproductive efficiency (King *et al.*, 1972).

### Diet prior to conception

#### Diet and fertility

The effect of malnutrition, and in particular undernutrition, on a woman's ability to conceive is probably unimportant as suggested by the high birth rates among Asian and African women living in very deprived circumstances (Davidson *et al.*, 1979).

The acute food shortage suffered by the Dutch and Russians in World War II did, however, appear to affect fertility rate. Antonov (1947) reported that in Leningrad (where the siege lasted from August 1941 to January 1943) in the first and second halves of 1942, 414 and 79 women respectively entered the maternity clinic to have their infants. Amenorrhoea was widely prevalent. This drop in the birth rate was almost certainly due to psychological as well as nutrition stress.

**The influence of maternal size prior to conception on the outcome of pregnancy**

In the many studies published concerned with the health of the neonate, maternal nutritional status and body size have shown a positive correlation with fetal size and vitality. Fig. 1.1 shows such a relationship of mean maternal height and mean birthweight among populations from Scotland, Hong Kong and India.

One interpretation that can be made from these types of results is that small infants are proportionate to the small size of their mothers. In well-nourished women the shape of the pelvic brim is round. In short, stunted women the posterior segment of the brim is flattened. A lighter, smaller fetus would certainly make delivery easier in these women (Davidson *et al.*, 1979).

It has been advocated (Nutrition Reviews, 1979) that there is a need to consider a woman's pre-pregnant weight in evaluating weight gain during pregnancy. Thus the optimal weight gain which was associated with reduced perinatal mortality rates has been reported at 13.6 kg for very thin mothers compared with 7.3 kg for overweight mothers (see p. 10).

**The influence of periconceptional vitamin supplementation in the development of specific birth deformities**

Amongst possible birth defects those of the neural tube (spina bifida and anencephaly) have been the object of intense epidemiological study (Smithells, 1982). Over the last 20 years, evidence has been accumulating that there may be a nutritional component in the environment contributing to these defects (Schorah *et al.*, 1983). Recently the specific effect of preconceptional

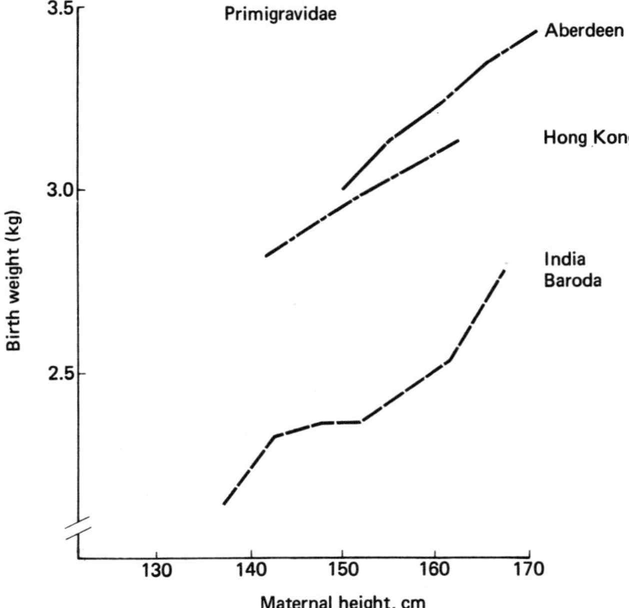


Fig. 1.1 Mean birthweight (kg) by maternal height (cm) in primigravidae women living in Aberdeen, Hong Kong and Baroda, India.

supplementation of certain vitamins (particularly of the B group) in women at risk of giving birth to a baby with a neural tube defect (NTD) has been investigated. Professor Smithells and colleagues (Smithells *et al.*, 1980) reported from five centres that of 178 infants of the multivitamin supplemented high risk mothers only one had a NTD; the proportion in the controls was 13 out of 260.

However, there exists real doubt that vitamin supplementation can prevent NTD and indeed supplementation could possibly be harmful (Lancet, 1984). A multicentre (16 UK centres, 11 overseas centres) randomized study (The MRC Vitamin Study) is to investigate the effect of extra vitamins around the time of conception on a mother's chance of having a baby with a NTD (Lancet, 1984).

## Diet from conception to birth

### Assessment of nutritional status

A balanced picture of nutrition in relation to human pregnancy can be obtained from four general categories of observation: records of large population groups; data from subjects who are hospitalized or attend clinics regularly; extrapolation from animal studies; controlled prospective studies of patients receiving prescribed diets.

To obtain accurate dietary data that reflect true intakes throughout pregnancy is a difficult task and large epidemiological studies rely on 24 hour recall which is of limited value. Smaller controlled studies are often conducted in artificial circumstances, e.g. hospitals, where subjects are 'abnormal' physiologically speaking. Animal studies have also been criticized – rodents and ruminants obviously cannot mimic the human being. There is, however, value in extrapolation from one species to another if the limitations are recognized, as their contribution is fundamentally important in the understanding of complex biochemical and physiological processes. Thus our knowledge today is based on a combination of facts gathered from a variety of sources. As a result recommended daily allowances (RDA) for nutrients from various authorities differ and margins of safety vary (Table 1.1). From Table 1.1 it is apparent that recommendations by the expert committees are made for extra energy needs during pregnancy. These types of recommendations are based on the factorial approach. In other words the total energy cost of pregnancy is estimated to be 335 MJ (80 000 kcal), 12 per cent of which is accounted for by the products of conception, and the remainder divided between the 3.5 kg maternal fat deposition and energy cost of maintenance metabolism, estimated to be 150 MJ (36 000 kcal). This could be met by increasing food intake by an additional 1.2 MJ (290 kcal) per day. The daily increment recommended by the DHSS (1979) is 1.0 MJ (240 kcal), the NRC/NAS (1980) and the FAO/WHO/UNU (1985), 1.2 MJ (285 kcal). However, recent studies on well-nourished mothers do not indicate that these increased levels of intake were attained, though maternal weight gain and birthweight were well within the normal range (see p. 6).

### Weight gain during pregnancy

Conventional recommendation dictates that on average 12.5 kg is gained by the end of the 9 months. Gain in weight occurs slowly at first so that by the end

Table 1.1 Recommended intakes of food energy and nutrients from two authorities relating to non-pregnant and pregnant women

| | UK DHSS 1979 | | USA NRC/NAS 1980 | |
|---|---|---|---|---|
| | Non-pregnant | Pregnant | Non-pregnant | Pregnant |
| Weight (kg) | — | — | 55.0 | — |
| Weight gain (kg) | — | 12.5 | — | 10–12 |
| Total energy (MJ) | 9.0 | 10.0 | 8.4 | 9.6 |
| Protein (g) | 54.0 | 60.0 | 44.0 | 74.0 |
| Vitamin D ($\mu$g) | 10.0 | 10.0 | 7.5 | 12.5 |
| Folacin ($\mu$g) | No set recommendation | | 400 | 800 |
| Vitamin $B_{12}$($\mu$g) | No set recommendation | | 3.0 | 4.0 |
| Calcium (mg) | 500.0 | 1200* | 800 | 1200 |
| Iron (mg) | 10.0 | 13.0 | 18.0 | B |
| Zinc (mg) | No set recommendation | | 15.0 | 20 |

* Third trimester only
B Recommend 30–60 mg supplement (see 1980 report)

of the first 20 weeks 3.5 kg is gained. Thereafter a gain of 0.5 kg per week is usual up to the time of delivery. Fig. 1.2 shows the components of this weight gain. An estimate of the components of weight gain during pregnancy in rural women from Guatemala (Lechtig *et al.*, 1975) shows that 7.0 kg is gained – of which approximately 2.0 kg is fat.

More than one-third of the weight gain in normal pregnancy can be accounted for as fat (3.5 kg–4.0 kg; Davidson *et al.*, 1979). This has a dual role in the reproductive cycle. Firstly it can be regarded as a buffer against possible food shortage in the last trimester when the products of conception double in weight (from approximately 2530 g at 30 weeks to 4750 g at 40 weeks, Davidson *et al.*, 1979). Secondly, Naismith (1983) has postulated that the substantial fat reserve may have an important role in meeting the high energy costs of lactation.

The figures above should be seen as average values, the variation around the mean is wide. Excessive weight gain (i.e. greater than 50 per cent of the mean) or inadequate gains (i.e. 50 per cent less than the mean) could be incompatible with a healthy outcome to pregnancy. This will be discussed in the section on specific disorders (see p. 9).

**Energy requirements**

The concept of increased energy requirements in pregnancy to the order of 10 per cent above the recommendations for a non-pregnant woman has recently been under scrutiny (Naismith, 1983). There is now good evidence from longitudinal dietary surveys that well-nourished women on self-selected diets do not increase their food consumption above pre-pregnancy levels.

In the UK the assessment of dietary intakes of women has shown a consistent downward trend in recent years (Whitehead *et al.*, 1981). Furthermore, several studies have indicated that women can have normal pregnancies and breastfeed their children normally even though their energy and nutrient

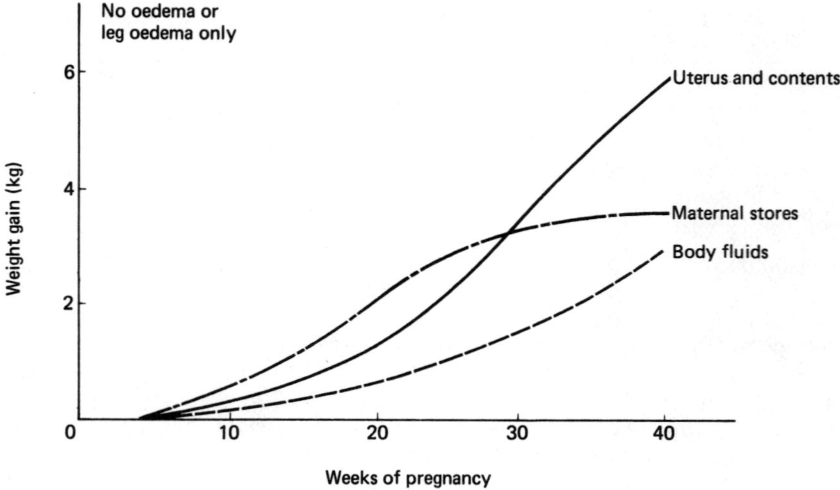


Fig. 1.2 The components of weight gain in normal pregnancy.

intake is far below recommended standards. There are data which suggest that because of cultural and physiological adaptations the extra energy requirements may be minimal.

In response to this situation a longitudinal multicentre study of the energy requirements of pregnant (and lactating) women was initiated in 1980 to allow the formulation of more realistic recommendations (Durnin *et al.*, 1985). Table 1.2 shows the results for energy intake data from one centre – Glasgow. A longitudinal study of 25 women from Cambridge has provided similar dietary data and is included in Table 1.2 (Whitehead *et al.*, 1981).

It is clear that the energy intake of the women involved in these two studies

Table 1.2 Mean daily energy intake (MJ (kcal)) and body weight changes (kg) for mothers reported by various investigators during 1st, 2nd and 3rd trimesters

| Study | Location | Weight gain (kg) | Energy intake MJ (kcal)/day Trimester 1st | 2nd | 3rd |
|---|---|---|---|---|---|
| Darby *et al.*, (1953) | Nashville, USA | 7.7* | 8.95 (2140) | 9.20 (2200) | 8.45 (2020) |
| Lunell *et al.*, (1969) | Stockholm, Sweden | 12.1 | 8.28 (1980) | 10.02 (2395) | 8.72 (2085) |
| Whitehead *et al.*, (1981) | Cambridge, UK | 12.6 | N/A | 8.16 (1950) | 8.39 (2005) |
| Durnin *et al.*, (1985) | Glasgow, Scotland | 11.9 | 8.80 (2100) | 8.80 (2100) | 8.93 (2400) |

* Calculated from authors data, baseline weight provided from first trimester only

N/A Not available

did not increase greatly during the course of pregnancy, and did not reach the levels recommended for pregnant women by the expert committees (see Table 1.1). Indeed they were comparable to values for the non-pregnant, non-lactating women. In spite of this the mean weight gain during pregnancy was within the normal range. The implication of these types of findings is that the additional needs for energy to support growth during pregnancy are satisfied by subtle changes in activity or by an enhanced efficiency of metabolism.

In the light of these findings, that in pregnancy there are energy conservation adaptations taking place, current recommendations may be set too high.

**Maternal energy balance – metabolic adaptation to conserve energy?**

During the 9 months of pregnancy certain adaptive mechanisms occur which have a major impact on maternal energy balance. First – fat storage and mobilization is under hormonal influence. For example, the accumulation of depot fat is under the control of the hormone progesterone secreted by the feto-placental unit and the corpus luteum. The hormone oestriol is believed to curtail fat deposition. During the third trimester when the fetus trebles in weight and the demands of pregnancy increase (i.e. extra maternal cardiac and respiratory work are required) the hormone placental lactogen is released. This mobilizes the stored fat which acts as a major source of energy during this period (Fig. 1.3).

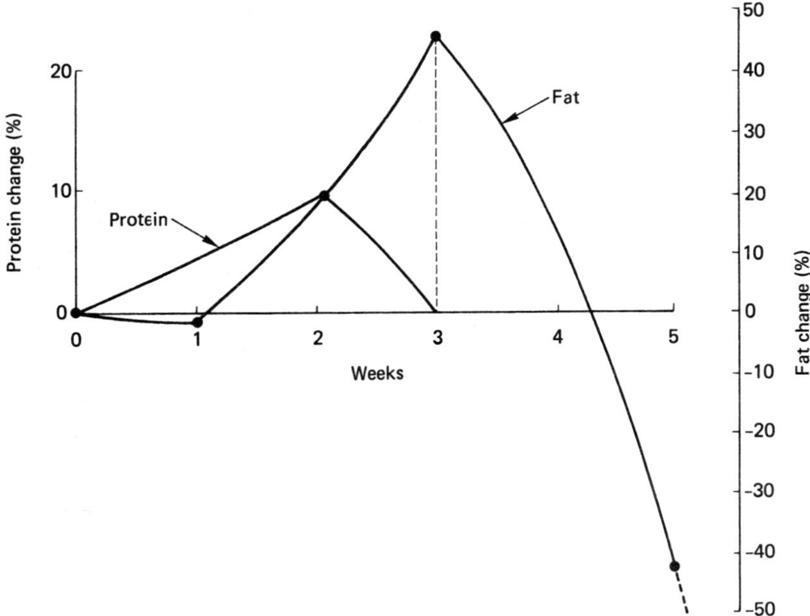


Fig. 1.3 Changes in the proportion of protein and fat in the carcasses of rats at different stages of reproduction.

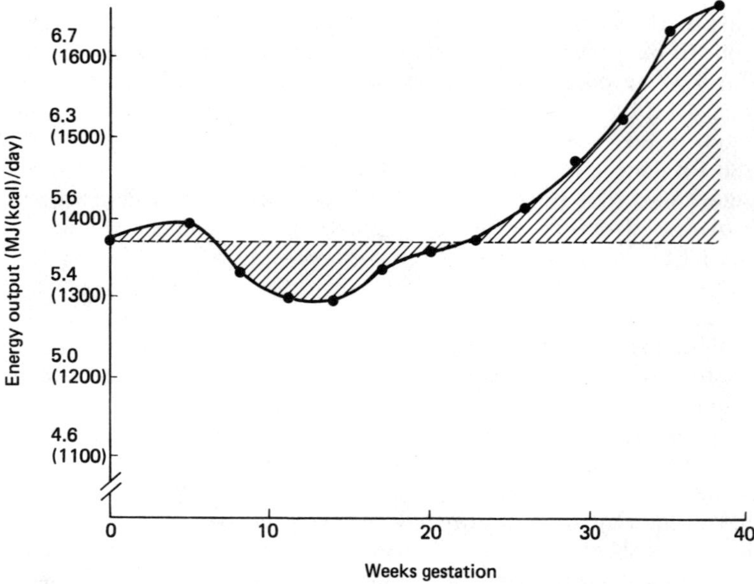


**Fig. 1.4** Changes in basal metabolic rate throughout pregnancy (MJ (kcal)/day). The dotted line represents pre-pregnancy value of 5.7 MJ (1365 kcal)/day.

In parallel with these phenomena is a substantial compensatory alteration in the non-pregnant component of the mother's physiology – she becomes a more efficient energy machine. Whitehead (1981) suggested from the results of their study (discussed in the previous section) that enhanced efficiency of metabolism occurs together with subtle changes in activity levels. Recently comprehensive data on energy expenditure in pregnant women have indicated that this might be the case. The preliminary data from Glasgow indicates that one component of energy expenditure – basal metabolic rate – is depressed in the first half of pregnancy (Durnin *et al.*, 1985). Figure 1.4 illustrates this. The authors reported that the physical activity of this group of pregnant women did not alter over the last few weeks of pregnancy. However, in the group of 67 women studied food intakes remained fairly constant and the total extra energy intake represented less than 84 MJ (20 000 kcal). Studies from the developing world add support to the argument that a normal pregnant woman does not require extra intake of food energy to match the theoretical cost of pregnancy. The pattern of change in resting metabolic rate measured in a group of rural Gambian women 'deviated substantially from that assumed in current theory', (Lawrence *et al.*, 1984) and the net extra cost of tissue maintenance was 4.2 MJ (1 000 kcal) – 3 per cent of the theoretical cost.

The third component of energy expenditure, diet-induced thermogenesis, where excess energy derived from food is converted to heat and dissipated, may be attenuated in the pregnant woman. Thus her thermic effect of feeding in response to a meal (Stock and Rothwell, 1982) may be reduced compared with her pre-pregnant state. Animal studies (the rat and mouse) have provided some evidence for this in pregnancy (Naismith and Brookes, 1983) and lactation (Trayhurn *et al.*, 1982).

These mechanisms of energy conservation are still in the early stages of investigation.

**Protein requirements and adjustments to protein metabolism**
It is generally accepted that total protein deposition at term is 925 g which corresponds to rates of 0.6, 1.8, 4.8 and 6.1 g/day over four stages of pregnancy. The factorial approach has been used to formulate recommendations which therefore provide a daily additional allowance (see Table 1.1). This allowance is assumed to cover the needs for both maternal physiological adjustments and growth and development of the conceptus. Recommendations from authorities vary, from 6.0 g/day in the UK (DHSS, 1979) to 30.0 g/day in the USA (NRC/NAS, 1980). It should also be noted that the USA recommendation for protein intake in non-pregnant women is 10 g/day less than the value of 54 g/day for women in the UK. Thus the extra protein allowance from USA recommendations seems more generous (see Table 1.1).

Just as energy metabolism adapts to pregnancy, so too does protein metabolism. Naismith (1983) has hypothesized from results of animal studies (principally the rat) that protein may be stored in the early gestational months (the anabolic phase) and then mobilized at the later stages (the catabolic phase) when the demands are greatest (see Fig. 1.3). These processes are probably under hormonal control, and progesterone appears to exert an anabolic effect by inhibiting the production of a catabolic hormone, corticosterone.

The implications of these findings of animal studies to the human situation are twofold. First, increased protein needs during pregnancy may be uniformly spread throughout the course of gestation. Secondly the influence of acute or chronic maternal undernourishment on the outcome of pregnancy is minimized by this mechanism.

The extra amount of protein recommended by the DHSS (1979) is equivalent to 10 per cent of the extra energy recommended in the same report. This supplement of protein from a mixed diet (which assumes the net protein utilization of 75) should be achieved with little difficulty by women consuming well-balanced diets. Indeed it could be argued that such women can readily provide the theoretical protein requirements for the fetus because of their habitual over-consumption of this nutrient along with most others.

## Nutrition and specific disorders

### Obesity and pregnancy

**Introduction**
Women do not begin pregnancy in a uniform state, nor does the course of pregnancy go forward in a uniform manner. For example, there will inevitably be a proportion of women who are overweight (110 per cent of ideal body weight) or obese (120 per cent of ideal body weight) at the onset of pregnancy, and a proportion of women who will gain excessive amounts of weight over the 9 months gestational period, thereby predisposing to obesity.

Indeed to be able to advocate the optimal weight gain that a mother should achieve during her pregnancy has exercised the minds of physicians for 150 years in an attempt to prevent excessive or inadequate weight gain. Both these circumstances would bring unacceptable consequences to the mother and her offspring.

Naismith (1983) has described the physiological changes that occur to a woman during her pregnancy as analogous to changes reported in obese people. Certainly changes already described relating to her adaptive mechanisms in energy balance can only predispose her to a tendency for rapid weight gain in pregnancy (see p. 7).

Two questions therefore need to be asked. First, should a woman who is already overweight at the onset of pregnancy be advised to restrict her diet in order to reduce the incidence of complications (e.g. pre-eclampsia, hypertension) and to enable her to achieve a more desirable body weight postnatally? Secondly, should a woman who appears to be gaining weight rapidly (particularly in the first 3 months of pregnancy) be advised to instigate an energy reducing diet to prevent the probability of finding herself obese at the completion of her reproductive cycle?

The answer to both questions appears to be no for physiological and psychological reasons.

**Abnormal weight gain, dietary restriction, and their consequences in pregnancy**

As there is strong evidence linking maternal diet, maternal weight gain and birthweight of the infant, one of the criteria used to assess normal weight gain is the incidence of abnormality in the newborn infant (Nutrition Reviews, 1979). A large scale study (Table 1.3) of 10 000 births indicates that women who gained more than 16.4 kg had fewer low birthweight infants than women who gained less than 6.8 kg. Similarly in a more recent study of 44 565 women (Naeye, 1979) the author reported that those who gained the least weight had twice the perinatal mortality rates compared with mothers with larger weight gains.

Compounding these observations, however, is the effect of the mother's pre-pregnancy weight, subsequent weight gain and the outcome of pregnancy. Table 1.4 provides information on a study conducted in the USA on approximately 4000 women where mothers had been selected into one of three body size categories. Wynn and Wynn (1975) concluded from this series that 'weight

Table 1.3 Influence of mother's weight gain during pregnancy on percentage of low birthweight babies born in the USA 1968 (10 000 births) (Wynn and Wynn, 1975)

| Pregnancy weight gain of mother (kg) | Percentage of infants born under 2500 g |
|---|---|
| 16.4+ | 3.0 |
| 11.8–16.4 | 4.3 |
| 7.3–11.7 | 8.2 |
| 0–6.8 | 15.2 |

Table 1.4 Proportion of low birthweight infants produced by mothers of different weights at the onset of pregnancy (3939 white mothers) (Wynn and Wynn, 1975)

| Weight at pregnancy onset (adjusted for height) | Percentage of infants with birthweight under 2500 g |
|---|---|
| Heaviest 10 % | 2.3 |
| Middle 10 % | 4.2 |
| Lightest 10 % | 7.8 |

before pregnancy is the second most important correlate of birth-weight after weight gain during pregnancy'. The Collaborative Perinatal Project reviewed by Naeye (1979) confirmed this – that a mother's optimal weight gain in pregnancy depends on her body build and that optimal weight gain of an overweight mother is about half that of a very thin mother. It should be noted that optimal weight gain for a normally proportioned woman was 9.1 kg in the aforementioned study compared with the conventionally accepted value of 12.5 kg.

The general consensus of opinion today seems to be that dietary restriction in pregnancy is not advisable and indeed to impose food intake limitations at a time when appetite is noticeably good is unnecessarily harsh. Results from animal studies have shown that to impose food restrictions on pre-existing obesity in a pregnant animal does impair fetal growth (Lederman and Rosso, 1981). This implies that the fetus cannot utilize maternal nutritional stores to prevent growth retardation even if the mother is obese.

Dietary restriction has in the past been recommended for two reasons; that the risks of middle aged obesity and the dangers of pre-eclampsia are minimized. In a review article Hytten (1979) states that there are no medical grounds to substantiate these claims. Furthermore the practicalities involved cannot be ignored. Women find restricting food intake during pregnancy a difficult task (Dieckmann, 1952), and frequently excessive weight is gained in the first trimester before antenatal clinics are routinely attended, therefore before practical advice can be given (Hytten, 1979). Perhaps only the grossly obese or those making excessive gains should be directed to curb their appetites.

To those women who purposefully restrict their intake to guarantee a quick return to their pre-pregnancy figure, the dire consequences of this practice should be emphasized, consequences that encompass not only the harmful effects on the maternal nutritional status, but to the unborn fetus (i.e. possible increased incidence of low birthweight).

Practical advice to women who are anxious to minimize or avoid obesity would be fruitfully directed towards the encouragement of breastfeeding for as long as possible, and then to consider sensible slimming at the completion of the reproductive cycle, if it is found to be necessary.

## Diabetes and pregnancy

The clinical management of diabetes has been discussed elsewhere (Chapter 8, p. 167).

## Hypertension associated with pregnancy

### Introduction

Classic books of nutrition in the 1960s from the UK (Davidson and Passmore, 1969) and the USA (Wohl and Goodhart, 1964) used the term 'toxemia of pregnancy' to describe disorders relating to high blood pressure, oedema and albuminuria which complicated the management of pregnancy. This term had been used for over a century (Gant and Worley, 1980) and covered a multitude of disorders including hyperemesis gravidarum (severe morning sickness) and acute yellow atrophy of the liver. Management included a strict dietary regimen, that is a restricted protein diet of 45–60 g/day and a restriction of sodium to 0.5 g/day (Davidson and Passmore, 1969), together with control of weight gain.

However, no toxin has ever been identified and the term 'toxemia' is no longer appropriate. Thus, the disorders relating to hypertension in pregnancy can be defined as follows (Gant and Worley, 1980).

A. Pregnancy-induced hypertension
   1. Pre-eclampsia
      a. mild
      b. severe
   2. Eclampsia

B. Chronic hypertension preceding pregnancy (any aetiology)
C. Chronic hypertension (any aetiology) with superimposed pregnancy-induced hypertension
   1. Superimposed pre-eclampsia or
   2. Superimposed eclampsia
D. Late or transient hypertension

The diagnosis of mild pre-eclampsia is traditionally based on mild hypertension (140/90) with proteinuria and/or oedema in the 20th week gestation. It is seen more commonly in primigravidae than multigravidae. The incidence reported from a Scottish survey was 24 per cent and 10 per cent respectively in the primi- and multigravidae (Davidson *et al.*, 1979). Anecdotal evidence from the USA suggests that pregnancy-induced hypertension (PIH) is seen more frequently in young black primigravidae from the lower social strata though race and socio-economic status *per se* cannot be directly linked to its aetiology (Chesley, 1971).

Severe PIH (severe pre-eclampsia) is diagnosed when blood pressure is raised over 160/110, with proteinuria of at least 5 g/24 hours together with oliguria, pulmonary oedema, and cerebral and visual disturbances. This condition is rare – 5 per cent and 1 per cent reported in primigravidae and multigravidae respectively from a Scottish survey (Davidson *et al.*, 1979).

Eclampsia is an extension of severe pre-eclampsia and is recognized by the onset of epileptic fits (grand mal in character).

For a full account of PIH see Gant and Worley (1980).

The pathogenesis of PIH is not known, but is almost certainly multifactorial, including trophoblastic, immunological, hormonal and nutritional in origin (Gant and Worley, 1980). Of the nutritional factors implicated the varied intake of protein, salt or even vitamin $B_6$ have been suspected as being causative from observations of epidemiological, clinical and laboratory studies (Wohl and Goodhart, 1964). More recently attention has been focused on the role of essential fatty acids, particularly arachidonic acid deficiency, as a causative factor (Gant and Worley, 1980). A strong association was reported between low plasma zinc levels and the incidence of PIH in a subgroup of 48 adolescent pregnant girls (Cherry *et al.*, 1981). The authors concluded that the influence of maternal zinc intake and plasma zinc levels on hypertension in pregnancy required further investigation (see also pp. 19 and 26).

**Weight and weight gain**

The interrelationship between the mother's pre-conceptual weight, her weight gain during pregnancy and PIH has been a matter of much debate and dispute. For example 'toxemia of pregnancy' was stated to be frequently seen in women who were overweight at the time of conception or who gained excessive weight from the second trimester onwards (Wohl and Goodhart, 1964). Women who were underweight at the onset of pregnancy were also said to be vulnerable to PIH.

Chesley (1976) in his comprehensive review 'Historical developments' states that it became the usual practice of American obstetricians to limit weight gain during pregnancy to 6.8–9.1 kg as a prophylaxis against pre-eclampsia. The practice of weight control during pregnancy, he states, is based on spurious data, and in PIH total gain during pregnancy is of no importance 'unless a large

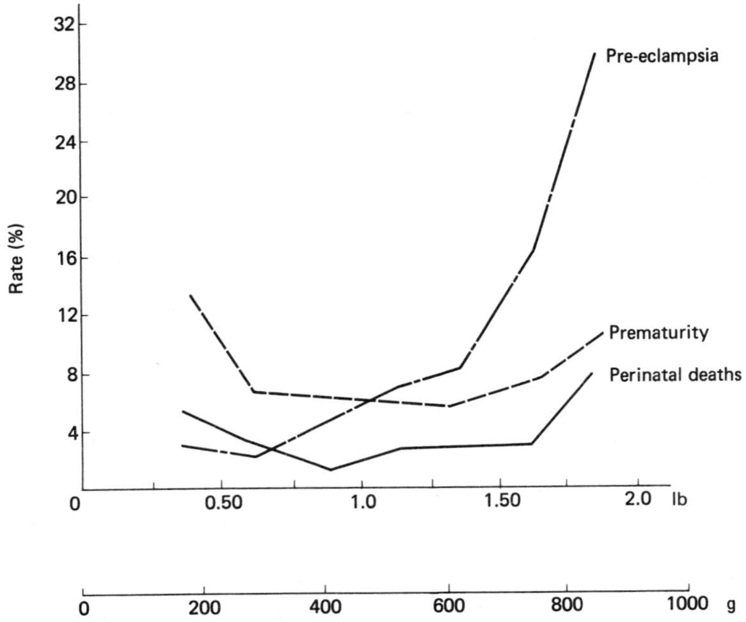


Fig. 1.5 Incidence of three major obstetric complications by mean weight gain between 20 weeks and delivery. (Prematurity = birthweight 2500 g or less).

component of the increment represents retention of fluid'. Indeed, excessive weight gain is a symptom used in the diagnosis of the disease (Fig. 1.5).

Pre-pregnancy maternal weight is, however, implicated (Gant and Worley, 1980). Obesity is second only to persistent hypertension through the 10th day after the previous delivery as an important factor determining the recurrence of PIH in subsequent pregnancies (note – as a predictive factor, not a causative one). Thus, the importance of pre-conceptional counselling regarding weight prior to conception is again emphasized, particularly in those known from previous pregnancies to be predisposed to this disorder.

**Does diet play a role in the management of pregnancy-induced hypertension?**
The answer to this question is probably no. It is unnecessary to restrict fluids or protein, certainly in mild pre-eclampsia. Nor is sodium restricted, although there is an element of self-induced restriction for patients with more severe forms, as illness prevents the consumption of solid foods. Protein intake should be reduced in patients with severe PIH who are hospitalized (Davidson *et al.*, 1979).

## Morning sickness (hyperemesis gravidarum) in pregnancy

The nutritional or clinical implications of morning sickness on the outcome of pregnancy are not a cause for concern unless the state persists. Certainly in the first trimester of pregnancy many women suffer as it is unpleasant, affecting over 50 per cent of pregnant women (Morgan, 1980). Although the specific cause is not known it is probably due to metabolic adaptations and changes in endocrine levels because of the growth of the fetus and placenta.

No better remedy has been suggested than dry toast and plain biscuits with tea early in the morning or when the sickness occurs. This practical advice together with the necessity to maintain a balanced and adequate food intake will ensure the mother does not suffer from nutritional deficiencies.

Occasionally the symptoms persist and worsen and a psychological component is suspected (Davidson *et al.*, 1979). In these cases hospitalization is necessary. Measures may be required to correct the metabolic imbalance that may have occurred as a result of the persistent vomiting, and the patient should receive fluids, electrolytes and vitamins (Davidson *et al.*, 1979).

## Pregnancy and alcohol intake

### Introduction

Alcohol and pregnancy do not mix (Nutrition Reviews, 1982c). For the mother who drinks moderately (10–50 g pure ethanol per day – 1 to 5 drinks) before or during pregnancy there are indications that this practice may be harmful to the outcome of pregnancy. It may retard intra-uterine growth, it may adversely affect fertility and the completion of pregnancy. In the mother addicted to alcohol it may cause the fetal alcohol syndrome (FAS) (Pratt, 1982). Both the Royal College of Psychiatrists in the UK and the Surgeon General in the USA recommend that women should abstain from all alcohol during pregnancy. Pratt (1982) has suggested that good motherhood begins at conception and it is not acceptable for any woman of child-bearing age to consume any alcohol unless she can be reasonably certain of not becoming pregnant. Heavy drinking or alcoholism prior to pregnancy affects fetal growth detrimentally, even with abstinence during pregnancy (Little *et al.*, 1980). This type of advice is controversial, and if there is a totally safe level of consumption it has yet to be ascertained.

Mothers who are chronic alcoholics are likely to suffer from various nutritional deficiencies and primary liver damage. Both these conditions may predispose towards the development of abnormalities.

**The fetal alcohol syndrome and intra-uterine growth retardation**

Few babies are born to the severely alcoholic woman. Therefore the incidence of FAS is correspondingly reduced and has been reported as 1 in 600 births (Table 1.5). Nearly all babies identified as having FAS are born to mothers who drink heavily on a daily basis, or certainly at frequent intervals. An amount of 90 ml ethanol per day has been stated as being a major risk to the infant, (Pratt, 1982).

Comprehensive reviews of the FAS have been given by Pratt (1982) and Nutrition Reviews (1982b). Weight and body length of the infants are less than the usual norms and poor growth is sustained postnatally. There are characteristic facial abnormalities including a short upturned nose, and the vernilion area of the upper lip is narrow. Mental retardation is common. Children aged 1–10 years with FAS have been shown to be immune deficient with an increased susceptibility to infection compared with matched controls (Nutrition Reviews, 1982d).

The mechanism which predisposes these effects is uncertain, but it seems likely that ethanol may exert a direct toxic or teratogenic effect upon the developing embryo in early pregnancy. Pratt (1982) has postulated three mechanisms.

Table 1.5 Increase in risk of abnormal fetal development from maternal alcohol consumption (as incidence %) (Pratt, 1982)

| Maternal alcohol intake g/day approx. | Congenital malformation | Abnormal behaviour (usually hyper-activity) | Mental deficiency IQ < 70 | Cerebral palsy | Small for gestational age (>2 SD below mean) | Characteristic fetal alcohol syndrome |
|---|---|---|---|---|---|---|
| 0–9 | 5 | 10 | 2–3 | 0.2 | 4 | 0 |
| Low | 9 | | | | 9 | |
| | 10 | | | | 9 | |
| 10–50 | 12 | 11 | | | 4 | |
| Moderate | 14 | | | | 9–11 | |
| >50 | 10 | 29 | 19 | 8 | 1 | 2.5 |
| heavy | 17 | 41 | 23 | | 15 | 13 |
| | 32 | | 44 | | 24 | 10–12 |
| | 38 | | 61 | | 29 | 25 |
| | | | | | | 26 |

IQ = Intelligence quotient

1. Pre-existing liver damage will make likely the circulation of poisonous metabolites of ethanol breakdown in quantities large enough to reach the developing fetal brain.
2. Liver damage may also disturb the balance of amino acids in the maternal and fetal circulation. There is evidence for this with the placental uptake and transfer of valine to the rat fetus (Patwardhan *et al.*, 1981). Thus, the inhibition of the accumulation of essential amino acids to the fetal circulation could contribute to the impairment of fetal growth as well as the dysgenesis associated with FAS.
3. There is the possibility that alcohol-induced hypoglycaemia may cause central nervous system dysfunction to which the fetus is susceptible.

Maternal nutritional deficiencies may be associated with FAS. Zinc deficiency may complicate alcoholism and could cause congenital defects (Nutrition Reviews, 1982a).

Growth retardation has been reported in infants of mothers consuming relatively small amounts of alcohol (see Table 1.5). In a study of 262 middle class women the author (Little, 1977) suggested that birthweight was reduced by 3 g for every 1 g of alcohol consumed in early pregnancy. Pratt (1982) has estimated that intra-uterine growth is retarded by 1 per cent for every 10 g alcohol consumed daily, during pregnancy.

A recent study by Wright and colleagues from London (Wright *et al.*, 1983), on 900 white women concluded that drinking more than 100 g alcohol per week, particularly at the time of conception, increased the risk of a low birthweight infant. Statistical adjustments were made for social class and cigarette smoking. Indeed the effect of alcohol was synergistic with that of smoking.

**Practical advice to women planning pregnancies**

Women should be encouraged to attend pre-conceptional clinics. There they should be advised to reduce their intake of alcohol to less than 100 g per week (10 drinks), prior to conception, and to give up smoking. To advocate total abstinence would be ideal as even the occasional drink may impose a minimal but preventable risk.

There appears to be no benefit to the fetus from a reduction of alcohol intake in the latter stages of pregnancy, though a mother should be encouraged to do so for her own wellbeing.

## Pregnancy and the occurrence of primary nutritional disease

### Introduction

To minimize the possible deleterious effects that pregnancy may impose on the nutritional status of the mother, changes occur in the mechanisms of absorption and utilization of specific nutrients which protect both the maternal physiology and the supply of nutrients to the fetus via the placenta. There is a general alteration in the level of circulating nutrients (particularly of iron) which has been termed haemodilution, but this term is now considered inappropriate (Thomson and Hytten, 1973). Plasma levels of retinol, ascorbic acid, biotin, folate and $B_{12}$ fall. However, those of carotene, tocopherols and cholesterol rise. Hytten and Chamberlain (1980) have hypothesized that the general lowering of nutrient levels in the blood produces a balance which favours transfer to the fetus rather than to the maternal tissues. Thus it has been stated that well-nourished women need not receive special supplements of minerals or vitamins, the exception to this state of affairs may be iron (see Thomson and Hytten, 1973).

The improved utilization of vitamins and minerals in pregnancy reflects an adjustment to the homeostatic mechanisms which are present in the non-pregnant state to prevent the excessive accumulation of nutrients. The mechanism controlling the absorption of calcium provides an example of this adjustment. The calculated daily accretion rate of calcium by the human fetus is 59 mg/day and 330 mg/day at 24 weeks and 36 weeks gestational age respectively (Shaw, 1973). The maternal absorption of dietary calcium (normally 20–30 per cent of an average intake of 500 mg/day) has been shown to increase in early pregnancy (Heaney and Skillman, 1971) in preparation for the high fetal demands in the third trimester (for details see below).

These types of adjustments are probably hormonally controlled (Hytten and Chamberlain, 1980; Naismith, 1983).

However, primary nutritional deficiencies do occur when these homeostatic mechanisms are not able to protect the maternal nutritional status through chronic deficiency, or increased requirement due to genetic predisposition.

## Calcium in pregnancy

### Requirement

The increment of calcium in the fetal skeleton is 30 g (Hytten and Chamberlain, 1980) which represents only 2.5 per cent of the calcium in the maternal skeleton. Hytten and Leitch (1971) have emphasized that lactation is a far more demanding process in terms of calcium depletion from the mother's own sources, (be it her diet or her skeletal stores) than is pregnancy. In a situation of plenty, not only will the fetal skeleton be calcified but there may be calcification of the maternal skeleton too.

Five hundred millilitres of milk provides 600 mg (15 mmol) calcium which is half the RDA (DHSS, 1979) for women in the third trimester. However these levels are achieved only in the Western world where calcium in the diet is plentiful. Reeve (1980) has estimated that the minimum intake below which calcium deficit is inevitable would be 400–600 mg (10–15 mmol) per day. Fifty per cent of dietary calcium has been shown to be absorbed by Indian women consuming these types of intakes.

### Deficiency of calcium and vitamin D

Epidemiological studies of customary food intakes of pregnant women living in the impoverished areas of the world have shown that intakes of calcium below 400 mg (10 mmol) are rare. Calcium deficiency therefore occurs only in a situation of poor absorption. Reeve (1980) has postulated that absorption fails because:

1. the gut is unresponsive to $1,25(OH)_2D_3$, for example in coeliac disease and
2. there is a lack of $1,25\ (OH)_2D_3$.

Marginal deficiency of vitamin D (for whatever reason) would result in maternal osteomalacia. Successive pregnancies would exacerbate the situation. Asian mothers living in the UK are vulnerable to this condition. Reeve (1980) has suggested a daily supplement of 10.0–12.5 μg cholecalciferol to those women at risk in the community (which would include women of Asian origin in Britain) should be routinely implemented.

## Iron in pregnancy

### Requirement

In pregnancy there is an increased requirement for iron. The mother acts as a 'hostess' to her fetus who can preferentially transfer iron across the placenta by active transport (mainly in the last 4 weeks of pregnancy) at the expense of the maternal stores. An infant born to an anaemic mother is rarely anaemic.

A mixed Western diet can supply approximately 14 mg iron per day (Chanarin, 1978). Absorption occurs along the upper 40 cm of the small intestine, and the mechanism is carefully controlled. Letsky (1980) provides a full account of the mechanism involved. The availability of iron from foods varies greatly. For example iron in cereals and eggs is poorly absorbed. Iron is well absorbed when it is present with meat, fish or liver.

Iron-deficiency anaemia is more common among pregnant women compared with non-pregnant women, and an incidence of 32 per cent was reported in a survey from Scotland among women who were described as being mildly anaemic (Davidson *et al.*, 1979).

The requirement for iron in pregnancy has been estimated by the factorial method. This requirement is derived from the expansion of the red cell mass (570 mg); the iron transferred to the fetus (200–370 mg); the iron content of the placenta (35–100 mg); blood loss in delivery (100–250 mg); and breast feeding (100–180 mg). This amounts to 700–1400 mg per pregnancy (Letsky, 1980). There is a saving of 240–480 mg iron because of amenorrhoea. This increased demand corresponds to a requirement of 4 mg per day in the second half of pregnancy compared with the non-pregnant state of 1–2 mg/day. During the second half of pregnancy absorption may reach 40 per cent of intake.

The RDA (DHSS, 1979) for iron in pregnancy is raised above that in the non-pregnant state to 13 mg/day (see Table 1.1); 'this would often be sufficient but some women become anaemic and need medical supplements of iron' (DHSS, 1979).

### Deficiency

Iron-deficiency anaemia is characterized by a fall in haemoglobin. In a healthy non-pregnant woman the lowest normal level of haemoglobin is accepted to be 12.0 g/100 ml; for the healthy pregnant woman the lowest acceptable value should be 10.6 g/100 ml (Letsky, 1980). Although gestation may run its course with no complications in women whose haemoglobin levels are below 11.0 g/100 ml, a number will be shown to be iron or folate deficient. Anaemia leads to tiredness and shortness of breath.

Prophylactic supplementation with elemental iron has been recommended for all women with haemoglobin levels of less than 12.0 g/100 ml when examined at the initial antenatal visit (Davidson *et al.*, 1979). The iron content of the supplement does vary, that is from 180 mg/day (Davidson *et al.*, 1979),

30–60 mg/day to pregnant women with iron stores, or 120–240 mg/day to those with none (Letsky, 1980). If 60–80 mg/day is taken by women consuming a Western-type diet, the haemoglobin level will be maintained within the normal range, but iron stores will not be replenished.

A supplementation trial on 647 pregnant women in India, 80 per cent of whom had haemoglobin levels less than 11.0 g/100 ml, was conducted to evaluate the impact of iron (the amount varying from 30 mg to 240 mg/day), folic acid and $B_{12}$. The results were disappointing, and 59 per cent of the women remained anaemic at the conclusion of the trial (Nutrition Reviews, 1975).

Ideally, women who are at particular risk in developing iron deficiency anaemia should receive medication, probably by the daily administration of ferrous iron. This category includes women with a history of anaemia, multiple births or frequent pregnancies. Less easy to identify but certainly as vulnerable are women who require a higher than average intake. Certainly iron supplementation to all those women should be routine.

**Iron supplementation and zinc status**

Meadows *et al.* (1981) have suggested that iron supplementation in pregnancy may increase the requirement for zinc – a serious situation, as the same group have shown that maternal leucocyte zinc depletion is associated with impaired fetal growth (see below). However, results from studies on the rat have not confirmed these findings (Fairweather-Tait *et al.*, 1984).

## Zinc in pregnancy

**Requirement**

The healthy adult human body contains 2.0 g of zinc.

Dietary zinc is essential to man as it is an integral part of enzymes involved in most major metabolic pathways. Recent studies on rats have indicated that maternal dietary zinc intake during pregnancy has a protective role for the fetus against toxic levels of lead (Nutrition Reviews, 1980).

Dietary zinc deficiency in pregnancy, on the other hand may have profound effects on the successful outcome of pregnancy (Nutrition Reviews, 1976; Cherry *et al.*, 1981).

Dietary intake of zinc for an adult female consuming a Western-type diet has been reported to be 7.6 mg/day (Lyon *et al.*, 1979) of which approximately 40 per cent is absorbed (Stamp, 1978).

The USA have included zinc in their table of recommended allowances. In pregnancy the RDA is increased from 15.0 mg/day to 20.0 mg/day (NRC/NAS, 1980). This increased recommendation is based on the estimated fetal requirement of 0.75 mg/day, with a generous safety factor included. In fact two-thirds of the fetal zinc requirement is acquired in the last trimester of pregnancy (Widdowson *et al.*, 1974) and this is therefore the time when the mother is particularly vulnerable to dietary deficiency.

**Deficiency**

Experimental zinc deficiency in pregnant animals (e.g. the rat) has profound effects on the developing fetus including decreased DNA replication in the brain and decreased total body and liver zinc content (Nutrition Reviews, 1976). At birth physical malformations have been described in the offspring together with behavioural disturbances.

The third trimester appears to be the vulnerable period in relation to these changes, as it is the period of 'extreme sensitivity' in the fetal requirement for zinc (Nutrition Reviews, 1976). A few days' deficiency appears to precipitate serious and lasting effects on the fetus.

It is possible, therefore, that maternal zinc deficiencies may cause similar changes in the human fetus (Meadows *et al.*, 1981) though at present there are few studies to support such hypotheses.

## Vitamins in pregnancy: folate and $B_{12}$

### Requirement

Vitamin $B_{12}$ or cobalamin is required together with folate for the formation of red blood cells. Man obtains preformed $B_{12}$ from foods of animal origin, and folate from a wide variety of foods. Deficiency of folate and more rarely vitamin $B_{12}$, for whatever cause, gives rise to megaloblastic anaemia, and a mild temporary form develops in about 2 per cent of pregnant women in the UK (Chanarin, 1978).

$B_{12}$ absorption in pregnancy is unaltered and most $B_{12}$ in food is available for absorption. Muscle, red cell and serum $B_{12}$ concentrations fall during pregnancy (205–1025 μg/l to 20–510 μg/l at term) and lower levels are found with multiple pregnancies (Letsky, 1980). Low levels seen in strict Hindu vegetarians affect serum fetal content adversely. Maternal $B_{12}$ stores appear to be unaffected by pregnancy.

Plasma folate levels fall as pregnancy advances (Letsky, 1980). However, there is no change in its absorption during pregnancy despite early reports to the contrary. The fall in serum folate from 6.0 μg/l in the non-pregnant state to 3.5 μg/l in pregnancy may be advantageous to both the maternal and fetal well-being. Firstly the lower levels may be protective against raised maternal glomerular filtration rate, i.e. urinary losses would be minimized. Secondly, placental transfer may be more efficient at these levels.

The non-pregnant adult requires 400 μg folate per day and this figure is doubled in pregnancy (NRC/NAS, 1980). Adequate intake can be guaranteed by daily supplementation of 300–500 μg, which is usually given in conjunction with iron.

Recommended daily intake of vitamin $B_{12}$ is raised from 2.0 μg in the non-pregnant state to 3.0 μg in pregnancy (DHSS, 1979). This should be met in all but those consuming vegan diets. Strict vegetarians and vegans would be well advised to supplement their diet during pregnancy.

### Deficiency

The cause of megaloblastic anaemia in pregnancy is almost always due to long standing folate deficiency in the Western world, and there is a marked increase in its incidence (10 per cent) in multiple pregnancy. Symptoms include tiredness, lassitude, shortness of breath and a sore mouth or tongue. Chanarin (1978) has a full account of the clinical features.

Pregnant women who have megaloblastic anaemia usually suffer from iron deficiency – and both are invariably due to poor nutrition. These cases respond dramatically to oral ingestion of 10 mg folic acid (Davidson *et al.*, 1979), and iron supplementation.

On a world-wide scale megaloblastic anaemia is seen more frequently in areas where malnutrition is prevalent. Here supplementation (possibly not selective) throughout the course of gestation is indicated.

# Nutrition and vulnerable groups in the community

## Nutrition and intervention programmes

### Introduction

Birthweight has an important influence on the health and survival of the infant. The incidence of low birthweight infants is high among women who live in environmentally and economically deprived conditions. Wharton (1978) estimates that in Britain 7 per cent of infants are born 2.5 kg or less, in Nigeria the figure is 20 per cent and in India 35 per cent. Birthweight is affected by social class and birth order (Table 1.6).

One of the several factors associated with impaired fetal growth, or shortened length of gestation, or both, is inadequate maternal food intake (Nutrition Reviews, 1984). Other factors associated with low birthweight are multiple pregnancies, high altitude residence, poor hygiene and low socio-economic status. These factors are either non-interventional or influenced by long-term intervention only, i.e. they are not cost-effective. Nutrition intervention to pregnant women whose dietary intake is limited by poverty or food shortage could be cost effective, thus the addition of food to these women's customary diet is an attractive proposition.

There are now a number of supplementation trials which have evaluated the effectiveness of improved maternal nutrition on subsequent birthweight (Table 1.7).

Projects have been conducted in the developing (Guatemala, Columbia, Mexico, India, Taiwan, The Gambia) and the developed (New York, USA, and Birmingham, UK) world. Naismith (1983) has summarized in detail three intervention studies, from Guatemala, Columbia and Taiwan. A comprehensive review is also to be found of the studies from The Gambia and New York in Nutrition Reviews (1984).

Table 1.6 Mean birthweights by social class and birth order with adjustment to maternal height (Hytten and Leitch, 1971)

| Birth rank | Social class I + II | III IV V | Difference in birthweight (kg) |
|---|---|---|---|
| First | | | |
| Mean birthweight (kg) | 3.23 | 3.14 | 0.09 |
| 2nd and 3rd | | | |
| Mean birthweight (kg) | 3.34 | 3.28 | 0.06 |

Table 1.7 Effect of maternal dietary supplementation on birthweight

| | Total supplement | | | | Customary |
|---|---|---|---|---|---|
| | Energy | Protein | Birthweight | | diet |
| Population(n) | MJ (kcal) | g | Mean g | <2500 g % | Mean MJ (kcal) |
| Guatemala | | | | | |
| (A)(192) | 30.12 (7200) | 506 | 2997 | 18 | 6.52 (1560) |
| (B)(165) | 175.73 (42 000) | 2953 | 3114 | 9 | N/A |
| Colombia | | | | | |
| (C)(200) | 0 | 0 | 2927 | 11 | 6.69 (1600) |
| (D)(207) | 58.99 (14 100) | 1 865 | 2978 | 9 | N/A |
| Taiwan | | | | | |
| (E)(111) | <41.84 (10 000) | 0 | 3067 | 7 | 8.37 (2000) |
| (F)(114) | 937.22 (224 000) | 11 200 | 3111 | 3 | N/A |
| The Gambia | | | | | |
| (G)(Dry)(42) | 1,112.94 (266 126) | 9800 | 2892 | 8 | 6.20 (1485) |
| (H)(Wet)(51) | 1,288.67 (308 146) | 11 480 | 3030 | 5 | 5.45 (1305) |
| New York | | | | | |
| (J)(102-985) | 1,240.00[a] (296 510) | 4760‡ | 3193* | 10 | 7.23 (1730) |

‡ WIC Programme food provided not as a supplement but as a 'substitution'.
Nutrient values calculated from authors' information
* No supplementation – birth weight 3057, 136 g impact

**The supplements used – which nutrient?**

The primary consideration which determines the nutrient of most importance for supplementation is the diet of the pregnant women (Lechtig *et al.*, 1975). For example if the limiting factor in the diet is protein, increasing protein intake alone without increasing energy intake may result in an increase in birthweight.

Because of this, and because of the differing circumstances of the women in the various studies that have been undertaken the nutrient content of the supplement differed, but usually contained energy or protein or both. For example The Gambian supplement consisted of 4.0 MJ (950 kcal) and 3.5 g protein/day in the dry season and 4.6 MJ (1100 kcal) and 41 g protein/day in the wet season in the form of groundnut-based biscuits and vitamin fortified tea drinks (Prentice *et al.*, 1983). In the Bacon Chow Study in Taiwan (McDonald *et al.*, 1981) on 294 women the supplemented group received 3.3 MJ (790 kcal) and 40 g protein/day as a sweetened liquid in a can. The supplement which was introduced into the mother's diet also differed, at various stages, for example from before conception and throughout pregnancy (Taiwan Study) or restricted to the third trimester only (Columbian Study).

It was apparent from the results of the studies described above that a lack of energy rather than protein was the factor most likely to limit fetal growth and that there existed a nutritional threshold below which intervention would benefit the outcome of pregnancy. This threshold appears to be 7.0 MJ (1680 kcal) per day (Naismith, 1983).

The effectiveness of the supplementation programme on birthweight was disappointing. Naismith (1983) has commented that marginally nourished mothers recruited into supplementation trials have infants whose birthweights 'remain stubbornly below those of infants born in Europe and the USA' (see Table 1.7). For example, increments of 117 g in Guatemala, and 44 g in Taiwan were reported. In The Gambia an increase of 186 g was achieved in the wet season, with no effect in the dry season. The authors (Prentice *et al.*, 1983) concluded that in the dry season the pregnant women consumed less than 6.3 MJ (1500 kcal) per day but gained 1.3 kg per month and that therefore they were in positive energy balance due to high metabolic efficiency. The result of this was that the supplement was ineffectual. Factors such as maternal stature and level of energy output must also have an impact on the effectiveness of the supplement. Lechtig *et al.* (1975) calculated that the anticipated input of a nutritional intervention on birthweight should range between 25 to 84 g of birthweight per 42 MJ (10 000 kcal) ingested during pregnancy.

The question must therefore be asked, do these types of programmes benefit the mother? The answer is probably yes, i.e. increased weight gain in pregnancy will probably improve lactational performance. Assessing results in this manner has not apparently been performed as a priority.

**Are the supplements utilized as the programmes intended?**

Traditional customs and taboos limit the impact of supplements in some cultures (Nutrition Reviews, 1984). Some pregnant women purposely limit their food intake to reduce the size of their infant at birth. The supplements can be shared out to other members of the family, or of the total supplement given only a small proportion is consumed by the women. In the women, infants and children (WIC) programme conducted in the USA in the 1970s (Edozien *et al.*, 1979) the supplement provided to pregnant women (31 qt milk, 54 eggs, 32 oz cereal and 6 × 46 oz fortified fruit juice per month) was used as a substitute for and not an addition to existing energy intakes, although protein intakes were increased compared with control values. Overall weight gain in pregnancy was greater compared with controls (no figures provided). Thus existing attitudes and actual needs within the community are prerequisites to the success of any programme.

In adequately fed women there is a lack of association between food intake (particularly energy intake) and birthweight due to the wide individual variation in both parameters within the biological norm. Results from the intervention programme indicate that food supplementation should be targetted to those most at risk, because unless a woman is in negative energy balance the supplement will prove ineffectual. This is because of the existence of the minimum (threshold) level of intake required to obtain an adequate birthweight (Lechtig *et al.*, 1975). Above this level pregnant women can adapt successfully to a wide range in energy intake (see p. 7) without affecting birthweight. Within a community some individuals respond to the supplement more successfully than others. In the selective supplementation study of 45 pregnant Asian mothers (Viegas *et al.*, 1982) living in Birmingham, UK, the nutritionally at-risk mothers produced heavier infants than their well-nourished sisters provided with a similar supplement. Thus poor nutrition contributed to poor growth even in a developed country.

Results from epidemiological studies in human populations, together with data from animal studies and experiments on nitrogen balance of pregnant women led Lechtig and colleagues to conclude that nutrition intervention during pregnancy, and not pre-conceptually, has a greater impact on improvement in birthweight (Lechtig *et al.*, 1975). The long-term benefits of a short-term cost effective programme may only become apparent in the next generation, for improving the health and nutritional status of infants and should lay the foundation for improved reproductive performance in later life.

## Nutrition and the pregnant adolescent

**Introduction**

Young, physiologically immature, primigravidae (less than 17–18 years of age) are a subgroup within the pregnant community who can be described as being at risk in many aspects of pregnancy not least being their nutritional status. Their social and economic circumstances are frequently inadequate. Their food habits will reflect that of any adolescent – thus they will be in the habit of:

1. bizarre eating periods;
2. slimming fads;
3. irregular meals; and
4. living on snacks and convenience foods.

A comprehensive review of teenage food habits is provided by Truswell and Darton-Hill (1981).

The pregnant teenager is at risk nutritionally for two important reasons. First she is biologically still immature and her requirements for certain nutrients are higher than those of the adult because of extra growth demands. Secondly she may not have the reserves of nutrients required to meet the impact of pregnancy. However, these concepts have recently been challenged (Rosso and Lederman, 1982). In their review 'Nutrition in the pregnant adolescent' they argue that pregnant teenagers are not necessarily biologically immature, the secular trend in the average age of menarche having fallen in the USA so that now it is 12.5 years. Secondly the concept of 'competition between the needs for maternal growth and fetal growth' should be reconsidered in the light of present day knowledge.

A longitudinal study over 30 years of 56 women conducted in Harvard ('The Longitudinal Studies of Child Health and Development of the Harvard School of Public Health') (Valadian, 1981) has shown that women who consumed diets high in protein during early adolescence were more likely to have successful and uncomplicated pregnancies compared with the remainder. Teenage multiparas are at even greater risk as the physiological stress imposed by the state of pregnancy is inevitably compounded.

**Birthweight**

Hytten and Chamberlain (1980) reported that age does have a slight effect on birthweight i.e. within parities birthweight is reduced with increased maternal age. This may be because young women tend to gain more weight than do older women (Nutrition Reviews, 1979). In fact parity appears to exert a greater effect on birthweight than age *per se* – first babies being, on average, 100 g heavier than second and subsequent parities. (For a full account, refer to Hytten and Leitch, 1971 Chapter 10). Data from the USA suggests that the pregnant adolescent has a high risk of giving birth to a low birthweight infant (<2 500 g), and the incidence of neonatal mortality is greater than in the older age groups. Under 15 years of age the neonatal mortality rate is 41.2 per 1000 live births compared with 17.3 per 1000 live births for women 30–34 years of age (Rosso and Lederman, 1982).

Further insight into the determinants of fetal maturation of infants born to young adolescent mothers is provided by a study on 412 young girls in Lima, Peru (Frisancho *et al.*, 1984). A reduction in birthweight of the order of 114 g was reported in infants born to young (13–15 years) 'still-growing' teenagers compared with mothers who had completed their expected growth in height.

**Energy requirements, vitamin and mineral status**

Studies on the requirement for energy and for nutrients in pregnant teenagers 'are most often reported from the US, probably because of the high incidence of women under 20 years of age who become pregnant' (twenty per cent compared with 7 per cent in Sweden) (Rosso and Lederman, 1982). The subjects tend to be located in low income groups, are unmarried, and from various racial backgrounds.

Teenagers who are pregnant have been described as being a sedentary group of girls – spending 90 per cent of their time lying down or seated (Blackburn and Calloway, 1974)! King *et al.*, (1972) reported in their study from California that no nutrient examined in 18 subjects was 'adequately supplied' when compared with the USA recommended allowances. Mean daily energy intake was reported as 7.95 MJ (1900 kcal). With the recent scrutiny of energy allowances it is possible that these values are indeed adequate. However, even if the quantity of the diet does not give cause for concern the quality almost certainly does.

Little data is available on energy output in this group. Blackburn and Calloway (1974) reported a 17 per cent rise in RMR in the third trimester compared with post-partum values in 8 women participating in their study. This is close to other reports. The calculated daily energy requirement in this group of women (by the factorial method) was 10.0 MJ (2400 kcal).

Zinc and vitamin $B_6$ status have been studied in depth in the pregnant teenager (Cherry *et al.*, 1971; Schuster *et al.*, 1981). The authors from both studies reported cause for concern with respect to these nutrients and the possible detrimental effects to the outcome of pregnancy.

King *et al.* (1972) measured the intakes of a number of nutrients by 18 pregnant teenagers, and reported that the intake of no nutrient met the recommended allowance. The intakes of iron, calcium and vitamin A were particularly at risk. Five of the girls had iron deficiency anaemia. Zinc intakes were not recorded. The authors noted that although some pregnant girls did attempt to improve their intake, many did not. Vitamin and mineral supplements were not taken and much of the medical advice went unheeded.

**Practical measures**

Generally the pattern of life in this group of teenagers reflects that from the disadvantaged section of the community. In any evaluation of their nutritional and clinical state the effect of alcohol, smoking and other drugs must be included as these substances have a profound effect on the outcome of pregnancy.

The pregnant adolescent frequently consumes the same low intake of certain nutrients as her non-pregnant sister. Pre-conceptual advice (at school) on sound nutritional guidelines may help to improve this situation, and should be followed up and reinforced at antenatal clinics. Whether the pregnant teenager chooses to comply with such advice has yet to be evaluated.

## References

Antonov, A.N. (1947). Children born during the siege of Leningrad in 1942. *J. Pediatr.*, **30**, 250–59.

Baird, D. (1945). The influence of social and economic factors on stillbirths and neonatal deaths. *J. Obstet. Gynaec. Brit. Cwlth.*, **52**, 217–34.

Blackburn, M.L. and Calloway, D.H. (1974). Energy expenditure of pregnant adolescents. *J. Am. Diet Ass.*, **65**, 24–30.

Blackwell, R.Q., Chow, B.F., Chinn, K.S.K., Blackwell, B. and Hsu, S.C. (1973). Prospective maternal nutrition study in Taiwan: rationale, study design, feasibility and preliminary findings. *Nutrition Reports International*, **7**, 517–32.

Chanarin, I. (1978). Anaemias and coagulation disorders of nutritional origin. In *Nutrition in the Clinical Management of Disease*, pp. 236–45. Eds. Dickerson, J.W.T. and Lee, H. Edward Arnold: London.

Cherry, F.F., Bennett, E.A., Bazzano, G.S., Johnson, L.K., Fosmire, G.J. and Batson, H.K. (1981). Plasma zinc in hypertension/toxaemia and other reproductive variables in adolescent pregnancy. *Am. J. Clin. Nutr.*, **34**, 2367–75.

Chesley, L.C. (1971). Hypertensive disorders in pregnancy. In *Williams Obstetrics* 14th ed., p. 721. Eds. Hellman, L.M. and Pritchard, J.A. Appleton: New York.

Chesley, L.C. (1976). Historical developments. In *Blood Pressure, Edema and Proteinuria in Pregnancy*, pp. 45–7. Ed. Friedman, E.A. Alan R. Liss Inc.: New York.

Darby, W.J., McGanity, W.J., Martin, M.B. Bridgforth, E., Densen, P.M., Kaser, M.M., Ogle, P.J., Newbill, J.A., Stockell, A., Ferguson, M.E., Touster, O., McClellan, G.S., Williams, C. and Cannon, R.O. (1953). The Vanderbilt Cooperative Study of maternal and infant nutrition. IV. Dietary, laboratory and physical findings in 2129 delivered pregnancies. *J. Nutr.*, **51**, 565–98.

Davidson, S. and Passmore R. (1969). *Human Nutrition and Dietetics* 4th ed., pp. 801–803. Churchill Livingstone: Edinburgh.

Davidson, S., Passmore, R., Brock, J.F. and Truswell, A.S. (1979). *Human Nutrition and Dietetics* 7th ed. Churchill Livingstone: Edinburgh.

DHSS (1979). *Recommended Daily Amounts of Food Energy and Nutrients for Groups of People in the United Kingdom*. HMSO: London.

Dieckmann, W.J. (1952). *The Toxemias of Pregnancy* 2nd ed. Kimpton: London.

Durnin, J.V.G.A., McKillop, F.M., Grant, S., Fitzgerald, G. (1985). Is nutritional status endangered by virtually no extra intake during pregnancy? *Lancet*, **ii**, 823–5.

Edozien, J.C., Switzer, B.R. and Bryan, R.B. (1979). Medical evaluation of the special supplemental food program for Women, Infants and Children. *Am. J. Clin. Nutr.*, **32**, 677–92.

Fairweather-Tait, S.J., Payne, V. and Williams, C.M. (1984). The effect of iron supplements on pregnancy in rats given a low-zinc diet. *Br. J. Nutr.*, **52**, 79–86.

FAO/WHO/UNU. (1985). *Energy and protein requirements.* Report of a joint FAO/WHO/UNU Expert Consultation (WHO Technical Report Series no. 522 and FAO Nutrition Meetings Report Series no. 724) Geneva.

Frisancho, A.R., Matos, J. and Bollettino, L.A. (1984). Influence of growth status and placental function on birth weight of infants born to young still-growing teenagers. *Am. J. Clin. Nutr.*, **40**, 801–807.

Gant, N.F. and Worley, R.J. (1980). *Hypertension in Pregnancy. Concepts and Management.* Appleton and Lange: New York.

Heaney, R.P. and Skillman, T.G. (1971). Calcium metabolism in normal human pregnancy. *J. Clin. End. Met.*, **33**, 661–70.

Hytten, F.E. (1979). Restriction of weight gain in pregnancy. Is it justified? *J. Hum. Nutr.*, **33**, 461–3.

Hytten, F.E. and Chamberlain, G. (1980). *Clinical Physiology in Obstetrics.* Blackwell: Oxford.

Hytten, F.E. and Leitch, I. (1971). *The Physiology of Human Pregnancy* 2nd ed. Blackwell: Oxford.

Jelliffe, D.B., Gurney, M. and Jelliffe, E.F.P. (1975). *Unsupplemented human milk and the nutrition of the exterogestate fetus.* Proc. 9th Int. Congr. Nutr. Mexico 1972, vol. 2, pp. 77–85, Karger, Basel.

King, J.C., Cohenour, S.H., Calloway, D.H. and Jacobson, H.N. (1972). Assessment of nutritional status of teenage pregnant girls. I. Nutrient intake and pregnancy. *Am. J. Clin. Nutr.*, **25**, 916–25.

Lancet (1984). *Medical Research Council Vitamin Study*, **1**, 1308.

Lawrence, M., Lawrence, F., Lamb, W.H. and Whitehead, R.G. (1984). Maintenance energy cost of pregnancy in rural Gambian women and influence of dietary status. *Lancet*, **1**, 363–5.

Lechtig, A., Yarbrough, C., Delgado, H., Habicht, J.P., Martorell, R. and Klein, R.E. (1975). Influence of maternal nutrition on birthweight. *Am. J. Clin. Nutr.*, **28**, 1223–33.

Lederman, S.A. and Rosso Pedro (1981). Effects of obesity, food restriction and pregnancy on fetal and maternal weight and on body composition in rats. *J. Nutr.*, **111**, 2162–71.

Letsky, E. (1980). *The Haematological System in Clinical Physiology in Obstetrics.* Eds. Hytten, F.E. and Chamberlaine, G. Blackwell: Oxford.

Little, R.E. (1977). Moderate alcohol use during pregnancy and decreased infant birthweight. *Am. J. Pub. Health*, **67**, 1154–6.

Little, R.E., Streissguth, A.P., Barr, H.M. and Herman, C.S. (1980). Decreased birthweight in infants of alcoholic women who abstained during pregnancy. *J. Pediatr.*, **96**, 974–7.

Lunell, N.O., Persson, B. and Sterky, G. (1969). Dietary habits during pregnancy. *Acta Obstet. Gynec. Scand.*, **48**, 187–94.

Lyon, T.D.B., Smith, H. and Smith, L.B. (1979). Zinc deficiency in West Scotland? A dietary intake study. *Br. J. Nutr.*, **42**, 413–16.

McDonald, E.C., Pollitt, E., Mueller, W., Hsueh, A.M. and Sherwin, R. (1981). The Bacon Chow study: maternal nutritional supplementation and birthweight of offspring. *Am. J. Clin. Nutr.*, **34**, 2133–44.

Meadows, N.J., Ruse, W., Smith, M.F., Day, J., Keeling, P.W.N., Scopes, J.W., and Thompson, R.P.H. (1981). Zinc and small babies. *Lancet*, **ii**, 1135–7.
Mora, J.O., de Paredes, B., Wagner, M., de Navarro, L., Suescun, J., Christiansen, N. and Herrera, M.G. (1979). Nutritional supplementation and the outcome of pregnancy. I. Birthweight. *Am. J. Clin. Nutr.*, **32**, 455–62.
Morgan, J.B. (1980). Nutrition and pregnancy. The mother and her fetus. *Br. Nutr. Found. Bull.*, **5**, 300–308.
Naeye, R.L. (1979). Weight gain and the outcome of pregnancy. *Am. J. Obstet. Gynecol.*, **135**, 3–9.
Naismith, D.J. (1983). Maternal nutrition and fetal health. In *Recent Advances in Perinatal Medicine (1)*. Ed. Chiswick, M.L. Churchill Livingstone: Edinburgh.
Naismith, D.J. and Brookes, R.H. (1983). Energetic efficiency during pregnancy. *Proc. Nutr. Soc.*, **42**, 79A.
NRC/NAS (1980). *Recommended dietary allowances*. 9th ed. Committee on dietary allowances Food and Nutrition Board. National Academy of Sciences Publication: Washington D.C.
Nutr. Rev. (1975). Iron supplementation for gestational anaemia: A model field trial. **33**, 332–4.
Nutr. Rev. (1976). Zinc deficiency in pregnant, fetal and young rats. **34**, 84–6.
Nutr. Rev. (1979). Maternal weight gain and the outcome of pregnancy. **37**, 318–21.
Nutr. Rev. (1980). Effects of dietary lead and zinc on pregnancy in the rat. **38**, 129–130.
Nutr. Rev. (1982a). The role of zinc deficiency in foetal alcohol syndrome. **40**, 43–5.
Nutr. Rev. (1982b). Immune deficiency and apparently increased susceptibility to infection in children with fetal alcohol syndrome. **40**, 45–7.
Nutr. Rev. (1982c). Impact of maternal alcohol intake on birthweight. **40**, 48–9.
Nutr. Rev. (1982d). The fetal alcohol syndrome and placental transport of valine. **40**, 61–3.
Nutr. Rev. (1984). Nutrition intervention in pregnancy. **42**, 42–4.
Patwardhan, R.V., Schenker, S., Henderson, G.I., Abou-Mourad, N.N. and Hoyumpa, A.M. Jr. (1981). Short-term and long-term ethanol administration inhibits the placenta uptake and transport of valine in rats. *J. Lab. Clin. Med.*, **98**, 251–62.
Pratt, O.E. (1982). Alcohol and the developing fetus. *Br. Med. Bull.* **38**, 43–52.
Prentice, A.M., Whitehead, R.G., Watkinson, M., Lamb, W.H. and Cole, T.J. (1983). Prenatal dietary supplementation of African women and birthweight. *Lancet*, **i**, 489–92.
Reeve, J. (1980). Calcium Metabolism. In *Clinical Physiology in Obstetrics*. Eds. Hytten, F.E. and Chamberlaine, G. Blackwell: Oxford.
Rosso, P. and Lederman, S.A. (1982). Nutrition in the pregnant adolescent. *Current Concepts in Nutrition*. **11**, 47–62.
Schorah, C.J., Weld, J., Hartley, R., Sheppard, S. and Smithells, R.W. (1983). The effect of periconceptual supplementation on blood vitamin concentrations in women at recurrence risk from neural tube defect. *Br. J. Nutr.*, **49**, 203–212.
Schuster, K., Bailey, L.B. and Mahan, C.S. (1981). Vitamin $B_6$ status of low-income adolescent and adult pregnant women and the condition of their infants at birth. *Am. J. Clin. Nutr.*, **34**, 1731–5.
Shaw, J.C.L. (1973). Parenteral nutrition in the management of sick low birthweight infants. *Ped. Clin. Nut. Am.*, **20**, 333–49.
Smithells, R.W. (1982). Neural tube defects: Prevention by vitamin supplements. *Pediatrics*, **69**, 498–9.
Smithells, R.W., Sheppard, S., Schorah, C.J., Seller, M.J., Nevin, N.C., Harris, R., Road, A.P. and Fielding, D.W. (1982). Possible prevention of neural tube defects by periconceptional vitamin supplementation. *Lancet*, **1**, 339–40.

Stamp, T.C.B. (1978). Mineral metabolism. In *Nutrition in the Clinical Management of Disease*, pp. 268–70. Ed. Dickerson, J.W.T. and Lee, H.A. Edward Arnold: London.

Stock, M.J. and Rothwell, N.J. (1982). *Obesity and Leanness. Basic Aspects*. John Libbey & Co. Ltd: London.

Thomson, A.M. and Hytten, F.E. (1973). Nutrition during pregnancy. *Wld. Rev. Nutr. Diet*, **16**, 22–45, Karger:Basel.

Trayhurn, P., Douglas, J.B. and McGuckin, M.M. (1982). Brown adipose tissue is 'suppressed' during lactation in mice. *Nature*, **298**, 59–60.

Truswell, A.S. and Darnton-Hill, I. (1981). Food habits of adolescents. *Nutr. Rev.*, **39**, 73–88.

Valadian, I., Berkey, C. and Reed, R.B. (1981). Adolescent nutrition as it relates to cardiovascular disease and reproductive capacity later in life. *Nutr. Rev.*, **39**, 107–111.

Viegas, O.A.C., Scott, P.H., Cole, T.J., Eaton, P., Needham, P.G. and Wharton, B.A. (1982). Dietary protein energy supplementation of pregnant Asian mothers at Sorrento, Birmingham. II: Selective during third trimester only. *Br. Med. J.*, **285**, 592–5.

Wharton, B.A. (1978). Childhood. In *Nutrition in the Clinical Management of Disease*, p. 12. Ed. Dickerson, J.W.T. and Lee, H.A. Edward Arnold: London.

Whitehead, R.G., Paul, A.A., Black, A.E, and Wiles, S.J. (1981). *Recommended dietary amounts of energy for pregnancy and lactation in the United Kingdom*. U.N. University Food and Nutrition Bulletin Suppl. 3, pp. 259–64.

Widdowson, E.M., Dauncey, J. and Shaw, J.C.L. (1974). Trace elements in fetal and early postnatal development. *Proc. Nutr. Soc.*, **33**, 275–91.

Wohl, M.G. and Goodhart, R.S. (1964). *Modern Nutrition in Health and Disease*. 3rd ed. pp. 1109–10. Lea and Febiger: Philadelphia.

Wright, J.T., Waterson, E.J., Barrison, I.G., Toplis, P.J., Lewis, I.G., Gordon, M.G., MacRae, K.D., Morris, N.F. and Murray-Lyon, I.M. (1983) Alcohol consumption, pregnancy and low birthweight. *Lancet*, **1**, 663–5.

Wynn, M. and Wynn, A. (1975). *Nutrition counselling in the prevention of low birthweight*. Foundation for education and research in childbearing. London. S.W.3.

# 2 Childhood

Elizabeth M.E. Poskitt



## Introduction

Children differ from adults in their growth, body composition and dependence on others for food. Nutritional problems are most likely in infancy and adolescence when growth is rapid and nutrient demands high. Young children are prone to infection and their response to infection both modifies, and is modified by, nutritional status. Their dependence on adults makes knowledge of normal nutrition more important in the clinical management of disease in infancy than in later childhood. In consequence, a large proportion of this chapter deals with infant nutrition and associated problems. Protein-calorie malnutrition, the major nutritional problem affecting both infants and older children in many parts of the world, is dealt with elsewhere.

Table 2.1 outlines age-related changes in body composition. In fetal life the percentage of body water, particularly extracellular water, is high and remains above adult levels until about 3 years of age. Before 34 weeks gestation the fetus contains little fat, but from 34 weeks onwards fat deposition is vigorous. By the time the full term infant has doubled birthweight at 4 to 5 months, the weight of fat in the body has trebled. The velocity of total bodyweight gain slows dramatically from 36 weeks gestation and growth rates continue to fall rapidly in the first 6 months of postnatal life. Growth accelerates again during puberty and the acceleration is greater and more prolonged in boys than girls. Food requirements per kilogramme bodyweight decline with age but less dramatically than growth rates. Over 25 per cent of

Table 2.1 Approximate body composition related to age*

| | Fetus Weeks | | | | Child Months | | Child Years | | Adult |
|---|---|---|---|---|---|---|---|---|---|
| Age | 26 | 32 | 35 | term | 5 | 12 | 5 | 10 | |
| *Whole body composition*: | | | | | | | | | |
| Weight (g) | 1000 | 2000 | 2500 | 3500 | 7000 | 10 000 | 19 000 | 30 000 | 70 000 |
| Water % | 85 | 80 | 77 | 71 | 60 | 59 | 60 | 60 | 60 |
| Fat % | 2 | 6 | 8 | 14 | 26 | 24 | 18 | 17 | 12 (men) 25 (women) |
| *Fat free mass*: | | | | | | | | | |
| Water % | 87 | 84 | 84 | 84 | 82 | 78 | 74 | 72 | 72 |
| Protein‡% | 8.5 | 12.5 | 12.5 | 13 | 15 | 19 | 20 | 20 | 20.5 |

* Fomon 1974; Widdowson 1981b
‡ Total N × 6.25

the energy intake of newborn infants is utilized in growth. At 6 months only 7 per cent of energy intake is required for growth and this proportion falls further with age (Widdowson, 1981a).

Table 2.2 illustrates the changing nutrient needs of infants and children. At any age there is a two-fold difference in energy intake by children of the same sex and age, which is not closely related to size for age (Widdowson, 1947). Mean energy intakes of British children have declined recently perhaps in association with reduced exercise (Durnin *et al.*, 1974; Whitehead *et al.*, 1981). Requirements for energy are very high for the first 2 months of life, dropping to levels of only 378 kJ (90 kcals)/kg/day at 4 to 6 months, and then rising again as the infant increases activity at the end of the first year. It may be that the fat deposited in the first 5 months of life allows this early fall in energy requirements since it is usual for there to be a gradual reduction in percentage bodyweight as fat over the second 6 months as weaning occurs.

In childhood, growth rates provide useful indicators of the adequacy of nutrition but weight and linear growth must be assessed in relation to one another and to values expected for age from reference standards (Tanner *et al.*, 1966; Gairdner and Pearson, 1971). Young children and adolescents grow rapidly. Some gain in weight does not necessarily mean satisfactory growth, particularly for children recovering from periods of poor nutrition and requiring accelerated or 'catch up' growth to achieve normal nutritional status. In adolescence individual size and growth rates are determined not only by age and sex but also pubertal status. Throughout childhood boys tend to have higher intakes of nutrients than girls but differences are small until early adolescence when they become more noticeable (Widdowson, 1947).

## Infancy

Infant feeding practices have changed greatly over the past 15 to 20 years (DHSS, 1974; DHSS, 1980c, Taitz and Lukmanji 1981). In the late 1960s the majority of British infants were fed reconstituted dried cows' milk with added sucrose. Recognition that high solute feeds encouraged the development of hypernatraemic dehydration in young infants led to withdrawal of all unmodified cows' milk infant formulas in Britain in 1974–5. Associated campaigns to increase the prevalence of breast-feeding have been fairly effective amongst well educated women but less effective in deprived areas of Britain. Contaminated water supplies and ignorance about how to mix feeds make bottle-feeding and infant formulas major health risks for young infants in developing countries (Anon, 1983). Widespread international concern over infant feeding practices has led both WHO and the babymilk manufacturers to publish codes of practice for the marketing of breast-milk substitutes (Anon, 1981).

### Breast-feeding

Perhaps it is unnecessary to extol the advantages of this natural physiological method of infant feeding. Many of the advantages of breast-feeding are self evident.

Table 2.2 Estimated requirements of infants and children according to age[1]

| | Fetus Weeks | | Child Months | | Years | | 15 years | | Adult | |
|---|---|---|---|---|---|---|---|---|---|---|
| Age | 28[3] | Term | 5 | 12 | 5 | 10 | Male | Female | Male | Female |
| *Total per kg per day*[2] | | | | | | | | | | |
| Energy | | | | | | | | | | |
| kJ | 630 | 530 | 378[8] | 420 | 340 | 260 | 252 | 231 | 180 | 180 |
| kcal | 150 | 126 | 90 | 100 | 80 | 62 | 60 | 55 | 46 | 46 |
| Protein g | 3.0 | 1.5 | 1.4 | 1.2 | 1.0 | 0.8 | 0.7 | 0.6 | 0.5 | 0.5 |
| Water ml | 200 | 150 | 120 | 100 | 80 | 50 | 30 | 30 | 30 | 30 |
| Sodium mmol | 3.0–4.0 | 2.5 | 1.0 | 1.0 | 0.5 | 0.5 | 0.5 | 0.5 | 0.5 | 0.5 |
| *Total per day* | | | | | | | | | | |
| Calcium mg[4] | 250 | 388 | 289 | 309 | 256 | 200 | 210 | 110 | 210 | 110 |
| Iron mg[5] | 6 | 7 | 8 | 8 | 8 | 10 | 12 | 18 | 12 | 18 |
| Vitamins[6] | | | | | | | | | | |
| A μg | 150 | 85 | 85 | 120 | 120 | 120 | 120 | 120 | 120 | 120 |
| C mg | 30 | 20 | 20 | 10 | 10 | 10 | 10 | 10 | 10 | 10 |
| D μg[7] | 10 | 10 | 2.5 | 2.5 | 2.5 | 2.5 | 2.5 | 2.5 | 2.5 | 2.5 |

1. Fomon 1974; Widdowson 1981a
2. Recommended allowances are usually at least 20 % higher than estimated requirements for major nutrients other than water and energy
3. Requirements vary enormously depending on clinical state. Full volume fluid intake should only be achieved over 10 days or more in sick infants
4. Values refer to calcium retention in infants and adolescents. Values in adolescence vary with growth spurt and may reach 400 mg per day for boys and 240 mg per day for girls. Recommended intakes are considerably higher due to variable absorption of calcium
5. Assuming 10 % absorption of iron intake
6. Recommend intakes for vitamins may be 100 % greater than estimated requirements
7. Requirements for vitamin D uncertain, particularly in presence of adequate sunshine – see text
8. Whitehead *et al.*, 1981

**Establishing breast-feeding**

Breast-feeding is most likely to succeed when the infant is suckled frequently in the first days of life. This requires a healthy infant with the ability to suck and a relaxed, healthy mother who is keen to breast-feed. In many societies and in some British maternity units, particular women are chosen to help new mothers with the techniques of breast-feeding.

Good maternal nutrition is important for successful lactation. Much of the energy in human milk can be derived from maternal fat stored during pregnancy but poor maternal nutrition results in secretion of small volumes of milk of low fat content (Jelliffe and Jelliffe, 1978). Mineral, trace element and vitamin content are also affected by maternal nutrition. Frequent suckling probably helps maintain adequate milk production when maternal energy intakes are low through stimulating high circulating prolactin levels (Davies, 1981a; Lunn *et al.*, 1984). The convenience of breast-feeding depends on social attitudes and maternal lifestyle. Unlike some mammals, which 'store' milk in the mammary glands, lactating women only continue to produce milk if the breast is emptied at frequent intervals. Lactation will not be established successfully unless the infant is suckled or milk expressed, at least five to six times a day.

One often quoted advantage of breast-feeding is the close human contact (bonding) that develops with successful breast-feeding (Klaus and Kennell, 1976). It is unlikely that the emotional interactions that occur between mother and breast-fed child are unique. However, successful breast-feeding is clinical evidence of appropriate mother–child interaction since the neurohumoral reflexes that stimulate milk production and milk ejection are readily inhibited by emotions such as fear, disgust, apprehension and pain (Jelliffe and Jelliffe, 1978).

**Composition of breast milk**

Table 2.3 outlines the approximate composition of colostrum, mature human milk, babymilk formulas and cows' milk.

*Colostrum*

Secretion of small quantities of colostrum starts before delivery. After birth the composition of colostrum changes rapidly as milk secretion begins. Colostrum has a very high protein content. In the first 24 hours post-partum more than 50 per cent of colostral protein is secretory immunoglobulin A (sIgA). Nucleotides, sodium and trace elements are also present in higher concentrations than in mature breast milk. Colostral and mature milk sIgA contribute little to protein nutrition since sIgA is resistant to digestion and can be recovered from infants' stools. Sulph-hydryl oxidase and antiproteases in milk may protect human milk proteins from digestion in the infant's gastrointestinal tract. After early infancy, intestinal secretion of sIgA has an important role in protecting infants from colonization by gastrointestinal pathogens. Many intestinal pathogens only cause symptoms when they adhere to intestinal mucosa. Intestinal secretion of sIgA is very low in early infancy, thus secretory sIgA from milk coats the mucosa and prevents adherence by potential pathogens. In the first 2 days of life some colostral sIgA crosses the gastrointestinal mucosa and reaches the circulation, although human neonates derive most circulating

Table 2.3 Approximate composition of colostrum, breast milk, babymilk formulas and cows' milk (per 100 ml as consumed)[1]

| | | Colostrum | Breast milk | Formulas[2] | Cows' milk |
|---|---|---|---|---|---|
| Energy[3] | | | | | |
| kJ | | variable | 294 | 272–294 | 291 |
| kcal | | variable | 70 | 65–70 | 67 |
| Total protein g | | 10 | 1.1 | 1.5–1.9 | 3.5 |
| sIgA g | | 5.4 | 0.15 | – | – |
| lactoferrin g | | 1.4 | 0.15 | – | – |
| casein:whey ratio | | 16:84 | 40:60 | 82:18–32:68 | 82:18 |
| Total fat g | | 2.9 | 4.2 | 2.4–3.8 | 3.6 |
| saturated:unsaturated | | 41:59 | 50:50 | 48:61–29:54 | 63:37 |
| Carbohydrate g | | 5.3 | 7.0 | 6.9–8.6 | 4.9 |
| Electrolytes | | | | | |
| sodium | mg | 48 | 15 | 15–31 | 52 |
| chloride | mg | 59 | 43 | 40–58 | 98 |
| calcium | mg | 31 | 35 | 36–71 | 120 |
| phosphate | mg | 14 | 15 | 31–55 | 95 |
| iron | μg | ? | 76 | 650–700 | 50 |
| Vitamins | | | | | |
| A | μg | 126 | 60 | 61–100 | 40 |
| C | mg | 4.4 | 3.8 | 5.5–6.9 | 1.5 |
| D | μg | 1.8 | 0.6 | 1.0–1.1 | 0.02 |

1. Fomon (1974); DHSS (1980c)
2. Composition varies with manufacturers
3. 1 kcal = 4.2 kJ; 1 kJ = 0.24 kcal

immunoglobulin transplacentally in late fetal life (Vukavic, 1983; Weaver *et al.*, 1984). About 100 ml of colostrum is secreted per day. Frequent suckling in the first days post-partum leads to earlier secretion of transitional and mature milk (Salariya *et al.*, 1978).

*Mature milk*

The composition of mature milk varies with both the gestational and postnatal age of the infant, the time of day, the stage in the feed and the nutritional state of the mother.

*Protein* Mature human milk contains approximately 11 g/litre protein and amino acids and about 460 mg/litre of urea and non amino acid nitrogen. About half the protein is in the form of lactalbumins. Human milk protein amino acids are present in more or less the proportions necessary for tissue synthesis although cysteine, taurine and tryptophan are present in higher concentrations. Neonates are unable to convert methionine to cysteine due to absence of cystathionease and relative deficiency of cystathione synthetase (Raiha, 1971). Cysteine is an essential amino acid for young infants although not for older children or adults in whom cysteine can be synthesized from methionine. In breast-fed neonates bile acids are all conjugated with taurine although even immature infants conjugate bile acids with glycine if there is insufficient taurine (Brueton *et al.*, 1978). Taurine is important for normal retinal development in kittens (Knopf *et al.*, 1978) but its importance for human retinal development is not established. The relatively high proportion of tryptophan in human milk is interesting but unexplained.

*Fat* The fat content of human milk varies enormously (Jelliffe and Jelliffe, 1978). In European women it is highest in the middle of the day, towards the end of a feed and early in lactation. The timing of the peak fat concentration may reflect the timing of the main meal of the day (Harzer *et al.*, 1983). In poorly nourished African women total fat content is less and tends to be highest in feeds given early in the day (Prentice *et al.*, 1981).

Full term infants absorb more than 90 per cent of the fat from human milk, only about 70 per cent of the butter fat in babymilk formulas based on cows' milk and probably an intermediate percentage of the mono- and polyunsaturated fats in the more modified modern formulas (Widdowson, 1981a; Brooke *et al.*, 1979). Pancreatic lipase secretion is low in neonates but fat absorption is aided by intragastric lipolysis with lingual lipase (Lebenthal *et al.*, 1983; Fink *et al.*, 1984). The composition of the fats and the presence of lipases in human milk also aid absorption.

Breast milk contains many enzymes the importance of which is not fully understood (Heitlinger, 1983). Bile salt stimulated lipase (BSL) constitutes about 1 per cent of the protein in human milk, is comparatively acid stable and has low substrate specificity. It is active in lipolysis since it is protected from proteolytic digestion by bile salts which act as catalysts (Hamosh, 1982).

The small fat droplet size in human milk allows rapid lipolysis. The nature of the fatty acids released by lipolysis encourages fat absorption. Mono- and polyunsaturated fatty acids are the predominant fatty acids in human milk. Saturated fatty acids are mostly in the $\beta$ position of the triglyceride molecule and are well absorbed in the monoglyceride form (Fomon, 1974; Lebenthal *et al.*, 1983).

*Carbohydrate* Lactose is the sole carbohydrate in human milk. Intestinal lactase develops late in fetal life and only reaches optimal levels around term but healthy infants, even the immature, have no difficulty digesting lactose. Despite being the only milk sugar, lactose is not essential for normal growth and development. Infants fed lactose free diets synthesize sufficient galactose for brain lipid production and normal brain development.

*Electrolytes* The bio-availability of electrolytes and trace elements in human milk is high. Calcium concentration in human milk is low compared with requirements but its distribution and the high lactose content facilitate absorption (Fransson and Lonnerdahl, 1984). Zinc binding ligands facilitate zinc absorption (Duncan and Harvey, 1978) and lactoferrin binds iron and facilitates absorption provided copper nutrition is satisfactory (Lee *et al.*, 1976).

*Vitamins* The vitamin content of human milk reflects maternal vitamin status (Rothberg *et al.*, 1982).

Human milk contains about 1 $\mu$g/litre of active vitamin D of which more than 90 per cent is fat soluble vitamin D or 25 hydroxyvitamin D (Reeve *et al.*,

1982). Infants are thought to require 2.5–10 μg/day but this figure is somewhat arbitrary. Rickets is common in breast-fed infants of osteomalacic women but the initial vitamin deficiency of these infants probably dates from intra-uterine life. Rickets is not common in young breast-fed infants of healthy, well nourished women despite the low vitamin D content of milk. Thus there may be other factors besides vitamin D accounting for the anti-rachitic effect of human milk (Makin *et al.*, 1983). Infant rats absorb calcium and phosphate in large quantities on diets containing no vitamin D and have fairly satisfactory bone mineralization (Halloran and de Luca, 1981). Initial calcium absorption of rats is by a passive system. At weaning calcium absorption changes gradually to an active vitamin D dependent process (Ghishan *et al.*, 1984). Perhaps human infants are similarly less dependent on vitamin D in the immediate postnatal period than later. Certainly *prolonged* breast-feeding without adequate exposure to summer sunlight and without vitamin supplementation predisposes infants to vitamin D deficiency rickets.

*Anti-infective properties of human milk*
Table 2.4 lists anti-infective factors in human milk. The relative protection from infection provided by breast-feeding has been recognized for a long time. Breast-fed infants have a lower incidence of gastroenteritis and upper respiratory tract infections including otitis media and bronchiolitis, than formula fed infants (Gerrard, 1974; Downham *et al.*, 1976).

*Cellular factors* Colostrum contains about 4000 cells/mm$^3$. Mature milk contains fewer cells. Macrophages, neutrophils, T and rosette forming lymphocytes are all present in milk and have different functions (Jelliffe and Jelliffe, 1978; Rolles and Cussens, 1980). The introduction of specific *E. coli* strains into the maternal gastrointestinal tract is followed rapidly by the secretion of strain specific sIgA in the milk. Presumably sensitized lymphocytes in maternal intestinal Peyer's patches migrate to the breast and into the milk carrying the information necessary to produce sIgA against organisms which the infants may acquire by contact with their mothers. Macrophages and

Table 2.4 Anti-infective factors in human milk

| |
|---|
| *Cellular factors* |
| Lymphocytes |
| Macrophages |
| Neutrophils |
| *Humoral factors* |
| Secretory Immunoglobulin A |
| Lactoferrin |
| Other nutrient binding proteins |
| Lysozyme |
| Interferon |
| Polyunsaturated fatty acids |
| $C_3$ and $C_4$ complement |
| Antistaphylococcal factors |

neutrophils in milk act as scavengers by ingesting and destroying bacteria already harmed by the humoral factors in the infant's jejunum and ileum.

*Humoral factors* SIgA, which forms about 10 per cent of the total protein in mature milk, is the main anti-infective humoral component of human milk. Other proteins, most notably lactoferrin, inhibit bacterial multiplication in the infant gut by binding specific nutrients such as iron, folate, $B_{12}$ and zinc thus making them unavailable to bacteria.

The low buffering capacity and high lactose content of human milk result in stools of low pH due to the volatile acids produced by bacterial fermentation. This encourages growth of *Lactobacillus bifidus* and discourages colonization by pathogenic bacteria. Long chain polyunsaturated fatty acids, lysozymes, interferon, antistaphylococcal factor and $C_3$ and $C_4$ complement fractions also discourage colonization by pathogenic organisms in the infant gut and contribute to the anti-infective properties of human milk (Yoshioka *et al.*, 1983; Goldman and Garza, 1983).

## Clinical problems associated with breast-feeding

### *Inadequate milk intake*

Most breast-fed infants thrive and thus provide evidence of the adequacy of their mothers' milk supply. When breast-fed infants fail to thrive, it may be difficult to determine whether or not inadequate milk intake is the cause. Not all underfed infants cry with hunger. Some become quiet and sleepy and appear content and well fed. Their behaviour is deceptive. Mothers' beliefs that they have sufficient milk do not mean that the babies are ingesting sufficient milk (Evans and Davies, 1977). Weighing infants before and after feeds without nappy changes (test weighing) is the method generally adopted to determine breast milk intake. Infants should be test weighed over 24 hours before the adequacy of intake can be reasonably assessed since intakes of milk vary during the day. More accurate methods than test weighing have been developed, but they have little clinical application (Whitfield *et al.*, 1981; Stothers, 1982).

### *Breast-milk jaundice*

This is probably the commonest clinical problem caused by breast-feeding. Infants who are breast-fed might be expected to be slightly more prone to physiological jaundice than formula-fed infants since the low fluid and energy intakes that result from receiving colostrum and small quantities of transitional milk rather than larger volumes of formula in the first days could exacerbate 'physiological' jaundice. Clinical studies fail to show correlations between weight loss and early jaundice in breast-fed infants and it is unnecessary to supplement breast-fed infants with water in normal temperate environments (de Carvalho *et al.*, 1981; Maisels and Gifford, 1983). Some breast-fed infants develop, or continue, significant unconjugated hyperbilirubinaemia in the second week of life. This 'breast milk' jaundice (BMJ) may persist for the duration of breast-feeding and often resolves gradually over the first 2 months of life even if breast-feeding continues. Plasma bilirubin rarely rises above 300 $\mu$mol/litre and usually falls to 150 $\mu$mol/litre or less after the first weeks. These infants thrive, thus distinguishing BMJ from more serious causes of late neonatal jaundice, namely hypothyroidism, infection and the neonatal hepatitis syndrome.

Mothers of infants with BMJ have a high breast milk lipase content and unusual long chain fatty acid triglycerides in their milk. It is thought that breast milk lipase leads to rapid breakdown and absorption of these fatty acids which then inhibit bilirubin uptake by the liver (Odell, 1981). Recent work has suggested an alternative explanation, namely that mothers of infants with breast milk jaundice have high enzymatic activity in their milk, which breaks down bilirubin glucuronide complexes in the infant's intestine allowing increased enterohepatic circulation of bilirubin and consequently increased bilirubin load for the immature liver to clear (Gourley and Arend, 1986).

### *Haemorrhagic disease of the newborn*

All infants are liable to vitamin K deficiency in the newborn period (Shearer *et al.*, 1982) and may present in the first week of life with bruising or haemorrhage, commonly from umbilical stump or gastrointestinal tract. In Britain all standard babymilks are now supplemented with vitamin K.

Haemorrhagic disease of the newborn (HDNB) used to be a common problem. Its prevalence declined in the 1960s and early 1970s when the majority of infants were formula fed and when premature, sick or asphyxiated infants were given vitamin K intramuscularly at birth. Recently haemorrhagic disease has reappeared following the increase in breast-feeding. It is not clear why breast-fed infants should be more prone to vitamin K deficiency than formula-fed infants although the rate and nature of gut bacterial colonization may affect absorption of vitamin K synthesized by intestinal bacteria and these may be influenced by the milk ingested. This is questionable (Shearer *et al.*, 1982). Since it is difficult to predict which infants are at particular risk of HDNB it seems reasonable to recommend that *all* infants receive 1 mg of vitamin K intramuscularly at birth. Verity *et al.* (1983) described HDNB apparently due to vitamin K deficiency in normal infants beyond the newborn period. This is disturbing. The possibility of vitamin K deficiency should be considered in all infants with bruising or bleeding episodes.

### *Drugs in breast milk*

There is a lot of concern and relatively little knowledge about the transmission of drugs in breast milk (Szefler, 1983). In general, lactating women should be advised to avoid all drugs. The presence of a drug in the milk in small quantities is not necessarily contraindication to breast-feeding. The concentration of the drug in milk and its effect (or likely effect) on the fetus needs considering (Committee on Drugs, 1983). Chloramphenicol, $^{131}I$ and thiouracil are examples of drugs which are present in quite high concentration in milk and, because of their effects, contraindicate breast-feeding. Antifolate and anticancer drugs are present in lower concentrations but their effects are such that they also contraindicate breast-feeding. Phenytoin, phenobarbitone and diazepam are secreted into milk in significant amounts. These drugs are relatively harmless to infants in small quantities and it is generally not practical for mothers on these drugs to stop treatment in order to breast-feed. It seems reasonable to observe each individual situation and assess whether or not the infant is being affected by drug ingestion and particularly whether sucking and mental state are impaired. Without evidence of drug effect, breast-feeding may continue.

*Infections transferred by breast milk*
Breast milk is not sterile but cells and humoral factors in milk protect the infant against many of the organisms transferred in the milk. Cytomegalovirus, hepatitis B and HIV amongst other viruses, may be transferred to infants in breast milk, particularly if the milk is not their own mother's milk and has not been pasteurized (Dworsky *et al.*, 1983).

## Formula feeding

Infants who are not breast-fed require infant formula (babymilks) instead. Nearly all standard British formulas use cows' milk as their base although over 10 per cent of artificially fed North American infants receive soya protein containing milks from birth (Committee on Nutrition, 1983). The recent history of baby milk development is summarized elsewhere (Foman, 1974; Wharton and Berger, 1976).

Unmodified cows' milk (and goats' milk) presents many hazards for young infants (see below) and should not be fed for the first 6 months of life at least.

### Formula composition

Recent DHSS recommendations are that the total protein of formula milks should not exceed 20 g/litre, but should be at least 15 g/litre if the casein:whey ratio follows that of cows' milk. This provides sufficient cysteine and taurine for infants' needs despite the relatively low proportions of these amino acids in cows' milk protein. Where the protein in the formula follows a casein:whey ratio similar to that of human milk, total protein can be as low as 12 g/litre without nutritional risk. Reconstituted formula should also contain 6.5–15 mmol/litre sodium, 13–26 mmol/litre potassium and 11–23 mmol/litre chloride. Calcium:phosphate ratio should be between 1.2:1 and 2.2:1 with calcium 30–120 mg/100 ml and phosphate 15–60 mg/100 ml reconstituted feed (DHSS, 1980a).

Several babymilk formulas now have modified fat content so the ratio of saturated to polyunsaturated fatty acids resembles that of human milk. DHSS recommendations are that linoleic acid and $\alpha$-linolenic acid (essential fatty acids in infants) should together form at least 1 per cent of the total energy and that linoleic acid should provide not more than 20 per cent of the total fatty acid (DHSS, 1980a).

All baby milks for full term infants now contain added vitamins and iron.

### How much should infants be fed?

Normal healthy newborns should be fed a few hours after birth. Initial feeds should offer about 60 ml/kg/day as six feeds. Feed volumes are increased until the infants are taking about 150 ml/kg/day by the end of the first week. Small or sick infants should be offered smaller volumes more frequently. After the first days or weeks, most infants settle to a regime of five feeds a day with one night feed omitted. Around 6 weeks old infants often seem very hungry and may demand, and take, considerably more than 150 ml/kg/day for a while and gain weight at rates greater than the expected 30 g per day without necessarily becoming overfat (Wickes, 1952).

**Problems arising from formula feeding**

Mothers often attribute problems such as 'colic', 'wind', green stools, 'not satisfied' and constipation to particular brands of formula. These problems resolve with a change of feed, perhaps chiefly because the mothers have decided that a change of milk is needed. It is difficult to attribute most of these symptoms to features of particular formulas although it is possible that milks containing high casein and high butter fat may be more slowly digested and thus more 'satisfying'. There is little clinical evidence for this.

Several conditions associated with cows' milk formula feeding have almost disappeared due to major modifications in formula composition. Description of these problems serves as a reminder of how easily an inappropriate diet can affect health in infancy.

*Hypernatraemic dehydration*

The renal solute load (RSL) is that part of the nitrogenous and electrolyte content of the diet which is not utilized in metabolism and must be excreted via the urine. In the late 1960s and early 1970s, hypernatraemic dehydration was a common problem in young infants who were receiving feeds with a high RSL. These infants were receiving unmodified cows' milk feeds sometimes together with high protein, high salt, weaning foods from a few weeks old.

The RSL for a 7 kg infant taking 1000 ml/day of cows' milk has been estimated at 221 mmol/day. (An equivalent volume of human milk would provide only 79 mmol/day.) The addition of high protein and high salt weaning foods increases the renal solute load further (Fomon, 1974). High solute feeds, reduced fluid intake with, or without, increased extra-renal fluid loss (as might happen in minor infection) present the kidney with a high RSL in a low urine volume. Blood urea and sodium rise and hypernatraemic dehydration develops. Infants with hypernatraemic dehydration often present only when circulatory collapse occurs since their blood volume is maintained until severe intracellular fluid loss has occurred (Taitz and Byers, 1972). The condition still carries a high morbidity and mortality.

*Hypocalcaemia*

Hypocalcaemia is common in neonates, particularly those who are sick or immature. The relative unresponsiveness of the neonatal parathyroids to falls in serum calcium is generally given as the explanation for hypocalcaemia but recent studies show that the majority of hypocalcaemic neonates have elevated parathyroid hormone (Hillman *et al.*, 1977; Atkinson, 1983). Occasionally hypocalcaemia develops in neonates who are otherwise well and thriving. These infants present towards the end of the first week with jitteriness, tetany or convulsions. This 'late' hypocalcaemia was common when infants were fed high phosphate, unmodified cows' milk, formula. Calcium absorption from cows' milk is relatively poor whereas phosphate absorption is good. Healthy infants absorbed excess phosphate and plasma phosphate rose whilst plasma calcium fell to balance the calcium–phosphate product. Jitteriness and hypocalcaemic convulsions developed. Oral or intravenous calcium and low phosphate formula feeds usually cured the problem. Late hypocalcaemia has almost disappeared since the introduction of low phosphate formulas.

*Hypercalcaemia of infancy*
Enthusiastic supplementation of babymilks and other infant foods with vitamin D in the 1950s led to an outbreak of failure to thrive, vomiting, constipation, polyuria, mental retardation, sometimes associated with supravalvular aortic stenosis and a typical 'elfin' facies amongst young infants (British Paediatric Association, 1964). Hypercalcaemia developed in response to excessive vitamin D consumption. Symptomatic infants had usually received over 100 $\mu$g vitamin D/day in infancy. Controlled supplementation of babymilks and infant weaning foods has eliminated hypercalcaemia secondary to excessive vitamin D intake but sporadic cases of idiopathic infantile hypercalcaemia (William's syndrome) still occur. In William's syndrome a presumed congenital hypersensitivity to vitamin D produces similar symptoms to acquired hypervitaminosis D. Hypercalcaemia is often shortlived and is controlled by low calcium, low vitamin D diet. The overall outlook for growth and intelligence does not seem to be improved by the diet.

*Vitamin E deficient haemolytic anaemia*
Vitamin E and selenium are important in maintaining the stability of cell membranes through their antioxidant effect. Newborn infants have low vitamin E levels. The introduction of milks with a high concentration of polyunsaturated fatty acids relative to the vitamin E content led to an increase in vitamin E sensitive haemolytic anaemia in infants, particularly amongst the premature. Supplementation of babymilks with vitamin E seems to have eliminated this problem. DHSS (1980a) recommendations are that the $\alpha$tocopherol (vitamin E) content of infant formula should amount to at least 0.3 mg $\alpha$tocopherol per 100 ml reconstituted feed with a ratio of $\alpha$tocopherol (mg) to polyunsaturated fatty acids (g) of 0.4:1.0.

*Milk intolerance*
Table 2.5 lists the main features of milks commonly used to manage disaccharide and/or cows' milk protein intolerance in infancy and early childhood.

*Lactose intolerance* Lactose intolerance due to primary alactasia is a very rare inborn error of metabolism. Secondary lactose intolerance is common, usually temporary and acquired during gastrointestinal stress.

Infants with hypolactasia secondary to gastrointestinal insult or malnutrition, present with the explosive passage of profuse watery, frothy stools, abdominal distension and weight loss. Bacterial digestion of unabsorbed lactose in the large bowel leads to production of acids, intestinal gas and intestinal hurry secondary to hyperosmolar colonic contents. Frequent acid stools cause perianal excoriation. Stools have pH$<$6 and usually show reducing substances which can be demonstrated as lactose on electrophoresis. Jejunal lactase levels are low. Lactose should be excluded from the diet until normal

Table 2.5 Lactose and/or cow milk protein free formulas available in Britain[1]

| Formula | Manufacturer | Protein source | Carbohydrate source |
|---|---|---|---|
| Formula MCT 1 | Cow and Gate | Cow milk | Glucose |
| [vm]Galactomin 17 | Cow and Gate | Cow milk | Glucose and maltodextrins |
| Portagen | Mead Johnson | Cow milk | Corn syrup solids, sucrose |
| Nutramigen | Mead Johnson | Hydrolysed casein | Sucrose, maltodextrins |
| Pregestimil | Mead Johnson | Hydrolysed casein | Corn syrup solids, maltodextrins, modified tapioca |
| Prosobee | Mead Johnson | Soya + methionine | Corn syrup solids |
| Velactin | Wander | Soya + methionine | Glucose, hydrolysate of soya flour and maize |
| Wysoy | Wyeth | Soya + methionine | Sucrose, glucose and maltodextrins |
| Formula S | Cow and Gate | Soya + methionine | Glucose, hydrolysed starch |
| [vmc]Comminuted Chicken meat | Cow and Gate | Chicken | None |

v additional special vitamin supplement required
m mineral supplement required
c carbohydrate source required
1 data from: manufacturers' information; Wharton (1982). Composition liable to change

weight is regained and intestinal symptoms have resolved. Small quantities of dilute lactose containing feed are then introduced into the diet and the infant or child gradually weaned back on to full strength formula or cows' milk over a few days.

Other disaccharide and even monosaccharide intolerances do occur in infants and older children. Usually these develop following periods of gastro-intestinal stress or malnutrition. The rapid turnover of intestinal cells makes them highly sensitive to nutritional deficiency. Occasionally, therefore, intravenous nutrition is necessary to restore the child's nutritional state and mucosal activity to a state in which enteral feeding is tolerated before the vicious circle of intestinal damage and malnutrition is broken.

*Cows' milk protein intolerance (CMPI)* This condition is greatly over-diagnosed. However, CMPI does occur and is often secondary to gastrointestinal insult or malnutrition. Infants present with a wide variety of symptoms but most commonly with intractable diarrhoea. Unfortunately there are no diagnostic features except that the condition resolves, usually within 48 hours, on removal of cows' milk protein from the feed and usually recurs within 48 hours on reintroduction of cows' milk protein a short while later. Since several cows' milk protein free formulas are also free of lactose (and since both lactose intolerance and CMPI may occur together) it is sometimes difficult to distinguish the two conditions unless jejunal lactase levels are measured. Intestinal biopsy and immunological studies are not particularly helpful in making a diagnosis of CMPI since the histological appearances in CMPI, lactose intolerance and normality overlap. Affected infants and children should be allowed to regain lost weight and lose their abnormal symptoms before cows' milk protein is restarted. Since some children show an anaphylactoid response and/or catastrophic diarrhoea in association with the reintroduction of cows' milk, the first reintroduction should be of a very small quantity (e.g. 5–10 ml) of cows' milk. The volume of cows' milk or formula offered can then be increased gradually (provided there are no ill effects) until full feeding is achieved.

Infants with CMPI can be fed either formula containing hydrolyzed cows' milk protein which does not seem to have significant allergenic effect; formula with non cow milk base such as a soya; or a comminuted chicken base with added carbohydrate, fat, vitamin and mineral source. Soya protein intolerance is fairly common, so hydrolyzed cows' milk protein formulas are probably the most satisfactory feed for CMPI infants. Soya flour is deficient in methionine and it is important that soya preparations fed to infants contain supplemental methionine (Committee on Nutrition, 1983).

Where milk intolerance occurs, mothers must be advised on suitable weaning foods if the infants are likely to be weaned before getting back on to normal formula. The composition of infant foods is liable to variation. The only way to be sure foods are free of milk or lactose is by consulting manufacturers or reading the list of contents on the packet. Pills may contain lactose as a filler and thus provide unexpected hazards.

## Nutrition of low birthweight (LBW) infants

Low birthweight infants (LBW) can be divided into those born before 37 weeks gestation (short gestation or true premature (SG)) and those weighing less than the 10th centile for the gestational age at any gestation (light for gestational age (LGA)). Some infants are both SG and LGA. There are many practical difficulties associated with maintaining adequate nutrition in these infants yet normal brain growth, the maintenance of the internal environment and the ability to combat infection are dependent on satisfactory nutrition.

### Requirements

Table 2.1 (p. 31) indicates the different body composition of immature infants. SG infants have higher respiratory rates, more permeable skin and larger surface area/volume relationship than full term infants. Renal function is immature and they retain sodium and excrete hydrogen ions less well. Therapeutic measures such as phototherapy (which increases stool fluid loss) and nursing under radiant heaters also increase fluid loss. Yet, if growth of SG infants is to resemble that which might have occurred *in utero*, growth rates must be above those of term infants and more fluid and nutrients per kg will be needed. LGA infants have fewer problems than SG infants due to greater maturity for weight, but they still require extra nutrients to allow for catch up growth (Widdowson, 1974; Atkinson, 1983).

The exact nutrient requirements of these infants are uncertain, partly because needs are affected radically by size and maturity. Feeding, either intravenously or enterally, is often a compromise between what is thought to be required and what can be fed with safety.

## Growth of LBW infants

### *SG*

Initially most SG infants have considerable weight loss and delayed weight gain. Extracellular fluid losses after birth are high and there are often problems achieving adequate nutrient intake. Once adequate nutrition is established, growth accelerates with skull circumference growing proportionately more rapidly than weight and length (Davies, 1981b). Weight and length usually accelerate across the centiles after the expected date of delivery to achieve a growth curve of between the tenth and fiftieth centiles for gestational age. Maximum growth in skull circumference occurs around 19 days for SG infants of 32–34 weeks gestation with few medical problems and at about 32 days for those with severe respiratory problems. Food intake is not necessarily less in the sick infants with slower growth rates, so presumably the energy costs of illness, particularly respiratory illness, contribute to the growth delay (Davies, 1981b).

### *LGA*

The growth velocity and growth outcome for LGA infants depend on the aetiology of the intra-uterine growth retardation and the maturity of these infants at birth. Term LGA infants usually show early catch up growth. Davies (1981b) has suggested that newborn infants who show marked wasting with low ponderal indices attributable to intra-uterine malnutrition have marked early catch up growth. Infants who are overall small but not wasted may be growth retarded for reasons other than intra-uterine malnutrition and show variable degrees of catch up, or no catch up at all.

## Enteral feeding

Swallowing and sucking movements occur *in utero* from 18–24 weeks gestation but these actions are weak and poorly co-ordinated before 34 weeks gestation. Sucking is associated with decreased ventilation and may be inadvisable in infants with significant respiratory problems (Shivpuri *et al.*, 1983). Infants who are unable to suck but able to tolerate enteral feeding require feeding by gavage. Small bolus feeds are given nasogastrically or orogastrically (as oral tubes obstruct respiration less) from a few hours after birth provided the infant's condition warrants this. If feeding is not possible due to extreme immaturity or severe respiratory or gut problems, 10 per cent dextrose solution is given intravenously. Neonatal glycogen stores are rapidly exhausted and LBW infants have little fat to mobilize as an alternative energy source. Early feeding, enteral or parental is very important since hypoglycaemia is common in all sick, SG and LGA infants. Oral or nasogastric feeding may precipitate a fall in arterial oxygen concentration and a rise in blood pressure, bradycardia and apnoea (Shivpuri *et al.*, 1983). Very small volume feeds or slow continuous nasogastric drip may be tolerated better.

The frequency of regurgitation and aspiration of feed have led some units to develop nasojejunal feeding for small, sick newborns enterally (Dryburgh, 1980). Gastric reflux is less likely, but it takes time for the feeding tube to pass into the jejunum and meanwhile these infants have to be fed gastrically or intravenously. Jejunally administered feeds must be isosmolar or rapid shifts of fluid across the jejunal wall embarrass the circulation. The weight gain of jejunally fed infants is slower than nasogastrically fed infants, possibly because important gastrointestinal hormone effects are not being stimulated (Whitfield, 1982). The importance of the gastrointestinal hormone responses to feeding on normal gut maturation is not certain (Lucas, 1981).

Small infants have proportionately higher nutrient requirements than normal full term infants. How suitable is human milk for them? The milk of term mothers may be low in protein, minerals and vitamins for the needs of LBW infants but the sodium, energy and protein content of the milk of mothers delivering prematurely is higher than that of mothers delivering at term (Atkinson *et al.*, 1978; Gross *et al.*, 1980; Schonler and Oh, 1980; Anderson *et al.*, 1983).

One of the dilemmas raised by feeding breast milk to LBW infants is the inability of the smaller and more immature infants to suck. These infants receive stored, pooled, pasteurized or deep frozen milk which is qualitatively less satisfactory than milk direct from the breast. How should human milk be collected and stored for these infants? Pasteurization reduces the anti-infective properties and lipolytic activity of milk to an extent which varies with the time and temperature at which pasteurization takes place. Lipase activity and humoral antibacterial effects are retained fairly well by deep freezing over some weeks although freezing reduces the bile salt sensitivity of the lipase and may reduce its efficiency (Hamosh, 1982). Lipase is present in the milk of mothers delivering as early as 25 weeks gestation. Reduction in milk lipase activity may explain the reduced weight gain of premature infants fed pasteurized human milk (Williamson *et al.*, 1978) compared with those fed formula. Fresh maternal milk is probably the ideal food for LBW infants since it contains lipase and has intact antibacterial mechanisms. Frozen maternal milk is probably the next most suitable food (DHSS, 1981). Recent concern over the transmission of HIV virus in breast milk has led to recommendations that infants should only receive unpasteurized milk from their own mothers.

*How much?*

It is usually recommended that SG and LGA infants need 180–200 ml/kg/day of standard formulas for optimal growth. This provides about 140 kcals/kg/day. In early life fluid overload predisposes LBW infants, particularly those with respiratory distress, anoxia and poor perfusion, to patent ductus arteriosus, bronchopulmonary dysplasia and necrotizing enterocolitis (Bell and Oh, 1983). Feed volumes must be built up slowly. Full volume feeds should not be achieved before 10 days of age and for sick infants it may be many weeks before they can tolerate full oral feeding. Initially small feeds are given hourly so respiratory embarrassment is minimized (Shivpuri *et al.*, 1983). In practice many low birthweight or sick infants require periods of intravenous feeding before oral feeds can be attempted safely.

*Special LBW infant formulas*

The difficulties of providing LBW infants with sufficient volume of milk to provide the nutrients needed for rapid growth has led to the development of special LBW infant formulas of increased energy density, increased protein and mineral content and supplemented with carnitine. Table 2.6 lists the particular compositional changes of some of these 'low birthweight' formulas.

It is not yet clear whether these formulas have advantages for growth over infants' own fresh mothers' milk (Atkinson *et al.*, 1983; Chessex *et al.*, 1983) but it seems likely that they have advantages over pooled term breast milk particularly if this has been pasteurized and has lost its main advantage of anti-bacterial effects (Brooke *et al.*, 1982; Williamson *et al.*, 1978). Studies using one particular low birthweight formula appear to show that infants fed this formula have a lower incidence of metabolic bone disease and more rapid gain in weight, length and skull circumference than infants fed banked breast milk (Lucas *et al.*, 1984).

**Intravenous feeding**

Intravenous feeding is not a practice to be undertaken lightly in any age group and this is particularly true for neonates. Neonates have difficulty coping with high infusion rates for amino acids, glucose and fat; and hyper-ammonaemia, hyperglycaemia and lipid deposits in brain, lungs and kidneys have all been attributed to intravenous feeding (Friedman *et al.*, 1978; Johnson *et al.*, 1972; Levene *et al.*, 1980). If Intralipid is not infused, other sources of essential fatty acids – such as plasma – should be given. Carnitine deficiency may occur (Schmidt-Sommerfeld *et al.*, 1982). Despite the difficulties, intravenous feeding is lifesaving for many seriously ill LBW infants and is the method of choice for initial feeding of infants less than 1000 g in many neonatal intensive care units. It is specialized management that should be administered only by the experienced. Details of intravenous feeding for neonates can be obtained from specialist neonatal texts and other sources (Fanaroff and Klaus, 1979; Grotte *et al.*, 1982; Kanarek *et al.*, 1982; Hughes, 1982; Forsyth, 1983; Insley, 1986; Yu, 1986).

**Specific nutritional problems of LBW infants**

*Acidosis*

Acidosis used to be a common problem amongst premature infants fed unmodified cows' milk formula. It probably reflected infants' inability to excrete the acid load presented by high protein, high phosphate feeds. It remains a problem in infected or stressed LBW neonates who are unable to utilize ingested amino acids for growth or tissue deposition. Infants present with poor feeding, increased respiratory rate, lethargy and poor weight gain. Age, renal maturation and improvements in general health usually allow the problem to resolve gradually (Berger *et al.*, 1980).

*Vitamin deficiencies*

Low birthweight infants need more vitamins than they are likely to receive in the small quantities of milk they ingest. Vitamin supplementation is desirable for all infants of birthweight less than 2 kg (DHSS, 1980a; Orzalesi, 1982). Newborn infants have low levels of vitamin E. In full term infants, levels rise to normal over the first few weeks of life. Levels in SG infants may remain low for months. It has been suggested that supplementing SG infants with vitamin E from birth protects against intraventricular haemorrhage and retrolental

Table 2.6 LBW formulas available in Britain

| Milk | Manufacturer | Energy kJ | Energy kcal | Protein g | Sodium mg | Calcium mg | Phosphorus mg | Vitamin D μg | Osmolality mosmol/litre |
|---|---|---|---|---|---|---|---|---|---|
| | | | | Composition/100 ml feed | | | | | |
| Nenatal | Cow and Gate | 319 | 76 | 1.8 | 20 | 100 | 50 | 3.0 | 340 |
| Prematalac | Cow and Gate | 332 | 79 | 2.4 | 60 | 67 | 53 | 1.1 | 342 |
| *SMA LBW* Formula | Wyeth | 336 | 80 | 2.0 | 32 | 75 | 40 | 1.3 | 268 |
| Oster-Prem | Farley Glaxo | 336 | 80 | 2.0 | 45 | 70 | 35 | 8.0 | 300 |
| Pre-Aptamil | Milupa | 311 | 74 | 2.1 | 35 | 60 | 45 | 1.1 | 350 |
| Mature breast milk | | 294 | 70 | 1.1 | 15 | 35 | 14 | 0.6 | 290 |

fibroplasia (Chiswick *et al.*, 1984; Finer *et al.*, 1984). Occasional infants present with vitamin E responsive haemolytic anaemia in the first month of life. Routine supplementation of VLBW infants is advisable.

*Bone disease of prematurity*

Bone disease is common in VLBW infants. Although usually described as 'rickets' of prematurity, vitamin D deficiency is only one of several precipitating factors and the condition is probably more appropriately termed metabolic bone disease of prematurity. Supplementation of VLBW infants with 10–12.5 μg (400–500IU) vitamin D per day achieves normal circulating 25 hydroxy and 1–25 dihydroxy vitamin D (Markestad *et al.*, 1984) but bone disease may present despite adequate vitamin D.

The fetus retains about 300 mg calcium per day in the last trimester (Widdowson, 1979). Neither breast milk nor modern low phosphate formulas for term infants provide sufficient calcium or phosphate for retention of bone mineral at the rate occurring *in utero* (Atkinson *et al.*, 1983). Acidosis and diuretics induce renal calcium loss. 'Rickets' of prematurity is probably a reflection of inadequate phosphate and calcium retention (Callenbach *et al.*, 1981; Sagy *et al.*, 1980; Yuen *et al.*, 1979) although protein deficiency and other mineral deficiency may also contribute. Supplementary phosphate or formulas with increased phosphate – with or without calcium – promote bone mineralization and should be considered for all VLBW infants, (Minton *et al.*, 1979; Callenbach *et al.*, 1981; Senterre *et al.*, 1983; Lucas *et al.*, 1984).

*Anaemia of prematurity*

*Early anaemia* Many LBW infants develop severe anaemia in the first weeks of life. The haemoglobin of newborn infants is 18–20 g/dl. Blood volume is about 80 ml/kg body weight. High tissue oxygen tension in postnatal, compared with intra-uterine, life produces a relative depression of bone marrow function and a fairly rapid fall in haemoglobin to 10–12 g/dl in all infants. Haemoglobin remains within this 'normal' range until about 5 years of age. Bone marrow immaturity, rapid growth, respiratory and other illness and frequent venepunctures contribute to more dramatic falls in haemoglobin in LBW infants. With haemoglobin levels below 10 g/dl some small infants feed poorly, seem lethargic and even develop cardiac failure. Treatment of this anaemia is by transfusion of 'partially packed' blood (Shaw, 1982).

*Late anaemia* LBW infants are at risk of iron deficiency anaemia from the second half of the first year. All infants have a predisposition to iron deficiency but the fortification of baby milk formulas has reduced the prevalence of iron deficiency in normal weight, full term infants. LBW premature infants have less opportunity to receive stores of iron *in utero* since much of the iron is transferred to the fetus in the last trimester. Postnatally their rapid growth rates demand more iron than provided by the relatively small volumes of milk ingested and the introduction of iron sources in weaning foods is likely to be at a chronologically greater age than in the normal newborn.

Iron increases red cell membrane instability through anti-oxidant effects. Low vitamin E levels in LBW newborn suggest that iron supplementation should not be given to formula-fed infants before 4 weeks of age. Iron also modifies the antibacterial effects of lactoferrin and transferrin. It is arguable that iron should be avoided in wholly breast-fed infants unless there is clear evidence of iron deficiency or until feeding with foods other than breast milk has begun. However, since prolonged breast-feeding predisposes to iron deficiency, iron should probably be given to all breast-fed premature infants after 6 months, even if they are still wholly breast-fed. By this time infants' iron stores are likely to be low.

Significant folate deficiency is also common in LBW infants (especially LGA infants) and may show itself as abnormal morphological changes in the peripheral blood even without significant anaemia. Daily requirements of folic acid have been estimated as 50–70 μg/day. Folic acid supplementation of 500–1000 μg/week should be given to LBW infants for the first year or until the infants are on a full mixed diet (Strelling *et al.*, 1979).

## Weaning

### Why?

Protein requirements per kg body weight fall rapidly in the first months of life. Energy requirements per kg also fall, but proportionately less. By the time infants have doubled birthweight at 4 to 5 months, the volumes of milk necessary to meet energy requirements may exceed a litre, although protein requirements can be met by considerably smaller volumes of milk. Thus the need for energy is one of the main reasons for weaning. Further, by 4 to 6 months, iron, trace elements and vitamins have often reached low levels. Weaning diets should be energy rich and should supply a wide variety of other nutrients. Provided infants continue to take 500–700 ml of milk a day, protein is not a major priority of weaning foods.

### When?

Some mothers are able to sustain excellent growth in their totally breast-fed infants for most of the first year (Ahn and MacLean, 1980). These mothers are usually those who have maintained high frequency of suckling throughout lactation and who are themselves very well nourished. In most women breast milk output fails to meet infants' needs from about 6 months onwards. DHSS (1974) recommendations are that weaning should be delayed until infants are 4 months but these recommendations should not be applied rigidly (DHSS, 1980c) if there is evidence that infants are unable to take or receive sufficient milk to maintain optimal growth at slightly younger ages (Waterlow and Thomson, 1979; Whitehead and Paul, 1981). In developed countries there is little reason to recommend weaning before 3 months for normal infants. Where mothers cannot provide sufficient milk to enable their infants to grow normally at this age, breast-feeding is probably failing and supplementary bottle feeds or a change to full formula feeding should be instituted instead. Reducing the fluid intake by satisfying infants with solid foods instead of milk risks dehydration in the very young.

Delaying weaning until after 6 months post-term predisposes to vitamin, trace element or iron deficiency. Around 6 months infants develop their first teeth and will chew if they are given objects to chew. There seem good reasons to introduce mixed feeding at this age. Weaning later when infants have learnt to refuse food by closing their mouths, shaking their heads or pushing the spoon away makes weaning a more troublesome process.

**How?**
New foods should be introduced gradually. They should be selected to provide a variety of nutrients. Cereals are the usual first weaning foods. Gluten containing cereals could precipitate early coeliac disease in susceptible individuals so rice based cereals are often recommended as first solids. This is probably a counsel of perfection. Wheat and rye cereals are widely used.

Other early weaning foods include egg yolk, well chopped and mashed vegetables such as spinach and carrot, liver preparations and fruit dishes such as stewed fruit. Many of these foods are now available as powders which only require the addition of water, or as tinned, pureed 'infant dinners' and 'infant puddings'.

As the weaning diet is introduced, one or more milk feeds are withdrawn and replaced by vitamin C containing infant fruit juice preparations. By 1 year of age, infants should be taking mixed diets similar to those of the rest of the family but well chopped up and with small energy rich snacks in between main meals so they do not go without food for more than about 4 hours during the day. They should continue to consume about a pint of milk and this seems a reasonable milk intake to recommend throughout childhood, since milk remains a major source of calcium and protein for many children. This author would recommend babymilks being fed until a year because of the added vitamins and iron and lower renal solute load. Other policies regard 'doorstep' milk as safe from 6 months (DHSS, 1980c; Committee on Nutrition, 1983).

'Follow on' milks have been introduced by some formula manufacturing firms as providing transitions between formula and cows' milks for weaning infants. These milks seem unnecessary. Since they contain much higher renal solute load than standard formulas and since they are recommended by manufacturers for 4 month old infants and upwards, they may even increase the risks of hypertonic dehydration. Standard infant formulas with weaning foods, provide adequate nutrition, vitamins and minerals to meet the needs of 6 to 12 month old infants. 'Follow on' milks add to the confusing profusion of formulas available for mothers to buy and if used before the recommended age their high protein and low fat content may even present nutritional risks.

## Vitamin supplementation in infancy

Standard British babymilks are all supplemented with vitamins and iron. Normal healthy term infants who feed well are unlikely to come to harm if they rely on the vitamins contained in their formula. Cows' ('doorstep') milk contains relatively little vitamin C and is also low in vitamin D and iron. The iron in cows' milk is less well absorbed than that in human milk. If the infant is on a good mixed weaning diet and receiving reasonable exposure to summer sunshine, iron and vitamin deficiencies are unlikely to arise. In Britain, relatively sunless summers can put the child population at risk of vitamin D deficiency, so vitamin D supplementation is advisable for all infants and young children. Vitamin A is not widely available in foods and should also be supplemented. Vitamin C is widely available in fruits and preserved foods but scurvy was once a major problem in British infants and children's vitamin supplements contain vitamin C also. DHSS recommendations are that children from 1 month to 2 years, and preferably 5 years, should receive Children's Vitamin Drops or a proprietary preparation containing vitamin A 200 μg, vitamin C 20 mg, vitamin D 7 μg daily, (DHSS, 1980c).

Breast milk from well nourished women has higher vitamin C and D content than cows' milk but breast-feeding by D deficient mothers can exacerbate the poor vitamin D status of infants born to such mothers. Vitamin D deficiency and osteomalacia are common in Asian women in Britain. Breast-fed Asian and African infants (in whom skin pigmentation may reduce vitamin D synthesis in a poor summer) should receive supplementary vitamin D 10 μg daily.

### Immigrant, vegetarian and 'cult' diets

Clearly, generalization cannot be made about the dietary practices of the many different immigrant groups in Britain. Poverty, ignorance of locally available foods for young infants, and linguistic difficulties are common to many of these groups and probably account for the development of the nutritional problems seen fairly frequently in young immigrant children. Prolonged breast-feeding or, alternatively, weaning diets consisting of 'doorstep' milk and little else, predispose to failure to thrive and iron deficiency. Vegetarian weaning diets may contribute to failure to thrive but rarely seem to cause protein deficiency, perhaps because these diets are usually accompanied by a good milk intake. Community programmes aimed at helping immigrant facilities to provide adequately for their children in an unfamiliar environment seem effective, (Jivani, 1978; Goel *et al.*, 1978).

Cult diets and elimination diets are more concerning than immigrant weaning practices in nutrition of young children. Religious groups with strict and wide ranging food avoidance may be particularly damaging for small children who need a variety of foods if requirements are to be met. It may be difficult to persuade parents in these groups to modify their diets for the nutritional safety of their children (Shinwell and Gorodischer, 1982; Shull *et al.*, 1977; Committee on Nutrition, 1977).

Modern interest in the widely published, but not well substantiated, risks of food allergens and additives (see later) is likely to increase the numbers of young children who are weaned on to diets containing a limited range of foods. Such diets will have to be assessed individually for nutritional adequacy and should only be adopted 'on doctor's advice' (David *et al.*, 1984). There is no conclusive evidence that prolonged breast feeding without weaning has long term effects in preventing eczema, asthma or other allergy in children from atopic families.

## Nutritional problems affecting young children

Minor feeding problems are common in young children. Generally, they do not affect growth or nutrition. Poor appetite is a common complaint. Frequently, parental anxiety arises because the child is small, perhaps because familial size is small. A careful dietary history usually shows that the child eats little at mealtimes, but has a high consumption of sweets, biscuits, crisps and fruit juice in between meals. Clinical examinations show no abnormality and the child usually follows a normal growth velocity. Parents should be advised to confine food to meals and recognized snack periods only. Young children quickly learn to manipulate their parents by being 'difficult' with food.

## Failure to thrive

Failure to thrive (FTT) implies failure to gain in height and weight at the expected rate. Its causes are numerous; a clinical classification of these is found in Table 2.7. The categories listed are not always distinct. For example, chronic infection may cause anorexia and reduced intake, failure to absorb due to lactose intolerance, failure to utilize due to the toxic effects of infection, and increased requirements due to the increased metabolic rate that accompanies pyrexia. Frequent acute infections may lead to FTT if there is insufficient time or inadequate food for catch up growth in between episodes of infection.

Some children with FTT appear to eat sufficient food for normal growth but grow inadequately nevertheless. This group includes many of the children with major congenital abnormalities, severe intra-uterine growth retardation or chromosomal abnormalities. Forced feeding is rarely successful in inducing catch up growth in this group. Presumably food not utilized in growth is expended in heat or activity.

Amongst this group of children who fail to thrive despite adequate food intake are some whose inappropriate nurturing appears to inhibit normal utilization of food for growth. Altering the psychological environment of these children usually results in rapid catch up growth (Widdowson, 1951). Reversible growth hormone and other hormone deficiencies in these children probably reflect the inhibitory effects of emotional stress on hypothalamic function and may be relevant to their FTT (Patton and Gardner, 1962; McCarthy, 1981).

Children with severe brain damage, particularly those with cerebral palsy, commonly FTT. For some, mental retardation and bulbar palsy affect the ability to suck, swallow and chew. Other children with severe spastic cerebral palsy or choreoathetosis waste energy in voluntary and involuntary movement.

Some children with FTT and feeding difficulties are helped by early weaning. Weaning can increase the energy density of the diet without increasing the weight and volume of intake. A semi-solid diet is often easier to feed by spoon to children who cannot suck. Semi-solids are commonly equally

Table 2.7 Clinical classification of causes of failure to thrive

| |
|---|
| Inadequate energy intake |
| Malabsorption |
| Increased energy loss |
| Failure to utilize absorbed energy |
| Increased energy requirements |

low in energy as milk unless supplemented with a fat source. Thus, where handicap is severe and feeding with semi-solid or monotonous diets prolonged, the nutritional adequacy of such diets, particularly for energy and vitamins, needs frequent checking since children grow and their requirements change. Housebound and institutionalized children are particularly liable to vitamin D deficiency due to lack of exposure to summer sunshine, especially if their vitamin D requirements are increased by anticonvulsant therapy.

Infants and toddlers with congenital heart disease fail to thrive for a variety of reasons. Some have low energy intake secondary to cardiac failure and breathlessness. Others have inefficient metabolism due to severe anoxia. Those with persistent cardiac failure or pulmonary hypertension may have raised metabolic rates and an increased need for energy (Menon and Poskitt, 1985). Growth may be improved by increasing the energy content but not the volume of the feed, by early weaning.

Children with renal failure commonly fail to thrive. In early stages of renal failure this may result in children growing along the third centile. Appetites are poor and supplementing the diet with high energy foods often results in the children eating less of other foods (Betts and Magrath, 1974). End stage renal failure is usually associated with very poor growth and the onset of renal osteodystrophy. Low plasma levels of a wide variety of nutrients may result from poor dietary intake and absorption and metabolic abnormalities. Elemental diets may be helpful. Supplementary one-hydroxylated versions of vitamin D are necessary. Much wider use of peritoneal and haemo-dialysis and even renal transplant has reduced the need to provide artificial diets for children with chronic renal failure. Dialysis often requires a higher protein intake than is usually expected.

## Children with a predisposition to obesity

Table 2.8 lists children with increased predisposition to obesity not associated with other significant pathology. Despite theories which were popular a few years ago, fat infants show only slight predisposition to later obesity. This probably relates to an inherent predisposition to obesity rather than feeding and nutrition in early infancy acting as the determinants of later obesity. Most fat infants slim to normal weight young children. Obesity is, however, very prevalent in the children of obese parents. Eighty per cent of older children presenting to obesity clinics have one obese parent and about forty per cent have two obese parents.

Most of these children are above average stature prepubertally. Some show early puberty and early growth spurt and are average or below average stature

Table 2.8 Risk factors for obesity in childhood

| |
|---|
| Obese parent |
| Single parent family |
| Single child or long gap between this and previous child |
| Large family |
| Low social class |

Table 2.9 Pathological conditions predisposing to obesity in childhood

| | |
|---|---|
| Endocrine causes: | Hypothyroidism |
| | Growth hormone deficiency |
| | Cushing's syndrome |
| Hypothalamic causes: | Prader–Willi syndrome |
| | Laurence Moon Biedl syndrome |
| | Craniopharygioma |
| | Perinatal or postnatal 'brain damage' |
| Immobility: | Meningomyelocele, with or without hydrocephalus |
| | Duchenne muscular dystrophy |
| Skeletal causes: | Achondroplasia |
| Drug treatment: | Corticosteroids |
| | Sodium valproate |
| Chromosomal causes: | Down's syndrome |
| | Klinefelter's syndrome |

in adult life. Prepubertally, however, tall stature distinguishes children with simple obesity from those with underlying pathology predisposing to obesity. Most of these latter children have short stature and usually other abnormal clinical features (Table 2.9).

In childhood the effect of growth means that slimming and loss of fat are not necessarily associated with loss of weight since lean body mass increases whilst fat loss occurs. If diets are very strict, intakes of energy and other nutrients may be insufficient to maintain normal growth rates and too rapid weight loss may be associated with slowing of growth. Most obese children require dietary intakes of 3.4–5.0 MJ (800–1200 kcal) per day although adolescent boys with very rapid growth may slim on considerably higher energy intakes.

Dietary control is difficult in childhood since children may not understand the need for control. This is particularly so for children with mental retardation and obesity. Children with spina bifida, Duchenne type muscular dystrophy and other causes of mental handicap and physical immobility frequently become obese. Inactivity, poor self control due to mental retardation, and edible 'treats' from well meaning, but unwisely indulgent, relatives all contribute to obesity. Physical handicap makes a reduced energy intake the only feasible way obesity can be controlled in these children (Guy, 1978). Parents should be advised on feeding at the time a child's condition is diagnosed.

Children with Prader–Willi syndrome (Table 2.10) present a major problem for dietary management. In early infancy these children commonly fail to thrive due to hypotonia and feeding difficulties. After the first year of life appetites may become enormous but even without excessive intakes, obesity develops rapidly and excessively. Overall short stature and poor prepubertal growth spurt coupled with low energy expenditure in activity because of the mental retardation, contribute to the development of obesity. In addition these children have abnormally low basal energy requirements (often only fifty per cent of expected values) providing the main explanation for their obesity. Weight reduction can be achieved by very strict dietary control but the parent–child conflict that may be associated with such control makes it difficult for families to pursue strict diets successfully (Holm and Pipes, 1976).

Table 2.10 Main clinical features of Prader–Willi syndrome

| | |
|---|---|
| Facial features: | Reduced biparietal diameter<br>Micrognathia<br>Carp-like mouth |
| Skeletal problems: | Short stature noticeable after infancy<br>Small hands and feet with tapering digits<br>Straight ulnar border to hand<br>Scoliosis |
| Neuromuscular problems: | Hypotonia in infancy<br>Mental retardation<br>Behavioural problems often with insatiable appetite<br>Convulsions |
| Endocrine: | Hypogonadism: micropenis, hypoplastic scrotum, cryptorchidism<br>Delayed puberty<br>Gross obesity with reduced basal energy requirements<br>Insulin resistant diabetes mellitus |

## Iron deficiency in childhood

All young children are at risk of iron deficiency since even in health, intake and absorption barely exceed requirements. Iron deficiency is particularly common amongst children from socio-economically deprived circumstances when prematurity and early weaning on to unsupplemented cows' milk may be contributory factors. Frequent infections encourage iron deficiency since iron absorption is inhibited by pyrexia (Beresford *et al.*, 1971). Levels of haemoglobin above 10.5 g/dl are usually accepted as satisfactory in preschool children since their haemoglobin is lower than adult levels perhaps because of the rapid growth of young children. However, iron deficiency may present before anaemia develops with anorexia, behavioural disturbances, apathy, misery and pica.

Iron deficiency may be a presentation of coeliac disease in childhood. Toddlers who fail to respond to oral iron or who have gastrointestinal symptoms or growth retardation deserve further investigation as do all children in whom there is inadequate explanation for iron deficiency.

## Vitamin deficiencies

Tables 2.11 and 2.12 outline briefly the main conditions and precipitating situations associated with vitamin deficiencies in childhood. For diagnosis and treatment larger texts should be consulted. The only likely vitamin deficiency to occur in this country in otherwise normal children is rickets which is described below.

### Rickets

Rickets used to be common in British children. Environmental improvements as a result of the Clean Air Act (1956) and supplementation of baby foods have

Table 2.11 Vitamin deficiencies in childhood: clinical features and predisposing causes

| Vitamin | Clinical features of deficiency | Predisposing causes |
|---|---|---|
| A – retinol | Night blindness, xerosis conjunctivae, keratomalacia, blindness<br>Follicular hyperkeratosis<br>Failure to thrive; anaemia; hepatosplenomegaly<br>Susceptibility to infection | Low fat diet; fat malabsorption; protein energy malnutrition; infection; chronic diarrhoea; stress<br>Deficiency of dark green leafy vegetables and highly coloured vegetables (tomatoes, peppers) |
| B group (see Table 2.12) | Deficiencies often occur together | Diets lacking in variety; over-cooked and over-refined foods; famine conditions; protein energy malnutrition |
| C – ascorbic acid | Scurvy: bleeding; bruising; reduced resistance to infection; osteoporosis; subperiosteal haemorrhages; anaemia; poor scar tissue formation | Artificial diets; overcooked foods; infection; stress; cold; tissue damage; malabsorption; lack of fruit and vegetables |
| D – calciferol | Rickets: see text | Sunlight deficiency, dark skin,<br>Lack of oily fish, animal liver, eggs, margarine in diet<br>Rapid growth: prematurity, adolescence<br>Drug therapy, anticonvulsants |
| E – tocopherol | See text. Haemolytic anaemia in premature<br>Progressive neurological degeneration in malabsorption syndromes | High essential fatty acid in diet<br>Premature<br>Fat malabsorption: cystic fibrosis abetalipoproteinaemia |
| K | Prolonged bleeding and clotting times; reduced factors II, VII, IX and X | Newborn, especially breast fed<br>Malabsorption<br>Liver disease; gut sterilization |

reduced the prevalence of rickets enormously. Exposure to summer sunlight (wavelength $\simeq$ 300 nm) is more important for maintenance of normal plasma 25 hydroxy vitamin D levels than dietary intake of vitamin D. Seaside summer holidays may be important in providing this exposure since British summers are so unpredictable (Poskitt *et al.*, 1979).

The late 1960s saw a resurgence of nutritional rickets in Britain amongst immigrants from India, Pakistan and Bangladesh. Inadequate sunlight exposure due to inner city life, skin pigmentation, traditional dress, the tradition of women and young children staying indoors and low intakes of vitamin D, probably all contributed to the resurgence. Unrefined chapatti flour

Table 2.12 Clinical features and predisposing causes for deficiency of B vitamins in childhood

| Vitamins | Clinical features | Predisposing causes |
|---|---|---|
| $B_1$ – thiamine | High output cardiac failure; cardiac arrhythmias; restlessness; encephalopathy | Polished rice diet; breast-fed infants of thiamine deficient mothers; chronic diarrhoea |
| $B_2$ – riboflavin | Angular stomatitis; glossitis; magenta tongue; normochromic anaemia | Protein – energy malnutrition; biliary atresia; chronic hepatitis |
| niacin | Light sensitive dermatitis; alternating diarrhoea and constipation; neuronal degeneration | Maize diets when not milled with alkali; diets low in tryptophan; high leucine diets: sorghum vulgare |
| $B_6$ – pyridoxine | Convulsions: hypochromic anaemia; seborrhoeic dermatitis; glossitis; peripheral neuritis | Inborn errors of metabolism with pyridoxine dependency; high maternal intake of pyridoxine in pregnancy; drug therapy: isoniazid; artificial diets without pyridoxine supplementation |
| folic acid | Failure to thrive; megaloblastic anaemia; thrombocytopenia; neutropenia | Overcooked foods; infants fed goat milk; prematurity; rapid cell turnover or regeneration; protein energy malnutrition; malabsorption; drug therapy; anticonvulsants |
| $B_{12}$ – cobalamin | Megaloblastic anaemia; subacute combined degeneration of the cord; dementia | Congenital abnormalities of intrinsic factor or transport proteins; strict vegans: no dairy products, no eggs; disease or resection of terminal ileum: especially ileo-caecal Crohn's disease |

consumption which reduces intestinal reabsorption of 25 hydroxy vitamin D secreted into the gut via the bile may also be relevant. Concern with Asian rickets, changing immigrant lifestyles and some supplementation of chapatti flour probably explain recent falls in the prevalence of rickets in this group of children. Rickets now seems commoner in immigrant children from the Horn of Africa and the Middle East. Supplementation with vitamin D is advisable for breast-fed infants from these families since the mothers are often deficient in vitamin D.

In early infancy, rickets presents with craniotabes (bulging forehead due to soft skull bones), hypotonia, and FTT. Hypocalcaemia and hypocalcaemic convulsions are common. Older children usually maintain normocalcaemia by secondary hyperparathyroidism but present with bone pain, misery, malaise, hypotonia, short stature, recurrent chestiness and bone deformity. Typically there is bowing of the legs and swelling at the metaphyses of bones and costochondral junctions giving the rickety 'rosary'. Indrawing of the lower chest due to the softness of the bones creates Harrison's sulcus around the attachment of the diaphragm. Plasma calcium is usually in the low normal range, phosphate very low and alkaline phosphatase – which is very variable in normal children – markedly raised. X-rays show widening of the epiphyseal plate, splayed shaggy ends to the metaphyses and bending of the bones. Treatment of nutritional rickets is with vitamin D 100 $\mu$g (4000 units) daily. Supplementation with 10 $\mu$g (400 units) for infants and 2.5 $\mu$g (100 units) for older children should be sufficient prophylaxis.

## Trace element deficiency

Deficiencies in trace elements can inhibit growth but they are rare except in children on artificial diets. Zinc deficiency is manifest in acrodermatitis enteropathica, where an inherited disorder of zinc metabolism leads to chronic diarrhoea, failure to thrive, mucocutaneous ulceration and dermatitis and ultimately death. The condition resolves completely with oral zinc supplementation. Many severely ill children have low plasma levels of trace elements, but the significance of these is usually not clear. Where there is malabsorption or tissue loss these may be relevant. Zinc deficiency is associated with a syndrome of delayed puberty and short stature in boys in Iran and Egypt. Accelerated growth and pubertal development occur with zinc supplementation (Sandstead *et al.*, 1967). Selenium deficiency presents as a cardiomyopathy (Keshan disease) over a wide belt of China where soil selenium content is extremely low. Keshan disease is found in no other selenium deficient area of the world.

## Nutrition in infective diarrhoea

Diarrhoea, usually secondary to infection, is very common in childhood. Appropriate management is important if chronic nutritional disturbances are to be avoided. The majority of cases of diarrhoea are self limiting. Temporary replacement of feeding by clear fluids orally settles most cases quickly. It may not be necessary to stop feeding in all cases and this will lessen the nutritional stress (Rees and Brook, 1979). Sodium ion absorption is linked with glucose transport mechanisms. Mixtures of 2 per cent glucose and saline will allow maximum opportunity for sodium and water absorption and minimum problems from the osmolar effects of unabsorbed glucose in the gut. Recognition of this has made it possible to treat most diarrhoeas with oral rehydration.

WHO recommendations for the composition of oral rehydration solutions are 111 mmol/litre glucose (2 per cent solution), sodium 90 mmol/litre and 20 mmol/litre potassium together with base. The high sodium concentration presents a possible risk of hyperosmolar dehydration for infants with their higher water requirements than adults. Solutions containing glucose 111 mmol/litre, sodium 50–60 mmol/litre, chloride 30–50 mmol/litre and bicarbonate or citrate 30 mmol/litre may be used instead (Finsberg *et al.*,

1982). Twenty-four hours of clear fluids in this form followed by regrading on to milk and diet over the course of some days is the traditional method of managing diarrhoea. Over this period the child's intake will be less than requirements and nutrition, and consequently gut function, may deteriorate further so the child is precipitated into the vicious downward spiral of deteriorating gut function and deteriorating nutrition. Feeding full strength milk from the day refeeding is started is not associated with greater complication rates amongst those children with uncomplicated diarrhoea (Brown and MacLean, 1984).

## Chronic nonspecific ('Toddler') diarrhoea

Persistent watery stools without other symptoms or evidence of illness are a common problem in the toddler (1–3 year old) age group. These children have good, although sometimes fussy, appetites and thrive. Stool examination shows no infection, infestation, malabsorption or lactose intolerance.

Toddler diarrhoea may have no direct connection with the diet, but it has been suggested that it results from the high carbohydrate, low fat, low roughage diet of many young children. Fussy appetites often cause the children to live off fruit drinks, sweets, biscuits, with little fruit, vegetables or fat. Increasing the fat content of the diet and reducing the carbohydrate intake may relieve the symptoms in some children. Time usually cures the others (Cohen *et al.*, 1979).

## Dental caries

The prevalence of dental caries is attributed to the high refined carbohydrate content of most young children's diets. Dummies containing sweetened solutions and putting children to bed with bottles of sweetened fruit juice contribute to the development of the 'nursing bottle syndrome' with carious destruction of the first incisors as they erupt. Supplementation of water supplies with fluoride to a concentration of 1 mg/litre reduces the prevalence of childhood dental caries. Where water supplies contain less fluoride than this, fluoride tablets can be given instead.

Enamel deposition takes place in the first dentition from the fourth month of gestation. Premature infants in Sweden with enamel defects and a liability to caries are more likely to be born in winter months and have usually received less breast milk in the first weeks of life than infants without enamel defects. Marginal vitamin D deficiency in the mother may make the newborn infant unable to absorb calcium or mobilize calcium from bone sufficiently well to maintain normal enamel formation (Mellander *et al.*, 1982).

## Food additives

There has been a lot of anxiety about the effects of 'unnatural' additives and preservatives in food on children's behaviour. Hyperactivity, poor school progress and behaviour disorders are attributed to these products. Trials of elimination diets have suggested impressive improvements in children's behaviour. Such trials have not always had proper control studies. Definite evidence that food additives have any effect on cerebral or other physiological function is lacking (Bierman and Furukawa, 1978; Stare *et al.*, 1980). Nevertheless, it is advisable that substances are not added to foods simply to make them more colourful or attractive in other ways. It seems likely that the present public fascination with elimination diets as treatment for a variety of conditions will increase. There are grounds for using such diets in certain recognized allergic conditions but whether or not elimination diets are scientifically proven to be helpful in a condition, it is important that their use does not result in nutritional deprivation. Vitamin deficiencies can be avoided by supplementation, but potential calcium deficiency is more worrying since a low calcium intake will reduce the amount of calcium laid down in bone. The effects of this may only become apparent in senile osteoporosis many years later (David *et al.*, 1984).

## Adolescence

Adolescence is a troublesome background against which to place any ill health. A growing desire for independence, strong peer group influences, demands from school and family, and changing physical and hormonal constitution all provide physical and emotional stresses additional to those of disease.

The main nutritional problems of adolescents in the developed world are obesity and anorexia nervosa. Both these conditions are discussed elsewhere in this book. Rapid growth and pubertal development affect the nutritional control of chronic conditions such as diabetes and cystic fibrosis and the instabilities of the adolescent lifestyle are likely to exacerbate any clinical deterioration. Thus the management of adolescents with chronic disease requires both sympathetic understanding and clinical skill.

It is impossible to be specific about the nutritional needs of adolescents. Mean estimates for age and sex obscure the enormous variation in individual requirements in this group of young people. Requirements are affected by the age of onset and the size of pubertal growth spurt as well as by age, sex and activity. Girls have earlier onset of puberty and smaller, briefer growth spurt so peak nutritional intake is in early adolescence. Boys have later, greater and more prolonged growth spurt. Peak nutritional requirements may be very high. Moreover the hormonal changes of puberty lead to development of lean rather than fat tissue, so boys who were previously overweight often slim spontaneously at puberty. Girls tend to deposit fat at puberty and unless their intake is well matched to their growth spurt, may become quite markedly obese once growth slows again. Both boys and girls have much greater energy intakes than adults around the time of peak height velocity and their erratic activity and eating patterns can result in huge intakes for one particular day, or one mealtime. This needs to be remembered before assessing adolescents' diets from brief records.

Truswell and Darnton-Hill (1981) have highlighted some of the common dietary habits which put otherwise normal adolescents at nutritional risk or complicate management of conditions where dietary therapy is important. These include preferences for 'fast', 'take-away' or 'carry-out' foods; the habit of missing meals; frequent snacking, with particularly high consumptions of sweets; unconventional meals; the start (or at least one hopes only the start) of alcohol consumption; high consumption of soft or other 'fun' drinks; strong food likes and dislikes; periods of high energy intakes; low intakes for some nutrients, and dieting crazes. In view of this long list of disturbing problems it is perhaps surprising that major nutritional problems are not more common in adolescence. Our adult concern is often directed more at the aesthetic and social effects of adolescent eating patterns than their nutritional effects. Adolescent intakes of calcium, iron, vitamin C, vitamin A, vitamin D and sometimes riboflavin and zinc are frequently below recommended levels (Truswell and Darnton-Hill, 1981) but clinical deficiency of any of these nutrients is rare. Perhaps this only illustrates the wide safety margin incorporated into most dietary recommendations! Vitamin D deficiency can be avoided provided the adolescent has adequate exposure to summer sunshine but Asian immigrants in urban areas, particularly girls who tend to live more secluded lives, are prone to nutritional rickets in adolescence. Iron deficiency is less common than might be expected from estimated intakes but this may relate to the fact that iron absorption varies with food mixtures and with body iron stores. If health is good, the proportion of iron absorbed from a low intake is high thus preventing clinical deficiency.

Pregnancy is an increasingly frequent feature of adolescence. The frequently low calcium, iron and vitamin D intakes which do not produce clinical deficiency in non-pregnant girls present nutritional risks for the pregnant adolescent and her fetus. This may be particularly so if long standing calcium fortification of flour in Britain ceases. Sixteen per cent of the calcium intake of British adolescents derives from flour and removal of this means that without alternative sources of calcium, over half the teenage girls will have calcium intakes below recommended levels (Hackett *et al.*, 1984).

Adolescence is not only the time when individuals test all kinds of foods and eating habits, but also the time when adult eating habits are established. Enlightened nutrition education is particularly important for this age group. Dietary habits and lifestyle that tend to minimize ill health in adult life should be emphasized. School canteens and snack bars should support nutrition education programmes by providing a variety of attractive whole foods, fruit, vegetables and salads, as well as the high energy foods so desired – and needed – by rapidly growing adolescents.

It would be satisfactory to end with clear guidelines on the diet an adolescent should adopt in order to maintain good health in adult life. Sadly knowledge in this field is too uncertain for us to be specific on this. Nevertheless, a varied diet with unrefined cereals; fruits and vegetables; modest intakes of meat, saturated fat and salt; low intakes of refined sugar and modest total energy would meet most nutritionists' views for a healthy diet. This coupled with advice against smoking and alcohol (pointing out the particular problems for women in their childbearing years) and encouragement to regular activity would seem the best recommendations present knowledge can provide.

## References


Ahn, C.H. and MacLean, W.C. (1980). Growth of the exclusively breast fed infant. *Am. J. Clin. Nutr.*, **33**, 182–92.

Anderson, D.M., Williams, F.H., Merkatz, R.B., Schulman, P.K., Kerr, D.S. and Pittard, W.B. (1983) Length of gestation and nutritional composition of human milk. *Am. J. Clin. Nutr.*, **37**, 810–14.

Anon. (1981). International code of marketing of breast milk substitutes. *WHO Chronicle*, **35**: 112–17.

Anon. (1983). The dynamics of breast feeding. *WHO Chronicle*, **37**, 6–10.

Atkinson, S.A. (1983). Calcium and phosphorus requirements of low birth weight infants: a nutritional and epidemiological perspective. *Nutr. Rev.*, **41**, 69–78.

Atkinson, S.A., Bryan, M.H. and Anderson G.H. (1978). Human milk: difference in sodium concentration in milk from mothers of term and premature infants. *J. Pediatr.*, **93**, 67–9.

Atkinson, S.A., Radde, I.C. and Anderson, G.H. (1983). Macromineral balances in premature infants fed their own mothers' milk or formula. *J. Pediatr.*, **102**, 99–106.

Bell, E.F. and Oh, W. (1983). Water requirements of premature newborn infants. *Acta Paediatr. Scand. (Supplement)*, **305**, 21–6.

Beresford, C.H., Neale, R.J. and Brooke, O.G. (1971). Iron absorption and pyrexia. *Lancet*, **1**, 568–72.

Berger, H.M., Scott, P.H. and Wharton, B.A. (1980). Metabolic acidosis, diet and growth. In *Topics in Perinatal Medicine*, pp. 88–97. Ed. Wharton, B.A., Pitman Medical Limited: Tunbridge Wells.

Betts, P.R. and Magrath, G. (1974). Growth pattern and dietary intake of children with chronic renal insufficiency. *Br. Med. J.*, **2**, 189–93.

Bierman, C.W. and Furukawa, C.J. (1978). Food additives and hyperkinesis: are there nuts among the berries? *Pediatrics*, **61**, 932–4.

British Paediatric Association. (1964). Infantile hypercalcaemia, nutritional rickets and infantile scurvy in Great Britain. *Br. Med. J.*, **1**, 1659.

Brooke, O.G., Alvear, J. and Arnold, M. (1979). Energy retention, energy expenditure and growth in healthy immature infants. *Pediatr. Res.* **13**, 215–20.

Brooke, O.G., Wood, C. and Barley, J. (1982). Energy balance, nitrogen balance and growth in preterm infants fed expressed breast milk, a premature infant formula and two low-solute adapted formulae. *Arch. Dis. Child.*, **57**, 898–904.

Brown, K.H. and MacLean, W.C. Jr. (1984). Nutritional management of acute diarrhoea. *Pediatrics*, **73**, 119–25.

Brueton, M.J., Berger, H.M., Brown, G.A., Ablitt, L., Iyngkaron, N. and Wharton, B.A. (1978). Duodenal bile acid conjugation patterns and dietary sulphur amino acids in the newborn. *Gut*, **19**, 95–8.

Callenbach, J.C., Sheehan, M.B., Abrahamson, S.J. and Hall, R.T. (1981). Etiologic factors in rickets of low birth-weight infants. *J. Pediatr.*, **98**, 800–805.

De Carvalho, M., Hall, M. and Harvey, D. (1981). Effects of water supplementation on physiological jaundice in breast fed babies. *Arch. Dis. Child.*, **56**, 568–9.

Chessex, P., Reichman, B., Verellen, G., Putet, G., Smith, J.M., Heim, T. and Swyer, P.R. (1983). Quality of growth in premature infants fed their own mother's milk. *J. Pediatr.* **102**, 107–112.

Chiswick, M.L., Johnson, M., Woodhall, C., Gowland, M., Davies, J., Toner, N. and Sims, D. (1984). Protective effect of vitamin E on intraventricular haemorrhage in the newborn. In *Biology of Vitamin E*, Ciba Foundation Symposium number 101, pp.186–200. Pitman Medical: Tunbridge Wells.

Cohen, S.A., Hendricks, K.M., Mathis, R.K., Laramee, S. and Allan Walker, W. (1979). Chronic nonspecific diarrhoea: dietary relationships. *Pediatrics*, **64**, 402–407.

Committee on Drugs. (1983). The transfer of drugs and other chemicals into human milk. *Pediatrics*, **72**, 375–83.

Committee on Nutrition. (1977). Nutritional aspects of vegetarianism, health foods and fad diets. *Pediatrics*, **59**, 460–64.

Committee on Nutrition. (1983). Soy-Protein Formula: Recommendations for use in infant feeding. *Pediatrics*, **72**, 359–63.

David, T.J., Waddington, E. and Stanton, R.H.J. (1984). Nutritional hazards of elimination diets in children with atopic eczema. *Arch. Dis. Child.*, **59**, 323–5.

Davies, D.P. (1981a). The physiology of lactation and its clinical implications. *J. Maternal and Child Health*, **6**, 212–17.

Davies, D.P. (1981b). Physical growth from fetus to early childhood. In *Scientific Foundations of Paediatrics* 2nd ed., pp. 303–30. Eds. Davis, J.A. and Dobbing, J. William Heinemann Medical Books Ltd: London.

DHSS. (1974). *Present day practice in infant feeding*. Report on Health and Social Subjects No. 9. HMSO: London.

DHSS. (1980a). *Artificial feeds for the young infant*. Report on Health and Social Subjects No. 18. HMSO: London.

DHSS. (1980b). *Rickets and osteomalacia*. Report on Health and Social Subjects No. 19. HMSO: London.

DHSS. (1980c). *Present day practice in infant feeding* (1980). Report on Health and Social Subjects No. 20. HMSO: London.

DHSS. (1981). *The collection and storage of human milk*. Report on Health and Social Subjects No. 22. HMSO: London.

Downham, M.A.P.S., Scott, R., Sims, D.G., Webb, J.K.G. and Gardner, P.S. (1976). Does breast feeding protect against respiratory syncytial virus? *Br. Med. J.*, **2**, 274–6.

Dryburgh, E. (1980). Transpyloric feeding in 49 infants undergoing intensive care. *Arch. Dis. Child.*, **55**, 879–82.

Duncan, J.R. and Harvey, L.S. (1978). Intestinal absorption of zinc: a role for a zinc-binding ligand in milk. *Am. J. Physiol.*, **235**, E556–9.

Durnin, J.V.G.A., Lonergan, M.E., Good, J. and Ewan, A. (1974). A cross-selectional nutritional and antropometric study with an interval of 7 years on 611 young adolescent school children. *Br. J. Nutr.*, **32**, 169–79.

Dworsky, M., Yow, M., Stagno, S., Pass, R.F. and Alford, C. (1983). Cytomegalovirus infection of breast milk and transmission in infancy. *Pediatrics*, **72**, 295–9.

Evans, T.J. and Davies, D.P. (1977). Failure to thrive at the breast: an old problem revisited. *Arch. Dis. Child.*, **52**, 974–5.

Fanaroff, A. and Klaus, M. (1979). The gastro intestinal tract – feeding and selected disorders. In *Care of the high risk neonate*, pp. 113–45. Eds. Klaus, K. and Fanaroff A.W. B. Saunders and Co.: Philadelphia.

Finsberg, L., Harper, P.A., Harrison, H.E. and Bradley Sack R. (1982). Oral rehydration for diarrhoea, *J. Pediatr.* **101**, 497–9.

Finer, N.N., Peters, K.L., Schindler, R.F. and Grant, G.D. (1984). Vitamin E and retrolental fibroplasia: prevention of serious ocular sequelae. In *Biology of vitamin E*, Ciba Foundation Symposium number 101, pp. 147–64. Pitman: London.

Fink, C.S., Hamosh, P. and Hamosh, M. (1984). Fat digestion in the stomach: stability of lingual lipase in the gastric environment, *Pediatr. Res.*, **18**, 248–53.

Fomon, S.J. (1974). *Infant Nutrition* 2nd ed. W.B. Saunders Company: Philadelphia.

Forsyth, J.S. (1983). Nutritional problems in the low birth weight baby. *Maternal and Child Health*, **8**, 305–308.

Fransson, G.B. and Lonnerdahl, B. (1984). Iron, copper, zinc, calcium and magnesium in human milk fat. *Am. J. Clin. Nutr.*, **39**, 185–9.

Friedman, Z., Mark, K.H., Maisels, M.J., Thorson, R. and Naeye, R. (1978). The effect of parenteral fat emulsion on the pulmonary and reticulo-endothelial systems in the newborn infant. *Pediatrics*, **61**, 694–8.

Gairdner, D. and Pearson, J. (1971). A growth chart for premature and other infants. *Arch. Dis. Child.*, **46**, 783–7.
Gerrard, J.W. (1974). Breast feeding: second thoughts. *Pediatrics*, **54**, 757–64.
Ghishan, F.M., Parker, P., Nichols, S. and Hoyumpa, A. (1984). Kinetics of intestinal calcium transport during maturation in rats, *Pediatr. Res.*, **18**, 235–9.
Goel, K.M., House, F. and Shanks, R.A. (1978). Infant feeding practices among immigrants in Glasgow. *Br. Med. J.*, **2**, 1181–3.
Goldman, A.S. and Garza, C. (1983). Immunologic components in human milk during the second year of lactation. *Acta Paediatr. Scand.*, **72**, 461–2.
Gourley, G.R. and Arend, R.A. (1986). $\beta$ glucoronidase and hyperbilirubinaemia in breast-fed and formula-fed babies. *Lancet*, **i**, 644–6.
Greene, H.L., Hazlett, D. and Demares, R. (1976). Relationship between Intralipid, induced hyperlipemia and pulmonary function. *Am. J. Clin. Nutr.*, **29**, 127.
Gross, S.J., David, R.T., Baumann, M.S. and Tomarelli, R.M. (1980). Nutritional composition of milk produced by mothers delivering preterm. *J. Pediatr.*, **96**, 641–4.
Grotte, G., Muerling S. and Wretlind, A. (1982) Parenteral Nutrition. In *Textbook of Paediatric Nutrition* 2nd ed. pp. 228–58. Eds. McLaren, D.S., and Burman, D. Churchill Livingstone: Edinburgh.
Guy, R. (1978). The growth of physically handicapped children with emphasis on appetite and activity. *Public Health* (London), **92**, 145–54.
Hackett, A.F., Rugg-Gunn, A.J., Allinson, M., Robinson, C.J., Appleton, D.R. and Easthoe, J.E. (1984). The importance of fortification of flour with calcium and the sources of calcium in the diet of 375 English adolescents. *Br. J. Nutr.*, **51**, 193–7.
Halloran, B.P. and De Luca, H.F. (1981). Effects of vitamin D deficiency on skeletal development during early growth in the rat. *Arch. Biochem. Biophys.*, **209**, 7–14.
Hamosh, M. (1982). Lingual and breast milk lipases. *Adv. Pediatr.*, **29**, 33–67.
Harzer, G., Haug, M., Dieterich, I. and Gentner, P.R. (1983). Changing patterns of human milk lipids in the course of the lactation and during the day. *Am. J. Clin. Nutr.*, **37**, 612–21.
Heitlinger, L.A. (1983). Enzymes in mother's milk and their possible role in digestion. *J. Pediatr.Gastroenterol. Nutr.*, **2**: (suppl. 1) S113–19.
Hillman, L.S., Rojanasathit, S., Slatopolsky, E. and Haddad, J.G. (1977). Serial measurements of serum calcium, magnesium, parathyroid hormone, calcitonin and 25 hydroxy vitamin D in premature and term infants in the first week of life. *Pediatr. Res.*, **11**, 739–44.
Holm, V.A. and Pipes, P.L. (1976). Food and children with Prader-Willi syndrome. *Am. J. Dis. Child.*, **130**, 1063–1067.
Hughes, C.A. (1982). Parenteral nutrition in preterm infants – personal practice. In *Topics in Perinatal Medicine II* pp. 87–102. Ed. Wharton, B.A. Pitman Medical: London.
Insley, J. (1986). *A Paediatric Vade-Mecum.*, pp. 53–67. Lloyd-Luke: London.
Jelliffe, D.B. and Jelliffe, E.F.B. (1978). *Human milk in the modern world.* Oxford University Press: Oxford.
Jivani, S.K.M. (1978). The practice of infant feeding among Asian immigrants. *Arch. Dis. Child.* 53, 69–73.
Johnson, J.D., Albritton, W.L. and Sunshine, P. (1972). Hyperammonaemia, accompanying parenteral nutrition in newborn infants. *J. Pediatr.*, **81**, 154–61.
Kanarek, K.S., Williams, P.R. and Curran, J.S. (1982). Total parenteral nutrition in infants and children. *Adv. Pediatr.*, **29**, 151–81.
Klaus, M.H. and Kennell, J.H. (1976). *Maternal – infant bonding.* C.V. Mosby Co: St. Louis.
Knopf, K., Sturman, J.A., Armstrong, M. and Hayes, K.C. (1978). Taurine: an essential nutrient for the cat. *J. Nutr.*, **108**, 773–8.

Lakdawala, D.R. and Widdowson, E.M. (1977). Vitamin D in human milk. *Lancet*, 1, 167–8.

Lebenthal, E., Lee, P.C. and Heitlinger, L.A. (1983). Impact of development of the gastrointestinal tract on infant feeding. *J. Pediatr.*, **102**, 1–9.

Lee, G.R., Williams, D.M. and Cartwright, G.E. (1976). Role of copper in iron metabolism and heme biosynthesis. In *Trace Elements in Human Health and Disease I*, pp. 373–90. Eds. Prasad, A.S. and Oberlas, D. Academic Press: New York.

Levene, M.I., Wigglesworth, J.S. and Desai, R. (1980). Pulmonary fat accumulation after Intralipid infusion in the preterm infant. *Lancet*, **ii**, 815–18.

Lucas, A. (1981). Gut hormones and infant feeding. In *Scientific Foundations of Paediatrics* 2nd ed., pp. 87–91. Eds. Davis, J.A. and Dobbing, J. William Heinemann Medical Books: London.

Lucas, A., Gore, S.M., Cole, T.J., Bamford, M.F., Dossetor, J.F.B., Barr, I., Dicarlo, L., Cork, S. and Lucas, P.J. (1984). Multicentre trial on feeding low birth weight infants: effects of diet on early growth. *Arch. Dis. Child.*, **59**, 722–30.

Lunn, P.G., Austin, S., Prentice, A.M. and Whitehead, R.G. (1984). The effect of improved nutrition on plasma prolactin concentrations and postpartum infertility in lactating Gambian women. *Am. J. Clin. Nutr.*, **39**, 227–35.

Maisels, M.J. and Gifford, K. (1983). Breast feeding, weight loss and jaundice. *J. Pediatr.*, **102**, 117–18.

Makin, H.L.J., Seamark, D.A. and Trafford, D.J.H. (1983). Vitamin D and its metabolites in human breast milk. *Arch. Dis. Child.*, **58**, 750–53.

Markestad, T., Aksnes, L., Finne, P.H. and Aarskog, D. (1984). Plasma concentrations of vitamin D metabolites in premature infants. *Pediatr. Res.*, **18**, 269–72.

McCarthy, D. (1981). The effects of emotional disturbance and deprivation on somatic growth. In *Scientific Foundation of Paediatrics* 2nd ed. pp. 54–73. Eds. Davis, J.A. and Dobbing, J. William Heinemann Medical Books Ltd: London.

Mellander, M., Noren, J.G., Feren, H. and Kjellmer, I. (1982). Mineralisation defects to deciduous teeth of low birth weight infants. *Acta Paediatr. Scand.*, **71**, 727–33.

Menon, G. and Poskitt, E.M.E. (1985). Why does congenital heart disease cause failure to thrive? *Arch. Dis. Child.*, **60**, 1134–9.

Minton, S.D.M., Steichen, J.J. and Tsang, R.C. (1979). Bone mineral content in term and preterm appropriate for gestational age infants. *J. Pediatr.*, **95**, 1037–42.

Odell, G.B. (1981). *Neonatal hyperbilirubinaemia*, pp. 67–9. Grune and Stratton: New York.

Orzalesi, M. (1982). Do breast and bottle fed babies require vitamin supplements? *Acta Paediatr. Scand.* (Suppl). **299**, 77–82.

Patton, R.G. and Gardner, L.I. (1962). Influence of family environment on growth: the syndrome of 'maternal deprivation'. *Pediatrics*, **30**, 957–62.

Poskitt, E.M.E., Cole, T.J. and Lawson, D.E.M. (1979). Diet, sunlight and 25 hydroxy vitamin D in healthy children and adults. *Br. Med. J.*, **1**, 221–3.

Prentice, A., Prentice, A.M. and Whitehead, R.G. (1981). Breast milk fat concentration of rural African women. 1. Short term variations within individuals. *Br. J. Nutr.*, **45**, 483–94.

Raiha, N.C.R. (1971). The development of aminoacid metabolism in the human liver. In *Metabolic processes in the fetus and newborn infant*. 3rd Nutricia Symposium, p. 26. Ed. Jonxis, J.H.P., Visser H.K.A., and Troelstra J.A. Stenfart Kroese: Leiden.

Rees, L. and Brook, C.G.D. (1979). Gradual reintroduction of full strength milk after acute gastroenteritis in children. *Lancet*, **i**, 770–71.

Reeve, L.E., Chesney, R.W. and de Luca, H.F. (1982). Vitamin D of human milk: identification of biologically active forms. *Am. J. Clin. Nutr.*, **36**, 122–6.

Rolles, C.J. and Cussens, L. (1980). Cells in human milk, *Arch. Dis. Child.*, **55**, 969–72.

Rothberg, A.D., Pettifor, J.M., Cohen, D.F., Sonnendecker, E.W.W. and Ross, F.P. (1982). Maternal-infant vitamin D relationships during breast feeding. *J. Pediatr.*, **101**, 500–503.

Sagy, M., Birembaum, E., Balim, A., Orda, S., Barzilay, Z. and Brish, M. (1980). Phosphate depletion syndrome in a premature infant fed human milk. *J. Pediatr.*, **96**, 683–5.

Salariya, E.M., Easton, P.A. and Cater, J. (1978). Duration of breast feeding after early initiation and frequent feeding. *Lancet*, **ii**, 1141–3.

Sandstead, H.H., Prasad, A.S., Schulert, A.R., Farid, Z., Miale, A. (Jr.), Bassilly, S. and Darby, W.J. (1967). Human zinc deficiency, endocrine manifestations and response to treatment. *Am. J. Clin. Nutr.*, **20**, 422–42.

Schmidt-Sommerfeld, E., Penn, D. and Wolf, H. (1982). Carnitine blood concentrations and fat utilisation in parenterally alimented premature newborn infants. *J. Pediatr.*, **100**, 260–64.

Schonler, R.J. and Oh, W. (1980). Composition of breast milk obtained from mothers of premature infants as compared to breast milk from donors. *J. Pediatr.*, **96**, 679–81.

Senterre, J., Putet, G., Salle, B. and Rigo, J. (1983). Effects of vitamin D and phosphorus supplementation on calcium retention in preterm infants fed banked human milk. *J. Pediatr.*, **103**, 305–307.

Shaw, J.C.L. (1982). Iron absorption by the premature infant. *Acta Paediatr. Scand. (Suppl)*, **299**, 83–9.

Shearer, M.J., Barkhan, P., Rahim, S. and Stimmler, L. (1982). Plasma vitamin K, in mothers and their newborn babies. *Lancet*, **ii**, 460–63.

Shinwell, E.D. and Gorodischer, R. (1982). Totally vegetarian diets and infant nutrition. *Pediatrics*, **70**, 582–6.

Shivpuri, C.R., Martin, R.J., Carlo, W.A. and Fanaroff, A.A. (1983). Decreased ventilation in preterm infants during oral feeding. *J. Pediatr.*, **103**, 285–9.

Shull, M.W., Reed, R.B., Valadian, I., Palombo, R., Thorne, H. and Dwyer, J.T. (1977). Velocities of growth in vegetarian preschool children. *Pediatrics*, **60**, 410–17.

Stare, F.T., Whelan, E.M. and Sheridan M. (1980). Diet and hyperactivity: is there a relationship? *Pediatrics*, **66**, 521–5.

Stothers, J.K. (1982). Accuracy of routine clinical test weighing. *Arch. Dis. Child.*, **57**, 810.

Strelling, M.K., Blackledge, D.G. and Goodall, H.B. (1979). Diagnosis and management of folate deficiency in low birth weight infants. *Arch. Dis. Child.*, **54**, 271–7.

de Swiet M. (1982). Blood pressure, sodium and take away food. *Arch. Dis. Child.*, **57**, 645–6.

Szefler, S.J. (1983). Drug excretion in human breast milk: potential effect on infant development. *J. Pediatr. Gastroenterol. Nutr.*, **2** (Suppl. 1) S120–6.

Taitz, L.S. and Byers, H.D. (1972). High calorie/osmolar feeding and hypertonic dehydration. *Arch. Dis. in Child.*; **47**, 257–60.

Taitz, L.S. and Lukmanji, Z. (1981). Alterations in feeding pattern and rates of weight gain in South Yorkshire infants, 1971–1977. *Human Biology*, **53**, 313–20.

Tanner, J.M., Whitehouse, R.H. and Takaishi, M. (1966). Standards from birth to maturity for height, weight, height velocity and weight velocity for British children in 1965. *Arch. Dis. Child.*, **41**, 454–71.

Truswell, A.S. and Darnton-Hill, I. (1981). Food habits of adolescents. *Nutr. Rev.*, **39**, 73–87.

Verity, C.M., Carswell, F. and Scott, G.L. (1983). Vitamin K deficiency causing infantile intracranial haemorrhage after the neonatal period. *Lancet*, **i**, 1439.

Vukavic, T. (1983). Intestinal absorption of IgA in the newborn. *J. Pediatr. Gastroenterol. Nutr.*, **2**, 248–51.

Waterlow, J. and Thomson, A.M. (1979). Observations on the adequacy of breast feeding. *Lancet*, **ii**, 238–42.

Weaver, L.T., Laker, M.F. and Nelson, R. (1984). Intestinal permeability in the newborn. *Arch. Dis. Child.*, **59**, 236–41.

Wharton, B.A. (1982). Nutrition. In *A Paediatric Vade Mecum*, pp. 21–50. Eds. Insley, J. and Wood, B. Lloyd-Luke: London.

Wharton, B.A. and Berger, H.M. (1976). Bottle-Feeding. *Br. Med. J.*, **1**, 1326–31.

Whitehead, R.G. and Paul, A.A. (1981). Infant growth and human milk requirements. *Lancet*, **ii**, 161–3.

Whitehead, R.G., Paul, A.A. and Cole, T.J. (1981). A critical analysis of measured food energy intakes during infancy and early childhood in comparison with current international recommendations. *J. Hum. Nutr.*, **35**, 339–48.

Whitfield, M.F. (1982). Poor weight gain of the low birth weight infant fed nasojejunally. *Arch. Dis. Child.*, **57**, 597–601.

Whitfield, M.F., Kay, R. and Stephens, S. (1981). Validity of routine clinical test weighing as a measure of the intake of breast fed infants. *Arch. Dis. Child.*, **56**, 919–21.

Wickes, I.G. (1952). Rate of gain and satiety in early infancy. *Arch. Dis. Child.*, **27**, 449–56.

Widdowson, E.M. (1947). *A study of individual children's diets*. MRC Special Reports Series No. 257. HMSO: London.

Widdowson, E.M. (1951) Mental contentment and physical growth. *Lancet*, **i**, 1316–18.

Widdowson, E.M. (1965). Absorption and excretion of fat, nitrogen and minerals from 'filled' milks by babies one week old. *Lancet*, **ii**, 1099–105.

Widdowson, E.M. (1974). Nutrition. In *Scientific Foundations of Paediatrics*, pp. 44–55. Eds. Davis, J.A. and Dobbing, J. William Heinemann Medical Books: London.

Widdowson, E.M. (1979). Nutritional needs of the foetus and young child. In *The Mother–Child Dyad*. pp. 35–9. Eds. Hambraeus, L. and Sjolin, S. XIV Symposium of Swedish Nutrition Foundation.

Widdowson, E.M. (1981a) Nutrition. In *Scientific Foundation of Paediatrics* 2nd ed., pp. 41–53. Eds. Davis, J.A. and Dobbing, J. Heinemann Medical Books Ltd: London.

Widdowson, E.M. (1981b). Changes in body proportions and composition during growth. In *Scientific Foundations of Paediatrics* 2nd ed., pp. 330–42. Eds. Davis J.A. and Dobbing J. William Heinemann Medical Books Ltd: London.

Williamson, S., Finucane, E., Ellis, H. and Gamsu, H.R. (1978). Effect of heat treatment of human milk on absorption of nitrogen, fat, sodium, calcium and phosphate by preterm infants. *Arch. Dis. Child.*, **53**, 555–63.

Yoshioka, H., Iseki Ken-ichi and Fujita, K. (1983). Development and differences of intestinal flora in the neonatal period in breast fed and bottle fed infants. *Pediatrics*, **72**, 317–21.

Yu, V.Y.H. (1986). Parenteral Nutrition. In *Textbook of Neonatology*, pp. 211–22. Ed. Roberton, NRC. Churchill Livingstone: Edinburgh.

Yuen, P., Lin, H.J., and Hutchinson, J.A. (1979). Copper deficiency in a low birth weight infant. *Arch. Dis. Child.*, **54**, 553–4.

# 3 Inborn errors of metabolism in children

J.E. Wraith and Jennifer Coutts



## Introduction

Over the last 30 years the application of new, sophisticated laboratory techniques and the introduction of large scale screening have led to the description of an ever-growing list of inborn errors of metabolism. Emphasis on the investigation of the biochemical abnormality has often overshadowed the fact that for the majority of such conditions curative treatment is not available. In a small number of disorders amplification of enzyme activity can be achieved by the administration of the appropriate cofactor, usually a vitamin. These disorders are termed vitamin-responsive. In homocystinuria due to cystathionine synthase deficiency, for example, oral administration of large doses of pyridoxine (vitamin $B_6$) produces marked biochemical improvement in about 50 per cent of affected individuals (Barber and Spaeth, 1967). Attempts have been made to replace the missing enzymes in a number of conditions and this work has been reviewed in a recent publication (Watts, 1982). Specific dietary restriction is the only effective method of treatment for some inborn errors of metabolism. These diets are often complex and exacting for the affected individual and family and there is the risk of inducing nutritional deficiencies in the growing infant and child.

## Phenylketonuria

Dietary treatment for phenylketonuria (PKU) was first described by Bickel *et al.*, in 1953. Since that time the condition has been subjected to intense study. PKU is one of the few causes of mental retardation for which effective medical treatment is available (Smith and Wolff, 1974). Newborn screening programmes have detected a spectrum of various hyperphenylalaninaemias. In classical PKU the concentration of phenylalanine in the blood is greater than 1800 $\mu$mol/litre (although it may be somewhat lower with the low protein intake of the breast fed infant, or those on a modified whey based formula), plasma tyrosine is not raised and metabolites of phenylalanine are present in the urine. The phenylalanine hydroxylating system which catalyzes the conversion of phenylalanine to tyrosine is a complex system located in the liver (Scriver and Clow, 1980). Tetrahydrobiopterin ($BH_4$) is the natural cofactor for phenylalanine hydroxylase (PH). The initial reduction of dihydrobiopterin ($BH_2$) to $BH_4$ requires dihydrofolate reductase. Once in the tetrahydro-form the biopterin 'shuttles' between $BH_4$ and $BH_2$ through the mediation of dihydropteridine reductase. Biopterins are synthesized initially from guanosine triphosphate and this step requires dihydropterine synthetase. The study of the hydroxylating system in humans has been hampered by the ethical problems associated with performing liver biopsy on children with PKU, who generally respond well to dietary treatment. From the various reports (Friedman *et al.*, 1973; Bartholome *et al.*, 1975; Berry *et al.*, 1982; Hsieh *et al.*, 1983) it can be concluded that classical PKU is associated with either zero or minute residual enzyme activity whereas in the hyperphenylalaninaemias considerable residual enzyme activity may be found (9–24 per cent, Hsieh *et al.*, 1983). Hydroxylase activity has been demonstrated in human serum and fibroblasts (Hoffbauer and Schrempf, 1976) but as considerable activity has also been found in PKU patients the significance of this finding is open to question.

Several variants of PKU associated with progressive neurological disease have been described (Smith *et al.*, 1975). These defects are rare, comprising 1–3 per cent of hyperphenylalaninaemias requiring treatment (Danks *et al.*, 1978; Danks *et al.*, 1979). It is now clear that these patients have deficient activity of tetrahydrobiopterin either due to a deficient synthesis (Kaufman *et al.*, 1978) or defective 'shuttling' due to a deficiency of dihydropteridine reductase (Kaufman *et al.*, 1975a). As tetrahydrobiopterin is the coenzyme of tyrosine and tryptophan hydroxylase a deficiency results in a deficient synthesis of the neurotransmitters dopamine and serotonin and hence the progressive neurological disease unresponsive to phenylalanine restriction alone. A logical treatment for these variants would be to administer the deficient cofactor. It has been suggested, however, that peripherally administered biopterins did not penetrate the blood brain barrier (Danks *et al.*, 1979) and therefore treatment was aimed at replacing the missing neurotransmitters with L-dopa, carbidopa and 5-OH tryptophan. Recent evidence, however (Kaufman *et al.*, 1982; Kaufman *et al.*, 1983), suggests that these compounds can enter the brain after peripheral administration if given in large enough doses and therefore the approach to treatment of these variants may have to be reconsidered.

The cause of the mental retardation in PKU is not known. Studies on affected children have shown that raised phenylalanine levels induce a modification in brain uptake of amino acids (Comar *et al.*, 1981) and animal work suggests that the amino acid imbalance leads to faulty brain protein synthesis (Agrawal *et al.*, 1970). Hyperphenylalaninaemic rats have reduced yields of myelin but the chemical content of the myelin is not different from normals and in some ways the brains are similar to those seen in malnourished animals (Heuther *et al.*, 1982a; Heuther *et al.*, 1982b). It is likely that the amino acid imbalance within the cells plays a central role in the aetiology of the mental retardation.

Treatment should be aimed at lowering phenylalanine levels to a value slightly above that found in normal subjects. There is no general agreement about the plasma level of phenylalanine for which treatment is required. Some centres would treat infants with plasma concentrations greater than 750 μmol/litre, but there is a view that treatment is not required below 1000 μmol/litre (Levy, 1983). If the plasma concentration is between 750–1200 μmol/litre the clinician may try to lower the phenylalanine level by using a whey based modified milk formula. This should be given in volumes supplying approximately 2 g protein/kg/day and with adequate energy of 480 + / – 65 KJ (115 + / – 15 kcal)/kg/day during the neonatal period (Forsum and Hambreu, 1972; Hambreu *et al.*, 1974). These children require close follow up and supervision over several months.

Ideally the children should be treated in centres where there is a team comprising a paediatrician, paediatric dietitian, specialist nurse and clinical psychologist. It is advantageous to have a laboratory concerned with the investigation of metabolic disorders attached or in close proximity to the centre. In this way the staff become very skilled at caring for these children, laboratory facilities can be geared to their needs and proper dietary supervision can be provided. Although there are exceptions, the single patient with PKU at a hospital does not usually obtain this type of service. These views on centralization are shared by many workers (Komrower, 1977; Raine, 1977) and are in accordance with the views of the Public Health Committee, Council of Europe (Bickel *et al.*, 1981).

Classical PKU is treated by a controlled low phenylalanine diet which should be started as early in life as possible in order to prevent brain damage. Once the diagnosis is established careful dietary treatment is of utmost importance to ensure normal physical and mental development. The diet requires biochemical monitoring of the concentration of phenylalanine in the blood.

## Protein

Any diet must provide the minimum requirement of essential amino acids and total nitrogen. The restriction of natural protein in order to control the phenylalanine concentration in the blood compared with the total range and intake of amino acids required necessitates the use of a protein substitute low in phenylalanine to correct the imbalance of plasma amino acids (Berry *et al.*, 1971). A variety of suitable products is available and they vary enormously in their content. It is necessary to understand their nutritional role if they are to be used safely. The quantity prescribed, together with the natural protein allowance supplying the essential phenylalanine required for growth, must provide the appropriate amount of protein and nitrogen for the age and weight of the child. The protein substitutes are based on hydrolysates of natural protein from which most of the phenylalanine has been removed (Albumaid XP, Minafen, Lofenalac) or are mixtures of synthetic l-amino acids (Aminogran, P.K.Aid 1, Maxamaid XP). Any of these preparations can be used successfully in the treatment of PKU provided that the differences in their composition are recognized and the total diet is modified accordingly. Some protein substitutes are particularly suitable for infants because they are almost complete foods providing energy, minerals and some vitamins e.g. Minafen and Lofenalac. Others are more suited to older children because they are concentrated sources of nitrogen and are taken in smaller amounts which may be regarded as medicine (Aminogran, P.K.Aid 1); and there are new preparations becoming available which are more palatable and which, as well as providing the necessary amino acids, also contain the required amounts of vitamins and minerals, e.g. Maxamaid XP.

## Phenylalanine

The most usual reason for phenylalanine deficiency is underprescription in the first weeks of life. Frequent plasma phenylalanine estimations are essential. If the method of estimation is one which shows the levels of all amino acids, a raised level of methionine in conjunction with a very low or undetectable level of phenylalanine indicates that an increase in the phenylalanine intake is urgent. Most children tolerate 200 mg phenylalanine or more. A few may only tolerate 150 mg but if the plasma levels are not satisfactory on an intake as low as this another reason for the high level should be considered before any further reduction of the phenylalanine intake. First, the total protein intake should be assessed; in these situations this is often found to be low because the baby is refusing the protein substitute or insufficient is being offered. An increased intake usually brings down the phenylalanine level. Failing this there may be some underlying infection producing a catabolic state and appropriate treatment of the infection will bring down the phenylalanine levels; in this situation the rapid catch-up in growth means that extra phenylalanine will be needed.

Generally, a raised phenylalanine level in a normally well controlled child means that the child has an infection and is therefore in a catabolic state or the diet does not provide enough energy and therefore protein is being used for energy and not synthesis of new tissue incorporating phenylalanine or too little protein substitute is being taken which again leads to failure to grow and poor utilization of phenylalanine. From the toddler stage pinching of forbidden foods can also be a problem and some parents become careless about measuring the diet. Infections do not require any emergency regime as the abnormal metabolites so formed are not toxic. The child's appetite should be used as a guide to dietary intake. It is most important to provide energy in the form of protein-free drinks and as the appetite improves gradually return to the normal dietary regimen.

## Energy intake

Adequate energy from carbohydrate and fat must be provided. Lack of these nutrients means that the protein substitute is used for energy resulting in a failure to grow and reduction in the utilization of phenylalanine which is evident in raised serum phenylalanine levels. In infancy the protein substitutes Minafen and Lofenalac provide adequate energy in relation to their nitrogen content. Older children need ample amounts of low protein bread, biscuits and pasta; cakes and biscuits made with low protein flour; sugar, sweets and sugary drinks and fats in the form of butter, margarine and cooking oils and fats.

## Minerals

The diet must contain all the minerals known to be required; calcium, sodium, potassium, phosphorus, chloride, magnesium and iron together with the trace elements copper, zinc, manganese, iodine, cobalt, molybdenum, chromium and nickel (Westall, 1963; Alexander *et al.*, 1974). Some protein substitutes such as Lofenalac, Minafen and Maxamaid XP contain the required amounts of minerals but others, particularly the pure amino acid preparations Aminogran and P.K.Aid 1, need to be supplemented. Aminogran Mineral Supplement or Metabolic Mineral Mixture are suitable supplements and should be given in doses of 1.5 g/kg/day up to a maximum of 8 g daily. The fruit, vegetables and cereals included in the diet will provide additional minerals.

## Vitamins

The amount of natural food tolerated in phenylketonuria is so restricted that severe vitamin deficiency can occur unless adequate supplements are given (Royston and Parry, 1962). Some of the protein substitutes such as Lofenalac and Maxamaid XP supply ample amounts of all vitamins but most of the other preparations are inadequately fortified and require supplementation. Three Ketovite tablets plus 5 ml Ketovite liquid supplement will provide the daily vitamin needs.

## Breast feeding

A mother who has been enjoying breast feeding her baby will find the diagnosis of PKU especially upsetting if it means that she has to entirely bottle feed. Fortunately it has been found to be possible to manage PKU during the first months of life and to continue with some breast feeding (Francis and Smith, 1981). The amount of breast milk the baby takes is regulated by complementary feeding of Minafen or Lofenalac. If the serum level of phenylalanine is too high more Minafen is prescribed and if the levels are lower than desired the volume of Minafen is reduced. On diagnosis the baby is fed entirely on Minafen or Lofenalac for 3 or 4 days depending on the initial serum phenylalanine level, while the mother expresses her milk to maintain lactation. Prescribed volumes of Minafen are then given 5 or 6 times daily followed by as much milk from the breast as the baby demands (Table 3.1).

Blood levels must be closely monitored, daily during the first week then twice weekly until the phenylalanine levels are satisfactory, thereafter weekly tests should be carried out. Subsequent adjustments to the phenylalanine intake from breast milk are achieved by increasing or reducing the volume of complementary feed prescribed as in Table 3.2.

Table 3.1 Initial breast feeding regimen for infants with PKU (Francis *et al.*, 1981)

| Initial blood phenylalanine ($\mu$m/litre) | Minafen (15 % solution) | Breast feeds |
|---|---|---|
| 2000 | 150–200 ml/kg wt/day followed by 60 ml × 5 feeds | Nil for 3 days* on demand (×5+) |
| 120–2000 | 150–200 ml/kg wt/day followed by 45 ml × 5 feeds | Nil for 2 days* on demand (×5+) |
| 1200 | 30 ml × 5 | On demand (×5+) |
| 900 | ? | On demand (×5+) |

* Mother expresses her milk to maintain lactation

Table 3.2 Adjusting phenylalanine intake in response to monitoring of serum levels

| Blood phenylalanine $\mu$mol/litre | Volume Minafen/day compared to previous intake | Breast feeds |
|---|---|---|
| 480 | + 75 ml | On demand: baby should take less |
| 180/litre | – 75 ml | On demand: baby should take more |
| 180–480 | no change | On demand |

Vitamin supplements of Ketovite liquid and tablets should be given, but other fluids, such as water or fruit juices and sucking a dummy, should be avoided as these will result in less stimulation of the mother's milk and hence may lead to a phenylalanine deficiency.

Around the fourth month solids can be introduced. Fifty milligrams of phenylalanine as baby rice or rusk mixed with drip breast milk or water should be given *before* the Minafen and breast feeds. Free food such as puree fruits and vegetables may be introduced later *after* Minafen and breast feeds.

At about 6 months, extra protein will be required and a small amount of Aminogran Food Supplement or P.K.Aid 1 mixed to a paste should be started. Five grams of Aminogran should be mixed with half a scoop of Aminogran Minerals and made into a paste with fruit juice. At first 1 teaspoon of this paste is given before one feed, gradually increasing to 1 teaspoon three times daily and then to the full dose of 3 g Aminogran Food Supplement/kg body weight/day plus 8 g Aminogran Minerals (3 scoops) per day. Breast feeds and Minafen should be proportionally reduced and finally stopped while the amount of solids is increased as appropriate for the child's age and phenylalanine tolerance. It is only when the baby is fully weaned that the actual tolerance for phenylalanine will be known.

There is divided medical opinion as to how long dietary treatment is necessary. Intellectual impairment occurs if the diet is stopped before the age of 2 years (McBean and Stephenson, 1968). In older children, 50 per cent of affected children showed a significant decrease in their IQ when the strict diet was changed to an unrestricted one at 7–8 years (Smith *et al.*, 1978). Subtle changes in cerebral function were found in children stopping the diet at 6 years when compared with another group who continued on the diet (Koch *et al.*, 1982). It is recognized that the strict diet can itself cause severe emotional and social problems and therefore risks have to be balanced.

The success of neonatal screening for PKU has meant that an increasing number of healthy, intelligent women with PKU are reaching child bearing age. In 1956 Dent reported three non-phenylketonuric, mentally retarded offspring of a PKU mother. This was followed in the 1960s by a number of reports of serious congenital abnormalities in a high proportion of children born to affected mothers (Denniston, 1963; Mabry *et al.*, 1965; Mabry *et al.*, 1966; Fisch *et al.*, 1966) as well as an increased risk of spontaneous abortion (Stephenson *et al.*, 1967). An international survey of maternal PKU and hyperphenylalaninaemia (Lenke and Levy, 1979) confirmed that women with PKU had a very high risk of bearing offspring with mental retardation and microcephaly and a lower, but still increased risk of having children with congenital heart disease and low birthweight. The data were insufficient to give a definitive risk in women with hyperphenylalaninaemia. The actual cause of the embryopathy is unknown. It has been suggested (Bessman *et al.*, 1978) that tyrosine depletion rather than phenylalanine excess causes the fetal damage. This, however, is questionable as there is no correlation between plasma tyrosine concentration in the mother and IQ in the offspring (Lenke and Levy, 1982). There is, however, a significant correlation between IQ and maternal phenylalanine level (Levy and Waisbren, 1983).

Attempts to treat after conception have been disappointing (Lenke and Levy, 1982), perhaps related in some cases to late initiation of the diet or poor compliance as a result of low IQ in the mother. In view of this it is ideal for treatment to start before pregnancy. As PKU children grow up, therefore, it is vital that the girls and their parents are well informed of the implications of PKU in pregnancy. Should a girl decide she wants children she must return to a strict diet and the plasma phenylalanine kept in the region of 400 $\mu$mol/litre. Once she is pregnant all the dietary requirements must be met. A generous protein intake is important, 80–100 g phenylalanine-free amino acid supplement such as P.K.Aid 1 or Aminogran should be taken from the 10th week of pregnancy. Blood levels need careful monitoring as the phenylalanine requirement will be greater than normal during pregnancy, with a sudden increase at about 20 weeks gestation. An adequate energy intake is important and women who are obese should try to lose their excess weight before they become pregnant, as it is difficult to keep their phenylalanine levels down on a low energy diet (Komrower *et al.*, 1979). Additional calcium and iron should be given during the second half of pregnancy.

## Maple syrup urine disease

Maple syrup urine disease, first described by Menkes *et al.*, in 1954, is a disorder of catabolism of the branched chain amino acids leucine, isoleucine and valine. It is known to occur in a number of phenotypic variants, one of which appears to be responsive to treatment with thiamine (Scriver *et al.*,

1971). In the classic type, the infant is normal at birth, but between the fourth and seventh day, fails to thrive, feeds poorly and vomits. Abnormal neurological behaviour such as convulsions and rigidity appear followed by stupor, hypotonia and irregular respirations. Untreated, the patient becomes progressively comatose and usually dies; if he survives this period severe mental retardation develops.

In affected individuals an absence of branched-chain-ketoacid-dehydrogenase activity can be demonstrated in white blood cells. The enzyme deficiency leads to an elevation of leucine, isoleucine, alloisoleucine and valine in both blood and urine. Abnormal excretion of the ketoacid derivatives gives the infant and his urine the characteristic smell.

At post-mortem a deficiency of myelin is found and this myelin has an abnormal protein and lipid concentration (Taketomi *et al.*, 1983). Work with experimental animals suggests that proteolytic degradation by a direct toxic effect of some of the metabolites may be responsible for faulty myelin production (Tribble and Shapira, 1983).

The treatment of maple syrup urine disease can be considered in two phases. Firstly, the treatment of the acute episode, either in a newborn or in an older child who has become ketoacidotic as a result of infection or illness and secondly chronic dietary treatment once the acute episode has been brought under control. Treatment of the acute episode requires a skilled team with excellent backup laboratory facilities for rapid measure of branched chain amino acid levels. It has been shown that both exchange transfusion (Hammerson *et al.*, 1978) and peritoneal dialysis (Gaull, 1969) are effective in clearing branched chain amino and keto acids. Adequate calories are required to limit the catabolic state and Clow *et al.*, (1981) have suggested the use of intralipid in the acute phase to try and induce anabolism. Other workers (Wendel *et al.*, 1982) have used infusion of dextrose with subcutaneous insulin, and total parenteral nutrition (lacking valine, leucine and isoleucine) to produce lowering of branched chain amino acids (Townsend and Kerr, 1982).

The aim of long term dietary treatment is to limit the intake of the amino acids leucine, isoleucine and valine to the amount which will keep the serum levels rather higher than in the normal individual. In our experience this has been the amounts contained in 3–5 g natural protein, therefore a protein substitute free from these amino acids is necessary to make up the total protein requirement. MSUD aid (Scientific Hospital Supplies) is a suitable preparation. Vitamins, minerals, carbohydrate and fat must also be included in forms appropriate to the child's age. Table 3.3 gives a suitable infant formula. It is impractical to adjust the level of one of the affected amino acids on its own using natural foods. If, for example, the level of valine remains low while the levels of leucine and isoleucine are satisfactory, a carefully measured amount of valine should be given with the MSUD aid. The dose, measured in multiples of 25 mg, will have to be weighed out by a pharmacist.

Adequate energy intake is very important at all times in this condition especially during infections. Catabolism leading to severe acidosis may arise from quite slight infections and parents must therefore be told to discontinue the natural protein whenever the child appears off colour. They should also ensure that the energy intake from carbohydrate is maintained probably using a high energy fluid such as 25 per cent glucose polymer solution with flavouring.

Table 3.3 Formula for an infant feed using an amino acid based protein substitute e.g. MSUD aid, Albumaid RVHB. This should be fed in volumes appropriate to the age and weight of the infant

| | Protein g | Fat g | Carbohydrate g | Energy kJ | kcal |
|---|---|---|---|---|---|
| Amino acid mixture (2.5 g) | 2.0 | – | – | 34 | 8 |
| Glucose polymer (8.0 g) | – | – | 8.0 | 128 | 32 |
| Arachis oil (8 ml) | – | 4.0 | – | 108 | 36 |
| Emulsion | – | – | – | – | – |
| Water (90 ml) | – | – | – | – | – |
| *Minerals | – | – | – | – | – |
| †Vitamins | – | – | – | – | – |
| | 2.0 | 4.0 | 8.0 | 320 | 76 |

* Metabolic Mineral Mixture or Aminogran Minerals at the rate of 1.5 g/kg body weight/day to a maximum 8 g should be added to the total
† Ketovite tablets and liquid vitamin supplement

The outcome in maple syrup urine disease appears to be directly related to the time taken to make the diagnosis after the appearance of the symptoms (Naughten *et al.*, 1982). This stresses the importance of considering metabolic disease as a cause of abnormal neurological behaviour in the newborn period. With intensive early treatment, long term results are improving (Committee for Improvement of Hereditary Disease Management, 1976; Clow *et al.*, 1981).

## Homocystinuria

Homocystinuria due to cystathionine synthase deficiency was first described by Carson *et al.*, (1963) as a result of screening mentally retarded individuals for inborn errors of metabolism. The deficiency of the enzyme causes an accumulation of homocystine and methionine in the plasma and an increase in their excretion in the urine. In addition, plasma levels of cystine are very low. In the classic, untreated patient, the clinical picture is one of lens dislocation, premature arterio-venous thrombosis, mental retardation and osteoporosis leading to spinal deformity. The patients tend to be tall and have arachnodactyly, resembling therefore, patients with Marfan's syndrome.

It was shown by Barber and Spaeth (1967) that marked biochemical improvement occurred in some patients after large doses of pyridoxine (vitamin $B_6$). There are, therefore, two variants of cystathionine-synthase deficient homocystinuria – pyridoxine responsive and pyridoxine unresponsive. The aim of treatment in both groups is to remove homocystine from the plasma and at the same time restore methionine and cystine concentrations to normal. This can be achieved by large doses of pyridoxine in the responsive group or by a low methionine diet supplemented with cystine in the unresponsive group.

For responsive patients the dose of pyridoxine varies from patient to patient but is usually between 400–750 mg/day (Sardharwalla, 1980). Folate deficiency has been observed in several patients on pyridoxine and hence supplements of this vitamin should be given routinely.

Newborns found to have homocystinuria on screening and confirmatory testing, should be assessed for pyridoxine-responsiveness by giving them 200–300 mg pyridoxine for 7–10 days whilst on milk feeds. If there is no response a low methionine diet should be introduced.

The principles of diet in the pyridoxine-resistant form of this condition are similar to those for the management of phenylketonuria. The amount of methionine tolerated is supplied by natural protein, usually 6.0 g and a methionine-free amino acid mixture such as Albumaid RVBH (Scientific Hospital Supplies) used to make up the protein requirement. The formula given in Table 3.3 is suitable for an infant feed.

The diet must be life-long if the patient is to avoid the complications of homocystinuria. Occasionally patients present when older, usually referred by ophthalmologists because of dislocated lenses. It is unreasonable to expect strict control in these patients because of the unpalatable nature of the diet. Attempts to treat this group, however, can be rewarding (Grobe, 1980) in preventing further deterioration especially of the eye problems.

## Organic acidaemias

The organic acidaemias are a group of disorders characterized by the accumulation in the plasma and excretion in the urine of low molecular weight, water soluble, carboxylic acid metabolites of amino acids, carbohydrates or fats. The introduction of gas-liquid-chromatography mass spectrometry have led to the discovery of a number of new conditions. Clinical presentation can be very variable. In the neonatal period, the infant may present with tachypnoea or apnoeic attacks associated with progressive neurological deterioration ultimately leading to coma. Biochemical investigation shows a marked metabolic acidosis often associated with massive ketonuria. Infants and children who avoid or survive this acute neonatal course may present later either with an acute episode of acidosis associated with a minor illness, unexplained mental retardation or failure to thrive. The management in the newborn period needs a specialized team, as described for maple syrup urine disease and therapeutic manoeuvres used to remove the offending metabolites are the same – exchange transfusion, peritoneal dialysis and glucose with insulin infusion. Several of the conditions respond to large doses of vitamins, for example methylmalonic and propionic acidaemia (Scriver and Rosenberg, 1973).

In patients with vitamin unresponsive disorders, treatment is by dietary protein restriction together with calorie supplements, vitamins, minerals and trace elements. Biochemical monitoring is necessary and again this is best achieved by a laboratory experienced in the diagnosis of metabolic disorders. Acute exacerbations may occur as a result of infections and other catabolic states; these need to be treated as aggressively as the acute neonatal illness.

## Hyperammonaemia

Hyperammonaemia occurs in several clinical situations in paediatrics and its treatment ultimately depends on the underlying cause. It is important to differentiate biochemically inborn errors of the urea cycle from other conditions associated with a high blood ammonia, such as Reye's syndrome, liver failure and various transport defects of the amino acids arginine and ornithine (Bachmann, 1982).

As with organic acidaemias the clinical presentation of urea cycle defects may be very variable and non specific with vomiting, hypotonia, seizures, coma and ultimately death. Older children may have intermittent episodes of severe vomiting, ataxia and clouding of consciousness as well as developmental delay. Treatment of urea cycle disorders is based on the removal of precursors, reducing the requirement for waste nitrogen excretion and correcting arginine deficiency, when present. Blood ammonia can be reduced by exchange transfusion, peritoneal dialysis or haemodialysis (Batshaw and Brusilow, 1980). By utilizing alternative pathways for ammonia removal, such as by the conversion to hippuric acid with sodium benzoate, chronic treatment is available (Batshaw *et al.*, 1982; Takeda *et al.*, 1983). The use of low protein diets, often supplemented with non-nitrogen containing analogues of essential amino acids results in a reduction in waste nitrogen production. N-carbamyl glutamate, an analogue of N-acetyl glutamate, is an activator of mitochondrial carbamyl phosphate and may help to reduce ammonia levels in infants with urea cycle defects.

A low protein diet is required for organic acidaemias and hyperammonaemia. The amount tolerated varies but it is important not to unnecessarily restrict it as this will inhibit growth. Ample energy from carbohydrate and fat should be supplied to ensure optimum use of protein for synthesis of new tissue. Infants should be given a modified formula such as Gold Cap SMA (Wyeth) to provide the required amount of protein. The volume of SMA tolerated is unlikely to be adequate on its own and should be supplemented with fat, carbohydrate and water. For every additional 100 ml add 10 ml arachis oil emulsion, 10 g glucose polymer and 90 ml water. Care should be taken to see that the mineral and vitamin requirements are met. If the volume of milk tolerated is very small, minerals and vitamin supplements should be added in appropriate amounts. Suitable preparations include Aminogran Mineral and Ketovite tablets and liquid.

Catabolism produced by infections can quickly upset the biochemical state of these children. When the children show signs of infection the protein intake must be stopped and energy intake maintained by giving high carbohydrate fluids such as Hycal (Beechams) or 25 per cent glucose polymer solution flavoured with fruit juice.

## Hyperlipoproteinaemias

This is a group of heterogenous disorders with different aetiologies, symptoms, prognoses and responses to treatment. Of the inherited disorders, in childhood, familial hypercholesterolaemia, inherited as an autosomal dominant trait is the most common. Hypercholesterolaemia is apparent in cord blood in homozygous infants, cutaneous xanthomata usually appear within the first four years of life and death frequently occurs before the age of 20 years from coronary artery disease (Goldstein and Brown, 1983). Heterozygotes manifest a similar pattern of disease but at a later age. Because of the poor prognosis associated with this condition attempts have been made to lower cholesterol levels by a variety of means and these have been reviewed in a number of publications (Fredrickson and Levy, 1970; West and Lloyd, 1973). Diet remains the cornerstone of therapy but in those who do not respond to diet alone a number of lipid-lowering drugs have been tried. More aggressive treatments have involved frequent plasma exchange (Thompson, 1981), which will induce regression of xanthomata but may not cause regression of atheroma (Leonard *et al.*, 1981), and ileal bypass surgery (Buchwald *et al.*, 1969).

With the other types of hyperlipoproteinaemias (Type I, III, IV and V), diet again is the main therapy and the degree of restriction in all cases depends on the severity of the condition. In familial hypercholesterolaemia the diet is very restrictive. Saturated fats must be kept to a minimum 10–20 g daily according to age with polyunsaturated fat in the form of corn oil or sunflower oil to add energy and palatability. It must be remembered that margarines contain more saturated fatty acids than the oils from which they are made and therefore only limited amounts should be used for spreading on bread and all fat used for cooking should be polyunsaturated oil.

Skimmed milk, white fish and pulses should be used regularly to provide an adequate protein intake since only small portions of lean meat and poultry can be eaten. In Type I hyperlipoproteinaemia a minimum fat diet may also be required but medium chain triglycerides (MCT) oil may be used to provide energy and improve palatability. These diets are very difficult to maintain as the ill effects of non-compliance are not noticeable in the short term and therefore the child cannot see any reason to keep to a diet which excludes crisps, biscuits, chocolate and ice cream and all convenience foods such as sausages, beefburgers and chip shop fish and chips.

A beta lipoproteinaemia is characterized clinically by fat malabsorption, ataxic neuropathy, retinitis pigmentosa and acanthocytosis. Triglycerides have to be restricted and MCT is contraindicated; carbohydrate supplements are therefore required. Vitamin E has been reported to induce clinical improvement in both the retinal and neuromuscular abnormalities (Muller *et al.*, 1970).

## Glycogen storage disease

There are a number of inherited disorders associated with the enzymes involved in the synthesis and degradation of glycogen. Diagnosis is suggested by the demonstration of a raised concentration of glycogen in the blood and tissues and is confirmed by specific enzyme assay in leucocytes, muscle or liver. Of those types requiring or amenable to treatment the commonest is type I (Von Gierke's disease) due to a deficiency of glucose-6-phosphatase (type Ia) or a defect in the transport enzyme glucose-6-phosphatase translocase (type Ib). The clinical features of both types are identical. An affected individual presents in early infancy with hepatomegaly, growth retardation, bleeding tendency, hypoglycaemia, hyperlacticacidaemia, hyperuricaemia, hyperlipaemia and impaired platelet function (Howell and Williams, 1983). In older patients the ultimate development of hepatic adenoma and carcinoma are potential serious problems (Howell *et al.*, 1976). Treatment is geared to maintaining glucose homeostasis throughout the 24 hour period; if this can be achieved, growth improves, hepatomegaly recedes, acidosis lessens, uric acid and lipid levels fall and potentially serious hypoglycaemia is avoided. Efforts to achieve this surgically, in the past, have included total parenteral nutrition (Folkman *et al.*, 1972), portal diversion (Starzl *et al.*, 1973) and recently liver transplantation (Starzl *et al.*, 1982). The technical problems associated with this surgery limit its application to a very few specialized centres. Dietary manipulation is the mainstay of treatment for most patients. The results of treatment with frequent daytime feeding and continual nocturnal nasogastric feeding are often dramatic, especially on growth (Greene *et al.*, 1976; Grobe and Ullrich, 1983). Galactose and fructose should be avoided as these carbohydrates are converted to glycogen and lactic acid. Fat should be restricted and a typical diet would consist of 60–70 per cent of the total calories as carbohydrates, 12–15 per cent as protein and 15–20 per cent as fat. When using nocturnal nasogastric feeding one-third of the total calories are given as an infusion over 12 hours at night and the other two-thirds by frequent day-time feeds. In case the tube slips at night an alarm system can be attached to prevent possible aspiration (Fernandes *et al.*, 1979).

In children with debranching enzyme deficiency (type III) and liver phosphorylase deficiency (type VI), the clinical features are similar to type I but much milder. These children require only frequent daytime feeds with a single feed in the middle of the night to prevent hypoglycaemia.

## Galactosaemia

Two inherited disorders of galactose metabolism, galactokinase deficiency and galactose-1-phosphate uridyl transferase deficiency have been studied in detail. A third variety, uridine diphosphate-4-epimerase deficiency, whilst being rare, can also present with features of 'classical' galactosaemia (Holton *et al.*, 1981). In galactokinase deficiency there is failure to form galactose-1-phosphate from galactose (Gitzelman, 1965). The only significant problem with this disorder appears to be the development of nuclear cataracts, although a number of other abnormalities have been found in individual patients (Gitzelman and Hansen, 1980). In galactosaemia due to galactose-1-phosphate uridyl transferase deficiency ('classical' galactosaemia), a more severe illness occurs once milk feeds have been introduced in the newborn period. Characteristically the infants are normal at birth and symptoms appear during the second week of life with jaundice, vomiting, lethargy, oedema, ascites, diarrhoea and hepatomegaly. If milk feeds are continued the disease can be rapidly fatal. Cataracts appear after days or weeks and there is a particular susceptibility to septicaemic illness e.g. *E. coli* (Levy *et al.*, 1977). If an infant survives the severe neonatal illness, mental development is retarded. Many enzymatic variants have been described since the description of the Duarte variant (Mathai and Beutler, 1966) and compound heterozygosity is common with variable clinical importance.

A galactosaemia workshop (Clothier and Davidson, 1983) attempted to establish dietary guidelines and correlate clinical data with dietary control. Evidence suggests that diet must be life long if patients are to avoid intellectual deterioration, hepatic cirrhosis and hepatic carcinoma (Brandt, 1980). A number of female infants are at risk from hypergonadotrophic hypogonadism associated with 'streak' ovaries (Kaufman *et al.*, 1981). Unfortunately, although early treatment prevents serious illness in the newborn period and ensures normal physical growth, intellectual impairment often persists (Donnell *et al.*, 1980).

All sources of lactose must be avoided i.e. cows' and other mammalian milks, cheese and butter and foods which have milk added to improve the texture and flavour such as breads and margarine. Another important source of galactose is the lactose used in pharmaceutical tablets and powders, for example proprietory brands of monosodium glutamate and some artificial sweetening tablets and powders. A recent development is the production of galactose by hydrolyzation of whey, which could in future be used in sugar confectionery. The exclusion of galactosides from legumes and gums is considered unnecessary since the alpha bonds linking galactosides in the main raffinoses and stachyoses of fruits and vegetables require alpha galactosidases for their digestion which are not present in the human intestinal mucosa (Clothier and Davidson, 1983). Suitable milk substitutes may be any one of the soya based infant formulas: Formula S, Prosobee and Wysoy which are completely lactose free and fully fortified with vitamins and minerals. Even if supplied with a list of manufactured foods by a dietitian it is essential that parents are instructed to read the labels on packages of food and to avoid any item containing milk, whey, casein, caseinate or milk sugar and of course lactose. They should also be told to ask the pharmacist to check that any medicines prescribed are lactose free. Occasional dietary indiscretions are inevitable but providing they are only occasional there is no evidence that such lapses are harmful.

## Avoidance of behavioural and psychological problems associated with dietary restriction

Most parents will understand at least a simplified explanation of the diet required for their child and be capable of following instructions so that the child receives the correct amounts and types of food but keeping a child to a very restricted diet, day in and day out indefinitely, must put a great strain on any family (Clothier, 1977). Separation of mother and baby at the time of diagnosis, which is sometimes inevitable, upsets the natural bonding process and families also suffer from feelings of isolation. They find that no one has heard of the condition from which their child suffers and may never meet another family with the same problem.

These stresses are bound to have some psychological effect but given the support of professional advisers who appreciate the difficulties the majority of families cope amazingly well. Most normal children go through phases of rebellion in their development and parents should be given the assurance, when the child on a diet is rebellious that this is a normal stage of development, and it should not last long or be damaging if properly handled. The most common problem, in disorders such as phenylketonuria, is refusal to take the protein substitute. This is natural, since most of these products are unpleasant tasting and parents feel guilty about making their child take something which they themselves dislike. Fortunately the newer preparations have a much improved flavour and fewer protracted periods of refusal are being encountered with their use. The professional team should advise the parents that pinching forbidden foods and refusal to take special foods and supplements are best handled calmly with rewards for compliance rather than punishment for non-compliance. It should, however, be realised that, while most parents tend to be over anxious, some will take the line of least resistance with their children and will need constant urging to be firmer.

Separation of mother and child at the time of diagnosis should be as short as possible. Centres specializing in the management of inborn errors of metabolism may not admit children found on screening to have phenylketonuria. The diagnosis can be confirmed and the special diet instituted on an outpatient basis. Hospitalization should be the last resort in overcoming feeding problems in phenylketonuria or homocystinuria. It can be justified occasionally in these conditions to give the parents a rest from the daily battle and to show that their child can take the diet if handled correctly. However, with reassurance and encouragement, home visits from a specialist nurse, health visitor or dietitian, hospital admission can usually be avoided. In those inborn errors of metabolism, such as organic acidaemias, where the effect of biochemical imbalance is acute, hospital admission cannot be avoided. Feelings of isolation can be helped if the child is brought to a clinic specializing in the particular condition and some families will find it helpful to belong to a group such as the National Society for Phenylketonuria and Allied Disorders which provides support for families in the United Kingdom who have a child with phenylketonuria. For other conditions the Research Trust for Metabolic Diseases in Children can be a point of contact.

## References


Agrawal, H.C., Bone, A.H. and Davidson, A.N. (1970). Effect of phenylalanine on protein synthesis in the developing rat brain. *Biochem. J.*, **117**, 325–31.

Alexander, F.W., Clayton, B.E. and Delves, H.T. (1974). Mineral and trace metal balances in children requiring normal and synthetic diets. *Q.J. Med.*, **43**, 89–112.

Bachman, C. (1982). *Hyperammonaemia in paediatrics: A challenge to clinical chemists.* XI International Congress of Clinical Chemists. Eds. Kaiser, E. and Gatt, F., Muller, M.M., Bayer, M. Walter de Gruyter & Co.: Berlin, New York.

Bartholome, K., Lutz, P. and Bickel, H. (1975). Determination of phenyalanine hydroxylase activity in patients with phenylketonuria and hyperphenylalaninaemia. *Pediatr. Res.*, **9**, 899–923.

Barber, G.W. and Spaeth, G.L. (1967). Pyridoxine therapy in Homocystinuria. *Lancet*, **i**, 337.

Batshaw, M.L. and Brusilow, S. (1980). Treatment of hyperammonaemic coma caused by inborn errors of urea synthesis. *J. Paediatr.*, **97**, 893–900.

Batshaw, M.L., Brusilow, S., Waber, L., Blom, W., Brubak, A.M., Burton, B., Cann, M.M., Kerr, D., Mamanes, P., Matalon, R., Myerberg, D. and Schafer, I.A. (1982). Treatment of inborn errors of urea synthesis: activation of alternative pathways of waste nitrogen synthesis. *N. Engl. J. Med.*, **306**, 1387–92.

Berry, H.K., Hunt, M.M. and Sutherland, B.S. (1971). Amino acid balance in treatment of phenylketonuria. *J. Am. Dietet. Assoc.*, **58**, 210–14.

Berry, H.K., Hsieh, M.H., Bofinger, M. and Scubert, W.K. (1982). Diagnosis of phenylalanine hydroxylase deficiency (phenylketonuria). *Am. J. Dis. Child.*, **136**, 111–14.

Bessman, S.P., Williamson, M.L. and Koch, R. (1978). Diet, genetics and mental retardation: Interaction between phenylketonuria heterozygous mother and fetus to produce non-specific diminution of I.Q. Evidence in support of the justification hypothesis. *Proc. Nat. Acad. Sci. U.S.A.*, **75**, 1562–6.

Bickel, H., Bachmann, C., Beckers, N.J. *et al.* (1981). Neonatal mass screening for metabolic disorders. Summary of recent session of the Committee of Experts to Study Inborn Errors of Metabolic Diseases, Public Health Committee, Council of Europe. *Eur. J. Pediatr.*, **137**, 133–9.

Bickel, H., Gerard, J. and Hickmans, E.M. (1953). Influence of phenylalanine intake on phenylketonuria. *Lancet*, **ii**, 812–13.

Brandt, N.J. (1980). How long should galactosaemia be treated. In *Inherited Disorders of Carbohydrate Metabolism* pp. 103–115. Eds. Burman, D., Holton, J.B. and Pennock, C.A. MTP Press: Lancaster.

Buchwald, H. (1969). Five years experience with the use of partial ileal bypass in the treatment of hypercholesterolemia and atherosclerosis. *Israel J. Med. Sci.*, **5**, 760–65.

Committee for Improvement of Hereditary Disease Management. (1976). Management of Maple Syrup Urine Disease in Canada. *Can. Med. Ass. J.*, **115**, 1005–1013.

Carson, N.A.J., Cusworth, D.C., Dent, C.E., Field, C.M.B., Neill, D.W. and Westall, R.G. (1963). Homocystinuria a new inborn error of metabolism associated with mental deficiency. *Arch. Dis. Child.*, **38**, 425–36.

Clothier, C.M. and Davidson, D.C. (1983). Galactosaemia workshop report. *Human Nutr. Appl. Nut.*, **37A**, 483–90.

Clothier, C. (1977). Management of Dietary Treatment in the Home. In: *Proceedings of 13th Symposium of Society for Studies of Inborn Errors of Metabolism*. Ed. Raine, D. N. MTP Press: Lancaster.

Clow, C.C., Reade, T.M. and Scriver, C.R. (1981). Outcome of early and long-term management of classical maple syrup urine disease. *Pediatrics*, **68**, 856–61.

Comar, D., Saudubray, J.M., Duthilleul, A., Delforge, J., Maziere, M., Berger, G., Charpentier, C., Todd-Pokrapek, A. (1981). Brain uptake of 11C-methionine in phenylketonuria. *Eur. J. Pediatr.*, **136**, 13–19.

Danks, D.M., Bartholome, K., Clayton, B.E., Curtius, H. Grobe, H., Kaufman, S., Leeming, R., Pffeideron, W., Pembold, H., and Rey, F. (1978). Malignant hyperphenylalaninaemia – current status. *J. Inherited Metab. Dis.*, **1**, 49–53.

Danks, D.M., Cotton, R.G.H. and Schlesinger, P. (1979). Diagnosis of malignant hyperphenylalaninaemia. *Arch. Dis. Child.*, **54**, 329–30.

Dent, C.E. (1956). Discussion of Armstrong: Relation of biochemical abnormality to development of mental defect in phenylketonuria in etiological factors in mental retardation, Report of 23rd Conference, Columbus, Ohio.

Denniston, J.C. (1963). Children of mothers with phenylketonuria. *J. Pediatr.*, **63**, 461–2.

Donnell, G.N., Koch, R., Fishler, K., Ng, W.G. (1980). Clinical aspects of galactosaemia. In *Inborn Errors of Metabolism* pp. 103–115. Eds. Burman, D., Holton, J.B. and Pennock, C.A. M.T.P. Press: Lancaster.

Fernandes, J., Jansen, H. and Jansen, T.C. (1979). Nocturnal gastric drip feeding in glucose-6-phosphatase deficient children. *Pediatr. Res.*, **13**, 225–9.

Fisch, R.O., Walker, W.A. and Anderson, J.A. (1966). Prenatal and postnatal developmental consequences of maternal phenylketonuria. *Paediatrics*, **37**, 979–86.

Folkman, J., Phillipart, A., Tze, H.J. and Crigler, J.J. (1972). Portal caval shunt for glycogen storage disease: value of prolonged intravenous hyperalimentation before surgery. *Surgery*, **72**, 306–14.

Forsum, E. and Hambreus, L. (1972). Biological evaluation of a whey protein fraction with special reference to its use as a phenylalanine low protein source in the dietary treatment of PKU. *Nutr. Metab.*, **14**, 48–62.

Francis, D. and Smith, I. (1981). Breast feeding regime for the treatment of infants with phenylketonuria. *Applied Nutrition: I*, Ed. C. Bateman. John Libbey: London.

Fredrikson, D.S. and Levy, R. (1970). Treatment of essential hyperlipaemia. *Lancet*, i, 191–2.

Friedman, P.A., Fisher, D.B., Kang, E.S. and Kaufman, S. (1973). Detection of hepatic phenylalanine 4-hydroxylase in classical phenylketonuria. *Proc. Nat. Acad. Sci. USA.*, **70**, 552–6.

Gaull, G. (1969). Pathogenesis of Maple Syrup Urine Disease, observations during dietary management and treatment of coma by peritoneal dialysis. *Biochem. Med.*, 3, 130–49.

Gitzelman, R. (1965) Deficiency of erythrocyte galactokinase in a patient with galactose diabetes. *Lancet*, **II**, 670–71.

Gitzelman, R. and Hansen R.G. (1980) Galactose metabolism hereditary defects and clinical significance. In *Inherited Disorders of Carbohydrate Metabolism* pp. 61–9 Eds. Burman, D., Holton, J.B. and Pennock, C.A. M.T.P. Press: Lancaster.

Goldstein, J.L., Kita, T. and Brown, M.S. (1983). Defective lipoprotein receptors and atherosclerosis. Lessons from an animal counterpart of familial hypercholesterolemia. *N. Engl. J. Med.*, **309**, 288–96.

Greene, H.L., Stonin, A.E., O'Neill, J.A. and Burr, I.M. (1976). Continuous nocturnal intra gastric feeding for the management of type I glycogen storage disease. *N. Engl. J. Med.*, **294**, 423–5.

Grobe, H. (1980). Homocystinuria (Cystathionine synthase deficiency) results of treatment in late diagnosed patients. *Eur. J. Pediatr.*, **135**, 199–203.

Grobe, H. and Ullrick, K. (1983). Glycogen Storage Disease Type I results of treatment with frequent daytime feeding combined with nocturnal intragastric feeding and with administration of a glucosidase inhibitor. *Eur. J. Pediatr.*, **140**, 102–4.

Hambreus, L.I., Forsum, E. and Lorenson, R. (1974). Use of a formula based on whey protein concentrate in the feeding of an infant with hyperphenylalaninaemia. *Nutr. Metabol.*, **17**, 84–90.

Hammerson, G., Wille, L., Schmidt, H., Lutz, P. and Bickel, H. (1978). Maple Syrup Urine Disease: Treatment of the acutely ill newborn. *Eur. J. Pediatr.*, **129**, 157–65.

Heuther, G., Kaus, R. and Neuhoff, V. (1982a) Brain development in experimental hyperphenylalaninaemia: myelination. *Neuropediatrics*, **13**, 177–82.

Heuther, G., Kaus, R., Neuhoff, V. (1982b). Brain development in experimental hyperphenylalaninaemia: disturbed proliferation and reduced cell numbers in the cerebellum. *Neuropediatrics*, **14**, 12–19.

Hoffbauer, R.W. and Schrempf, G. (1976). Phenylalanine hydroxylation in cultured fibroblasts from patients with phenylketonuria, *Lancet*, **ii**, 194.

Holton, J.B., Gillett, M.G., MacFaul, R. and Young, R. (1981). Galactosaemia: A new severe variant due to uridine diphosphate galactose-4-epimerase deficiency. *Arch. Dis. Child.*, **56**, 885–7.

Howell, R.R., Stevenson, R.E., Ben-Menachem, Y., Phyliky, R.L. and Berry, H.D. (1976). Hepatic adenomata with Type I glycogen storage disease. JAMA, **236**, 1481–4.

Howell, R.R. and Williams, J.C. (1983). *The Glycogen Storage Diseases: The Metabolic Basis of Inherited Metabolic Disease.*, pp. 141–66. Eds. Stanbury, J.B. Wingarde, I.B., Fredrickson, D.S., Goldstein, J.L. and Brown, M.S. McGraw Hill: New York.

Hsieh, M.C., Berry, H.K., Bofinger, M., Phillips, P., Guilfoile, M.B. and Hunt, M. (1983). Comparative diagnostic value of phenylalanine challenge and phenylalanine hydroxylase activity in phenylketonuria. *Clinical Genetics*, **23**, 415–21.

Kaufman, S., Holtzman, N.A., Milstein, S., Butler, I.J. and Krumholz (1975a). Phenylketonuria due to deficiency of dihydropteridine reductase. *N. Engl. J. Med.*, **93**, 785–90.

Kaufman, S., Max, E.E., and Kang, E.S. (1975b). Phenylalanine hydroxylase activity in liver biopsies from hyperphenylalanine heterozygotes: deviation from proportionality with gene dosage. *Pediat. Res.*, **9**, 632–4.

Kaufman, S. (1978). The enzymes of the hepatic phenylalanine hydroxylating system. *J. Inher. Metab. Dis.*, **1**, 63–5.

Kaufman, F.R., Kogut, M.D., Donnell, G.N., Goebelsmann, U., March, C. and Koch, R. (1981). Hypergonadotrophic hypogonadism in female patients with galactosaemia. *N. Engl. J. Med.*, **304**, 994–8.

Kaufman, S., Kapatos, G., McInnes, R.R., Schulman, J.D., and Rizzo, W.B. (1982). The use of tetrahydropterins in the treatment of hyperphenylalaninaemia due to defective synthesis of tetrahydropterins: Evidence that peripherally administered tetrahydropterins enters the brain. *Pediatrics*, **70**, 376–80.

Kaufman, S., Kapatos, G. Rizzo, W.B., Schulman, J.D., Tamarkin, L. and Van Loon, G.R. (1983). Tetrahydropterin therapy for hyperphenylalaninaemia caused by defective synthesis of tetrahydropterins. *Ann. Neurol.*, **14**, 308–15.

Koch, R., Azen, C.G., Friedman, E.G. and Williamson, M.L. (1982). Preliminary report on the effects of diet discontinuation in PKU. *J. Pediatr.* **100**, 870–75.

Komrower, G.M. (1977). The role of the hospital in primary care for the child in the community. *Br. Med. J.*, **2**, 787–9.

Komrower, G.M., Sardharwalla, I.B., Coutts, J.M.J., and Ingham, D. (1979). Management of maternal phenylketonuria: an emerging problem. *Br. Med. J.* **1**, 1383–7.

Lenke, R.R. and Levy, H.L. (1979). Maternal phenylketonuria and hyperphenylalaninaemia: an international survey of the outcome of untreated and treated pregnancies. *N. Engl. J. Med.*, **303**, 1202–8.

Lenke, R.R. and Levy, H.L. (1982). Maternal phenylketonuria: results of dietary therapy. *Am. J. Obstet. Gynaecol.*, **142**, 548–53.

Leonard, J.V., Clarke, M., Macartney, F.J. and Slack, J. (1981). Progression of atheroma in homozygous familial hypercholesterolaemia during regular plasma exchange (letter). *Lancet*, **ii**, 811.

Levy, H.L., Sepe, S.J., Shih, V.E., Vawter, G.F. and Klein, J.C. (1977). Sepsis due to Escherichia Coli in neonates with galactosaemia. *N. Engl. J. Med.*, **297**, 823–5.

Levy, H.L. and Waisbren, S.E. (1983). Effects of untreated maternal phenylketonuria and hyperphenylalaninaemia on the fetus. *N. Engl. J. Med.*, **309**, 1269–74.

Mabry, C.C., Denneston, J.C., Nelson, T.L. and Son, C.D. (1965). Maternal phenylketonuria: A cause of mental retardation in children without metabolic defect. *N. Engl. J. Med.*, **269**, 1404–8.

Mabry, C.C., Denneston, J.C. and Coldwell, J.G. (1966). Mental retardation in the children of phenylketonuric mothers. *N. Engl. J. Med.*, **275**, 1331.

McBean, M.S. and Stephenson, J.B.P. (1968). Treatment of classical phenylketonuria. *Arch. Dis. Child.*, **43**, 1–7.

Mathai, C.K. and Beutler, E. (1966). Electrophoretic variation of galactose-1-phosphate uridyl transferase. *Science*, **154**, 1179–80.

Menkes, J.H., Hurst, P.L. and Craig, J.M. (1954). A new syndrome of progressive infantile dysfunction associated with unusual urinary substance. *Pediatrics*, **14**, 462–6.

Muller, D.R., Harries, J.T. and Lloyd, J.K. (1970). Vitamin E therapy in abetalipoproteinaemia. *Arch. Dis. Child.* **45**, 715.

Naughten, E.R., Jenkins, J., Francis, D.E.M., and Leonard, J.V. (1982). Outcome of maple syrup urine disease. *Arch. Dis. Child.* **57**, 918–21.

Raine, D.N. (1977) The need for a national policy for the management of inherited metabolic disease. In *Proceedings of 13th Symposium of Society for the Study of Inborn Errors of Metabolism*. Ed. Raine, D.N. MTP Press: Lancaster.

Royston, N.J.W. and Parry, T.E. (1962). Megablastic anaemia complicating dietary treatment of phenylketonuria in infancy. *Arch. Dis. Child.* **37**, 430–35.

Sardharwalla, I.B. (1980). Management of homocystinuria. In *Topics in Paediatrics 2: Nutrition in Childhood*. pp. 110–18. Ed. B.A. Wharton, Pitman Medical: Tunbridge Wells.

Scriver, C.R., Mackenzie, S., Clow, C.L. *et al.* (1971). Thiamine-responsive maple syrup urine disease. *Lancet*, **i**, 310–12.
Scriver, C.R. and Rosenburg, L.E. (1973). Vitamin responsive amino acidopathies. In *Amino Acid Disorders*. pp. 453–78. Saunders: Philadelphia.
Scriver, C.R. and Clow, C.L. (1980). Phenylketonuria: Epitome of human biochemical genetics. *N. Engl. J. Med.* **303**, 1336–42; 1394–1400.
Simon and Gibson. (1980). Lipid Lowering Drugs.
Smith, I. and Wolff, O.H. (1974). Duration of treatment of phenylketonuria. *Lancet*, **i**, 1229–30.
Smith, I., Clayton, B.E. and Wolff, O.H. (1975). New variant of phenylketonuria with progressive neurological illness unresponsive to phenylalanine restriction. *Lancet*, **i**, 1108–11.
Smith, I., Lobascher, M.E., Stevenson, J.E., Wolff, O.H., Schmidt, H., Guibel-Kaiser, S. and Bickel, J. (1978). Effect of stopping low phenylalanine diet on intellectual progress of children with phenylketonuria. *Br. Med. J.* **2**, 723–6.
Starzl, T.E., Putman, C.W., Porter, K.A. *et al.* (1973) Portal diversion for the treatment of glycogen storage disease in humans. *Ann. Surg.*, **178**, 525–39.
Starzl, T.E., Iwatsuki, S., Van Thiel, D.H. *et al.* (1982). Evolution of liver transplantation. *Hepatology*, **2**, 614–36.
Stephenson, J.P.B. and McBean, M.S. (1967). Diagnosis of phenylketonuria (Phenylalanine hydroxylase deficiency, temporary and permanent). *Br. Med. J.*, **2**, 579.
Takeda, E., Kuroda, Y., Toshima, W., Watanabe, T., Naito, E., and Miyao, M. (1983). Effect of long-term administration of sodium benzoate to a patient with partial ornithine carbamoyl transferase deficiency. *Clin. Paediatr.* (Phila.) **22**, 206–8.
Taketomi, T., Kunishita, T., Hara, A. and Mizushima, S. (1983). Abnormal protein and lipid compositions of the cerebral myelin of a patient with maple syrup urine disease. *Japan J. Exp. Med.*, **53**, 109–16.
Thompson, G.R. (1981). Plasma exchange for hypercholesterolaemia. *Lancet* **i**, 1246–8.
Townsend, I. and Kerr, D. (1982). Total parental nutrition therapy of toxic maple syrup disease. *Am. J. Clin. Nutr.*, **36**, 359–65.
Tribble, D., Shapira, R. (1983). Degradation in rat brain initiated by metabolites causative of maple syrup urine disease. *Biochem. Biophys. Res. Communication*, **114**, 440–6.
Watts, R.W.E. (1982). The Treatment of Inborn Errors of Metabolism: Introduction and General Principles. In *Advances in Treatment of Inborn Errors of Metabolism*. pp. 1–6. Eds. d'A Crawfurd, M., Gibbs, D.A. and Watts, R.W.E. John Wiley: Chichester.
Wendel, V., Langerbeck, U., Lambeck, I. and Bremer, H.J. (1982). Maple syrup urine disease – therapeutic use of insulin in catabolic states. *Eur. J. Pediat.*, **139**, 172–5.
West, R.J., and Lloyd, J.K. (1973). The use of cholestyramine resin in treatment of children with familial hypercholesterolemia. *Arch. Dis. Child.* **48**, 370–74.
Westall, R.G. (1963). Dietary treatment of a child with maple syrup urine disease (branch chain ketoaciduria). *Arch. Dis. Child.* **38**, 485–91.

# 4 Marasmus and kwashiorkor

Michael H.N. Golden



## Introduction

Severe undernutrition, in its various forms, is undoubtedly the commonest of severe illnesses. In poor, technologically backward countries it is the major cause of death: it stunts the physical and mental development of the majority of the population.

It would be a mistake, however, to think that severe undernutrition is a problem confined to poor nations: it accompanies a wide variety of medical and surgical conditions common in industrialized societies, especially chronic illnesses. In the conditions associated with malnutrition, the nutritional state itself alters the expression and course of the 'primary' condition as well as its response to conventional treatment. Indeed, notwithstanding the diagnostic label attached to the patient, it is frequently the accompanying malnutrition that is the major cause of morbidity and mortality. A clinical history of severe weight loss or anorexia is not just a diagnostic pointer making a severe or chronic 'primary' diagnosis probable; rather, it is a signal both for the treatment of malnutrition, a harbinger of death, and for the modification of the treatment regimens used for the primary diagnosis.

The rational treatment of malnutrition depends upon a clear understanding of its pathogenesis: we do not yet have this full understanding. Nevertheless, over the past few years, there has been a complete revolution in our concepts of the mechanisms leading to the two major forms of malnutrition: marasmus and kwashiorkor. These are briefly reviewed here to provide the rationale for the treatment proposed; fuller accounts may be found in Jackson and Golden (1983), Golden and Jackson (1986) and Golden (1985).

## Pathogenesis of marasmus

The pathogenesis is illustrated schematically in Figure 4.1. We start from the point where the patient has a reduced total food intake. Reduced intakes secondary to psychiatric abnormality, infection, starvation, malabsorption, neoplasia or to an initial specific nutrient deficiency (such as protein or zinc deficiency, for example) are not different in principal although the details may differ. These patients all follow the same general path.

Children stop growing and then both children and adults lose weight. This is the most obvious abnormality clinically, and forms the basis for the various anthropometric classifications of malnutrition.

### Reduced requirement

As weight is lost the absolute nutritional requirements are reduced simply on

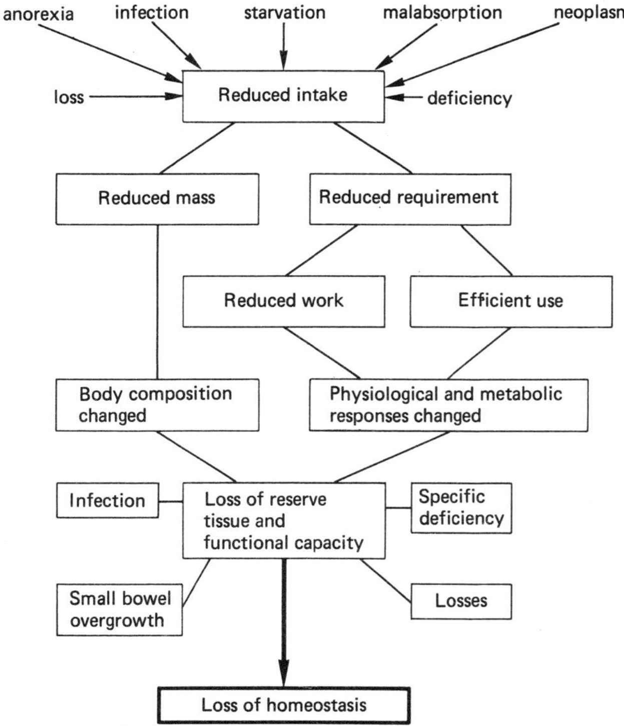


Fig. 4.1 Proposed pathogenesis of marasmus.

the basis of decreased mass. However, we find that there is also a relative reduction in requirement so that each gram of body tissue requires less energy. This comes about in two ways. First, there is more efficient utilization of ingested food. For example, dynamic measurements show that a much higher proportion of the amino acids released from protein during tissue breakdown are utilized to resynthesize tissue instead of being oxidized (Golden *et al.*, 1977). However, we normally utilize our food quite efficiently so that there is a relatively small absolute saving in this increased efficiency.

By far the most important adaptation is in the actual work performed by the body itself – its organs, tissues, cells, organelles and enzymatic machinery. All the processes of the body show this reductive adaptation: *no* physiological function has so far been studied in severe undernutrition and found to be normal. Some of these changes are shown in Table 4.1.

## Physiological and metabolic changes

One of the most fundamental reductive adaptations is a slowing of the activity of the sodium pump. Normally about one-third of basal energy requirements are consumed by this ion pump. Thus, this adaptation alone leads to a substantial saving in energy utilization, at the cost of allowing the intracellular sodium concentration to rise and potassium to fall. A further considerable saving in energy expenditure is achieved by a reduction in the intensity of protein turnover. Even mechanical work and spontaneous activity are severely curtailed in the malnourished individual.

Table 4.1 Physiological changes in malnourished children and in children after recovery to normal weight-for-height. (Data derived from: Alleyne, 1966a and b, 1967; Klahr and Alleyne, 1973; Brooke *et al.*, 1974b; Golden *et al.*, 1977; Patrick and Golden, 1977)

| Physiological change | Malnourished | Recovered | Mal–Rec % Rec |
|---|---|---|---|
| Metabolic rate (kJ/kg $0.75^{-1}$/day) | 315 | 417 | −24 |
| Sodium pump activity ($h^{-1}$) | 3.62 | 4.94 | −27 |
| Intracellular sodium (mM/kg DS) | 169 | 109 | +55 |
| Intracellular potassium (mM/kg DS) | 341 | 387 | −12 |
| Protein synthesis (g/kg/day) | 4.0 | 6.3 | −37 |
| Protein breakdown (g/kg/day) | 3.7 | 6.4 | −42 |
| Cardiac output (l/min/$m^3$) | 4.77 | 6.90 | −31 |
| Stroke volume (ml/beat/$m^3$) | 44.1 | 53.0 | −22 |
| Circulation time (s) | 13.7 | 10.5 | +30 |
| GFR (Cin-ml/min/$m^3$) | 47.1 | 92.4 | −41 |
| Renal blood flow (Cpah-ml/min/$m^3$) | 249 | 321 | −22 |
| H+ excretion after $NH_4Cl$ ($\mu$Eq/min) | 10.4 | 28.4 | −63 |
| Osmolal clearance rate (ml/min) | 0.20 | 0.66 | −70 |
| Percentage infused sodium excreted | 22.3 | 48.7 | −54 |
| Sodium excreted % of sodium filtered | | | |
| normal ECF | 0.50 | 1.23 | −59 |
| expanded ECF | 0.82 | 11.07 | −93 |
| Response to temperature change | poikilotherm | homeotherm | – |

The reduced work at every level of organization leads directly to alteration of physiological responses, many of which have important therapeutic implications.

There is a reduction in cardiac output due to both a lowered heart rate and stroke volume. The ventricular function curves (stroke work/pressure) are altered so that the point of maximum performance occurs at a lower mean pressure. These patients are thus easily precipitated into heart failure.

The maximum concentrating and diluting ability of the kidney is severely restricted. There is a very limited capacity to excrete free hydrogen ions, titratable acid and ammonia in response to an acid load. There is also a very severe limitation of the ability to excrete sodium, particularly in response to an expanded extracellular fluid volume. During the early phase of treatment, when the sodium pump is recovering and the excess intracellular sodium is being exported to the extracellular compartment, acute circulatory overload and sudden death can easily occur (Patrick, 1977).

There is a reduction in gastric acid output. The intestine is atrophic with a marked reduction in the pancreatic enzyme production and in the cellular enzymes and transport systems for nutrient absorption. The digestive and absorptive capacity is easily overwhelmed (James, 1970).

The malnourished patient becomes poikilothermic. Even a modest reduction to 25°C or elevation to 33°C in environmental temperature may lead to hypothermia or pyrexia respectively (Brooke *et al.*, 1973, 1974a). Malnourished patients reduce their oxygen consumption in response to a cool environment: they do not have a normal sweating response.

The inflammatory response and the immune system also partake in the reductive adaptation and are either absent or severely blunted in seriously malnourished patients. This adaptation has major implications for the recognition of infection and the altered relationship between the malnourished host and his flora.

## Body composition

There is a change in body composition. Most tissues contribute to the loss of weight; however, they do not contribute equally. Subcutaneous fat may virtually disappear and muscle mass is often reduced by more than half. Skin and intestine are also disproportionally affected whereas the viscera and central nervous system are relatively well preserved. The chemical composition of the whole body is not only altered because of the absolute and relative changes in the size of the organs within the body, but also as a consequence of the reductive adaptations themselves. Thus, the change in activity of the sodium pump invariably leads to an increased total body sodium and reduced total body potassium, irrespective of the patient's state of hydration, and the serum electrolyte concentrations.

The reduction in the metabolic activity of the cells leads to a reduction in the enzyme, soluble protein and RNA complement that is synthesized and maintained by the cell. Most of the trace elements are used by the body to form integral parts of these cell components. They cannot be retained in the tissues in isolation when the parent proteins are not required. There is thus a reduction in the tissue concentration of zinc, copper, manganese, magnesium and probably selenium (Golden and Golden, 1981). During reversal of the adaptation and 'catchup' from malnutrition the deficits of all these minerals have to be made good. Iron is the one exception. There is an increased concentration of tissue iron in most forms of severe malnutrition (Golden *et al.*, 1985a). As the soluble protein complement of the tissues falls there is a relative increase in structural proteins (Picou *et al.*, 1966) which leads to a change in the amino acid composition of the tissues, with a particular reduction in the essential amino acids.

## Loss of reserve

Normally the metabolic capacity greatly exceeds that which is required under normal circumstances. The cost of the reductive adaptations and the reduction in functional tissue mass is to dispense, to a greater or lesser extent, with the reserve capacity. The malnourished individual has a reduced capacity to respond appropriately to any perturbation.

## Vicious cycles

Superimposed upon the reduced ability to respond to metabolic perturbations and environmental changes are the pathological effects of the stresses themselves. The curtailment of the inflammatory and immune responses makes repeated or, more usually, chronic infections, ubiquitous. The lack of peristalsis, achlorhydria, poor secretion of IgA and bile salts combine to allow faecal bacteria and fungi to overgrow the small intestine and stomach.

The diarrhoea and repeated infections give rise to specific nutrient deficiencies, particularly of mineral elements. When the integrity of the skin is breached either from the burn-like lesions of severe childhood malnutrition, or from bed-sores and traumatic or surgical lesions which do not heal, blood and serum can be lost in considerable amounts.

All these consequences of being unable to cope with stress themselves give rise to anorexia, malabsorption and a reduced intake. The cycle is now complete. The debilitated patient will reach a self-perpetuating stage where deterioration, leading to death, is rapid.

## Loss of homeostasis

As the physiological and tissue reserve is whittled away and the effects of chronic infection and diarrhoea deplete the patient, he becomes more and more 'brittle', like a diabetic patient losing homeostatic control of his blood sugar. However, unlike the diabetic, in the severely malnourished patient it is not just one organ or system which is functionally deranged but all of them.

When treatment regimens are planned we must always work within the limited metabolic capacity of our patients whilst we reverse the reductive adaptations dietetically, and break the vicious cycles by replacing losses, treating infections, suppressing the overgrowth of intestinal flora and correcting any specific nutrient deficiencies.

## Pathogenesis of kwashiorkor

The clinical features of kwashiorkor are oedema, severe fatty liver, skin dyspigmentation and breakdown, hair colour changes, and very low levels of circulating hepatic export proteins. In contrast to marasmus, kwashiorkor has only once been convincingly reproduced in experimental animals (Coward and Whitehead, 1972). Why should kwashiorkor be so difficult to reproduce experimentally? Why have the applied programmes designed to prevent kwashiorkor been so uniformly unsuccessful? The obvious first answer to consider is that the hypotheses that have been proposed and that form the conceptual base to the experimental and applied studies, are incorrect. Certainly the extant hypotheses: protein deficiency (Williams, 1935); niacin deficiency (Gillman and Gillman, 1951); antidiuretic hormone like action of excess free ferritin (Srikantia, 1958); dysadaptation to a protein deficient diet (Gopalan, 1968); hormonal dysadaptation (Whitehead, 1979); or aflatoxicosis (Hendrickse, 1984) do not adequately explain more than a few of the features of kwashiorkor listed in Table 4.2. The features must all be reconciled in any unifying hypothesis of the aetiology and pathogenesis of kwashiorkor.

Table 4.2 Observations made that must be reconciled in any theory of the pathogenesis and aetiology of kwashiorkor

1. The association of oedema, fatty liver, skin lesions, hair discolouration and mental changes, suggesting a common mechanism.
2. The association with certain staple foods: cassava, yam, plaintain, rice, maize, cruciferae.
3. The lack of kwashiorkor in 'primitive' cultures where the staple foods, associated in other cultures with kwashiorkor, are prepared in the traditional manner such as fermentation (cassava, breadfruit), or by the addition of burnt plant ash (maize).
4. The precipitation of kwashiorkor by infection, particularly measles, tuberculosis, malaria and diarrhoea.
5. The almost universal presence of infection and overgrowth of bacteria in the small intestine.
6. The unpredictable fluctuation in prevalence from year to year.
7. The association with humid climates and wet seasons.
8. Occurrence predominantly in the newly weaned child.
9. The occasional occurrence of kwashiorkor in the very young or in the fully breast-fed child.
10. It is extremely difficult to produce under controlled, hygienic conditions with a full diet lacking single essential nutrients (or classes of nutrients).
11. Skin lesions are particularly florid in dark skinned patients in the tropics.
12. Associated with low levels of hepatic export proteins.
13. Associated with high levels of circulating ferritin and vitamin $B_{12}$.
14. Associated with low concentrations of vitamins E and A, carotene, zinc and selenium.
15. Usual response to admission to hospital with treatment of infection, provision of a hygienic environment and a milk based diet.
16. Usual complete recovery leaving no pathological lesions, with subsequent growth and metabolic responses that are not different from peers that never had kwashiorkor.

Recently it has been proposed that kwashiorkor results from an imbalance between the production of free radicals in the patient and their safe disposal (Golden, 1985, 1986). This mechanism would explain the features of kwashiorkor listed in Table 4.2. In this scheme kwashiorkor and marasmus are not seen as opposite ends of a spectrum going from pure energy deficiency (marasmus) to pure protein deficiency (kwashiorkor), to give a whole gradation of intermediate conditions termed 'protein-energy malnutrition' but as two aetiologically distinct conditions: marasmus being the condition produced by both energy and protein deficiency (*vide supra*) and kwashiorkor being secondary to the superimposition of various noxa. These noxa include various infections and toxins from contaminated food and are presented to a patient whose antioxidant and free radical protective mechanisms are compromised. There are thus two primary variables, the noxa and the diet-etically determined inability to respond. Because the diets that are low in the components necessary to maintain adequate free radical protection are frequently also low in energy and protein (many of these components are fellow-travellers of dietary protein such as the sulphur amino acids, zinc, copper and manganese), marasmus and kwashiorkor frequently coexist in the same subject and in the same population. However, there are populations where kwashiorkor is common and marasmus rare such as Uganda; the opposite pattern is found in Ethiopia, thus there is not a necessary association or graduation between the two conditions.

The theory of kwashiorkor is summarized in Figure 4.2 and the evidence for the theory in Figure 4.3. In essence all the conditions which precipitate kwashiorkor in a susceptible subject cause an increased flux of free radicals. In kwashiorkor we find a decrease in all the protective pathways: vitamins A, E,

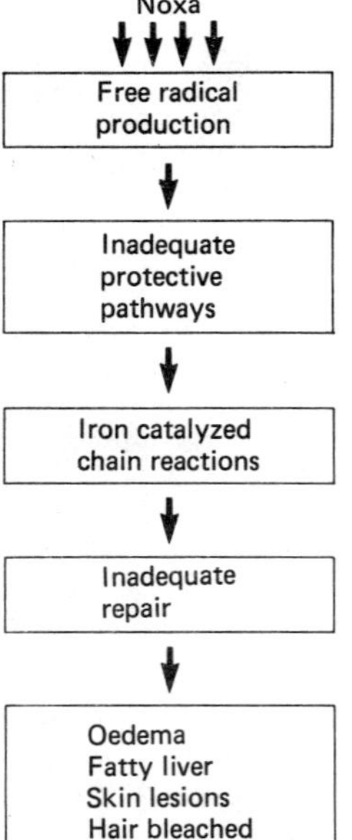


Fig. 4.2 Proposed pathogenesis of kwashiorkor.

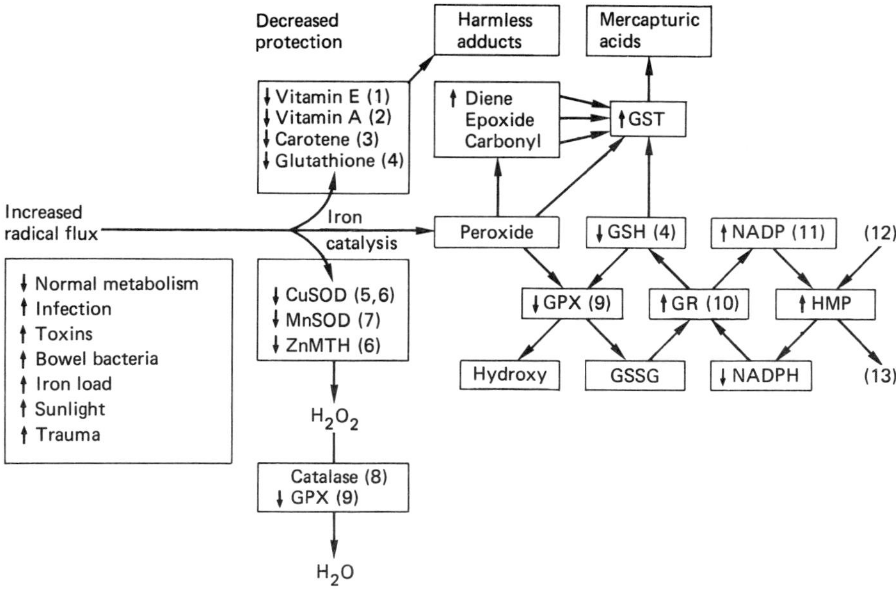


Fig. 4.3 Diagram showing the mechanisms of radical production and subsequent metabolism. The arrows *beside* the substrates, products and enzymes show whether they have been demonstrated to be increased or decreased in children with kwashiorkor. The numbers refer to the essential nutrients involved: (1) vitamin E: (2) vitamin A: (3) carotene: (4) sulphur amino acids, CYS: (5) copper: (6) zinc: (7) manganese: (8) iron: (9) selenium: (10) riboflavin: (11) nicotinic acid: (12) magnesium and phosphorus: (13) thiamine.
Abbreviations: CuSOD – Copper-zinc superoxide dismutase; MnSOD – Manganese superoxide dismutase; GST – Glutathione-S-transferase; GPX – Glutathione peroxidase; GSH – glutathione (reduced); GSSG – Glutathione (oxidized); GR – Glutathione reductase; NADP – Nicotine adenine dinucleotide phosphate (oxidized); NADPH – Nicotine adenine dinucleotide phosphate (reduced); HMP, Hexose-monophosphate-shunt (G6PD and 6-phosphogluconic acid dehydrogenase).

C and carotene, the superoxide dismutase enzymes and glutathione peroxidase. There is an increase in tissue iron, which by redox cycling will catalyze the generation of free radicals. Despite induction of the enzymes involved in glutathione reduction, glutathione reductase and the hexose monophosphate shunt, there is a decrease in reduced NADPH. Glutathione is present at very low levels in kwashiorkor (Fig. 4.4). We even find induction of the glutathione-S-transferase enzymes in red cells, evidence for an increased flux of products such as carbonyls, peroxides and epoxides – molecules with electrophilic centres.

At least 13 different nutrients: vitamin E; vitamin A; carotene; sulphur amino acids; copper; zinc; manganese; iron; selenium; riboflavine; nicotinic acid; magnesium and thiamine, are involved in this scheme. Clearly a compromised intake of even some of these nutrients could profoundly affect the body's ability to withstand radical producing stresses.

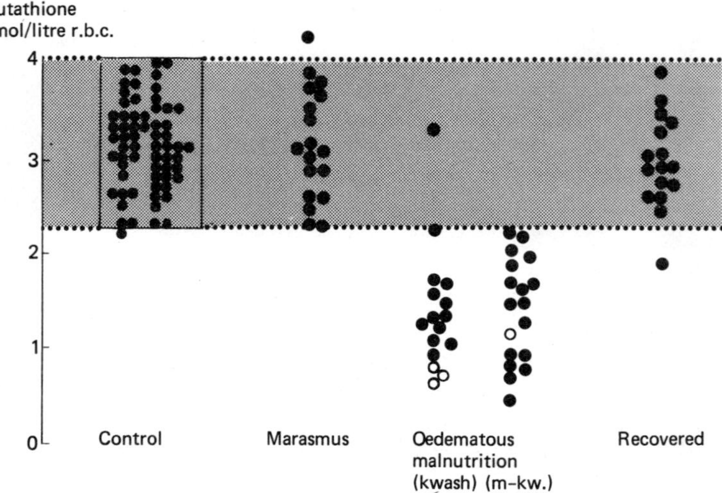


Fig. 4.4 Red blood cell glutathione concentration (GSH + GSSG) in control, malnourished and recovered children. Each point represents a separate child. The children depicted by open circles died.

## Principles of treatment

The approach to therapy must be holistic. All the various abnormalities have to be attended to, in a balanced way, relatively slowly at first, so that the child is able to correct his own disordered metabolism and to synthesize the metabolic machinery necessary to utilize the building blocks required for regrowth. The patient will signal his readiness to enter the intense anabolism of 'catch up' by developing a voracious appetite. The appetite is an extremely important barometer of metabolic wellbeing and must be relied upon and given priority when making clinical judgements.

At first, care must be taken not to overstep the patient's homeostatic capacity for it is at the early transition stage when patients die. The principal is best illustrated with an example. All children with malnutrition have low activities of intestinal lactase, sucrase and maltase when compared with normal individuals; however, the deficiency is not absolute, rather, it is one of reduced capacity. If a small amount of isotonic disaccharide is given to a malnourished patient it will be absorbed at the same rate as in a normal patient. However, as either the absolute amount or the tonicity of the disaccharide is increased the absorption rate falls further and further behind that of the normal subject (James, 1970). The actual level (amount or tonicity) at which the capacity is exceeded depends upon the severity of the individual case. The same considerations apply to the amount of other nutrients in the diet, in the loads presented to the liver for metabolic conversion, the heart for circulation and to the kidney for excretion. When the effects of infection, specific nutrient deficiencies, small bowel bacterial overgrowth, and gross changes in body composition are superimposed on this lack of homeostasis, it is apparent that the successful treatment of these patients requires attention to the individual details of each patient. Malnutrition should not be managed using a standard protocol, with important therapeutic decisions, such as the type and quantity of the diet, being left to a relatively inexperienced member of staff.

The residential management of malnutrition can be divided into four phases 1. Resuscitation; 2. Preparation for high energy feeding; 3. Rehabilitation; 4. Preparation for discharge. At each stage attention should be paid both to the physical and to the mental wellbeing of the child.

## Marasmus *vs* kwashiorkor

The question arises as to whether or not there should be a difference between the treatment of the child with marasmus and kwashiorkor. In the past we have used the same treatment for both conditions with moderate success – indeed many children have both conditions. In terms of reducing stress for the children with kwashiorkor, treating infections, looking after the children in hygienic surroundings and giving them food uncontaminated with bacteria or toxins, will do much, but this is simply standard practice for any patient. The repletion of specific nutrient deficits equally clearly should proceed in both marasmus and in kwashiorkor. However, the new insights into the pathogenesis of kwashiorkor immediately raise the possibility of giving specific treatment directed towards the underlying mechanisms of the disease. Such therapeutic manoeuvres could include specific antioxidant therapy with sulphydryls and natural or artificial antioxidants and free radical scavengers, provision of additional sulphur amino acids, iron chelation therapy, xanthine oxidase inhibitors and particular provision of additional supplements of those nutrients known to be important in the enzymes involved in protection from radical damage. None of these treatments have yet undergone formal therapeutic trial in kwashiorkor. It would therefore be premature to presume upon the results of such trials.

However, it has been established that it is dangerous to give the child with kwashiorkor iron supplements (McFarlane *et al.*, 1970) – and malnourished patients should never be given parenteral iron.

The last edition of this book advocated supplying the extra energy required by malnourished children in the form of vegetable oil. However, these oils contain high concentrations of polyunsaturated fatty acids. With their multiple double bonds they are substrates, *par excellence*, for peroxidation reactions. Indeed, in experimental animals where there is inadequate protection against free radical/peroxide formation, dietary vegetable oils can give an overwhelming stress leading to severe illness and death. We have preliminary data to show that diets high in these oils lead to a further lowering of the already depleted vitamin E and that the red cell glutathione concentration remains low or falls on these diets. This is clearly a dangerous situation which may provide the explanation for the clinical deterioration of some of the children after admission to the ward. Until more information becomes available it would be prudent to avoid diets rich in polyunsaturated fatty acids in patients showing features of kwashiorkor. Alternative sources of fat energy would be coconut oil or medium chain triglycerides.

The benefits observed originally from giving a milk based diet (Williams,

1935) may have been due to the sulphur amino acids that it contains together with selenium, vitamin E and other fellow-travellers. The possibility that the lactoferrin in the milk is of direct therapeutic benefit should also be considered, for this protein will chelate iron, even at low pH. From a pragmatic point of view, milk based diets should therefore continue to form the basis of the therapeutic diets for both kwashiorkor and marasmus; until much more is known of the details of pathogenesis so that formulae can be tailored to correct specific deficiencies, it would be unwise to alter a treatment which has been empirically successful. In the past year or so kwashiorkor has again become an area of intense investigation, after an eclipse in interest of almost twenty years; the recommended treatments are likely to change.

## Resuscitation

As we have seen all the physiological, biochemical and behavioural measurements that have been made in malnourished patients are abnormal. To single out a particular abnormality, usually because we have a laboratory that can perform the measurement, and to concentrate on treating that abnormality is fraught with danger. For example in the past, we have attempted to correct abnormal plasma sodium concentrations using standard therapeutic procedures, that have been formulated from experience in well nourished populations, only to find the response of the malnourished patient was opposite to that anticipated. Often there is a conflict between the specific treatments for different aspects of the child's condition. Thus oedema is associated with sodium retention, yet diarrhoea is known to be associated with sodium depletion. Which should take precedence in the treatment of the oedematous child with diarrhoea? The attempts to resolve this therapeutic dilemma by giving conventional treatment to one facet, guided by the serum sodium concentration, while ignoring the other facet of the illness lead to the death of many patients. We are still ignorant of the relative importance of the factors involved in deranged homeostasis. Many of the 'abnormalities' are in fact appropriate adaptations in response to the metabolic state. Hence, rather than attempting to correct the abnormality, it is better to remedy the basis for the adaptation. Reversal of the abnormality will follow. This is particularly true of the abnormal distribution of fluid and electrolytes between body compartments.

The guiding principles of the resuscitation period are: 1. to give supportive therapy to allow repair to proceed; 2. to keep within the functional capacity of the patient; and 3. to think in terms of balance of nutrients in the whole child and not in terms of concentrations. These guidelines can be viewed from the various aspects of treatment:

1. Control of infection and overgrowth of bowel flora.
2. Repletion of specific nutrient deficiencies.
3. Control of metabolic state through dietary energy intake.

### Control of infection and overgrowth of bowel flora

Patients with malnutrition should be presumed to have an infection until proven otherwise. Diligence and care should be exercised to identify the location and nature of the infection. In sick patients in whom a specific infection has not been identified it is reasonable to introduce therapy blindly, using powerful broad spectrum antibiotics active against anaerobic, Gram-negative and Gram-positive organisms. In practice, virtually all malnourished children receive antibiotic treatment. Giving antibiotics in this situation should be viewed as treatment of a presumptive infection: it is not prophylaxis!

The combination of either erythromycin or penicillin and gentamycin is particularly effective. When supplies of gentamycin are limited, chloramphenicol or tetracycline are relatively cheap alternatives which should be used.

In areas where malaria is prevalent all children should receive antimalarials unless a laboratory can confirm the absence of malarial parasites. Tuberculosis must be sought diligently and if there is any doubt, it should be assumed to be present and active.

A clinical diagnosis of small bowel overgrowth can be made on the basis of gaseous abdominal distension. These patients often have a history of chronic diarrhoea with offensive watery stools. Metronidazole often has a dramatic effect and should be continued until the patient has reached a stage of recovery where he can resist recolonization of his small intestine. In most situations it is wise to give metronidazole to all children with severe malnutrition.

Intestinal parasites are extremely common and if facilities are available stools should be examined for ova and cysts; if not, antihelminthics should be given routinely. Mebendazole (100 mg, twice daily for 3 days) is the best antihelminthic to use. Levamisol is a reasonable alternative which has the added advantage of stimulating the cell mediated immune system. Thiabendazole can be used, but as it often gives rise to nausea and vomiting, routine treatment is better delayed until after the acute phase of the illness is controlled. Piperazine is not adequate for most of the common worms. Giardiasis is treated with metronidazole.

Our knowledge of pharmacokinetics in malnutrition is very incomplete. Drugs like gentamycin which are distributed in the extracellular fluid, will have a larger volume of distribution in malnutrition; others which are fat soluble or which bind to albumin may have a smaller volume of distribution. Intestinal absorption of drugs may be impaired, as may the mechanisms of elimination. Furthermore, these determinants of pharmacokinetics are likely to change rapidly during resuscitation and growth. It is probably best to use standard therepeutic doses, until more information becomes available; however, the possibility of drug toxicity or inadequate dosage should be continually considered.

## Repletion of specific nutrient deficits

In normal clinical practice one is almost entirely dependent upon the identification of clinical signs to recognize the presence of specific nutrient deficits. There are nutrient deficits in three senses.

1. Loss of tissue leads to a balanced deficiency of all the normal constituents of that tissue. Repletion is accomplished by stimulating regrowth of the whole tissue. There is not necessarily a balance in terms of the whole

body because the tissue lost may, or may not, be normally rich in a particular component.

2. Within the tissue there may be unbalanced losses relative to the normal composition of that tissue. Some constituents may become much more depleted than others secondary to metabolic adaptation. The abnormal balance of nutrients has to be redressed before tissue synthesis can take place.
3. For many micronutrients there is a further unbalanced loss relative to the demands of the tissue. This is a pathological rather than a physiological deficit secondary to metabolic readjustment.

The nutrient which becomes limiting first for the adapted function of a particular tissue, will determine the pathological pattern displayed by that tissue. Other nutrients may thus be pathologically deficient without displaying specific physical signs. Their deficiencies will be unmasked if only the limiting nutrient is provided.

During the resuscitation phase, deficiencies of the third type have to be replaced: during the preparation for catch-up those of the second type are corrected, and during catch-up weight gain the first type of deficiency is corrected.

**Minerals (cations)**

Potassium and magnesium are invariably deficient in all tissues, and this may account for a wide range of the metabolic disturbances. Potassium should be given orally as potassium chloride, between 2 and 4 mmol/kg body weight/day once the patient has been seen to pass urine.

The potassium can only be effectively retained if magnesium deficiency is corrected and sufficient energy is given to supply the sodium pump with ATP. Between 0.5 to 1.0 mmol/kg body weight/day of magnesium should be given. Magnesium hydroxide is cheap; however, it is very insoluble and in the presence of achlorhydria is unlikely to be efficiently utilized. Magnesium chloride and sulphate may induce a metabolic acidosis in full therapeutic doses. We have recently used magnesium acetate; however, there may be an accumulation of acetate as it normally requires a kinase to initiate its metabolism. The safest approach is to give magnesium chloride with equimolar amounts of potassium citrate to prevent the metabolic acidosis of the chloride.

Correction of a pathological (type 3) deficiency of these two minerals, which occurs in at least half the children, may take several days. However, as potassium and magnesium losses are due to major reductive adaptations, they should be given routinely. Retention in excess of that required for new tissue may continue for several weeks.

Zinc deficiency is always present with chronic diarrhoea, skin atrophy or ulceration, or oedema, and is a potent cause of anorexia. Zinc plays an important role in maintaining the cell mediated immune response and in protein synthesis. Zinc (2 mg/kg/day) should be given as the acetate. Zinc sulphate can be used but is not as efficacious.

Copper tends to be deficient in diets based on cows' milk and so clinical deficiency commonly supervenes during recovery even in children replete on admission. Copper (0.2 mg/kg/day) can be given as the acetate, chloride or sulphate.

**Iron**

Anaemia is frequently present and serum iron is low, consequently iron has been included in most treatment regimens advocated in the past. However, iron is the biological catalyst of peroxidizing reactions, consequently trials of iron chelation therapy in the treatment of kwashiorkor are being conducted! Iron binding proteins are low and easily saturated, further they lose their bacteriostatic effects when the molecule is bound with iron. Iron should be withheld from the malnourished patient. Anaemia may be due to folic acid deficiency, copper deficiency, vitamin E deficiency or to the general depression of metabolism as well as due to iron deficiency. Anaemia is best treated with blood transfusion.

When the child has regained his appetite and started to grow rapidly, then additional dietary iron will be required at a dose of about 4 mg/kg/day.

Most milk based diets contain adequate calcium but supplementation may be required with diets formulated from local produce or based on other protein sources.

At the present time the situation is unclear about other cations. There is evidence that chromium, vanadium and manganese may be important.

**Minerals (anions)**

Phosphate depletion contributes to the limited ability of the kidney to excrete an acid load, and possibly to the gross osteopenia seen in the children. Intracellular levels of phosphate are deficient, which is of importance for energy production. The phosphate content of cows' milk is adequate for phosphate repletion. Diets in which the energy density is increased by the addition of (saturated) oil or carbohydrate may contain insufficient phosphorus.

Selenium deficiency is common (Golden *et al.*, 1985). It is an integral part of the enzyme glutathione peroxidase, an essential enzyme in the protective repertoire against peroxide and other oxidant damage. A supplement of 40–60 μg/day should be given where a deficiency is suspected.

Iodine should be given in areas where endemic goitre is encountered.

**Vitamins**

Deficiency of nearly all the vitamins has been described. A vitamin mix should be given routinely to all malnourished children. In some instances the quantities of vitamins in commercial supplements are insufficient and additional specific therapy is required. In rice eating areas additional thiamine should be given parenterally on admission. In most malnourished populations, oral folic acid (5 mg/day) should be given.

Vitamin A deficiency is very common: its level of deficiency correlates with the prognosis. The early manifestations are very slight loss of reflectivity of the conjunctiva. Bitot's spots are uncommon in young children and the other eye signs are late manifestations of deficiency. Even in areas without clinical vitamin A deficiency, plasma vitamin A and hepatic stores are low. Vitamin A 150 000 Units i.m. should be given routinely.

It is now clear that most children also have vitamin E deficiency: this also correlates with prognosis. Adequate vitamin E is usually not included in multivitamin preparations. A daily dose of 400 iu of vitamin E should be given.

The position of vitamin D in the malnourished child needs urgent investigation: we are not in a position to make recommendations.

As stated supplementation with the first limiting nutrient may unmask deficiencies in other nutrients. This is particularly likely to happen if more than maintenance energy and protein is given, so that the child attempts to synthesize new tissue before the imbalances are corrected.

## Control of energy intake

The recommended dietary allowance for energy has a narrow range. The energy required for maintenance varies with age and weight. In a child between 6 and 24 months about 400 kJ/kg body weight/day should be offered. A relatively small increase or decrease in energy intake leads to marked metabolic changes, and affects the requirements for other nutrients.

A patient remains in a steady state when he takes exactly enough energy to cover his needs. A small increase in energy intake leads to synthesis of new tissue, requiring all the essential building blocks (vitamins, minerals and amino acids) for building new tissue. In the absence of one essential nutrient protoplasm cannot be made and the extra energy, protein and minerals have to be disposed of harmlessly. If the excess is large it may overwhelm the existing metabolic machinery. Fortunately, the child develops anorexia, which functions as a protective mechanism in this respect. Conversely, the other nutrients cannot be utilized if the energy intake is insufficient, and weight loss will continue; the adaptive mechanisms will not be reversed, and the functional capacity will not be restored.

Thus, by regulating the dietary intake over quite a narrow range the metabolic status of the patient can be manipulated. In arriving at an approximate figure of 400 kJ/kg/day, allowance has been made for spillage (10 per cent) and for some malabsorption (10 per cent). If the child has increased intestinal losses the intake can be increased accordingly. A daily weight chart accurate to at least 20 gm is the most convenient way of adjusting the intake.

The requirement for protein is relatively small at this time and 0.6 gm/kg/day of milk protein covers all the needs. Diets supplying more protein than this can of course be given.

In an anorectic child a maintenance intake must be given by nasogastric tube. It is very dangerous to force feed a patient in excess of his requirements. Strict attention to detail is needed, with accurate recording and precise formulation of the feeds. Anorexia may be the response to excessive feeding, to an unfulfilled need for a specific nutrient, or to an undiagnosed or inadequately treated infection.

## Intravenous therapy

The use of intravenous therapy is to be avoided, and is only indicated where there is actual circulatory collapse. The loss of homeostasis makes the child very vulnerable to error, furthermore the risks of septicaemia are increased and the intestine is not stimulated to regrow.

The same fluids can be given cheaply, effectively and with greater safety with a nasogastric drip. Even the catastrophic watery diarrhoea of cholera can be successfully treated with oral fluids.

## Blood transfusion

In particularly ill patients who fail to respond to therapy, a blood transfusion may result in dramatic improvement. The blood is given as a non-specific source of nutrients or for its anti-infective proteins and cells and possibly for its transferrin, and not as a rule for anaemia. Whenever possible it is advisable to give whole fresh blood – rather than packed cells or plasma. A volume of 10 ml/kg usually suffices, but may have to be repeated in the most severely ill patients. It should be given slowly to minimize the risk of precipitating low output cardiac failure.

Transfusion should be given *before* the sodium pump is stimulated. When sodium is moving out of the cells, the vascular volume is increased and acute cardiac failure is easily precipitated. Transfusion should not be given to any patient who has received more than a maintenance intake of energy, until he is well into the rapid growth phase and his physiological responses to stress have been fully restored.

## Diarrhoea

The intestine has taken part in the process of reductive adaptation as well as being damaged by bacterial overgrowth. Treatment of the floral overgrowth will relieve much of the diarrhoea. Parenteral rather than oral feeding leads to rapid atrophy of the intestine (up to 50 per cent of intestinal weight in one week). The concept of 'resting the intestine to allow it to repair itself' is pernicious and only leads to more profound malnutrition. The intestine must be stimulated, within its absorptive capacity, to allow it to recover.

Undue emphasis has been placed upon acquired lactase deficiency as a cause for malnutrition: even though all these children will fail to meet the standards of normal lactase absorption set by severe stress tests, they can absorb lactose if given in small amounts and frequently. Many thousands of children have been successfully treated for severe malnutrition with cows' milk based diets. In malnutrition *all* the digestive enzymes are reduced in amount: *any* food which is presented in a bolus that is too large or too concentrated will cause diarrhoea, by exceeding the capacity for absorption. When the intestine is stimulated by food, and has its own infections and nutrient deficiencies treated, it is able to synthesize new enzymes and transport systems.

As the intestine synthesizes digestive and absorptive machinery the quantities and strength of food given in each bolus can be increased. Because there is a limitation on the amount and strength of each bolus given to the child, to give sufficient food it has to be given frequently. The principle is to give little, often and isotonically. If there is insufficient staff to give frequent feeds and the mother is not able to follow instructions precisely, it is often better to give the patient an intragastric drip.

Often it is necessary to start with 4.3 per cent dextrose/0.18 per cent sodium chloride, into which the other mineral supplements have been incorporated during formulation. This saves considerably on nursing time and obviates the problem of medicines being forgotten.

## Vomiting

Vomiting is seldom a major problem when small volumes of isosmotic feed are given and bacterial overgrowth treated. Occasionally stale curds in the stomach need to be removed by washing with isotonic clear fluid. Persistent vomiting may be due to regurgitation and rumination. This difficult physiological problem is best managed by loving firmness administered by a single, persistent, experienced nurse. If the child is very sick then a nasojejunal tube or the judicious use of very small doses of metoclopramide may be helpful. Metoclopramide causes extrapyramidal signs if given in standard (per kilo) doses to young children.

## Hypothermia and hypoglycaemia

These two conditions often occur together and are frequently caused by severe infection. However, the children are poikilothermic and even the tropical environment can be too cold for these patients. Hourly feeds throughout the night as well as during the day usually prevent hypothermia. Occasionally radiant heat from a lamp is required, or close nursing by the mother. Each child needs a blanket. In many hospitals undue emphasis is put on frequent washing of the patient; when a malnourished child is washed he must be carefully and thoroughly dried.

Occasionally unresponsive children improve with 50 per cent dextrose intravenously. It is not clear whether this is having its effect by supplying energy or by rapidly changing serum osmolality and thereby alleviating cerebral oedema. In careful studies of fasting in malnourished children, glucose fell to very low levels without any clinical alteration in the patients. The children do not produce the catecholamine response to hypoglycaemia, which is responsible for most of the clinical signs by which we recognize hypoglycaemia in normal patients.

## Conclusion of the resuscitation period

It is important to treat each patient individually and not according to a rigid protocol or time schedule. Nevertheless using the regimen outlined we have found that most metabolic derangements correct themselves within a week. In the sickest patients a longer period is required; this is often due to our failure to recognize a specific nutrient deficiency or an infection.

The successfully treated child manifests his improvement with a return of appetite. The disappearance of anorexia and the development of a voracious appetite marks the successful end of the resuscitation phase, notwithstanding biochemical derangements.

# Preparation for high energy feeding

The transition from a maintenance diet to an intake that allows for catch-up growth should be made gradually. If large energy intakes are introduced abruptly, some children get a syndrome which frequently results in death. The children who are intolerant to excess energy rapidly develop congestive cardiac failure, followed by profuse diarrhoea and circulatory collapse, at some time during the first four days of high energy feeding. At post mortem the condition can be recognized by the quantities of straw coloured clear fluid in the intestinal lumen. This condition is probably the same as the sudden death occurring in patients released from concentration camps and those following starvation for morbid obesity when they are refed. The patients at risk can be identified on admission because the sodium pump of their leucocytes responds *in vitro* to provision of energy with a rapid extrusion of sodium (Patrick, 1977). The exact mechanism of the salt and water shifts is not clear, but the syndrome can be prevented by the gradual introduction of high energy feeds. An increasing pulse and respiratory rate at this time are danger signals which should lead to a reduction in food intake.

## Catch up weight gain (rehabilitation)

In 1961 Waterlow demonstrated that the rate of weight gain during rehabilitation is directly proportional to the dietary energy intake. It is not related to the protein intake, once sufficient protein is given. Once maintenance energy requirements have been met the extra energy is available for tissue synthesis and deposition. Approximately 20 to 25 kJ are utilized to lay down one gram of new tissue. The theoretical implications that this has on the time taken for recovery is shown in Table 4.3. Relatively small increments in energy intake can have a profound effect on weight gain.

One of the main objectives during rehabilitation is to increase the energy intake to achieve maximum weight gain in the shortest possible time. Shortening the residential stay minimizes the psychological trauma of a strange environment, decreases cross infection risk, reduces hospital costs per patient and increases the numbers of children that can be treated.

Maximum energy intakes are achieved in two ways. Firstly, we have to increase the energy density of the feed by adding a concentrated source of energy to the diet. This is most easily done by modifying milk preparation, by addition of coconut oil or medium chain triglycerides and/or carbohydrate. Oil is particularly effective as it not only has over twice the energy density of carbohydrate, but also it does not increase the osmolality of the diet. In children with steatorrhoea medium chain triglycerides, which do not require bile salts for absorption, are particularly useful.

To get sufficient diet into the patient, he must be fed not less than four hourly through the whole twenty-four hour period. The volume of feed offered is increased progressively during the early phase of rehabilitation.

Secondly when the patient is growing rapidly he has to be fed truly *ad libitum*. The intake should not be restricted to comply with some preconceived idea of what the patient 'should' take. The patient himself should determine his intake. The only way to make sure that the patient is fed to appetite is to ensure that something is left from each feed. If the whole diet is being consumed not enough is being offered. At this stage as much as 1000 kJ or even

Table 4.3 Predicted effects of energy intake on the rate of weight gain, protein requirements and time for recovery from severe wasting

| Feed volume ml/kg/4h | Energy intake kJ/kg/day | Energy for growth kJ/kg/day | Rate of weight gain g/kg/day | Protein requirement g/kg/day | Protein energy ratio kJ/kJ% | Days to recovery days |
|---|---|---|---|---|---|---|
| 22.2 | 400 | 0 | 0 | 0.6 (0.8) | 2.6 (3.3) | – |
| 23.3 | 420 | 20 | 1 | 0.8 (1.0) | 3.1 (3.9) | 300 |
| 24.2 | 440 | 40 | 2 | 1.0 (1.2) | 3.6 (4.5) | 150 |
| 33.3 | 600 | 200 | 10 | 2.2 (2.7) | 6.1 (7.7) | 30 |
| 44.4 | 800 | 400 | 20 | 3.8 (4.7) | 7.9 (9.8) | 15 |

*Assumptions:*

1. Feed contains 300 kJ/100 ml: this is approximately the energy density of milk.
2. The energy requirement for maintainance is 400 kJ/kg body weight.
3. Weight gain assumed to be excess energy divided by 20 (g/day), i.e. one g tissue takes 20 kJ to synthesize.
4. Assumes maintenance nitrogen requirement of 100 mg/kg/day and a nitrogen retention of 25 mgN/g weight gained. Numbers in parenthesis show effect of a net protein utilization of 80 %.
5. Child starts at 70 % weight-for-height, and does not gain in height during gain in weight to 100 % weight-for-height.

1300 kJ/kg/day may be taken, and the patients gain weight at over twenty times the normal rate of weight gain.

Supplements of minerals and vitamins must be continued throughout this period. Not only are the requirements for these nutrients much higher in the rapidly growing child than in the child growing at a normal rate, but also the relative proportion of the various nutrients required is altered depending upon the particular tissue that the child is attempting to synthesize.

Unfortunately we do not know the precise dietary requirements for weight gain at a particular accelerated rate or for the synthesis of any particular tissue. In the past, use of diets low in trace elements, such as zinc, resulted in both a limitation in the absolute rate of weight gain and in the type of tissue the patient was able to synthesize. This resulted in the children becoming relatively obese during recovery with excess fat tissue and inadequate muscle. Theoretically the child must retain all the constituents of lean tissue: they must all be provided in the diet in adequate amounts.

During rapid weight gain any substantial lack in the diet is quickly translated into clinical deficiency. This is the one drawback to encouraging a very rapid rate of weight gain in circumstances of ignorance concerning the dietary requirements.

Progress is most easily followed if weights are regularly plotted on a chart. The standard growth chart is unsatisfactory for this as the intense changes that take place over a short period cannot be demonstrated on its compressed time axis.

It is possible to achieve rapid catch up growth on diets other than those based on cows' milk. Provided that the principles of energy density, *ad libitum* frequent feeding, and supplementation with protoplasmic constituents (principally minerals) are adhered to, diets can be formulated from many blends of locally available ingredients.

Once a child has corrected his wasting, his appetite decreases and he voluntarily ingests an amount that can be easily met on an ordinary diet.

Hospital type treatment is required during the resuscitation phase. Rehabilitation can be carried out successfully in some type of rehabilitation centre, indeed, this can be advantageous in that the educative experience for the mother can be much more profound if the setting is similar to her own dwelling, and similar cooking and washing facilities are used as she uses at home. Mothers who do not visit their children often do not recognize their own children after a few weeks; this is very bad psychologically for both mother and child. Most mothers are deeply affected by seeing the profound changes that diet produces in their children. Staff must both demand that the family visits and insist that the family assists actively in the care of their child.

## Preparation for discharge

It is desirable to do everything possible to prevent a child relapsing with another episode of malnutrition after discharge. A number of simple steps may help.

Delayed weaning and particularly improper feeding are usually associated with malnutrition. It is not infrequent to admit children who have never had any solid food, indeed who have had nothing but dirty dilute bottle feeds. After admission most children are fed formula feeds or thick porridges with a cup and spoon. It is important to ensure that all children are established on the type of mixed feeding that is recommended for the region before discharge. The transition from formula feed to solid food is more difficult the older the child gets. During the first day or so of the transition period, food is often refused and some weight loss takes place. The mother must be given practice in preparing the feed and giving the food to the child, so that she sees precisely the type, consistency and the way that the child takes the food.

Education of the mother as to feeding the child, what to do in case of intercurrent infection, the principles of hygiene and sanitation and how to mentally stimulate the child are an integral part of treatment. The child should not be discharged until they are accomplished.

Courses of immunization against poliomyelitis, tetanus, pertussis, diphtheria, measles and tuberculosis should be initiated before discharge.

After discharge the patient should be followed up at regular intervals. At each visit the education given to the mother must be reinforced; she must be encouraged and supported. The child should be weighed and measured and the results recorded on a graph. Any faltering in the normal growth pattern is then recognized early and appropriate remedial measures taken.

## Conclusion

The problems raised by malnutrition cover the whole spectrum of human experience, from that of the individual to that of society. Childhood malnutrition is the most common serious illness in the world today. Lessons learnt from the study and management of these children have relevance for malnourished individuals of all ages and for those whose malnutrition is secondary to a wide spectrum of disorders. A clear understanding of the aetiology and pathogenesis of these disorders is a prerequisite for designing effective intervention and prevention at an early stage.

## References

Alleyne, G.A.O. (1966a), Cardiac function in severely malnourished Jamaican children. *Clin. Sci.*, **30**, 553–62.

Alleyne, G.A.O. (1966b). The excretion of water and solute by malnourished children. *West Indian Med. J.*, **15**, 150–54.

Alleyne, G.A.O. (1967). The effect of severe protein-caloric malnutrition on the renal function of Jamaican children. *Pediatrics*, **39**, 400–11.

Brooke, O.G., Harris, M. and Salvora, C.B. (1973). The response of malnourished babies to cold. *J. Physiol.*, **233**, 75–91.

Brooke, O.G. and Salvora, C.B. (1974a). Response of malnourished babies to heat. *Arch. Dis. Child.*, **49**, 123–7.

Brooke, O.G., Cocks, T. and March, Y. (1974b). Resting metabolic rate in malnourished babies in relation to total body potassium. *Acta. Paediatr. Scand.*, **63**, 817–25.

Coward, D.G. and Whitehead, R.G. (1972). Experimental protein-energy malnutrition in baby baboons. *Br. J. Nutr.*, **28**, 223–37.

Gillman, J. and Gillman, T. (1951). *Perspectives in Human Malnutrition*. Grune and Stratton: New York.

Golden, M.H.N. (1985). The consequences of protein deficiency in man and its relationship to the features of kwashiorkor. In *Nutritional Adaptation in Man*, pp. 169–87. Eds. Blaxter, K.B. and Waterlow, J.C. John Libbey: London.

Golden, M.H.N. (1987). Free radicals in the pathogenesis of kwashiorkor. *Proc. Nutr. Soc.*, **46**, 53–68.

Golden, M.H.N. and Golden, B.E. (1981). Trace elements: potential importance in human nutrition with particular reference to zinc and vanadium. *Br. Med. Bull.*, **37**, 31–6.

Golden, M.H.N. and Jackson, A.A. (1986). Generalised malnutrition. In *Basic and Clinical Nutrition*, in press. Ed. Chandra, R.K. Lange Publishing Co: Cleveland.

Golden, M.H.N., Waterlow, J.C. and Picou, D. (1977). Protein turnover synthesis and breakdown before and after recovery from protein energy malnutrition. *Clin. Sci. Mol. Med.*, **53**, 473–7.

Golden, M.H.N., Golden, B.E. and Bennett, F.I. (1985a). Relationship of trace element deficiencies to malnutrition. In *Trace Elements in Nutrition of Children*, pp. 183–207. Ed. Chandra, R.K. Raven Press: New York.

Golden, M.H.N., Golden, B.E. and Bennett, F.I. (1985b). High Ferritin values in malnourished children. In *Trace Element Metabolism in Man and Animals-5*, pp. 775–9. Eds. Mills, C.F., Bremner, I. and Chesters, J.K. Commonwealth Agriculture Bureau: Aberdeen.

Gopalan, G. (1968). Kwashiorkor and marasmus: evolution and distinguishing features. In *Calorie Deficiencies and Protein Deficiency*, pp. 49–58. Eds. McCance, R.A. and Widdowson, E.M. Churchill Livingstone: London.

Hendrickse, R.G. (1984). The influence of aflatoxins on child health in the tropics with particular reference to kwashiorkor. *Trans. Roy. Soc. Trop. Med. Hyg.*, **78**, 427–35.

Jackson, A.A. and Golden, M.H.N. (1987). Protein Energy Malnutrition. In *Oxford Textbook of Medicine*, 2nd edition, pp. 812–23. Eds. Weatherall, D.J., Ledingham, J.G.G. and Warrell, D.A. Oxford University Press: Oxford.

James, W.P.T. (1970). Sugar absorption and intestinal motility in children when malnourished and after treatment. *Clin. Sci.*, **39**, 305–18.
Klahr, S. and Alleyne, G.A.O. (1973). Effects of chronic protein calorie malnutrition on the kidney. *Kidney International*, **3**, 129–41.
McFarlane, H., Reddy, S., Adcock, K.J., Adeshina, M., Cooke, A.R. and Akene, J. (1970). Immunity, transferrin and survival in kwashiorkor. *Br. Med. J.*, **1**, 268–72.
Patrick, J. (1977). Death during recovery from severe malnutrition and its possible relationship to sodium pump activity in the leucocyte. *Br. Med. J.*, **1**, 1051–54.
Patrick, J. and Golden, M.H.N. (1977). Leucocyte electrolytes and sodium transport in protein energy malnutrition. *Am. J. Clin. Nutr.*, **30**, 1478–81.
Picou, D., Halliday, D. and Garrow, J.S. (1966). Total body protein, collogen and non-collogen protein in infantile protein malnutrition. *Clin. Sci.*, **30**, 363–9.
Srikantia, S.G. (1958). Ferritin in nutritional oedema. *Lancet*, **1**, 667–8.
Williams, C.D. (1935). Kwashiorkor. *Lancet*, **ii**, 1151–2.
Whitehead, R.G. (1979). The relative roles of protein and energy deficiency in the pathogenesis of protein-energy malnutrition. *Z. Ernahrungswiss*, **23**, (Suppl), 72–84.

# 5 Nutrition in the elderly

A. Norman Exton-Smith



## Introduction

Although frank malnutrition has been largely eliminated from most sections of our population it is still occasionally found amongst the elderly. Malnutrition in the older groups is brought about by the changes in economic circumstances and way of life which often occur on retirement and by the increasing incidence of disease and disabilities which lead to alterations in dietary intake, absorption, and metabolism of nutrients occurring particularly during the eighth decade. In some instances there is an exaggeration in old age of faulty food habits which have been developed during earlier years. The First Report of the Panel on the Nutrition of the Elderly (DHSS, 1970) stated that 'there is little doubt that more is known of the nutritional state of our nation than of any other in the world, but in relation to the elderly the evidence is still inadequate.' The Panel recommended that the field surveys on which the Department of Health and its collaborators had already embarked should be complemented by longitudinal studies designed to detect changes in nutritional intakes with age and to determine the relationship between nutrition and health in old age.

# Physiology of ageing and nutrition

## Nutrition and the rate of ageing

The first experimental proof that restriction of food intake can influence the life-span of animals came with the work of McCay and his colleagues (1935) who showed that rats whose growth was almost completely arrested by a period of severe food restriction lived longer than those fed *ad libitum*. A more moderate restriction of food throughout life has also been shown to increase life expectancy (Berg and Simms, 1961). According to Miller and Payne (1968) when experiments have been repeated other observers have commented upon the miserable state of the long-living rats; they are seen to be underweight and in poor condition. These authors examined the longevity of animals whose nutrient intake was adjusted to growth rather than being fed with a dietary regime of constant composition throughout life. Five different regimes were used and the greatest prolongation of life was achieved in animals fed a stock diet until mature (120 days) and thereafter a mixture of 20 per cent stock diet and 80 per cent starch. Compared with animals on a stock diet throughout life these animals had a maximum life-span 100 days longer and their mean life expectancy was 28 per cent longer; moreover, they appeared healthy in old age. This extended life-span after maturity must be contrasted with the rats in the McCay experiments who had an extended juvenile life.

Ross and Bras (1974) have shown that the frequency of various types of tumour and several age-related diseases can be modified by dietary means. The rats under investigation were allowed a choice of three complete balanced diets differing only in the amounts of sugar and protein they contained; in this self-selection method (SS) each rat could eat as much or as little as it liked of each kind of food. As a control, three other groups of rats were fed on low, intermediate, and high protein diets. The rats on the SS regime grew more quickly than the others and reached higher body weights, but they had a far higher incidence of tumours and of renal, cardiac, and prostate gland diseases. Two-thirds of the SS rats had three or more diseases at the time of death, while of the rats fed low, intermediate, or high protein diets alone, only 9, 26 and 28 per cent respectively had multiple affections at the time of death.

Ross (1969) has shown that when the life-span of rats is prolonged, that is, the survival curves are displaced to the right on the time scale, several parameters of ageing are also shifted to the right; these include collagen changes, and hepatic enzyme patterns as well as the incidence of the diseases of ageing. These diseases according to Simms *et al.*, (1959) have certain similarities in rat and man and occupy comparable positions in the life-spans of the two species. In brief, the results of animal experiments indicate that overfeeding in earlier life hastens maturity and shortens life, and overfeeding after maturity shortens life and increases the incidence of certain diseases in old age.

There are several aspects in which experimental data from animals have direct relevance to the problems of ageing and human nutrition. The life-span of the rats in the experiments of Miller and Payne was only prolonged in the group that was prevented from reaching maximum weight and this corresponds to the similar inverse relationship between life expectancy and obesity in man. The high incidence of multiple pathology in old age in the SS rats of

Ross's experiments resembles that found in the human elderly population for whom Williamson and his colleagues (1964) have demonstrated that men of 65 years and over have a mean of 3.26 diseases and women a mean of 3.42 diseases. Nutritional factors influence not only growth and development before maturity but also, in consequence, the ageing of the mature individual, since certain attributes in old age depend on the status at the end of the period of growth. It has, for example, been shown (McCay, 1955) that rats fed from birth on a milk diet have denser bones with a higher calcium content when they die in old age than those fed on a mixed stock diet containing meat and many products commonly eaten by man. In old people it is often difficult to distinguish the effects of nutritional factors that are operating for the first time in old age and those that may have influenced nutritional status many years previously and in some instances even in childhood. This problem is clearly seen in relation to the development of bone rarefaction in old age. There is evidence (Garn *et al.*, 1967; Exton-Smith *et al.*, 1969) that the liability to osteoporosis is determined, at least in part, by the loss of bone which appears to be a universal phenomenon of ageing and by the skeletal status before maturity. Moreover, when the duration of operative factors is prolonged over many years as seems likely in many cases before the clinical syndrome of osteoporosis develops, it is inevitable that the disorder becomes more frequent with advancing age. In consequence, the process will appear as a manifestation of ageing, and the problem is to determine whether age-related changes are a universal phenomenon or whether they can be influenced by nutritional or other means.

## Physiological changes with age affecting nutrition

Ageing is associated with a decline in average values for many physiological functions. Shock and his colleagues of the Gerontology Research Centre, Baltimore, have investigated the changes which occur between the ages of 30 and 80 years (Shock, 1972). Thus resting cardiac output was reduced by 30 per cent, renal blood flow by 50 per cent, and the maximum breathing capacity and maximum oxygen uptake by 60–70 per cent over the age span of 30 to 80 years. Nevertheless a wide range of values was found among different subjects at each age decade and in some instances the difference in physiological performances became greater with advancing age. Thus the effects of age are highly individual and chronological age alone is a poor index of physiological function.

When extra demands are imposed on an organ system the age differences are more pronounced than when the measurements are made under resting conditions. Older individuals show a greater displacement and a slower rate of recovery in physiological function compared with the young. In consequence the greatest age decrements are found in tests which impose a stress on the organism and require the co-ordinated activity of a number of organ systems, for example, in physical exercise.

If standards of normality applicable to young people are adopted, many of the elderly are found to have low blood and tissue levels of nutrients; for example, red cell transketolase levels were found to be reduced in elderly patients admitted to a geriatric department and these levels could be increased by the administration of thiamine (Griffiths *et al.*, 1967). The real significance of low levels is uncertain since the metabolic expenditure in old people is diminished owing to decreased physical activity. It is clearly important to determine whether the low concentrations of certain nutrients in the blood and tissues represent subclinical malnutrition. As homeostatic mechanism becomes increasingly impaired, the precarious physiological balance may be upset by the operation of environmental and medical hazards to which the elderly are prone. Thus some cases of overt malnutrition which are seen in old people may be the result of stress due to pathological processes in those individuals whose nutrition is only marginally adequate.

## Metabolic rate

The total energy production per square metre of body surface area falls progressively with advancing age. According to Shock *et al.* (1963) there is an average decrement of about 12 kcal/m$^2$ per hour between the ages of 20 and 90 years. The fall is believed to be due to a loss of metabolizing tissue with age since animal experiments show that there is no decrease in oxygen uptake of tissue slices, homogenates, or isolated mitochondria from rat heart, liver and kidney (Barrows, 1966); nor is there any evidence that the thyroid gland shows any reduction in its capability to produce or release thyroxine with advancing age.

The total energy production per 24 hours is the sum of the basal energy production and that required for daily activities. McGandy and his colleagues (1966) have investigated the changes which occur with age in energy expenditure for daily activities and have related total energy production to caloric intake. The subjects studied were 167 men whose ages ranged from 20 to 99 years. The total caloric intake fell from a mean of 2688 kcal/day in subjects aged 20–34 years to 2093 kcal/day in the group aged 75–99 years. There was found to be a fairly close agreement between the caloric intakes and the energy expenditure at all ages. The calories required for activities fell more than the basal calories especially among the group of 80-year-old subjects. Thus the reduction in the energy metabolism of older subjects is a reflection of tissue loss and to greater extent, especially in the very old, of reduction in physical activity.

The importance of exercise is clearly seen in Durnin's study of elderly farmers (Durnin *et al.*, 1966). The lowest energy output was 2200 kcal/day and the highest was 4200 kcal/day. Thus in this small group of men from the same socioeconomic background engaged in the same occupation one man could expend almost twice as much energy as another. The considerable differences in energy expenditure observed in very old people can often be accounted for by complicating factors. For example, disease and disability are increasingly prevalent above the age of 75 and these may therefore affect the capacity for exercise. The main causes are degenerative joint disease, and disorders of the respiratory and cardiovascular systems. In some instances in order to overcome the effects of disability an individual must expend an amount of energy which is greater than average in performing specific tasks, for example, the elderly amputee who has been retrained in walking.

When the diet is balanced the dietary intake required to meet the energy expenditure in old people who maintain their activities will usually ensure an adequate intake of all nutrients. On the other hand, when physical activity is considerably curtailed, particularly in the housebound state (Exton-Smith *et al.*, 1972), the intake of many nutrients may be insufficient.

## Recommended intakes of nutrients

Many countries have formulated 'standards' for energy and nutrient intakes and the recommendations for the United Kingdom have been published by the Department of Health and Social Security (1969 and 1979a). The values for elderly people are shown in Table 5.1.

Table 5.1 Recommended daily intakes of energy and nutrients for elderly people in the UK (from DHSS Report, 1969 and 1979a)

| | Men | | Women | |
|---|---|---|---|---|
| | 65–74 | 75 and over | 55–74 | 75 and over |
| Energy (kcal) | 2350 | 2100 | 2050 | 1900 |
| (MJ) | 9.8 | 8.8 | 8.6 | 8.0 |
| Protein (g) | 59 | 53 | 51 | 48 |
| Calcium (mg) | 500 | 500 | 500 | 500 |
| Iron (mg) | 10 | 10 | 10 | 10 |
| Thiamine (mg) | 0.9 | 0.8 | 0.8 | 0.7 |
| Riboflavin (mg) | 1.7 | 1.7 | 1.3 | 1.3 |
| Nicotinic acid (mg) | 18 | 18 | 15 | 15 |
| Ascorbic acid (mg) | 30 | 30 | 30 | 30 |
| Vitamin A (μg retinol equi.) | 750 | 750 | 750 | 750 |
| Vitamin D (μg cholecalciferol) | 2.5 | 2.5 | 2.5 | 2.5 |

The values for energy are similar to those recommended by the FAO/WHO (1973), except the UK values for elderly women are considerably higher. The recommendations for the elderly, however, are based on estimates of the average rate at which activities decline, that is, they take account of the diminution in energy expenditure associated with the increasing incidence of physical infirmity with age. Nevertheless, as has been shown above, there are many individuals whose activities are well maintained in old age and whose calorie intakes are much greater than the recommended values.

## Nutritional surveys

Most of the nutritional surveys which have been made of the elderly population have been on the basis of cross-sectional studies. Age differences have been established by the comparison of the results of measurements made on individuals of various age groups. These surveys have usually revealed that a proportion of subjects have low intakes of certain nutrients. In order to assess the effects on health of these low intakes serial investigations on the same individual are required. Moreover such longitudinal studies are the only means of clearly identifying the changes which are due to ageing. Ideally the repeated measurements (which must include dietary intake, medical examination, and laboratory investigations) should be made on the same person at standardized intervals of time over as long a period as possible; for obvious reasons there have been few studies of this kind.

## Cross-sectional studies

There have been a number of nutritional surveys of random samples of old people at home and of the aged in hospitals and residential homes. In a survey sponsored by the King Edward's Hospital Fund for London (Exton-Smith and Stanton, 1965) an investigation was made of the diets of old people living alone at home in two North London Boroughs. The participants were 60 women whose ages ranged from 70 to 80 years (with the exception of three aged 89, 90, and 94 years). The mean daily intakes of nutrients were satisfactory and are shown in Table 5.2.

Few instances of malnutrition were revealed by the survey, but a proportion of the subjects had intakes of nutrients which were less than the recommended allowances, especially for iron and vitamin C. There was a striking correlation between diet and health; nearly all the subjects whose diet was better than average were judged on clinical assessment to be better than average in health. Although a good diet is undoubtedly one of the factors responsible for good health it is probably more likely that better health and greater physical activity are associated with good appetite and a larger intake of food.

When the 60 subjects were arranged in groups according to their ages a striking decrease in intakes of all nutrients with advancing age was found. Table 5.3 shows the percentage falls in mean intake for subjects in their late seventies compared with those in their early seventies.

The age differences in intake revealed by this cross-sectional study might be the result of several factors:

Table 5.2 Mean daily intakes of calories and nutrients for women in eighth decade

| | | | |
|---|---|---|---|
| Kilocalories | 1890 | Calcium (mg) | 860 |
| Protein (g) | 57 | Iron (mg) | 9.9 |
| Fat (g) | 74 | Vitamin C (mg) | 37 |
| Carbohydrate (g) | 221 | Vitamin D (IU) | 135 |

Table 5.3 Cross-sectional study: fall in mean intake of nutrients during the eighth decade

| Calories and nutrients | Fall in intake (%) |
|---|---|
| Kilocalories | 19 |
| Protein | 24 |
| Fat | 30 |
| Carbohydrate | 8 |
| Calcium | 18 |
| Iron | 29 |
| Vitamin C | 31 |

1. Reduction in basal metabolic rate and lean body mass leading to a fall in physiological requirements with advancing age. Thus the decrease in intake may represent true age changes affecting all individuals.
2. A reduction in appetite and energy expenditure in some of the older subjects due to the development of disease or disability as they enter the second half of the eighth decade. It is known that there is a striking increase in the prevalence of incapacity in the elderly population after the age of 75 (Sheldon, 1948).
3. Failure of certain individuals, notably the obese, to reach extreme old age. Thus the dietary intake of the thinner individuals of the late seventies group would be expected to be less.
4. Secular differences between the two groups in that the lifelong dietary pattern of the older group may have been different from that of the early seventies group. Indeed it is possible that the habitual dietary pattern may have been one of the factors responsible for the longevity of those who reach extreme old age.

This cross-sectional study must be interpreted as revealing interesting age differences between the two groups and it was not possible to determine the relative importance of the four factors. The most important, however, was believed to be the influence of disease and disability affecting particularly the older subjects. Further evidence that low intakes of nutrients are associated with impairment of health in old age was obtained from a study of the nutrition of housebound elderly people (Exton-Smith *et al.*, 1972). The intakes of the housebound were compared with age-matched active people, and for women the differences amounted to 15 per cent less for carbohydrate to 46 per cent less for vitamin C. For the housebound group as a whole there was no decline in intake with advancing age. This is because for the housebound, in contrast with the active group, disability was just as severe in the younger as in the older people. It can be concluded that disability has a greater influence on nutrient intake than the effects of increasing age alone.

## Longitudinal studies

The 60 women who participated in the first King Edward's Hospital Fund Survey were followed up to form a longitudinal study and the 22 women who were still alive and could be traced were re-examined 6.5 years later (Stanton and Exton-Smith, 1970). It was found that for those subjects who maintained their health (as assessed on clinical examination and by a scoring system recording physical disabilities) the intakes of nutrients in the two surveys were remarkably similar. But for those women whose health had declined there was considerable fall in intake amounting on average to 20 per cent for protein and 17 per cent for calories. From this limited study it was confirmed that nutrient intakes in old age are usually maintained provided the person remains active and fit, and that physical disability is the most likely cause of declining intakes in the elderly.

One of the first longitudinal studies designed to assess the nutritional status of the elderly was carried out in San Mateo, California. The initial survey on 577 subjects over the age of 50 was conducted in 1948–9 and all but 47 subjects lived in their own homes (Gillum and Morgan, 1955). When the data from the first survey were analyzed on a cross-sectional basis by comparing the nutrient intakes of subjects in the three age groups, 55–64, 65–74, and 75 years and over it was found there was a progressive fall in intakes with age especially after the age of 75 years. These results were similar to those found in the first survey of the King Edward's Hospital Fund. Further studies were conducted four, six and fourteen years later (Chope and Breslow, 1956; Steinkamp *et al.*, 1965) and there were 141 participants in all four surveys. Although a reduction in intake after the age of 75 occurred there was no significant difference between the four studies in the proportion of calories contributed by carbohydrate, protein, and fat for any of the groups. Moreover, there was little alteration with age in individual intakes of animal protein; those subjects with low intakes in 1948 tended to maintain the same pattern through to 1962. When interpreting these results it is still not possible to determine whether the lifelong nutritional pattern of those who reach extreme old age has contributed to their longevity or whether their heredity which has enabled them to survive has also in some manner characterized their nutrition (Watkin, 1968).

In a study carried out by the MRC Epidemiological Unit in a South Wales town (Burr *et al.*, 1982) 830 old people who were originally seen in 1971 were followed up after 8 years. The marked decline in body weight with age which was evident in the original cross-sectional data appeared to be due to a loss of weight in individuals rather than to any survival advantages of less obese persons. Indeed over the age of 70 (both males and females) tended to have been heavier when originally seen than those who died, even when those who died within the first year were excluded. Thus the prognostic significance of being above average weight, which is adverse in younger persons, paradoxically becomes a favourable influence in the elderly.

## The occurrence of nutritional deficiencies

Although the individual dietary pattern in the majority of old people remains similar to that which was established by habits acquired at a younger age, there are many factors that begin to operate more frequently with increasing age and these may lead to nutritional deficiencies. Malnutrition may be defined as a disturbance of form or function due to lack of (or excess of) calories or of one or more nutrients (DHSS, 1972). This definition includes both obesity and undernutrition. Obesity is a problem in old age and after the age of 75 it is much more common in women than in men, but it usually results from long-standing faulty eating habits. Undernutrition, on the other hand, results from environmental and physical factors which usually affect people in later life.

### Prevalence

The results of the nutrition survey of the elderly (1972) based on random samples of old people living at home in six areas of the United Kingdom show that malnutrition occurs in about 3 per cent of the population over the age of 65 years. This includes protein calorie malnutrition, iron deficiency and vitamin deficiencies. When the subjects who participated in this survey were followed up 5 years later the proportion with malnutrition had increased to 7 per cent

Table 5.4 Causes of nutritional deficiencies

| Primary | Secondary |
|---|---|
| Ignorance | Impaired appetite |
| Social isolation | Masticatory inefficiency |
| Physical disability | Malabsorption |
| Mental disturbance | Alcoholism |
| Iatrogenic | Drugs |
| Poverty | Increased requirements |

and the prevalence was found to be twice as high in those over the age of 80 compared with those aged 70–79 years (DHSS, 1979b).

## Causes

There are two main groups of factors that lead to nutritional deficiency in the elderly (Exton-Smith, 1971) and these are summarized in Table 5.4.

**Ignorance**
The King Edward's Hospital Fund Survey (Exton-Smith and Stanton, 1965) showed that ignorance of the basic facts of nutrition is prevalent in elderly women. Their views had often been formulated many years ago, and even in childhood, when dietary habits had been dictated by financial stringency. It is likely that in men ignorance is even more important, especially in certain sections of the elderly population. Thus a man who is recently widowed may have to fend for himself for the first time and he may have little idea of what constitutes a balanced diet. Widower's scurvy is seen most often in the man living alone and eating mostly packaged food, tea, bread, butter, and jam.

**Social isolation**
The Stockport survey of the social needs of the over-eighties (Brockington and Lempert, 1967) showed that dietary intake was related to the number of outside interests of old people. Dietary intake was found to be better in those old people who eat at clubs in the company of others. By contrast, for many old people living alone in social isolation there is loss of interest sometimes amounting to apathy and consequent neglect in the preparation of food. What food is eaten is usually taken in the form of snacks.

**Physical disabilities**
Elderly people with physical disorders such as hemiplegia, arthritis, and impairment of vision may have difficulty in getting and preparing food. This applies particularly to the housebound living alone without adequate support from others.

**Mental disturbances**
The unmet medical, nursing, and social needs of the elderly are greatest in those with psychiatric disorders (Stokoe, 1965). Malnutrition also occurs in this

group which consists mainly of old people suffering from chronic brain syndrome and confusional states. Perhaps even more important is the association between malnutrition and depressive illness, which leads to a disinclination to obtain, to cook and, even in severe cases, to eat food.

**Iatrogenic**
A badly planned dietary regime may lead to malnutrition, especially when it is continued longer than necessary. Thus cases of scurvy have been reported in patients having a 'gastric' diet for peptic ulcer since this is often deficient in vitamin C.

**Poverty**
The food eaten by pensioners is often dull, monotonous, and tasteless. Brockington and Lempert (1967) showed that old people who are able to supplement their income from savings or from part-time earnings have a better diet than those whose sole financial means is the old age pension. In the winter months many old people must make a choice between spending money on food or fuel. Thus poverty is a factor to be considered in the elderly more often than in other age groups.

**Impairment of appetite**
Both transitory and long-continued impairment of appetite are common in old age. The time taken for recovery of appetite following an infectious illness is longer than in a younger person; frank malnutrition may be precipitated in a person whose nutrition was previously only marginally adequate.

**Masticatory inefficiency**
A poor state of dentition, and especially ill-fitting dentures, often leads an elderly individual to select soft foods consisting mainly of carbohydrate and the more nutritious foods requiring mastication are avoided. Neill (1972) carried out masticatory studies in some of the participants in the DHSS Nutrition Survey of the Elderly. The relationship between the quality of the subjects' dentures and their masticatory performance was demonstrated. Those subjects who had few teeth remaining but no dentures performed about as well as those wearing dentures of indifferent quality.

**Malabsorption**
Mild degrees of malabsorption are not uncommon in the elderly. This may be due to small bowel ischaemia, gluten sensitivity, or other causes. The absorption of fat and fat-soluble vitamins and of folic acid and vitamin $B_{12}$ is mainly affected.

**Alcohol and drugs**
When alcohol intake is excessive, calorie needs may be derived mainly from this source and the intake of other nutrients may be curtailed. Folic acid metabolism is impaired in some alcoholics and megaloblastic anaemia can occur; it is also impaired in those taking barbiturates and anticonvulsant drugs and in those receiving cytotoxic agents, such as methotrexate. Enzyme induction by anticonvulsant drugs can also lead to vitamin D deficiency.

**Increased requirements**

Negative nitrogen balance and the breakdown of tissue protein can occur in patients who are immobilized in bed for long periods, in those who suffer from long-continued pyrexia, and as a result of extensive bed sores with the loss of protein-rich fluid. The extent to which this can be reversed by high supplemental intakes of protein is uncertain.

## Vulnerable groups

A combination of primary and secondary factors often operate together to produce malnutrition in the individual. Sometimes the factors are interrelated; for example, limited mobility, loneliness, social isolation, and depression are all found in housebound old people and make them especially liable to malnutrition when they are receiving insufficient support from others.

The housebound have been found to have nutrient intakes which are substantially lower than those of active people matched for age (Exton-Smith *et al.*, 1972). Since about 10 per cent of the elderly population are housebound, that is, about three-quarters of a million old people in Great Britain, this section of the population represents the largest single group vulnerable to malnutrition. Thus disability in old age not only affects the mode of living of those afflicted but it also has an adverse effect on dietary intakes and nutritional status.

**Risk factors**

In the second DHSS Survey (DHSS, 1979b) eleven risk factors (both medical and environmental) predisposing to malnutrition were identified. These were living alone, no regular cooked meals, receipt of supplementary benefits, social classes IV and V, reduced mental test score, depression, chronic bronchitis and emphysema, gastrectomy, poor dentition, difficulty in swallowing and the housebound state. There was a highly significant difference ($P < 0.001$) in the distribution of risk factors between the malnourised and non-malnourished; thus 27 per cent of the malnourished had 5 of these risk factors compared with 2 per cent of the non-malnourished. A striking feature of this survey was the much higher incidence of malnutrition in one of the survey areas (Sunderland). Fifteen per cent of the Sunderland sample had malnutrition compared with 7 per cent for all survey areas. Moreover the incidence of single risk factors such as low mental test score, depression, chronic bronchitis and emphysema, poor dentition and being housebound was much higher in Sunderland than in other areas and more of the subjects in Sunderland had several risk factors for malnutrition. The combination of poor health (mental and physical), poor dentition and poor social conditions appears to explain the high incidence of malnutrition. Chronic deprivation over many years and a hard life in an industrial northern conurbation may have contributed to some of the medical and social conditions which are conducive to malnutrition in old age.

**Detection of malnutrition**

The clinical significance of malnutrition is far greater than its incidence might suggest, since in almost every case it is treatable with excellent results. Difficulties in detection of the early signs of malnutrition are similar to those encountered in the early recognition of many diseases in old age. But in the case of nutritional deficiencies there are two further difficulties: for almost every nutrient there is a long latent period before a low intake leads to overt clinical manifestations and early diagnosis must depend upon the finding of abnormalities in special tests, including biochemical and haematological investigations; secondly, in the elderly the true significance of departures from normality revealed by these tests is unknown. Many of the abnormalities can be related to low intakes of certain nutrients, but in old age there is considerable variation between individuals. Some of these problems are discussed in greater detail in the next section dealing with specific nutritional deficiencies. In general, however, it should be remembered that in younger persons the margin of safety is wide, but in old age homeostatic mechanisms are often impaired and the precarious physiological balance may be upset by the operation of medical and environmental hazards to which the elderly are prone. Frank malnutrition may be precipitated by such stress in those individuals whose nutrition is only marginally adequate (Exton-Smith, 1968).

## Clinical nutritional deficiencies

The most comprehensive study of the nutritional status of the elderly population so far undertaken was the DHSS Nutrition Survey of 1972. Excluding obesity, 27 of the 879 subjects over the age of 65 participating in the survey were diagnosed by the clinicians as malnourished. In the following sections nutritional deficiencies which are to be found in the elderly population are described and the problems of diagnosis are discussed.

### Protein-energy malnutrition

#### Protein metabolism

The total amount of protein in the body declines with age. Forbes and Reina (1970) have studied the body composition of subjects at different ages between 25 and 75 years on a longitudinal basis. Using $^{40}$K counting it was found that the lean body mass (LBM) declines progressively after the age of 25, whereas body fat increases, so that the total body weight fails to reveal the continuous decrease in LBM. Men weighing approximately 75 kg at the age of 25 years have an average LBM of 61 kg and a fat content of 13 kg; at the age of 65 years, however, the LBM has declined by 12 kg (20 per cent) and the body fat has risen by 15 kg (120 per cent), without any marked change in total body weight. Although decline in LBM is continuous after the age of 25, the rate of loss is not constant and it appears to accelerate in old age.

Munro (1972) has calculated that a dietary allowance of 0.35 g of protein/kg body weight is adequate to maintain nitrogen balance in young subjects under ideal conditions; but for older subjects under less artificial conditions he considers the need to be 0.6 g/kg body weight. On this basis the DHSS recommendations (1969) for minimum protein requirements are 39 g and 38 g for men aged 65–75 years and over 75 years respectively, and 36 g and 34 g for women in the corresponding age groups. The actual recommended intakes (59 g, 53 g, 51 g, and 48 g respectively) are, however, considerably higher and are calculated on the basis that protein intake should provide 10 per cent of the energy requirements. For the normal utilization of dietary protein sufficient energy must be available, and the protein–energy relationship is more important than the absolute amount of protein. In the elderly it is also important to take into account the quality and amino acid composition of the dietary proteins; thus the needs for the essential amino acids, methionine and lysine which cannot be synthesized, rise sharply after the age of 50 years (Tuttle *et al.*, 1957, 1965).

Serum albumin concentration decreases with advancing age. Yan and Franks (1968) found that in the elderly the total intravascular albumin was 1.43 g/kg body weight and the interstitial albumin was 1.65 g/kg; these figures were significantly lower than those found in young subjects, namely, 1.60 g/kg and 2.20 g/kg respectively. Thus the total albumin pool is about 20 per cent lower in the elderly subjects. Since homeostasis of serum albumin levels in healthy individuals is maintained by a mechanism in the liver which is sensitive to osmotic pressure (Rothschild *et al.*, 1969) it is possible that the decrease in serum albumin with age is due to a decline in the sensitivity of this mechanism.

**Incidence**

In the DHSS Survey of 1972, a search for malnutrition was made in all subjects having low energy intakes; there were 41 men whose intake was less than 1500 kcal/day and 47 women with less than 1200 kcal/day. Of the 88 subjects, 14 (all women) were obese and were 'dieting', and 22 of the remaining 74 were assessed by the clinicians as better than average in health. It was considered that 8 of the 88 subjects could have protein–calorie malnutrition on the basis of the clinical assessment and the finding of serum pseudo-cholinesterase activity of less than 150 units [this enzyme is related to protein–energy nutrition (Hutchinson *et al.*, 1951)].

In the whole survey sample (879 subjects) 13 per cent had serum albumin levels of less than 3.5 g/100 ml, and 8 per cent had serum pseudo-cholinesterase activities of less than 150 units. There were some correlations between these variables and the clinicians' assessments of the state of health, and low activity of pseudo-cholinesterase was correlated with skinfold thickness.

**Relationship between physical state and protein intake**

From an analysis of the findings of the DHSS Survey of the Elderly, Anderson and his colleagues (1972) examined the association between inadequate protein intake and the depletion of the body reserves of protein. A slight but consistent relationship was found between intake of protein and the bulk of arm muscle (as measured by the arm circumference minus a value for surface fat based on the triceps skinfold thickness). This could partly be explained by larger individuals eating more food and hence more protein. A part of the relationship was also due to the percentage of energy derived from protein and this raised the possibility of a relationship between reserves of protein stored in muscle and protein intake as opposed to energy intake.

No consistent relationship was found between protein intake and serum albumin levels, but there was a significant relationship between serum albumin levels and oedema. Serum albumin was less than 3.5 g/100 ml in 48 subjects and 40 per cent had oedema; 22 per cent had oedema when the albumin was 3.5–4.49 g/100 ml, and 13 per cent when it was above 4.5 g/100 ml. It is considered that a possible explanation lies in the effects of stress; in this case the stress is non-nutritional disease (mainly cardiac failure) superimposed upon levels of serum albumin which in most cases would have been unassociated with oedema had it not been for the additional burden. Three of the forty-eight subjects with serum albumin levels of less than 3.5 g/100 ml were thought to have oedema due to protein deficiency; in the remainder, diseases such as congestive cardiac failure imposed a stress on already impaired homeostatic mechanisms. Since the stress could be diagnosed clinically and tended to mask the underlying protein deficiency it was concluded that a state of sub-clinical nutritional deficiency existed in many of the subjects.

The significance of a sub-clinical malnutrition, including protein deficiency, is difficult to assess. But it may be of greater importance in the elderly than at other ages since hoemostatic mechanisms are impaired and stress due to a variety of pathological processes, which are common in old age, may upset the precarious physiological balance. Phillips (1983) has measured total body protein turnover in a group of ill, elderly in-patients using a tracer dose of $^{15}N$ glycine. In comparison with normal elderly controls the ill subjects had significantly higher total body nitrogen flux, protein synthesis and breakdown rates and significantly lower plasma albumin. This increase in protein turnover in spite of a reduced muscle mass in the ill subjects appears to be due to the effects of tissue trauma and inflammation. It is not known, however, whether the failure to maintain the body pool of albumin in ill old people can be influenced by increased dietary intake. Moreover, it has yet to be established if a higher intake of protein and of other nutrients would confer benefits on the older individual who is in a state of sub-clinical malnutrition and enable him to resist more effectively the effects of stress due to non-nutritional disease.

## Anaemia and iron deficiency

The normal levels of haemoglobin (Hb) and erythrocytes (RBC) as defined by WHO study groups (WHO, 1959, 1968) are: for men, Hb 13 g/100 ml and RBC $4.7 \times 10^6$ per $mm^3$, and for women, Hb 12 g/100 ml and RBC $4.0 \times 10^6$ per $mm^3$. Normal old people are not anaemic; Hb and RBC levels below these limits should not be ascribed to 'old age'.

### Clinical features

Lack of iron leads to microcytic, hypochromic anaemia which, if sufficiently severe, produces symptoms such as tiredness, lack of energy, breathlessness on exertion, and palpitations. A milder degree of anaemia, particularly if it develops slowly, gives rise to few symptoms because of compensatory processes which lead to more efficient release of oxygen from the haemoglobin. Various tissue changes occur in iron deficiency and the most characteristic is koilonychia with spoon-shaped deformity of the nails. Patients often complain of a sore tongue which becomes smooth and redder than normal due to atrophy of the papillae. Difficulty in swallowing due to the Plummer–Vinson syndrome resulting from a web of mucosa in the post-cricoid region is rare. But lack of acid secretion in the stomach is common in iron deficiency and the gastric mucosa may show atrophic or inflammatory changes. Severe anaemia with typical manifestations is rarely due to poor dietary iron intake alone; in such cases there is nearly always occult gastrointestinal haemorrhage.

**Population studies**

In the DHSS survey of 1972 the over-all frequency of anaemia was 7.3 per cent and was about the same in the two sexes. The only factors for which a significant correlation with Hb was found were mode of living and serum iron (SI) concentration. When all persons were grouped together, those living alone had a higher incidence of anaemia ($P<0.01$); of the 165 subjects who lived alone 15 (9 per cent) were anaemic compared with 31 (6 per cent) of the 492 who lived with their spouse or relatives.

Analysis of the haematological data for anaemic subjects revealed that iron deficiency was the sole cause of anaemia in only 12.9 per cent. Iron deficiency associated with sub-normal serum folate levels was found in 22.6 per cent of anaemic subjects and iron deficiency with sub-normal serum vitamin $B_6$ in 8.1 per cent of anaemic subjects; in a further 19.3 per cent of anaemic subjects all three serum levels were sub-normal. A high proportion of old people with anaemia (35.5 per cent) had a normal serum iron concentration and in nearly half of these (14.6 per cent) the serum iron, folate, vitamin $B_6$, and vitamin $B_{12}$ levels were normal.

The relationship between Hb concentration and the serum iron concentration (SI) was significant (at 1 per cent level) when all subjects were grouped together. The assessment of body iron status was made by estimation of the SI and the total iron-binding capacity (TIBC), and for all persons grouped together a negative correlation was found between these variables. Overt iron deficiency as measured by SI of less than 60 μg/100 ml and TIBC higher than 400 μg/100 ml was found in 4.7 per cent of the elderly men and 13.2 per cent of the elderly women. The most likely explanation of this difference is the lower iron intake of most groups of women compared with those of the men; thus in the six areas surveyed in only one group of women (the 65–74-year age group in one area in Scotland) was the mean intake greater than the recommended allowance of 10 mg/day, whereas, by contrast, only one group of men (75 + age group in Sunderland) failed to meet the recommended intake for iron. It is also possible that certain chronic diseases, which are known to reduce TIBC, may have been responsible for masking iron deficiency in the men.

The conclusions drawn from the DHSS survey were that the mean values of serum iron, folate, vitamin $B_6$, and vitamin $B_{12}$ concentrations are lower in old people compared with the young, and a higher proportion of old people have sub-normal values than in the younger population. Very few old people with sub-normal values of these nutrients were anaemic and 14.6 per cent of the anaemic subjects had normal values for these nutrients. Thus it is possible that other factors may be of importance in suppressing haemopoiesis in old age.

**Hospital studies**

Investigations carried out on elderly patients in hospital show a much higher incidence of anaemia. In a study co-ordinated by the Department of Health and Social Security (1970), anaemia (based on an Hb of less than 12 g/100 ml) was found in 27 per cent of males and 32 per cent of females. Although nutritional iron deficiency may play a part the major cause is haemorrhage from the gastrointestinal tract due to haemorrhoids, hiatus hernia, peptic ulcer, diverticular disease, and carcinoma; gastric haemorrhage may also be induced by such drugs as aspirin and phenylbutazone.

**Significance of iron deficiency**

Ericsson (1972) has investigated in a double-blind study 45 clinically healthy persons (25 men and 20 women) aged 57 to 71 years. One group was given ferrous fumarate (60 mg $Fe^{++}$) twice daily for 3 months and the other a placebo. Iron deficiency was believed to exist in some individuals on the basis of low amounts of stainable iron in the marrow in association with high TIBC levels; a decrease in the TIBC occurred only when it was initially high and only in the group treated with iron. It was also found that subjects treated with iron had an increase in physical work capacity as measured on a bicycle ergometer. Elwood and Hughes (1970), however, were not able to demonstrate any benefits of iron supplementation in improving symptoms and psychomotor performance in younger subjects.

## Vitamin B complex deficiency

**Clinical manifestations**

The changes in the mucous membranes of the tongue and lips include:

*Cheilosis* – red, denuded, often scaly, epithelium at the line of closure of the lips;
*Angular stomatitis* – greyish white, sodden and swollen epithelium, progressing to fissuring, radiating outwards from the corners of the mouth;
*Nasolabial seborrhoea* – enlarged follicles around the sides of the nose, and plugged with sebaceous material;
*Glossitis* – bare, red, smooth tongue with loss of filiform papillae, sometimes associated with fissuring and enlargement of the fungiform papillae.

A high incidence of these changes, which have been attributed to deficiency of riboflavin, nicotinamide, and possibly pyridoxine, has been reported by some authors (Griffiths *et al.*, 1967; Taylor, 1968; and Brocklehurst *et al.*, 1968).

Brin (1964, 1968) has proposed five stages in the development of vitamin deficiency disease based on observations made on the development of human thiamine deficiency. It is noteworthy that the overt disease state is not manifest until stage four. During the 'physiological' stage three the symptoms are loss of appetite, general malaise, and increased irritability – all common complaints due to many other causes in the elderly. In stages four and five, thiamine deficiency leads to cardiac and neurological manifestations including bradycardia, cardiac enlargement, oedema, peripheral neuropathy, mental confusion, and ophthalmoplegia. Wernicke's encephalopathy is almost certainly due to thiamine deficiency; the clinical features include diplopia and nystagmus progressing to ophthalmoplegia and the mental changes of Korsakoff's psychosis – loss of memory, disorientation, confabulation, and hallucinations. In Britain and the United States it is usually associated with alcoholism, but Philip and Smith (1973) have described Wernicke's encephalopathy in old people with accidental hypothermia and it is possible that the poor nutritional status of many people who are admitted with hypothermia is responsible. Acute confusional states associated with toxic-infective processes, which account for one-third of cases of mental disorder in old people admitted to hospital (Hodkinson, 1964), may in some instances also be attributable to a relative thiamine deficiency. In these patients blood pyruvate levels are often elevated and fall again when the underlying process (for example, pneumonia) responds to appropriate treatment. Some confirmation of the importance of thiamine deficiency in the pathogenesis of confusional states has been obtained in an investigation of elderly orthopaedic patients (Older and Dickerson, 1982) – see below.

**B complex nutritional status**

There is conflict of opinion on the extent to which the tongue mucous membrane lesions reputed to be due to vitamin deficiency can be corrected by vitamin supplementation. Brocklehurst and his colleagues (1968) conducted a controlled trial on 80 elderly in-patients, the majority of whom had tongue signs. One group received a placebo and the other a daily vitamin supplementation of thiamine (15 mg), riboflavin (15 mg), nicotinamide (50 mg), pyridoxine (10 mg), and ascorbic acid (200 mg). In the treated group after one year the tongue appearance had returned to normal and there was a striking improvement in the general physical and mental condition of the patients. In the untreated group there was clinical evidence of deterioration in many cases. It was concluded that there is chronic vitamin deficiency in a large number of elderly people which can be reversed by large doses of vitamin supplements for long periods. Dymock and Brocklehurst (1973) repeated their earlier studies and used single vitamin supplementation on 77 old people in hospital who survived for one year's clinical trial. Riboflavin therapy was associated with significant improvement in cheilosis and possibly in angular stomatitis, nicotinamide produced a significant improvement in the dorsum of the tongue. MacLeod (1972) on the other hand failed to confirm these findings. In a series of 80 patients with abnormal tongue appearance, vitamin supplementation for one year had no effect on the tongue changes nor on the signs of angular stomatitis. Similar negative results were obtained in the series investigated by Berry and Darke (1972). Of the 27 patients who had lesions of the lip or angle of the mouth, 24 did not improve after one year's administration of riboflavin. Moreover in the 66 elderly patients who had abnormal appearances of the dorsum of the tongue there was no statistical difference in the response rate between those who received vitamin B supplementation and those who were treated with a placebo. In 90 per cent of the subjects who had changes in the dorsal surface of the tongue a fungal infection was found and Berry and Darke consider that this is the most likely cause of these changes.

In the DHSS Survey of 1972 a special attempt was made to relate changes in the mucous membranes to riboflavin deficiency. Of the 778 subjects examined 57 were diagnosed as having either angular stomatitis or cheilosis. There was no statistical difference in the mean riboflavin intakes in those with lip lesions compared with those without these lesions. Out of the 23 subjects who had very low intakes of riboflavin (less than 0.7 mg for males and 0.55 mg for females) 4 subjects had lip lesions. It was concluded that although there may be some element of clinical ariboflavinosis in the elderly population the number must be very small and in general the riboflavin status appears to be satisfactory.

**Significance of deficiencies**

Brin and his colleagues (Brin, 1964, 1968) have investigated the biochemical changes in thiamine deficiency. Thiamine adequacy was assessed by determining its urinary excretion level, by measurement of the erythrocyte transketolase (TK) activity and by calculation of the TPP effect. In the last test thiamine pyrophosphate (TPP), the coenzyme of thiamine, is added to the haemolysed cells and the TPP effect is calculated from the increment of TK activity due to the addition of TPP, expressing this as a percentage of the TK activity of unenriched blood. On a thiamine depleted diet urinary thiamine excretion is reduced to 50 μg daily after about 5 days; the TK activity is depressed with a positive TPP effect of about 15 per cent and the urinary thiamine is reduced to 25 μg after about 10 days, the third or 'physiological' stage is reached by 21 days when the urinary thiamine is 0–25 μg daily and the TK activity is reduced 15–25 per cent with a TPP effect up to 30 per cent. By the time clinical manifestations of deficiency appeared the TK activity was reduced more than 35 per cent and the TPP effect was in excess of 40 per cent. It was noted that the urinary thiamine excretion reached a minimum level in 12 days and once this level was reached it was not possible to differentiate between a pre-clinical deficiency state and severe disease by this measure alone. Values of TPP effect below 15 per cent were taken as normal; above this critical level there was found to be a definitive curve of relationship between TK activity and TPP effect.

In a study of 233 subjects aged 44 to 94 years, Brin and others (1965) found thiamine deficiency in 37 per cent as judged by reduced thiamine excretion and in 5 per cent if based on a TPP effect of greater than 15 per cent. In a study of 80 elderly long-stay patients, Griffiths (1968) found that only 21 were not thiamine-deficient based on a less strict criterion of a TPP effect of more than 10 per cent. The subjects were re-examined at 3, 6, 9, and 12 months after thiamine supplementation and only one failed to return to the normal level after one year. Baker and others (1979) investigated the vitamin status of non-hospitalized elderly North Americans and found thiamine deficiency to be the second most common vitamin deficiency, along with ascorbic acid.

Older and Dickerson (1982) have shown that in elderly patients undergoing elective hip replacement with pre-operative TPP effect of less than 10 per cent, a temporary post-operative thiamine deficiency occurred with a rise in TPP effect to 24 per cent and a return to baseline by 14 days. In patients requiring hemiarthroplasty for fracture of the femoral neck there were similar raised levels on the second post-operative day but these abnormal values were sustained until at least the 14th day. In both emergency and elective surgery patients those who were most confused had TPP effect values in the frank deficiency range.

The riboflavin status of 128 old people has been investigated by Thurnham (1972) in a study of accidental hypothermia based on a random sample of the elderly population in the London Borough of Camden. The erythrocyte glutathione reductase activity (EGR) and the percentage stimulation of EGR by flavin adenine dinucleotide (FAD) were measured. A stimulation of greater than 30 per cent (usually regarded as the upper limit of normal) was found in 18 per cent of the men and in 19 per cent of the women. Using these reference values, Vir and Love (1980) also found that the incidence of deficiency among the elderly at home was 18 per cent of men, 19 per cent of women and 25 per cent of those in sheltered dwellings. Thus it is considered that there may be marginal riboflavin deficiency in about one-fifth of the elderly population. Although the true significance of this marginal deficiency is at present unknown these laboratory tests serve to identify those individuals who might benefit from vitamin supplementation to prevent the appearance of acute deficiency disease.

Thurnham and others (1979) later showed that those old people who ate vitamin fortified breakfast cereals (VC) had better riboflavin (and thiamine) status than those not taking these cereals. Thus 27 per cent of the old people not eating VC had an EGR-AC $\geqslant$ 1.30 compared with only 9 per cent of those eating vitamin fortified cereals.

## Folate deficiency

**Clinical manifestations**

Although folate deficiency causes a general disturbance in which various tissues and organs are involved, the main clinical findings are anaemia, and changes in the nervous system and mucous membrane of the tongue. The anaemia is megaloblastic characterized by abnormal nucleated red cell precursors (megaloblasts) in the bone marrow and macrocytes in the peripheral blood. There is associated leucopenia with hypersegmentation of the neutrophils, and the number of platelets may be reduced. There may be the complaint of soreness or burning of the tongue and the surface may be red due to acute glossitis; but it is more commonly smooth, shiny, and atrophic. In patients with chronic neurological diseases, especially peripheral neuropathy, the changes including megaloblastic anaemia, are more often due to folate deficiency than to vitamin $B_{12}$ deficiency (Grant *et al.*, 1965). Mental changes may precede the anaemia; they are non-specific and include mild confusion, depression, apathy, and intellectual impairment. Cases of dementia due to folate deficiency have been reported and Strachan and Henderson (1967) noted a response in two patients with dementia to prolonged folate administration.

**Causes**

The main causes of folate deficiency in the elderly are inadequate intake, malabsorption, increased utilization, and impaired effectiveness. In contrast to vitamin $B_{12}$ deficiency, dietary inadequacy of folate is an important cause of deficiency. A mixed diet contains 500–800 $\mu$g folate per day; but as it is mainly in the reduced form, the folate is readily destroyed by sunlight, oxidation, and cooking. The minimum requirements are 50–100 $\mu$g/day, but many times this amount may be required if there is increased utilization. Dietary deficiency is often associated with mental and physical disorders interfering with shopping and cooking, as well as with poverty. Absorption of folate occurs in the upper small intestine and it may be impaired in gluten enteropathy and in other conditions giving rise to malabsorption syndrome. Folate requirements increase when cell turnover increases, e.g. in haemolytic anaemia, myeloproliferative syndromes, carcinoma, myeloma, and in certain chronic inflammatory diseases such as tuberculosis and Crohn's disease. Under certain conditions the effectiveness of available folate is impaired – vitamin C deficiency inhibits folate coenzymes and in scurvy impaired folate metabolism can lead to megaloblastic anaemia (*vide infra*); various drugs including methotrexate, anticonvulsants, and trimethoprim interfere with folate metabolism.

**Folate status in the elderly**

Herbert (1967) maintains that folate deficiency is the commonest vitamin deficiency in man. Although a folate-free diet quickly leads to lowering of serum folate levels, many months elapse before clinical or haematological changes develop. In a survey of elderly patients admitted to a geriatric department in a London hospital, Hurdle and Williams (1966) found low serum folate levels (less than 5 ng/ml) in one-third of the patients. A deficiency of body stores was indicated by a positive FIGLU test in 50 per cent of the patients with folate deficiency. A nutritional origin was suggested by the finding of an increase in the incidence with greater severity of disability; two-thirds of those unable to look after themselves were folate deficient. Read and his colleagues (1965) in Bristol found that 80 per cent of entrants to old people's homes had folate deficiency, based on a serum folate level of less than 6 ng/ml. Such a lower limit, however, does not represent a very strict criterion of deficiency. In the DHSS Survey of 1972 serum folate levels of less than 3 ng/ml were found in 14.6 per cent of the subjects living at home. Red cell folate levels of less than 150 ng/ml were found in 16.1 per cent indicating chronic folate deficiency; more severe degrees of deficiency with red cell folate concentrations of less than 100 ng/ml were found in 3.7 per cent of the subjects studied. There was a significant correlation between serum and red cell folate concentrations ($P<0.01$).

Batata and his colleagues (1967) in Oxford found that 10 per cent of patients over the age of 60 had serum folate levels of less than 2.1 ng/ml. A nutritional origin was suspected since with severe disability (and in consequence an inability of the patient to look after himself) the more likely was there to be folate deficiency; there was found to be a statistically significant relationship between organic brain disease and low folate levels. Girdwood (1968) adopting a similar criterion (serum levels less than 2.2 ng/ml) found that 8 per cent of elderly hospital patients in Edinburgh were deficient, although he was unable to trace any cases of megaloblastic anaemia in the elderly due to nutritional deficiency. He therefore concluded that there must be considerable variation in different parts of the country. In some parts, at least, megaloblastic anaemia certainly exists and there must be a reservoir of old people in Great Britain who suffer from a folate deficiency state without being significantly anaemic. Although anaemia is uncommon the extent to which these deficiency states have an adverse effect on health is uncertain.

Sneath and her colleagues (1973) examined the relationship between folate status and dementia in patients admitted to the geriatric department. In a series of 115 consecutive admissions 14 patients were diagnosed as having dementia. Their mean red cell folate concentration (279 ng/ml) was significantly lower than the mean (394 ng/ml) for the group as a whole and also significantly lower than that in 8 patients with carcinoma, 14 patients with congestive cardiac failure, and 23 patients with hemiplegia. There was also some correlation between intellectual function as assessed on a 16 point mental test score and the red cell folate concentration in those with low red cell folate levels (below 200 ng/ml). Thus the association between poor folate nutrition and dementia was confirmed in this study. It was thought that the dementia leads to inadequate dietary intake and in turn to folate deficiency, but the possibility that folate deficiency of itself leads to impaired mental function could not be excluded.

## Vitamin $B_{12}$ deficiency

### Clinical manifestations

The clinical features of vitamin $B_{12}$ deficiency include megaloblastic anaemia, glossitis, subacute combined degeneration of the cord, peripheral neuropathy, and mental changes. The onset of symptoms is usually insidious so that the anaemia may be severe when the patient first presents. The apathy, tiredness, weakness, and breathlessness due to the anaemia are difficult to evaluate in the elderly patient. The skin may have a yellow tinge. Although the classical raw 'red-beef' tongue can occur, the tongue surface is more often smooth, pale, and atrophic. Paraesthesiae in the hands and feet, unsteadiness on standing, and weakness of the legs occur in patients with peripheral neuropathy, and pyramidal and posterior column lesions. Mental changes may predominate; some may be due specifically to vitamin $B_{12}$ deficiency since it is known that the cortical degeneration occurring in $B_{12}$ deficiency is similar to that which occurs in the spinal cord. Shulman (1972) found a higher incidence of psychiatric symptoms in patients with anaemia due to $B_{12}$ deficiency than in those patients whose anaemia was due to other causes. He considers that psychiatrists should be aware of the possibility of $B_{12}$ deficiency in patients with anaemia or after gastrectomy or where fatigue, mental confusion, or dementia are of unknown origin. Cantor (1963) has emphasized that many old people with vitamin $B_{12}$ deficiency are labelled as 'senile' or 'arteriosclerotic'. Only 5 of his 13 patients were referred with the diagnosis of anaemia. The common presentations were congestive cardiac failure, neurological changes, and mental disturbances. Sedatives and hypnotics were tolerated badly, even when given in conventional doses.

### Causes

Vitamin $B_{12}$ occurs in most animal tissues but not in plants. It is absorbed in the ileum after binding with intrinsic factor (IF), a mucoprotein secreted by the gastric parietal cells. Apart from vegans, in whom dietary deficiency of vitamin $B_{12}$ may occur, the deficiency is due to malabsorption. This may be the result of gastric lesions as in pernicious anaemia, chronic atrophic gastritis, and after partial or total gastrectomy. It can also be the result of intestinal lesions in such conditions as gluten-sensitive enteropathy, jejunal diverticulosis, blind-loop syndrome, fistula, and also after ileal resection. The commonest cause is pernicious anaemia, in which the vitamin $B_{12}$ deficiency is secondary to lack of IF secretion. The gastric lesion is believed to be an autoimmune phenomenon, since antibodies to both IF and parietal cells have been found in the gastric juice of patients with pernicious anaemia (Fisher *et al.*, 1965, 1966), and it is thought that they interfere with the secretion and function of IF (Rose *et al.*, 1970).

*Vitamin $B_{12}$ status in the elderly*. Pernicious anaemia is a disease of later life occurring more frequently as age advances. The over-all prevalence in the United Kingdom is 0.1 to 0.2 per cent, but over the age of 60 it is about 1 per cent. MacLennan and others (1973) found an incidence of 2.5 per cent in two surveys of people aged 65 and over living at home in Glasgow and Kilsyth. The incidence of pernicious anaemia is higher in Scotland than in England, and it is higher in the North of England than in the South. In the general population the incidence of achlorhydria, chronic gastritis, and circulating antibodies to parietal cells rises steadily after middle age. These changes could account for the progressive fall in serum vitamin $B_{12}$ levels with advancing age which have been reported (Cape and Shinton, 1961). It is believed, however, that the serum levels of vitamin $B_{12}$ may also be affected by the tissue status of other haemopoietic nutrients, notably iron and folate. Thus low $B_{12}$ levels accompany iron deficiency and they rise following the administration of oral iron. Similarly, low serum $B_{12}$ levels are found in about one-third of patients with nutritional megaloblastic anaemia due to folate deficiency, and treatment with folic acid alone restores the serum $B_{12}$ level (Mollin *et al.*, 1963). It can be concluded that vitamin $B_{12}$ status cannot always be accurately assessed by measurement of serum levels.

## Ascorbic acid deficiency

### Clinical features

Scurvy has almost disappeared from our population, but it occasionally occurs in the elderly, especially in men. The manifestations include swelling and bleeding of the gums (not seen in edentulous individuals), weakness, anaemia, extensive haemorrhages in the skin of the legs and arms ('sheet' haemorrhages), and sometimes haemorrhages at other sites. Russell and his colleagues (1968) have shown that vitamin C deficiency may play a part in maintaining gastrointestinal haemorrhage which had been precipitated initially by gastric irritants such as aspirin. Sub-lingual 'petechiae' have been regarded by Taylor (1968) as an early sign of scurvy, but Andrews and others (1969) have shown by histological examination that the lesions are small aneurysmal dilatations of the minute vessels under the tongue. It is highly unlikely, therefore, that they can be caused by acute vitamin C deficiency; moreover, they do not disappear when ascorbic acid intake is increased.

Anaemia is common in scurvy; it is usually normocytic or macrocytic with normoblastic or macronormoblastic erythropoiesis, but cases of true megaloblastic anaemia have been reported (Hyams and Ross, 1963; Goldberg, 1963). The origin of anaemia is often multifactorial: haemolysis, bleeding, dietary deficiency of iron, and derangement of red cell metabolism have been incriminated (Cox, 1968). Megaloblastic change has been attributed either to an associated dietary folate deficiency or to impairment of folate metabolism in scurvy. Stokes and his colleagues (1975) have shown that megaloblastic anaemia of scurvy is caused in part by removal of tetrahydrofolates from the metabolic pool due to oxidation to 10-formylfolic acid. It is believed that an important role of ascorbic acid in metabolism is to prevent the oxidation of the tetrahydrofolates and thus to maintain the availability of the folate metabolic pool.

Mental changes are probably common in scurvy. Walker (1968) drew attention to depression associated with vitamin C deficiency, and Kinsman and Hood (1971) to personality changes in experimentally induced scurvy. It has been known for some time that wound healing may be delayed in vitamin C deficiency and the administration of vitamin C may promote the healing of pressure sores by increasing collagen formation (Burr and Rajan, 1972).

**Vitamin C status of old people**

Although overt manifestations of deficiency are rare the body stores of vitamin C in many old people are diminished. Low levels of leucocyte ascorbic acid (LAA) have been reported by several observers; the levels are lower in the elderly than in younger subjects (Bowers and Kubik, 1965; Andrews *et al.*, 1969), lower in winter than in summer (Andrews *et al.*, 1966), lower in men than in women (Milne *et al.*, 1971), and smokers have lower LAA levels compared with non-smokers (Brook and Grimshaw, 1968). Furthermore, diminished ascorbic acid levels have been reported in institutionalized old people (Kataria *et al.*, 1965; Andrews and Brook, 1966). They have been attributed to: the effects of cooking in institutions of such foods as potatoes, the delay in delivery of the meal to the recipient, and to an inadequate supply of fruit and fruit juices (Andrews, 1973). Similar factors may be responsible for the inferior vitamin C status of old people receiving meals-on-wheels, mainly the housebound. These meals are cooked in institutions and are kept hot for several hours in containers before they are delivered. Stanton (1971) has shown that 90 per cent of the vitamin C may be destroyed before the meal is served. Davies and others (1973), in a study of a meals-on-wheels service supplied on average two to three days per week, have demonstrated that the vitamin C intake may be considerably less on those days on which the old person receives a domiciliary meal compared with days on which he or she does the cooking at home. The low levels of LAA in certain old people are not a natural accompaniment of ageing since by feeding with ascorbic acid they can be brought to levels seen in younger people (Andrews *et al.*, 1966).

In a study in Edinburgh, Milne and his colleagues (1971) found that LAA levels were significantly higher in July to December compared with those in blood samples taken during the rest of the year. Slightly more than half the subjects had intakes of less than 30 mg/day and a significantly greater proportion had low intakes in the months October to March compared with the months April to September. Vitamin C intake was correlated with LAA level and it was found that LAA levels increased in parallel with, but lagged behind, seasonal increases in vitamin C intakes. Similar findings were reported in the Nutrition Survey of the Elderly (DHSS, 1972) and there was a correlation between LAA levels and vitamin C intake (Darke, 1972).

**Significance of low tissue stores**

The Edinburgh study and other dietary surveys disclose that there is a significant number of old people whose intake of vitamin C is less than 10 mg/day, which is known to be the amount required to prevent or cure scurvy (Bartley *et al.*, 1953). The recommended allowance of 30 mg daily (DHSS, 1969) takes into account the considerable individual variations in requirements, and increased requirements due to stress. Although a high proportion of the elderly population are consuming less than 30 mg per day the majority will not suffer any ill-effects. Our assessment of vitamin C requirements is handicapped by lack of knowledge of the tissue levels needed for health. Windsor and Williams (1970) by measuring total hydroxyproline excretion (THP) in response to vitamin C, found that THP increased when the initial LAA content was less than 15 $\mu$g/$10^8$WBC, but when the LAA level was higher than this the response to vitamin C supplementation failed to occur. Thurnham (1972) in an investigation of old people who participated in the Camden Survey of deep body temperatures in the elderly (Fox *et al.*, 1973) found that 28 per cent of the men and 10 per cent of the women had LAA levels of less than 15 $\mu$g/$10^8$WBC. The higher proportion of men with deficiency is in keeping with the findings of clinicians that scurvy is more prone to occur in men than in women.

Srikantia and his colleagues (1970) have re-examined the human requirements for vitamin C. They conducted longitudinal studies in 19 adult male volunteers in whom the levels of LAA were followed at intervals after fully saturating them with vitamin C. These authors showed that the maximum leucocyte concentration can be maintained by intakes of as little as 10 mg daily in some subjects and by intakes of less than 22 mg daily in all the subjects investigated. In very old people, however, individual variability may be greater. The scatter diagrams for LAA and average daily vitamin C intake based on data from the DHSS Nutrition Survey of the Elderly (Darke, 1972) show that there are some subjects, especially the men, who have high vitamin C intakes ($>50$ mg/day) yet have low LAA levels of less than 15 $\mu$g/$10^8$WBC.

Wilson and his colleagues (1972) have studied the relationship between LAA levels and mortality in aged hospital patients. The mortality was found to be 47 per cent within 4 weeks of admission for those whose initial LAA levels were less than 12 $\mu$g/$10^8$WBC compared with 10 per cent when the LAA was greater than 25 $\mu$g/$10^8$WBC ($P<0.01$). Subsequent investigation, however, showed that mortality was not directly related to LAA levels but to the severity of the illness which in turn, influenced the tissue stores of vitamin C (Wilson *et al.*, 1973). In the follow-up study administration of vitamin C failed to produce an increase in LAA levels in many of the subjects; nor did it influence mortality. Thus it is believed that many illnesses occurring in elderly patients depress LAA concentration; moreover, a number of drugs used in clinical practice, for example tetracycline (Windsor *et al.*, 1972), also depress LAA levels.

## Vitamin D deficiency and osteomalacia

Osteomalacia is a generalized disease of bone due to lack of vitamin D and is characterized by a deficient calcification of a normal bone matrix. Histological examination reveals an increase in the amount of osteoid, that is, non-calcified matrix around the bone trabeculae.

**Clinical manifestations**

In the early stages the patient often complains of vague pains in a variety of sites and these are usually dismissed as 'rheumatism'. Later the pain becomes more persistent and localized to the bones which are extremely tender to pressure. The patient becomes shorter owing to deformities of the trunk – usually kyphosis – and on radiography the intervertebral discs are often ballooned and the soft vertebral bodies become biconcave ('Cod-fish vertebrae'). Other bones may become deformed such as the sternum, the pelvis, and the femoral necks. Another characteristic finding on radiographic examination is the appearance of Looser zones or pseudo-fractures. These are bands of decalcification perpendicular or oblique to the surface of the bone and on either side of the translucency there may be a denser band of callus. They occur in only about one-third of cases of osteomalacia, but as they are pathognomonic of osteomalacia, a skeletal survey should be conducted in suspected cases, particular attention being paid to the pubic rami, the femoral neck, the ribs, the border of the scapula, the upper end of the humerus, and less frequently the shafts of the tibia, fibula, radius, and ulna. In addition to Looser zones true spontaneous fractures occur.

Muscular weakness is often striking. For many years this has been regarded as a typical feature of rickets, but only recently has it been recognized in osteomalacia. It usually takes the form of a proximal myopathy affecting the muscles of the pelvic and shoulder girdles. The patient may complain of difficulty in climbing stairs and in getting up from a chair; when walking the patient may have a typical 'waddling gait'. When the shoulder girdle muscles are involved the patient is unable to raise the arms and perform such activities as brushing the hair.

**Aetiology**

The vitamin D deficiency leading to osteomalacia in old people is often multifactorial in origin. It has been attributed to a fall in dietary intake of vitamin D (Exton-Smith *et al.*, 1966), a reduction in exposure to sunlight (Stamp and Round, 1974), malabsorption, including gluten enteropathy (Moss *et al.*, 1965), gastrectomy (Clark *et al.*, 1964), an increased physiological requirement for vitamin D (Dent, 1970), and impaired conversion of 25-hydroxycholecalciferol to the active 1,25-dihydroxycholecalciferol due to a decline in renal function in old age (Fraser and Kodicek, 1970; Lund *et al.*, 1975).

**Prevalence**

The many conditions which may give rise to vitamin D deficiency in old age account for the fact that osteomalacia is more common in the elderly than in younger age groups. Anderson and his colleagues (1966) have drawn attention to osteomalacia occurring in elderly women in Glasgow. They investigated a group of 100 women aged 68 to 93 years who had been newly admitted to a Geriatric Department and who had a possible clinical indication of osteomalacia (see Table 5.5).

In this group 16 cases of osteomalacia were discovered. Subsequently 4 per

Table 5.5 Possible clinical indications for osteomalacia

| |
|---|
| Vague and generalized pain |
| Low backache |
| Muscle weakness and stiffness |
| Waddling gait |
| Skeletal deformity |
| Bone tenderness |
| Malabsorption states |
| Long confinement indoors |
| Malnutrition |

cent of all elderly women admitted to the same department were found to have osteomalacia. Chalmers, an orthopaedic surgeon in Edinburgh, and his colleagues (Chalmers *et al.*, 1967) have described the clinical features of 37 cases of osteomalacia. Thirty-four of the patients were women, whose ages ranged from 39 to 89 years and the majority were over the age of 70. They consider that osteomalacia is not uncommon in elderly women among whom it is likely to be confused with senile osteoporosis and that there is a need for screening of all elderly patients presenting with weakness, skeletal pain, pathological fractures, or with diminished radiological density of bone.

In many cases the diagnosis of osteomalacia can be made on the basis of the history of bone pains and muscular weakness, the typical biochemical findings (low serum inorganic phosphorus, low or normal serum calcium, raised serum alkaline phosphatase, and diminished urinary excretion of calcium), and the radiological finding of Looser zones. But there are some suspected cases in which the diagnosis remains in doubt and bone biopsy will be necessary so that histological examination can be carried out on undecalcified sections. Diagnosis may also be confirmed by a therapeutic trial with vitamin D. Monitoring of treatment should be undertaken by such procedures as demonstrating the rise in total hydroxyproline excretion in response to vitamin D (Smith and Dick, 1968), the decreased proportion of osteoid with a calcification front and its increase with therapy (Bordier *et al.*, 1968) and the rise in serum inorganic phosphorus in response to intravenous vitamin $D_3$ (Whittle *et al.*, 1969).

**Vitamin D status of the elderly population**

Using radio-stereo-assay of 25-hydroxycholecalciferol levels, Stamp and Round (1974) have shown seasonal variations in vitamin D status in both young and old subjects. They conclude that summer sunlight is an important, and possibly the chief, determinant of vitamin D nutrition in Britain. In this study, the older people who participated in a nutrition survey in the London Borough of Camden, had significantly lower levels of 25-hydroxycholecalciferol than those found in the younger subjects.

The studies of vitamin D status of elderly people living at home conducted by Lawson and his colleagues (1979) have shown that the circulating levels of 25-hydroxyvitamin D (25-OHD) correlate with the amount of sunlight exposure and are independent of the vitamin D content of the diet, whereas in winter the levels correlate with dietary intake and the amount of sunlight exposure the previous summer. Stephen and Dattani (1980) have examined the effects of increasing age on 25-OHD levels. In subjects of both sexes there was a linear decline between the ages of 65 and 90; the winter levels were lower than the summer levels and both were lower in women than in men. The summer levels declined more rapidly than the winter levels and by the age of 90 in each sex the summer levels equalled the winter levels. This study clearly shows the effects of limitation of sunlight exposure due to reduction in out-doors activity which occurs in very old people. In this respect, housebound old people (Exton-Smith *et al.*, 1972) may be at the greatest disadvantage since they lack exposure to sunlight and often have very low dietary intakes; 48 per cent of housebound women aged 70 to 79 years had a dietary intake of less than 30 IU per day compared with 13 per cent of active women of similar age.

The question has recently arisen whether vitamin D deficiency is of clinical importance in the absence of the usual features of osteomalacia. Aaron and her colleagues (1974a) in Leeds have shown by histological methods that 20 to 30 per cent of women with fracture of the proximal femur and about 40 per cent of men had csteomalacia. Later they showed (Aaron *et al.*, 1974b) that the proportion with osteomalacia varied with the season. The highest frequency of abnormal calcification fronts (43 per cent) was observed in February to April and the lowest (15 per cent) in August to October. The highest frequency of abnormal osteoid covered surfaces (47 per cent) was observed in April to June and the lowest (13 per cent) in October to December. They concluded that variation in hours of sunshine is responsible for a seasonal variation in osteomalacia in femoral neck fractures and, possibly, in the elderly population as a whole. The significance of vitamin D deficiency as an important factor in the pathogenesis of fracture of the femoral neck has been confirmed by the study of Faccini *et al.*, (1976). The mean value of trabecular osteoid area in the fracture group was 4 per cent compared with 1 per cent in a control group. The difference was also striking in the proportion of trabecular surface covered by osteoid; the mean value for the fracture group was 24.5 per cent compared with 7.9 per cent for the control group.

Further analysis of the results (Cooke *et al.*, 1982) showed that 38 per cent of the fracture patients had histological evidence of osteomalacia based on a trabecular osteoid area of greater than 2.0 per cent and this proportion was significantly higher ($P<0.01$) than in the control group. Brown and his colleagues (1976) found significantly lower levels of 25-hydroxycholecalciferol in patients with fracture of the femoral neck compared with those in controls of similar age from whom blood samples were taken at the same time of year. This is believed to be a reflection of the decreased out-of-doors activity of the patients prior to their fracture.

It has been suggested by Bullamore and his colleagues (1970) that vitamin D deficiency may in part be responsible for the development of osteoporosis in old age. They have shown that lack of vitamin D further impairs calcium absorption which is already reduced in many older people. Calcium absorption can be increased by large doses of vitamin D. Thus in addition to severe vitamin D deficiency manifesting itself as osteomalacia, mild continued vitamin D deficiency may account for the increased porosity of bone and the liability to fracture especially in elderly women.

There is an obvious need for improvement of the vitamin D status in a considerable number of elderly people. This could be achieved by dietary supplementation or by exposure to ultraviolet light. Irrespective of whether vitamin D deficiency is concerned in the pathogenesis of osteoporosis these measures might be expected to reduce the fracture rate particularly in those individuals whose disabilities confine them to home or an institution.

## Prevention of malnutrition

The salient features of the nutritional deficiencies which have been described in the previous section and which are relevant to the problem of the prevention of malnutrition in the elderly population can be summarized as follows:

1. A significant proportion of older people have low dietary intakes and many of these are well below the recommended nutrient intakes for the United Kingdom. In some instances there is an association between low intakes and socioeconomic factors (for example, living alone) and with physical disorders, especially those which render the individual housebound.
2. Many old people have blood and tissue levels of nutrients that are below the arbitrarily defined limits adopted for younger people. The lowest levels are often found in those individuals with physical disorders.
3. Only rarely are the low intakes and abnormal biochemical findings associated with a disturbance of form or function that is required for the diagnosis of clinical malnutrition.
4. The significance of sub-clinical malnutrition and the extent to which the health of these old people would benefit from increased dietary intakes are unknown. Nevertheless it would seem prudent to attempt to raise the levels of nutrients in order to make these individuals more resistant to the effects of stress due to non-nutritional diseases which become increasingly common with advancing years.

In most forms of nutritional deficiency in the elderly the factors responsible can be identified. Malnutrition can occur in isolation but it is more often associated with other unmet medical and social needs. Thus a prime consideration in improving nutrition is the early ascertainment and correction of needs in vulnerable groups of the elderly population.

### Vulnerable groups

Old people especially at risk are the socially isolated, those with physical disability including impairment of the special senses which contribute to isolation, the recently bereaved, very old men living alone, and those with mental disorders, particularly depression. Unless these vulnerable groups can be identified, preventive measures would have to be applied to all old people irrespective of the fact that the majority will never suffer from malnutrition. The undesirability and the inefficiency of applying such procedures can be overcome only by the recognition of those especially at risk. The application of preventive measures to these smaller groups rather than to the entire elderly population becomes a manageable proposition.

The housebound, who account for nearly 10 per cent of old people living in their homes, constitute the largest group at risk. Physical and mental disorders in old age not only affect the mode of living and social relationships of those afflicted, but also the dietary pattern and nutritional status. Since the majority of the housebound are already known to the health and social services, the prevention of malnutrition in this group should present less difficulty than in other vulnerable groups who are not so readily identifiable.

## Assessment of nutritional status

When the groups of old people especially at risk have been identified the prevention of malnutrition is the responsibility of the primary medical care team. Although the assessment of dietary intakes should ideally be made by dieticians, their skills are not often available for old people at home. A rough guide to the quality of the diet can be obtained by health visitors using simple scoring systems (for example, the method designed by Marr *et al.*, 1961) which are based on the number of main meals and the frequency of consumption of certain foods containing protein (meat, bread, eggs, cheese, and milk). If the diet is found to be insufficient, means must be sought for improving nutritional intake; this may entail instruction by a dietician or health visitor either individually or when old people attend clubs or day centres. When clinical malnutrition is suspected the diagnosis can sometimes be confirmed by the general practitioner using appropriate biochemical and haematological investigations; in other instances, however, referral to hospital for more specialized investigations will be necessary, for example, for bone biopsy when there are clinical findings suggestive of osteomalacia.

## Club meals and meals-on-wheels

It has been shown that there is often an improvement in nutrient intake when old people eat at clubs in the company of others. Many find that it is more convenient to have a club meal since there is no shopping, cooking, or washing-up to be done. The King Edward's Hospital Fund Survey (Exton-Smith and Stanton, 1965) showed that in order to make an effective contribution to the total dietary intake at least four club meals a week should be eaten. The club or domiciliary meal must be as nutritious as possible since the recipient tends to regard it as the main meal of the day and often takes only snacks at other times.

About 1.5 per cent of old people receive meals-on-wheels (DHSS, 1970) but the real need is probably much greater than this. The meals service is usually provided by the WRVS and the regular visits to the homes of housebound old people do much to prevent social isolation. One of the disadvantages of the present system of delivery is that food must be kept hot for several hours after cooking before the meal reaches the old person's home. During this period at least some of the nutritive value is lost. There is need for experimentation in this field. In several areas the provision of frozen meals has been tried. The meal can be cooked immediately before it is eaten and since food is delivered only once a week the service is economical in personnel. The main disadvantages however, are that there may be no proper facilities for cold storage, the patient may be unable to cook the meal himself, and he is visited much less frequently by voluntary workers.

## Nutrient supplementation

The most satisfactory means of promoting good nutrition is by improving the quality, and in some cases the quantity, of the diet. Thus for those whose consumption of vitamin C is inadequate, intake could be improved by the addition of oranges, blackcurrant juice, rose hip syrup, or tomatoes. The alternative of prescribing ascorbic acid tablets is satisfactory, but less desirable. The very low intake of vitamin D by many old people must lead to consideration of supplementation. A means of increasing the intake would be by the fortification of milk which is a procedure adopted in the United States. In the first instance the distribution of fortified milk might best be restricted to housebound old people who tend to have the lowest vitamin D intakes and lack exposure to sunlight.

It is important that supplementation should only be introduced after the results of carefully controlled trials are available to assess the benefits derived from increased intakes. Once the practice of supplementation has become widespread it is difficult to prove the benefits. Moreover there is an understandable reluctance to withdraw a prophylactic measure on the basis of doubts about its value when it has been employed for several years.

## References


Aaron, J.E., Gallagher, J.C., Anderson, J., Stasiak, L., Longton, E.B., Nordin, B.E.C. and Nicholson, M. (1974a). Frequency of osteomalacia and osteoporosis in fractures of the proximal femur. *Lancet*, **i**, 229–33.

Aaron, J.E., Gallagher, J.C. and Nordin, B.E.C. (1974b). Seasonal variation of osteomalacia in femoral-neck fractures. *Lancet*, **ii**, 84–5.

Anderson, I., Campbell, A.E.R., Dunn, A. and Runciman, J.B.M. (1966). Osteomalacia in elderly women. *Scot. Med. J.*, **11**, 429–35.

Anderson, W.F., Cohen, C., Hyams, D.E., Millard, P.H., Plowright, N.M. Woodford-Williams, E. and Berry, W.T.C. (1972). Clincal and sub-clinical malnutrition in Old Age. In *Nutrition in Old Age*. Ed. Carlson, L.A. Almquist and Wiksell: Uppsala.

Andrews, J. (1973). Vitamin C status of elderly long-stay hospital patients. *Geront. Clin.*, **15**, 221–6.

Andrews, J. and Brook, M. (1966). Leucocyte vitamin C content and clinical signs in the elderly. *Lancet*, **i**, 1350–1.

Andrews, J., Brook, M. and Allen, M.A. (1966). Influence of abode and season on the vitamin C status of the elderly. *Geront. Clin.*, **8**, 257–66.

Andrews, J., Letcher, M. and Brook, M. (1969). Vitamin C supplementation in the elderly. *Br. Med. J.*, **ii**, 416–18.

Baker, H., Frank, O., Think, I.S., Jaslow, J.P. and Louria, D.B. (1979). Vitamin profiles in elderly persons living at home or in nursing homes, versus profile in healthy young subjects. *J. Am. Geriatr. Soc.*, **27**, 444–50.

Barrows, C.H. (1966). In *Perspectives in Experimental Gerontology*. Ed. Shock, N.W. C.C. Thomas: Springfield, Illinois.

Bartley, W., Krebs, II. A. and O'Brien, J.R.P. (1953). Vitamin C requirements of human adults. *MRC Special Report Series*, No. 280. HMSO: London.

Batata, M., Spray, G.H., Bolton, F.G., Higgins, G. and Wollner, L. (1967). Blood and bone marrow changes in elderly patients, with special reference to folic acid, vitamin $B_{12}$, iron and ascorbic acid. *Br. Med. J.*, **ii**, 667–9.

Berg, B.N. and Simms, H.S. (1961). Nutrition and longevity in the rat. III. Food restriction beyond 800 days. *J. Nutr.*, 74, 23–32.

Berry, W.T.C. and Darke, S. (1972). Nutrition of the elderly living at home. *Age Ageing*, **1**, 177–81.

Bordier, P., Matrajt, H., Hioco, D., Hepner, G.W., Thompson, G.R. and Booth, C.C. (1968). Subclinical vitamin D deficiency following gastric surgery. *Lancet*, **i**, 437–40.

Brin, M. (1964). Erythrocyte as a biopsy tissue for functional evaluation of thiamine status. *J. Am. Med. Ass.*, **187**, 762–6.

Brin, M. (1968). Biochemical methods and findings in US surveys. In *Vitamins in the Elderly*. Eds. Exton-Smith, A.N. and Scott, D.L. John Wright: Bristol.

Brin, M., Dibble, M.V., Peel, A., McMullen, E., Bourquin, A. and Chen, N. (1965). Some preliminary findings on the nutritional status of the aged in Onondaga County, New York. *Am. J. Clin. Nutr.*, **17**, 240.

Bowers, E.F. and Kubik, M.M. (1965). Vitamin C levels in old people. *Br. J. Clin. Pract.*, **19**, 141–7.

Brockington, F. and Lempert, S.M. (1967). *The Stockport Survey. The Social Needs of the Over 80s*. University Press: Manchester.

Brocklehurst, J., Griffiths, L.L., Taylor, G.F., Mark, J., Scott, D.L. and Blackley, J. (1968). The clinical features of chronic vitamin deficiency. *Geront. Clin.*, **10**, 309–20.

Brown, I.R.F., Bakowska, A. and Millard, P.H. (1976). Vitamin D status of patients with femoral neck fractures. *Age Ageing*, **5**, 127–31.

Brook, J. and Grimshaw, J.J. (1968). Vitamin C concentration of plasma and leucocytes as related to smoking habit, age and sex of humans. *Am. J. Clin. Nutr.*, **21**, 1254–8.

Buliamore, J.R., Gallagher, J.C., Wilkinson, R., Nordin, B.E.C. and Peacock, M. (1970). Effect of age on calcium absorption. *Lancet*, **ii**, 535–7.

Burr, M.L., Lennings, C.I. and Milbank, J.E. (1982). The prognostic significance of weight and of vitamin C status in the elderly. *Age Ageing*, **11**, 249–55.

Burr, R.G, and Rajan, K.T. (1972). Leucocyte ascorbic acid and pressure sores in paraplegia. *Br. J. Nutr.*, **28**, 275–81.

Cantor, A.M. (1963). A study of pernicious anaemia in elderly patients. *Geront. Clin.*, **5**, 23–9.

Cape, R.D.T. and Shinton, N.K. (1961). Serum vitamin $B_{12}$ concentration in the elderly, *Geront. Clin.*, **3**, 163–72.

Chalmers, J., Conacher, W.D.H., Gardener, D.L. and Scott, P.R. (1967). Osteomalacia a common disease in elderly women. *J. Bone Jt Surg.*, **49B**, 403–23.

Chope, H.D. and Breslow, L. (1956). Nutritional status of the ageing. *Am. J. Publ. Hlth.*, **46**, 61–7.

Clark, C.G., Crooks, J., Dawson, A.A. and Mitchell, P.E.G. (1964). Disordered calcium metabolism after Polya partial gastrectomy. *Lancet*, **i**, 734–8.

Cook, P.J., Exton-Smith, A.N., Brocklehurst, J.C. and Lempert-Barber, S.M. (1982). Fractured femurs, falls and bone disorders. *J. R. Coll. Phys. Lond.*, **16**, 45–9.

Cox, E.V. (1968). The anaemia of scurvy. *Vitams Horm.*, **26**, 635–52.

Davies, L., Hastrop, K. and Bender, A.E. (1973). Ascorbic acid in meals-on-wheels. *Mod. Geriat.*, **3**, 390–3.

Darke, S. (1972). Requirements for vitamins in old age. In *Nutrition in Old Age*. Ed. Carlson, L.A. Almquist and Wiksell: Uppsala.

Dent, C.E. (1970). Rickets (and osteomalacia) nutritional and metabolic 1919–69. *Proc. R. Soc. Med.*, **63**, 401–8.

DHSS. (1969). Recommended intakes of nutrients for the United Kingdom. *Report on Public Health and Medical Subjects*, No. 120. HMSO: London.

DHSS. (1970). First report by the panel on nutrition of the elderly. *Report on Public Health and Medical Subjects*, No. 123. HMSO: London.

DHSS. (1972). A nutritional survey of the elderly. *Report on Public Health and*

*Medical Subjects*, No. 3. HMSO: London.
DHSS. (1979a). Recommended daily amounts of food energy and nutrients for groups of people in the United Kingdom. *Report on Health and Social Subjects*, No. 15. HMSO: London.
DHSS. (1979b). Nutrition and health in old age. *Report on Health and Social Subjects* No. 16. HMSO:London
Durnin, J.V.G.A., Lonergan, M.E., Wheatcroft, J.J., Norgan, N.G., MacLeod, C.C., MacFarlan, M.R.S. and Chambers, M. (1966). The energy expenditure and food intake of middle-aged and elderly farmers. *Proc. VII. Int. Congr. Nutr.*, Hamburg.
Dymock, S.M. and Brocklehurst, J.C. (1973). Clinical effects of water-soluble vitamin supplementation in geriatric patients. *Age Ageing*, **2**, 172–6.
Elwood, P.C. and Hughes, D. (1970). Clinical trial of iron therapy on psychomotor function in anaemic women. *Br. Med. J.*, **iii**, 254–5.
Ericsson, P. (1972). Iron metabolism in the elderly. In *Nutrition in Old Age*. Ed. Carlson, L.A. Almquist and Wiksell: Uppsala.
Exton-Smith, A.N. (1968). The problem of subclinical malnutrition in the elderly. In *Vitamins in the Elderly*. Eds. Exton-Smith, A.N. and Scott, D.L. John Wright: Bristol.
Exton-Smith, A.N. (1971). Nutrition of the elderly. *Br. J. Hosp. Med.*, **5**, 639–45.
Exton-Smith, A.N., Hodkinson, H.M. and Stanton, B.R. (1966). Nutrition and metabolic bone disease in old age. *Lancet*, **i**, 999–1001.
Exton-Smith, A.N., Millard, P.H., Payne, P.R. and Wheeler, E.F. (1969). Pattern of development and loss of bone with age. *Lancet*, **ii**, 1154–7.
Exton-Smith, A.N. and Stanton, B.R. (1965). *Report on an Investigation into the Dietary of Elderly Women Living Alone*. King Edward's Hospital Fund: London.
Exton-Smith, A.N. Stanton, B.R. and Windsor, A.C.M. (1972). *Nutrition of Housebound Old People*. King Edward's Hospital Fund: London.
Faccini, J.M., Exton-Smith, A.N. and Boyde, A. (1976). Disorders of bone and fracture of the femoral neck. *Lancet*, **i**, 1089–92.
FAO/WHO (1973). *Expert Committee on Energy and Protein*. FAO–WHO, Geneva.
Fisher, J.M., Rees, C. and Taylor, K.B. (1965). Antibodies in gastric juice. *Science*, **150**, 1467–9.
Fisher, J.M., Rees, C. and Taylor, K.B. (1966). Intrinsic factor antibodies in gastric juice of pernicious anaemia patients. *Lancet*, **ii**, 88–9.
Forbes, G.B. and Reina, J.C. (1970). Adult lean body mass declines with age; some longitudinal observations. *Metabolism*, **19**, 653–63.
Fox, R.H., Woodward, P.M., Exton-Smith, A.N., Green, M.F., Donnison, D.V. and Wicks, M.H. (1973). Body temperatures in the elderly: a national study of physiological, social and environmental conditions. *Br. Med. J.*, **i**, 200–206.
Fraser, D.R. and Kodicek, E. (1970). Unique biosynthesis by kidney of a biologically active vitamin D metabolite. *Nature*, **228**, 764–5.
Garn, S.M., Rohmann, C.G. and Wagner, B. (1967). Bone loss as a general phenomenon in man. *Fed. Proc.*, **26**, 1729–36.
Gillum, H.L. and Morgan, A.F. (1955). Nutritional status of the ageing. *J. Nutr.*, **55**, 265–88.
Girdwood, R.H. (1968). Deficiencies of folic acid and vitamin $B_{12}$ in the elderly. In *Vitamins in the Elderly*. Eds. Exton-Smith, A.N. and Scott, D.L. John Wright: Bristol.
Goldberg, A. (1963). The anaemia of scurvy. *Q. J. Med.*, **32**, 51–64.
Grant, H.C., Hoffbrand, A.V. and Wells, D.G. (1965). Folate deficiency and neurological disease. *Lancet*, **ii**, 763–7.
Griffiths, L.L. (1968). Biochemical findings of the Farnborough survey. In *Vitamins in the Elderly*. Eds. Exton-Smith, A.N. and Scott, D.L. John Wright: Bristol.

Griffiths, L.L., Brocklehurst, J.C., Scott, D.L., Marks, J. and Blackley, J. (1967). Thiamine and ascorbic acid levels in the elderly. *Geront. Clin.*, **9**, 1–10.

Herbert, V. (1967). Biochemical and haematologic lesions in folic acid deficiency. *Am. J. Clin. Nutr.*, **20**, 562–72.

Hodkinson, H.M. (1973). Mental impairment in the elderly. *J. R. Coll. Phys.*, **7**, 305–17.

Hurdle, A.D.F. and Williams, T.C.P. (1966). Folic acid deficiency in elderly patients admitted to hospital. *Br. Med. J.*, **ii**, 202–5.

Hutchinson, A.O., McCance, R.A. and Widdowson, E.M. (1951). Serum cholinesterase. In *Studies of Undernutrition. Special Report Series, Medical Research Council, No. 285*. HMSO: London.

Hyams, D.E. and Ross, E.J. (1963). Scurvy, megaloblastic anaemia, osteoporosis. *Br. J. Clin. Pract.*, **17**, 332–40.

Kataria, M.S., Rao, D.B. and Curtis, R.C. (1965). Vitamin C levels in the elderly. *Geront. Clin.*, **7**, 189–92.

Kinsman, R.A. and Hood, J. (1971). Some behavioural effects of ascorbic acid deficiency. *Am. J. Clin. Nutr.*, **24**, 455–64.

Lawson, D.E.M., Paul, A.A., Black, A.E. Cole, T.J., Mandal A.R. and Davie, M. (1979). Relative contributions of diet and sunlight to vitamin D state in the elderly. *Br. Med. J.*, **ii**, 303–305.

Lund, B., Hjorth, L., Kjaer, I., Reimann, I., Friss, T., Anderson, R.B. and Sørenson, O.H. (1975). Treatment of osteoporosis of ageing with 1$\alpha$-hydroxycholecalciferol. *Lancet*, **ii**, 1168–71.

MacLennan, W.J., Andrews, G.R., MacLeod, C. and Caird, F.I. (1973). Anaemia in the elderly. *Q. J. Med.*, **42**, 1–13.

MacLeod, R.D.M. (1972). Abnormal tongue appearances and vitamin status of the elderly. *Age Ageing*, **1**, 99–102.

McCay, C.M. (1955). Bridging the gap between research and geontological nutrition. In *Old Age and the Modern World, Third Congr. Int. Ass. Gerontology*.

McCay, C.M. Crowell, M.R. and Maynard, L.A. (1935). Effect of retarded growth upon the length of life span and upon the ultimate body size. *J. Nutr.*, **10**, 63.

McGandy, R.B., Burrows, C.H., Spanias, A., Meredith, A., Stone, J.L. and Norris, A.H. (1966). Nutrient intakes and energy expenditure in men of different ages. *J. Geront.*, **21**, 581–7.

Marr, J.W., Heady, J.A. and Morris, J. (1961). Towards a method of large scale individual diet surveys. *Proc. Third Int. Congr. Dietetics.*

Miller, D.S. and Payne, P.R. (1968). Longevity and protein intake. *Expl. Geront.*, **3**, 231–5.

Milne, J.S., Lonergan, M.E., Williamson, J., Moore, F.M.L., McMaster, R. and Percy, N. (1971). Leucocyte ascorbic acid levels and vitamin C intake in older people. *Br. Med. J.*, **iv**, 383–6.

Mollin, D.L., Waters, A.H. and Harriss, E. (1963). Clinical aspects of the metabolic interrelationships between folic acid and vitamin $B_{12}$. In *Vitamin $B_{12}$ and Intrinsic Factor*, 2. Ed. Heinrich, H.C. Enke: Stuttgart.

Moss, A.J., Waterhouse, C. and Terry, R. (1965). Gluten sensitive enteropathy with osteomalacia, but without steatorrhoea. *N. Engl. J. Med.*, **272**, 825–30.

Munro, H.M. (1972). Protein requirements and metabolism in ageing. In *Nutrition in Old Age*. Ed. Carlson, L.A. Almquist and Wiksell: Uppsala.

Neill, D.J. (1972). Masticatory studies. In *A Nutrition Survey of the Elderly*. HMSO: London.

Older, M.W.J. and Dickerson, J.W.T. (1982). Thiamine and the elderly orthopaedic patient. *Age Ageing*, **11**, 101–107.

Philip, G. and Smith, J.F. (1973). Hypothermia and Wernicke's encephalopathy. *Lancet*, **ii**, 122–4.

Phillips, P. (1983). Protein turnover in the elderly: a comparison between ill patients and normal controls. *Clin. Nutr.* (submitted for publication).
Read, A.E., Gough, K.R., Pardoe, J.L. and Nicholas, A. (1965). Nutritional studies on the entrants to an Old People's Home, with particular reference to folic acid deficiency. *Br. Med. J.*, **ii**, 843–8.
Rose, M.S., Chanarin, I., Doniach, D., Brostoff, J. and Ardeman, S. (1970). Intrinsic factor antibodies in the absence of pernicious anaemia: 3 to 7 year follow-up. *Lancet*, **ii**, 9–12.
Ross, M. H. (1969). Aging, nutrition and hepatic enzyme patterns in the rat. *J. Nutr.*, **97**, 565.
Ross, M.H. and Bras, G. (1974). Dietary preference and diseases of age. *Nature*, **250**, 263–5.
Rothschild, M.A., Oratz, M., Mongelli, J. and Schreiber, S.S. (1969). Effects of albumin concentration on albumin synthesis in the perfused liver. *Am. J. Physiol.*, **216**, 1127–30.
Russell, R.I., Williamson, J.M., Goldberg, A. and Wares, E. (1968). Ascorbic acid levels in leucocytes in patients with gastrointestinal haemorrhage. *Lancet*, **ii**, 603–10.
Sheldon, J.H. (1948). *The Social Medicine of Old Age.* Oxford University Press: London.
Shock, N.W. (1972). Energy metabolism, caloric intake and physical activity of the ageing. In *Nutrition in Old Age.* Ed. Carlson, L.A. Almquist and Wiksell: Uppsala.
Shock, N.W., Watkin, D.M., Yiengst, M.J., Norris, A.H., Gaffney, G.W., Gregerman, R.I. and Falzone, J.A. (1963). Age differences in the water content of the body as related to basal oxygen consumption in males. *J. Geront.*, **18**, 1–8.
Shulman, R. (1972). Present status of vitamin $B_{12}$ and folic acid deficiency in psychiatric illness. *Can. Psych. Ass. J.*, **17**, 205–209.
Simms, H.S., Berg, B.N. and Davies, D.F. (1959). Onset of disease and the longevity of rat and man. *Ciba Foundation, Colloquia on Ageing*, Vol. 5. Eds. Wolstenholme, G.E.W. and O'Connor, M. Churchill: London.
Smith, R. and Dick, M. (1968). Total urinary hydroxyproline excretion after administration of vitamin D to healthy human volunteers and to a patient with osteomalacia. *Lancet*, **1**, 279–81.
Sneath, P., Chanarin, I., Hodkinson, H.M., McPherson, C.K. and Reynolds, E.H. (1973). Folate status on a geriatric population and its relationship to dementia. *Age Ageing*, **2**, 177–82.
Srikantia, S.G., Mohanram, M. and Krishanswamy, K. (1970). Human requirements of ascorbic acid. *Am. J. Clin. Nutr.*, **23**, 59–62.
Stamp, T.C.B. and Round, J.M. (1974). Seasonal changes in human plasma levels of 25-hydroxyvitamin D. *Nature*, **247**, 563–5.
Stanton, B.R. (1971). *Meals for the Elderly.* King Edward's Hospital Fund: London.
Stanton, B.R. and Exton-Smith, A.N. (1970). *A Longitudinal Study of the Dietary of Elderly Women.* King Edward's Hospital Fund: London.
Steinkamp, R.C., Cohen, N.L. and Walsh, H.E. (1965). Resurvey of an ageing population – 14 year follow up. *J. Am. Diet. Ass.*, **46**, 103–10.
Stephen, J.M.L. and Dattani, O. (1980). Decline in vitamin D status in old age, Personal communication.
Stokes, P.L., Melikian, V., Leeming, R.L., Portman-Graham, H., Blair, J.A. and Cooke, W.T. (1975). Folate metabolism in scurvy. *Am. J. Clin. Nutr.*, **28**, 126–9.
Stokoe, I.H. (1965). The physical and mental care of the elderly at home. In *Psychiatric Disorders of the Aged.* World Psychiatric Association Symposium: London.
Strachan, R.W., Henderson, J.G. (1967). Psychiatric syndromes due to avitaminosis $B_{12}$ with normal blood and marrow. *Q. J. Med.*, **34**, 303–12.
Taylor, G.F. (1968). A clinical survey of elderly people from a nutritional stand-point.

In *Vitamins in the Elderly*. Eds. Exton-Smith, A.N. and Scott, D.L. John Wright: Bristol.

Thurnham, D. (1972). Riboflavin status of the elderly, personal communication.

Thurnham, D.I., Hassan, F.M. and Powers, H.J. (1979). Effects of riboflavin deficiency on erythrocytes. In *The Importance of Vitamins to Human Health*. Ed. Taylor, T.G. M.T.P. Press: Lancaster.

Tuttle, S.G., Bassett, S.H., Griffith, W.H. Mulcare, D. and Swendseid, M.E. (1965) Further observations on the amino-acid requirements of older men. *Am. J. Clin. Nutr.*, **16**, 229–31.

Tuttle, S.G., Swendseid, M.E., Mulcare, D., Griffith, W.H. and Bassett, S.H. (1957). Study of the essential amino acid requirements of men aged over 50 years. *Metabolism*, **6**, 564–70.

Vir, S.C. and Love, A.H.G. (1980). Thiamine, riboflavin and vitamin $B_6$ status of the aged living at home and in institutions. *Irish J. Med. Sci.*, **149**, 107–16.

Walker, A. (1968). Chronic scurvy. *Br. J. Derm.*, **80**, 625–30.

Watkin, D.M. (1968). Nutritional problems today in the elderly in the United States. In *Vitamins in the Elderly*. Eds. Exton-Smith, A.N. and Scott, D.L. John Wright: Bristol.

Whittle, H., Blair, A., Neale, G., Thalassinos, N., McLaughlin, M., Marsh, M.N., Peters, P.J., Wedzicha, B. and Thompson, G.R. (1969). Intravenous vitamin D in the detection of vitamin D deficiency. *Lancet*, **i**, 747–53.

Williamson, J., Stokoe, I.H., Gray, S., Fisher, M., Smith, A., McGhee, A. and Stephenson, E. (1964). The unreported needs of the elderly at home. *Lancet*, **i**, 1117–20.

Wilson, T.S., Datta, S.B., Murrell, J.S. and Andrews, C.T. (1973). Relation of vitamin C levels to mortality in a geriatric hospital: a study of the effect of vitamin C administration. *Age Ageing*, **2**, 163–71.

Wilson, T.S., Weeks, M.M., Mukherjee, S.K., Murrell, J.S. and Andrews, C.T. (1972). A study of vitamin C levels in the aged and subsequent mortality. *Geront. Clin.*, **14**, 17–24.

Windsor, A.C.M., Hobbs, C.B., Treby, D.A. and Cowper, R.A. (1972). Effect of tetracycline on leucocyte ascorbic acid levels. *Br. Med. J.*, **i**, 214–15.

Windsor, A.C.M. and Williams, C.B. (1970). Urinary hydroxyproline in the elderly with low ascorbic acid levels. *Br. Med. J.*, **i**, 732–3.

WHO (1959). Iron deficiency anaemia. *Tech. Rep. Ser. Wld Hlth Org.*, No. 182.

WHO (1968). Nutritional anaemias. *Tech. Rep. Ser. Wld Hlth Org.*, No. 405.

Yan, S.H.Y. and Franks, J.J. (1968). Albumin metabolism in elderly men and women, *J. Lab. Clin. Med.*, **72**, 449–54.

# Obesity — management in the treatment of disease

B. Jacqueline Stordy



## Introduction

There is much confusion about how and when to treat obesity, partly because of the difficulty of defining and classifying the condition. Obesity is a heterogeneous condition not a single entity with a well known cause and an easy cure. There is doubt over the degree of health hazard and there is debate about appropriate treatments.

## Definition of obesity

Obesity is an increase in the body fat content which frequently results in impairment of health. The definition of obesity is dependent on deciding what is a normal (and desirable) body fat content and what is abnormal and undesirable. The diagnosis of obesity may be made on two entirely different definitions of excess, a statistical definition or an operational definition (Berger, 1981). Statistical definitions are based on an assessment of obesity or body fatness in populations, the average degree of obesity will then be regarded as normal and individuals whose adiposity is one or two standard deviations in excess of 'normal' would be regarded as obese. Such statistical definitions suffer from the disadvantage that relative weight has increased rapidly in Europe since the last war, today's average relative weight would be considered considerably overweight based upon 1940s relative weight standards. An ever changing standard of obesity is not very helpful. More often an operational definition is used, where obesity is defined as a body fat content which is associated with increased mortality, morbidity or a reduction in performance capacity.

## Measurement of body fat content

Adipose tissue mass can be determined by densitometric methods such as under water weighing, by the use of fat soluble gases or by measuring lean body mass by the natural gamma radiation from isotope K40 and then subtracting lean body mass from weight. More recently computerized tomography has been used to study the size of intra-abdominal and subcutaneous fat stores. These time consuming and technically demanding techniques are essential for the scientist as objective measures of body fat; however, the clinician, dietitian or epidemiologist requires simpler assessments of adipose tissue mass. Skinfold measurements are often suggested as a convenient and reliable technique. However, users of this technique require skill and training, observer error appears to become more significant with increasing adiposity and there is a tendency for body fatness to be underestimated. Moreover, skinfolds may not be valid as a measure of total body fat if, with increasing obesity, the proportion of fat that is subcutaneous changes. Skinfold measurements have been correlated with other methods for determining body fat and reviewed by Lohman (1981). The correlation coefficients obtained vary and are not particularly high. Womersley and Durnin (1977) achieved a value of 0.8 emphasizing the need for other more direct methods of determining adipose tissue mass.

For most purposes the most convenient methods of assessing body fatness depend on body weight measurement and the relationship of body weight to height. Many indices have been developed including the body mass index (Quetelet's index) – weight in kilogrammes/height in metres$^2$, the ponderal index – height$^3$/weight and the weight/height ratio. The most widely acceptable index at the time of writing is the body mass index because it is largely independent of height. Garrow's (1981) proposed classification of body mass index and grades of obesity has been widely accepted.

| *Grade of obesity* | *Body mass index* |
|---|---|
| Grade 1 | 20–24.9 |
| Grade 11 | 25–29.9 |
| Grade III | 30–40 |
| Grade IV | >40 |

In general terms it has been suggested that people with a body mass index exceeding 30 should be strongly recommended to lose weight, those with a body mass index of 25–29 should be encouraged to lose weight if they have any associated pathology, such as high blood pressure or Type II diabetes, and those with a body mass index less than 25 should be discouraged from losing weight, unless their body fat is centrally and more particularly intra-abdominally deposited.

# Classification of obesity

## Genetic obesity

**Constitutional obesity**
Obesity runs in families but until very recently it was not clear whether the genetic component is more important than the environmental component in determining body fatness. Studies of twins indicate that obesity is highly heritable (Fabsitz *et al.*, 1980; Feinleib *et al.*, 1977; Börjeson, 1976; Brook *et al.*, 1975), but studies of adopted children until recently were not conclusive. Some suggested heredity is more important than environment in determining body fatness (Annest *et al.*, 1983; Withers, 1964), others (Hartz *et al.*, 1977; Garn, 1977; Garn *et al.*, 1977) concluded family environment is more important than heredity. The matter appears to have been resolved by Stunkard *et al.*, (1986) in a large study of 5455 adoptees where details of biological as well as adoptive parents were known. Human fatness was assessed using body mass index and examined across a range from extreme thinness to severe obesity. This study found that there was a clear and close relationship between body mass index of biological parents and the weight class of adoptees and that there was no relationship between the body mass index of adoptive parents and the weight class of adoptees. These results suggest that childhood family environment alone has little effect on adult fatness and that genetic predisposition has a strong influence. However, genetic predisposition may well be influenced by environmental factors. It is much more likely for the genetic predisposition for obesity to be exposed where food is plentiful and attractive. As suggested by Taitz (1983) heredity may be responsible for the variation in adipose tissue size but environmental factors determine the incidence of obesity.

Genetic factors probably determine the site as well as the size of adipose tissue. Vague (1956) classified obesity as android when most of the fat was found around the waist and in the upper parts of the body, and gynoid when most of the fat was found distributed about the hips and thighs. As his terminology suggests android obesity is found mostly in men and gynoid obesity in women. He noted that diabetes and atherosclerosis are much more commonly associated with android than gynoid obesity. These ideas have been accepted more widely since Larsson *et al.*, (1984) demonstrated that the waist/hip circumference ratio is a much better predictor of heart disease than body mass index or skinfold thickness. The greater the ratio i.e. the greater the waist measurement, the greater the risk of heart disease, stroke and risk factors for heart disease. This type of obesity may be termed truncal or abdominal obesity. When the waist/hip ratio exceeds 1 for men and 0.8 for women, risks associated with obesity increase steeply even when the body mass index is low and indicates acceptable thinness. There is evidence of functional and biochemical differences in the adipocytes from different regions. Adipocytes from the gluteal and femoral regions are larger and have greater lipoprotein lipase activity and are resistant to lipolysis; intra-abdominal fat and central subcutaneous fat are much more sensitive to lipolytic stimuli such as catecholamines. It may become necessary to distinguish between intra-abdominal and subcutaneous central fat because the fatty acids from intra-abdominal fat can influence liver metabolism and reduce insulin clearance leading to the characteristic hyperinsulinaemia and insulin resistance found in some obese people; the central subcutaneous fat deposits cannot influence liver metabolism so directly.

**Somatic dysmorphic syndromes**
Obesity is a feature of certain recognizable patterns of malformations – somatic dysmorphic syndromes. Some of these syndromes are hereditary and all of them are rare. A summary of their features is given in Table 6.1. Detailed descriptions are given by Taitz (1983) in his book *The Obese Child*.

## Hypothalamic obesity

Tumours or inflammatory lesions of the hypothalamus associated with leukaemia, meningitis and tuberculosis can produce obesity. (Damage to either the paraventricular or the ventromedial region may be responsible.) The obesity is of acute onset and although hyperphagia is usually present it is not essential. High levels of insulin and impairment of control of insulin secretion are found.

## Endocrine obesity

Obesity may be found secondary to several endocrine disorders including hypothyroidism, insulinoma, B-cell hyperplasia, Cushing's disease (spontaneous and iatrogenic) and oestrogen administration.

Table 6.1 Somatic dysmorphic syndromes (adapted from Taitz, 1983)

| | |
|---|---|
| *Laurence Moon Biedl syndrome*<br>Retinitis pigmentosa<br>Hypogenitalism<br>Mental retardation<br>Polydactyly<br>Obesity | *Carpenter syndrome*<br>Acrocephaly<br>Abnormal facies<br>Brachysyndactyly and polydactyly<br>Hypogenitalism<br>Mental retardation<br>Obesity |
| *Prader–Willi syndrome*<br>Neonatal hypotonia<br>Typical facies<br>Hypogenitalism<br>Small hands and feet<br>Mental retardation<br>Obesity | *Summitt syndrome*<br>Acrocephaly<br>Brachydactyly and syndactyly<br>Genu valgum<br>Obesity |
| *Cohen syndrome*<br>Hypotonia<br>Hyperextensible joints<br>Odd facies<br>Mental retardation<br>Obesity | |

## The relationship of obesity to mortality and morbidity

The curve relating mortality to measures of body fatness such as body mass index and relative weight is characteristically U-shaped, with persons at the lowest and highest body mass index having increased mortality rates. The early studies (Society of Actuaries, Build and Blood Disease Study, 1959) based on the Life Insurance data have been criticized on the basis that the sample was self selected (mostly men) who self-reported their own weight and height (notoriously unreliable). The sample did not take into account weight changes during the life policy and was based on numbers of policies, not numbers of persons – some persons might have been represented more than once. The American Cancer Society (Lew and Garfinkel, 1979) and the Build Study, 1979 (Society of Actuaries and Association of Life Insurance Medical Directors, 1980) confirmed the original findings. Age has an important influence on the relationship, with the risk of overweight being much greater in young adult males. Life expectancy during childhood does not appear to be significantly affected by obesity (Taitz, 1983); however, the importance of childhood obesity in later life should be considered.

In middle and old age, obesity is bad for cardiovascular risk but less so with increasing age, but thinness is increasingly bad for non-cardiovascular risk. Smoking is a confounding factor in the relationship between mortality and body mass index, with mortality risk associated with smoking being much greater than that associated with obesity. Smoking in normal weight individuals is a greater hazard than Grade II obesity in patients who do not smoke (James, 1984).

Discussions about obesity and acceptable weight understandably focus on the upper limits and little consideration is given to the lowest desirable weights. The Royal College of Physicians' report (1983), and The Health Education Council's (1980) acceptable weight ranges for women overlap weights which are known to be associated with a high incidence of amenorrhoea or if women become pregnant with an increased risk of low infant birthweight with associated increased mortality risk and congenital malformation rate. Mean weight at onset of amenorrhoea in the UK is 53 kg (Crisp, 1978), in Sweden 52 kg (Fries, 1974), and in the USA the 50th percentile for onset of amenorrhoea is 55 kg for women 1.63 m tall (Frisch, 1977). Low prepregnancy weight may be associated with increased risk of cerebral palsy and other neurological disorders, as well as more reproductive illness in the mothers (Bjerre and Bjerre, 1976). Low weight may only be undesirable for those who achieve it by dietary restriction. The woman who stays slim while eating heartily and has no pathological condition is probably less likely to suffer the complications of low weight.

One of the unfortunate consequences of the life insurance studies was that a concept of 'desirable or ideal' weight developed; the ideal weight suggested was lower than average weight and was that weight associated with lowest mortality. Subsequent re-evaluation of the data has demonstrated there is no statistically significant increase in mortality until the relative weight exceeds the present average weight by approximately 25 per cent and the so-called desirable weight by 35 to 40 per cent (Berger, 1981). On the basis of mortality statistics there is little evidence that weight reducing regimes should be instigated unless the body mass index is above 30. Less than 10 per cent of British men and women fall into this category of obesity (Truswell, 1985).

Morbidity and quality of life may be just as important as length of life and obesity can contribute to a loss in quality of life because of obesity related conditions such as diabetes mellitus and hypertension, or because of the psychosocial sequelae of obesity, impairment of self image and economic and social discrimination.

The risk factors for coronary heart disease, hyperlipidaemia, hypertension, hyperuricaemia and low HDL cholesterol levels are more prevalent in the obese but there is debate about whether obesity itself is an independent risk factor in cardiovascular disease. Diabetes, arthritis (not only of the load bearing joints), breast cancer and pulmonary disorders are also more prevalent in the obese. The higher prevalence in the obese may not necessarily indicate causality; not every obese person is hypertensive or diabetic. However, weight reduction in people with obesity related disorders can improve their condition and may reduce the medication required to control diabetes, hypertension or pain associated with arthritis. Where obesity is associated with morbidity which will respond to weight loss there is a clear indication for treatment.

## The dietary management of obesity

There is no way round the laws of thermodynamics which indicate that in order to produce a reduction in the body energy stores, energy intake must be lower than energy output, but the question arises how much lower in order to get substantial, safe weight loss.

### Expected weight loss

One kilogramme of adipose tissue contains around 7000 kilocalories. Thus assuming adipose tissue is the only tissue lost on weight reducing regimes an energy deficit of 1000 kcal a day should achieve 1 kg weight loss in a week. Hence the traditional 1000 kcal slimming diet for women with a habitual energy intake of 2000 kcal should achieve weight losses of around 1 kg in a week. For a long time it has been known that when an individual restricts their food intake there is an adaptive reduction in metabolic rate (Benedict, 1915; Keys *et al.*, 1950; and Apfelbaum, 1971). Thus the theoretically predicted energy deficit and weight loss is not achieved. The adaptive reduction in metabolic rate can be as much as 15 per cent and is a reduction in metabolic rate during activity as well as at rest. Furthermore there must be obese women with habitual energy intakes of less than 2000 kcal/day who would not achieve such weight losses. In one study of 37 obese women on 800 kcal/day strictly supervized in a metabolic unit (Garrow, 1978), three women lost less than 2 kg in a 3 week period and the minimum weight loss observed was 1.5 kg. Obese people who apparently fail to lose weight or lose weight slowly on diets of 800–1500 kcal/day are not necessarily cheating. In normal subjects weighed under standardized conditions daily weight fluctuations of 0.5 kg are quite common. Weight gain prior to menstruation of around 0.5 kg may also be observed so that real adipose tissue losses may be masked by fluid retention.

Adipose tissue is not the only tissue lost on reducing diets. Fast weight losses may be due to a reduction in energy stored as glycogen. The muscles and liver of adult man contain varying amounts of glycogen (between 0 and 800 g). Associated with each gram of glycogen is 3 to 4 g of water. The energy store of glycogen is up to 3500 kcal (800 g of glycogen) but is more usually around 1600 kcal (400 g glycogen) and is used up after a few days total starvation. The associated weight loss would be 400 g (from glycogen) plus 1200 g of associated fluid loss. Even before glycogen reserves are depleted fatty acids from adipose tissue become the major body fuel.

James (1984) has devised a useful if laborious method of predicting weight loss. First energy requirement (R) is estimated from the table below.

*Children 10–18 years*
Boys R = 1.4 (0.074 wt + 2.8)
Girls R = 1.4 (0.056 wt + 2.9)
*Adults 18–30 years*
Men R = 1.4 (0.063 wt + 2.9)
Women R = 1.4 (0.062 wt + 2.0)
*Adults 30–60 years*
Men R = 1.4 (0.048 wt + 3.65)
Women R = 1.4 (0.034 wt + 3.5)
R is estimated in MJ per day and based on body weight in kg.

After one month's slimming the activity factor 1.4 should be reduced to 1.25 to take account of the adaptive fall in metabolic rate and weight loss is predicted as follows:

Dietary intake is specified I; Daily energy deficit = R – I. Assuming 1 kg of weight loss is equivalent to an energy deficit of 30 MJ; the predicted weight loss is $\frac{R-I}{30}$ kg/day or R – I in a 30 day month.

## Criteria for weight reducing diets

Many weight reducing diets have been devised by professional nutritionists and dietitians as well as lay personnel. Very few fulfil the criteria suggested in Table 6.2. Most do not fulfil even the most basic nutritional criteria of supplying recommended amounts of all essential vitamins and minerals (Fisher *et al.*, 1985; Stordy and Roberts, 1988).

Diets may be devised which provide a seven day cycle of set meals in which

Table 6.2 Criteria for weight reducing diets

1. The energy deficit should be large enough to achieve encouraging rates of weight loss. Deficits of 1000 kcal/day are needed.
2. The diet should fulfil recommended intakes of protein, related to target body weight (0.75 g/kg target weight minimum) WHO 1985.
3. The diet should supply recommended amounts of all essential vitamins and minerals.
4. The diet should fit in with the life style of the obese person and preferably be flexible allowing for social and business functions.
5. The dietary instructions should provide a sound basis for nutrition education.

the patient has no choice of food. Such diets can, with care, be designed to provide the recommended amounts of protein, minerals and vitamins but this becomes exceedingly difficult on diets providing less than 1000 kcal. When diets are based on self-selection from lists of foods in various categories the nutritional value of the diets cannot be assured. It is even difficult to ensure a so-called 1000 kcal diet does provide just that. In one study (Stordy *et al.*, 1988) of diets designed by dietitians energy intakes on self selected 1000 kcal diets were sometimes as high as 1700 kcal per day. It is not surprising if patients on such diets fail to lose weight.

Weight reducing diets based on conventional food only succeed if the obese person has the will power and determination to stick to the diet. This is often very difficult to achieve when the food supply is palatable and readily available. Strict dietary control is necessary for long periods of time, usually months, if substantial weight loss is to be achieved. This is exceedingly difficult in the face of social and physiological pressures to eat. A woman who keeps to a 1000 kcal reducing diet for 6 days but then eats a conventional Sunday lunch and drinks a small sherry beforehand and wine with the meal may well undo all the control achieved on the previous 6 days.

## Other factors influencing success

The empathy of doctors and dietitians towards the obese patient is vital to the success of a weight loss programme. Commercial slimming organizations who stand or fall by the success of their programme have found that dietary advice is more successful if given by someone who has previously been overweight. Financial penalty for failure to keep to a regime and financial cost of dietary advice may also improve compliance. Regular consultancies – at least once a fortnight, weighings under the same conditions on the same scale and family support can provide the best conditions for managing obesity (Truswell, 1985).

## Very low calorie diets (VLCDs)

Dietary restriction with conventional foods has been notoriously unsuccessful in the past. There are very few extensive detailed metabolic studies indicating the safety or otherwise of conventional dietary restriction. In contrast there are many such studies of very low calorie diets (300–500 kcal/day). Wadden *et al.*, (1983) in their review reported that not only were such regimes successful in achieving substantial weight loss (16–20 lb/month) but mortality is less than that predicted for patients with the same degree of obesity living their normal lives.

Very low calorie diets are usually formulae based on mixtures of milk and soya proteins together with carbohydrate and added vitamins, minerals and essential fatty acids. Sometimes conventional foods are used and vitamin and mineral supplements are taken separately. Very low calorie diets were brought into disrepute by the unscrupulous introduction of diets based on collagen and gelatin proteins (the liquid protein diets) which were also nutritionally inadequate in other respects and led to over 60 deaths. Cardiac arrythmias and myocardial degeneration were thought to be the cause of death. Modern well formulated VLCDs are not associated with such problems and there is some evidence that electrocardiographic abnormalities may even improve (James, 1984). VLCDs have been criticized because of the negative nitrogen balance observed in users. Experience indicates that after an initial period of negative nitrogen balance, usually of 2 to 3 weeks duration, users adapt and are subsequently only in slight negative nitrogen balance (Wynn, 1985). The obese have more lean body mass as well as adipose tissue (James, 1978), there is an increase in skin area, blood volume and muscle size. As adipose tissue is lost it is appropriate that some of the protein from lean tissues is lost as well. For example (assuming 10 per cent of total body nitrogen is in skin and overall body composition is 34 gN/kg body weight), an 80 kg woman 1.65 m tall has a surface area of 1.88 $m^2$ and has 231 g nitrogen in skin. If she loses 20 kg weight her skin area would decrease to 1.66 $m^2$ and the nitrogen content to 204 g. Thus a loss of 27 g nitrogen from skin associated with a weight loss of 20 kg would be appropriate. Furthermore (assuming red cell volume 25 ml/kg, plasma volume 45 ml/kg, protein content of RBC 35 g/100ml, protein content of plasma 70 g/ml), the woman at 80 kg would have 952 g protein in blood and at 60 kg, 714 g protein in blood. Thus a loss of 238 g protein (38 gN) from the reduction in cellular and plasma blood proteins would be appropriate and expected. There are other tissues where a similar protein loss would be appropriate.

## Behavioural weight control and cognitive restructuring

It would be difficult to improve the summary of the behavioural principles of weight loss provided by Stunkard and Berthold (1985) (see table 6.3).

Behaviour modification is probably more successful when practised on a one-to-one basis and can be very time consuming. Although it implies that behaviour of the obese is different from that of the slim that is not necessarily so. It was thought that the obese responded more to external cues to eat than internal cues of appetite but such ideas have largely been discounted.

## Long term weight maintenance

All too often the problems of long term weight maintenance are neglected, either because substantial weight loss is not achieved in the first place and therefore the 'problem' never arises, or because there is a glib assumption that once the poor eating habits of the obese have been re-educated there will be no further problem. As outlined earlier the obese person does not necessarily eat large quantities of food thus re-education involves educating the person with a tendency to obesity to consume less food permanently. Ravussin *et al.*, (1982) have demonstrated that obese people lack 'regulatory thermogenesis' and in the post-obese state show a decrease in energy expenditure of 16–20 kcal/kg of weight loss/day. Thus if the individual loses 20 kg the post-obesity energy intake should be 300–400 kcal less day in order to prevent weight gain. If the obese person was one of the unfortunate few who only eat small quantities of food in the first place, then the problem of weight maintenance is obviously very great. Preliminary reports suggest that weight maintenance, a problem with all therapies, also seems somewhat better with a very low calorie diet than conventional diets. Blackburn and Greenberg (1978) reporting on the use of a

Table 6.3 Behavioural principles of weight loss in five books (adapted from Stunkard and Berthold, 1985)

1. Stimulus control
   A. *Shopping*
      1. Shop for food after eating
      2. Shop from a list
      3. Avoid ready-to-eat foods
      4. Don't carry more cash than needed for shopping list

   B. *Plans*
      1. Plan to limit food intake
      2. Substitute exercise for snacking
      3. Eat meals and snacks at scheduled times
      4. Don't accept food offered by others

   C. *Activities*
      1. Store food out of sight
      2. Eat all food in the same place
      3. Remove food from inappropriate storage areas in the house
      4. Keep serving dishes off the table
      5. Use smaller dishes and utensils
      6. Avoid being the food server
      7. Leave the table immediately after eating
      8. Don't save leftovers

   D. *Holidays and parties*
      1. Drink fewer alcoholic beverages
      2. Plan eating habits before parties
      3. Eat a low-calorie snack before parties
      4. Practice polite ways to decline food
      5. Don't get discouraged by an occasional setback
2. Eating behaviour
   1. Put fork down between mouthfuls
   2. Chew thoroughly before swallowing
   3. Prepare foods one portion at a time
   4. Leave some food on the plate
   5. Pause in the middle of the meal
   6. Do nothing else while eating (read, watch television)

3. Reward
   1. Solicit help from family and friends
   2. Help family and friends provide this help in the form of praise and material rewards
   3. Utilize self-monitoring records as basis for rewards
   4. Plan specific rewards for specific behaviours (behavioural contracts)

4. Self-monitoring
   Keep diet diary that includes:
   1. Time and place of eating
   2. Type and amount of food
   3. Who is present/How you feel

5. Nutrition education
   1. Use diet diary to identify problem areas
   2. Make small changes that you can continue
   3. Learn nutritional values of foods
   4. Decrease fat intake; increase complex carbohydrates

6. Physical activity
   A. *Routine Activity*
      1. Increase routine activity
      2. Increase use of stairs
      3. Keep a record of distance walked each day

   B. *Exercise*
      1. Begin a very mild exercise programme
      2. Keep a record of daily exercise
      3. Increase the exercise very gradually

7. Cognitive restructuring
   1. Avoid setting unreasonable goals
   2. Think about progress, not shortcomings
   3. Avoid imperatives like 'always' and 'never'
   4. Counter negative thoughts with rational restatements
   5. Set weight goals

very low calorie diet as part of a weight loss programme stated that one out of three patients maintained their weight loss for 2 years. Similar results were reported by Cormillot *et al.*, (1981) whilst Bistrian and Sherman (1978) found that one-third of their patients maintained at least 9 kg (20 lbs) of weight loss for at least 4 years.

## Preventing obesity

The growing evidence that fatness is inherited and that the health hazards of obesity are more closely associated with some types of fat distribution suggests that prophylactic measures should be refocused on the most vulnerable. Such a policy could be more efficient and cost effective, moreover it might decrease any excessive concern about body fatness that is found in the community as a whole. For women, particularly, moderate overweight is a low health risk and there are health risks associated with thinness. However, it remains to be demonstrated convincingly that pre-obese persons can be taught habits of eating and exercise that will effectively reduce the size of their unwanted adipose legacy (Van Itallie, 1986).

## References

Annest, J.L., Sing, C.F., Biron, P. and Mongeau, J.G. (1983). Family aggregation of blood pressure and weight in adoptive families. III. Analysis of the role of shared genes and shared household environment in explaining family resemblance for height, weight and selected height/weight indices. *Am. J. Epidemiol.*, **117**, 492–506.

Apfelbaum, M., Bostsarron, J. and Lacatis, D. (1971). Effect of caloric restriction and excessive calorie intake on energy expenditure *Am. J. Clin. Nutr.*, **24**, 1405–1409.

Asher, W.L. and Dietz, R.E. (1972). Effectiveness of weight reduction involving 'diet pills'. *Curr. Ther. Res.*, **14**, 510–24.

Benedict, F.G. (1915). Factors affecting basal metabolism. *J. Biol. Chem.*, **20**, 263–99.

Berger, M., Berchtold, P., Greis, F.A. and Zimmerman, H. (1981). Indications for the treatment of obesity. In *Recent Advances in Obesity Research III*. Eds. Bjorntorp, Cairella and Howard. John Libbey: London.

Bistrian, B.R. and Sherman, M. (1978). Results of treatment of obesity with a protein sparing modified fast. *Int. J. Obesity*, **2**, 143–8.

Bjerre, B. and Bjerre, I. (1976) Significance of obstetric fatness in prognosis of low birthweight children. *Acta Paediat. Scand.*, **65**, 544–56.

Blackburn, G.L. and Greenburg, I. (1978). Multidisciplinary approach to adult obesity therapy. *Int. J. Obesity*, **2**, 133–4.

Börjeson, M. (1976). The aetiology of obesity in children: a study of 101 twin pairs. *Acta Paediat. Scand.*, **65**, 279–87.

Brook, C.G.D., Huntley, R.M.C. and Slack, J. (1975). Influence of heredity and environment in determination of skinfold thickness in children. *Br. Med. J.*, **2**, 719–21.

Cormillot, A., Zukerfeld, R., Olkies, A. *et al.*, (1981). A multiple approach to the treatment of obesity using total fasting or a very-low calorie diet. *Int. J. Obesity.*, **5**, 297–304.

Crisp, A.H. (1978). Psychopathology of weight related amenorrhoea. In *Adances in Gynaecological Endocrinology*. Royal College Obstetrics and Gynaecology: London.

Evans, F.A. (1938). Treatment of obesity with low calorie diets: report of 121 additional cases. *Int. Clin.*, 3, 19–23.

Evans, F.A. and Strang, J.M. (1929). A departure from the usual methods of treating obesity. *Am. J. Med. Sci.*, **77**, 339–48.

Fabsitz, R., Feinleib, M. and Hrbec. Z. (1980). Weight changes in adult twins. *Acta Genet. Med. Gemellol.*, **29**, 273–9.

Feinleib, M., Garrison, R.J., Fabsitz, R. *et al.*, (1977). The NHLBI twin study of cardiovascular disease risk factors: methodology and summary of results. *Am. J. Epidemiol.*, **106**, 284–95.

Fisher, M.C. and Lachance, P.A. (1985). Nutritional evaluation of published weight-reducing diets. *J. Am. Dietet. Ass.*, **85**, 450–54.

Fries, H. (1974). Secondary amenorrhoea, self-induced weight reduction and anorexia nervosa. *Acta Psychiat. Scand.*, (Suppl) **248**.

Frisch, R.E. (1977). Food intake, fatness and reproductive ability. In *Anorexia Nervosa*. Ed. Vigersky, R.A. Raven Press: New York.

Garn, S.M. (1977). Effect of parental fatness of biological and adoptive children. *Ecol. Food Nutr.*, **6**, 91–3.

Garn, S.M., Bailey, S.M. and Higgins, I.T. (1977). Fatness similarities in adopted pairs. *Am. J. Clin. Nutr.*, **29**, 1067–8.

Garrow, J.S. (1978). *Energy Balance and Obesity in Man*, p. 171. Elsevier: North Holland and New York.

Hartz, A., Giefer, E. and Rimm, A.A. (1977). Relative importance of the effect of family environment and heredity on obesity. *Ann. Hum. Genet.*, **41**, 185–93.

Health Education Council. (1980). *Looking After Yourself*. Health Education Council, London.

James, W.P.T. (1984). Treatment of obesity. The constraints on success. In *Clinics in Endocrinology and Metabolism*. **13**, No. 3.

James, W.P.T., Davies, H.L., Bailes, J. and Dauncey, M.J. (1978). Elevated metabolic rates in obesity. *Lancet*, 1, 1122–5.

Keys, A., Brozek, J., Henschel, A. *et al.*, (1950). *The Biology of Human Starvation*, Vols 1 and 2. University of Minnesota Press: Minneapolis.

Larsson, B., Suardsudd, K., Welin, L. *et al.*, (1984). Abdominal adipose distribution and risk of cardiovascular disease and death: A 13 year follow-up of participants in the study of men born in 1913. *Br. Med. J.*, **288**, 1401–1404.

Lew, E.A. and Garfinkel, L. (1979). Variations in mortality by weight among 750,000 men and women. *J. Clin. Diseases*, **32**, 563–7.

Lohman, T.G. (1981). Skinfolds and body density and their relation to body fatness. *Human Biol.*, **53**, 181–225.

Prentice, A.M., Black, A.E., Coward, W.A. *et al.*, (1986). High levels of energy expenditure in obese women. *Br. Med. J.*, **292**, 983–7.

Ravussin, E., Burnand, B., Schutz, Y. and Jequier, E. (1982). Twenty-four hour energy expenditure and resting metabolic rate in obese, moderately obese and control subjects. *Am. J. Clin. Nutr.*, **35**, 566–73.

Royal College of Physicians. (1983). *Report of a Working Party on Obesity*. Royal College Physicians: London.

Society of Actuaries and Association of Life Insurance Medical Directors (1980). *The Build Study 1979*. Recording and Statistical Corporation: Chicago.

Stordy, B.J. and Roberts, M.L. (1988). The nutrient composition of weight reducing diets recommended by dietitians. In Preparation.
Strang, J.M., McClugage, H.B. and Evans, F.A. (1930). The nitrogen balance during dietary correction of obesity. *Am. J. Med. Sci.*, **181**, 336–49.
Stunkard, A.J. and Berthold, H.C. (1985). What's behaviour therapy? A very short description of behavioural weight control. *Am. J. Clin. Nutr.*, **41**, 821–3.
Stunkard, A., Thorkild, I.A., Sorensen, *et al.*, (1986). An adoption study of human obesity. *N. Engl. J. Med.*, **314**, 193–8.
Taitz, L. (1983). *The Obese Child.* Blackwell Scientific Publications: London.
Truswell, A.S. (1985). Obesity: Diagnosis and risks. *Br. Med. J.*, **291**, 655–7.
Vague, J. (1956). The degree of masculine differentiation of obesities: a factor determining predisposition to diabetes, atherosclerosis, gout and uric calculous disease. *Amer. J. Clin. Nutr.* **4**, 20.
Van Itallie, T.B. (1986). Bad news and good news about obesity. *N. Engl. J. Med.*, **314**, 239–40.
Wadden, T.A., Stunkard, A.J. and Brownell, K.D. (1983). Very low calorie diets: their efficacy, safety and future. *Ann. Int. Med.*, **29**, 674–84.
W.H.O. (1985). *Energy and protein requirements.* WHO Technical Reports Series: Geneva.
Withers, R.F.J. (1964). Problems in the genetic obesity. *Eugen Rev.*, **56**, 81–90.
Womersley, J. and Durnin, J.V.G.A. (1977). A comparison of skinfold method with extent of 'overweight' and various weight/height relationships in the assessment of obesity. *Br. J. Nutr.*, **38**, 271–84.
Wynn, V., Abraham, R.R. and Densen, J.W. (1985). Method for estimating rate of fat loss during treatment of obesity by calorie restriction. *Lancet.*, **1**, 482–6.

# 7 Anorexia nervosa

M.A. Jackson and Harry A. Lee



## Introduction

Minor appetite disorders are quite a common occurrence at puberty although the fully developed syndrome of anorexia nervosa is much less common. There is a prevalence of about 1 in every 150 school girls between the ages of 16 and 18 years, the average age of onset being 17.6 plus or minus 5.1 years in females. It is less common in males with less than 10 per cent of anorectic patients being male with an average age of onset of 16.2 plus or minus 3.2 years. Anorexia is predominantly a disorder of young adults, in particular females, and rarely presents after the age of 30. However, when it does occur in later age groups, almost uniquely amongst females, it can be a very difficult condition to treat. The serious nature of this condition can be judged by the fact that in the more severely affected group there is a 10–15 per cent mortality rate.

The triggering mechanism for this disorder may well be a dietary behaviour problem in the young female, particularly one who has previously been overweight and then wants to reduce weight far in excess of what is required. Characteristically such patients conceal, resist and avoid all forms of treatment. It is, therefore, most important that any long-term dieting programme in adolescent girls should be carefully supervised both by a doctor and a dietitian. There can be no advocacy for fasting, for this may well lead to the establishment of a pattern of dietary deprivation which can lead to anorexia nervosa. It is well known that some patients oscillate between obesity and anorexia nervosa before finally establishing a so-called normal weight. Usually, rapid weight loss occurs for apparently no good reason although one must be mindful of the differential diagnosis for this condition (Table 7.1). Most anorexia nervosa patients are very clever at concealing their dietary habits, not only from their family but from the attendant doctor. They have a total obsession about food, their weight and body image and it is not unusual for anorectic patients to fall to weights around 30 kg before the then obviously clinical emaciation draws the attention of the immediate family and thereby medical attention. Usually these patients in spite of their severe emaciation claim they are feeling well and even on very careful questioning will deny any

Table 7.1 Differential diagnosis of anorexia nervosa

| |
|---|
| 1. Primary depressive illness |
| 2. Chronic drug abuse, e.g. Laxatives, diuretics |
| 3. Addison's disease |
| 4. Anterior pituitary insufficiency |
| 5. Tuberculosis (Generalized – not related to ethnic group) |
| 6. Crohn's disease |
| 7. Carcinoma of the pancreas |
| 8. Thyrotoxicosis |
| 9. Diabetes mellitus |
| 10. Carcinoma of the duodenum (rare) |

untoward symptoms or, indeed, any deviation from a normal eating pattern.

Anorectic patients remain surprisingly active even when they have lost a considerable amount of their body weight, often more than 50 per cent. Nevertheless, careful history taking soon reveals a pre-occupation with body weight and a morbid fear of overeating and the possible consequences of once again becoming obese. These patients initially may vacillate between overeating and vomiting and many will later resort to the use of laxatives or diuretics if they can obtain them.

The aim of this chapter is to deal with the purely nutritional aspect of these patients and their management rather than go into a lengthy psychiatric discussion about their problems. It is our view that many of these patients are best managed by psychiatrists with an interest in anorexia nervosa and also a physician who really understands their nutritional requirements. Anorexia nervosa is an overdiagnosed clinical condition and there are a number of diseases that must be considered and, indeed, excluded in the differential diagnosis before a conclusion of anorexia nervosa is reached (See Table 7.1). Most of the other conditions can be excluded clinically and with few investigations, but nevertheless, mistakes still occur. As indicated earlier, 90 per cent of anorexia nervosa patients when first diagnosed will be female and 85 per cent of these will be between the ages of 13 and 20 years. Most patients will have lost more than 25 per cent of their body weight (Crisp, 1965). Often the first complaint of many of these patients is secondary amenorrhoea. Most patients have a preoccupation with body weight and have a disturbed body image and often complain of severe abdominal pain and many suffer from constipation. On examination, most patients will be found to be emaciated with cold blue peripheries and have lanugo hair. If they are severely malnourished, they will have bradycardia and postural hypotension. Severely ill patients will also usually be hypothermic.

## Nutritional – metabolic changes

The nutritional–metabolic changes are due to weight loss which occurs mainly as a result of a low intake or avoidance of carbohydrates (Crisp, 1965; Russell, 1967) although a relatively high protein intake may be maintained until the disease is well advanced. Indeed, some patients may have such a high protein intake they develop a considerable blood urea: serum creatinine divergence, so that if only the blood urea were measured a diagnosis of uraemia might be falsely made (Richards, 1975). Unfortunately, few studies have been undertaken with respect to actual protein intake in these patients (Beaumont *et al.*, 1981). Many patients abuse laxatives and diuretics and indulge in vomiting which may result in a hypokalaemic alkalosis. The haemoglobin concentration is maintained until late in the course of the disease but a relative lymphocytosis with neutropenia is common (Rieger *et al.*, 1978). The fasting blood sugar is low in these patients and severe hypoglycaemia may be the presenting complication of anorexia nervosa (Zalin and Lant, 1984). Total body protein stores are depleted late on and serum albumin and globulin concentrations remain normal until the patient is severely malnourished. Interestingly, infection is rare in this group of patients (Bowers and Eckert, 1978). Cellular immunity assessed by skin testing correlates well with weight loss and anthropometric tests, anergy being observed in those patients below 60 per cent of ideal body weight. Anergy does not correlate with serum albumin, total iron binding capacity or transferrin (Pertschuk *et al.*, 1982). Patients with anorexia nervosa have reduced serum concentrations of IgG, IgM, transferrin, C1Q, $C_2$, $C_3$, Factor B, $\beta$ 1H, $C_3$B activator, properdin and $C_4$ binding protein (Wyatt *et al.*, 1982). The serum cholesterol is usually elevated (Crisp, 1970). Serum lactic dehydrogenase and oestrogen concentrations are usually low. Extra-cellular water is often increased but circulatory blood volume and plasma volume are decreased (Lefebvre, 1980). Hypophosphataemia only usually occurs during re-feeding. Serum alkaline phosphatase, even in these adolescent patients, is usually at the lower limit of normal.

Vitamin deficiency is rare unless the patient is severely malnourished but hypercarotenaemia may occur. Whether this is due to an excess ingestion of vitamin A contained in foods, e.g., carrots, or carotene that these patients may indulge in, is uncertain.

Serum concentrations of magnesium and iron are usually within the normal range. There is a disturbance of zinc metabolism (Jackson *et al.*, 1987) in anorexia nervosa patients resulting in a small rise in serum zinc concentration after a zinc supplemented food intake (Dinsmore *et al.*, 1985). Some anorexia nervosa patients have a low serum zinc concentration when initially diagnosed and others will develop a low serum concentration as they become anabolic during re-feeding if they are not given adequate zinc supplements. From our own observations the urinary zinc excretion falls in these patients in the first week or two of aggressive re-feeding. For this reason zinc supplements are always given to our patients.

At St. Mary's Hospital (Portsmouth) we measured the fasting plasma amino acid profiles in 13 female patients aged between 13 and 22 years with anorexia nervosa. All patients were referred by consultant psychiatrists for metabolic and nutritional assessment. All of the patients were at least 25 per cent below their ideal weight. The control group were adults between the ages of 20 and 35 years and who had normal nutritional status. All the plasma amino acid concentrations were lower in the anorexic patients compared to those in the control. The most significant differences were in the concentrations of all the essential amino acids (valine, leucine, isoleucine, lysine, threonine, methionine, tryptophan and phenylalanine) and also the semi essential amino acids, histidine and tyrosine (Fig. 7.1) (Jackson *et al.*,in preparation).

Nitrogen balance studies in these patients showed that they had adapted to

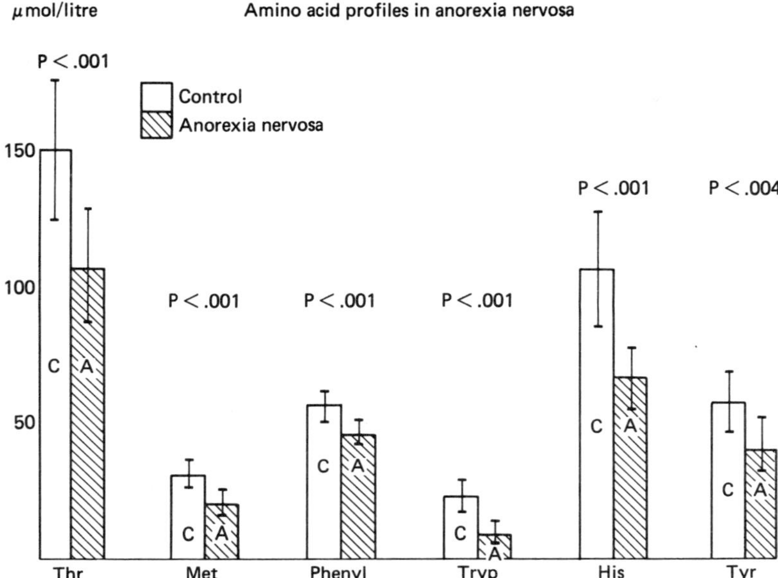


Fig. 7.1 Plasma amino-acids: *Control column* marked C; *Anorexia nervosa* column marked A. The height of the column is the mean and the vertical bar is the SD. (*Note*: Significantly low concentrations of all essential and semi-essential amino acids.)

their low protein intake. They had very low urinary and faecal nitrogen excretion values (Fig. 7.2).

## Dangers of re-feeding

One of the major dangers during re-feeding of these patients is heart failure (Powers, 1982). These severely malnourished patients have small hearts radiologically, often with abnormal electrocardiograms. The ECG may show bradycardia, 'U' wave, (Warren and Steinberg, 1979; Thurston and Marks, 1974) and lengthening of the QT interval and changes in the ST segment (Folhin, 1977; Thurston and Marks, 1974; Palossy, 1977). Sudden death due to dysrhythmias may occur during re-feeding (Isner *et al.*,1985). Patients often develop fluid retention during the first week of re-feeding and therefore the sodium intake must be carefully restricted, i.e., 30 mmol/day if possible. Such fluid retention may be due to the poor myocardial state of these patients or to some temporary impairment of renal function, i.e., diminished creatinine clearance approximately 45–50 ml/minute (Boag *et al.*, 1985).

In the severely malnourished patient, the 24 hour sodium intake should be kept below 30 mmol/day and if this is not achieved the patient is liable to become grossly oedematous (See Fig. 7.2 at day 18). If re-feeding is pursued too rapidly then electrolyte disturbances are increasingly common and dangerous. Should an anorexia nervosa patient be admitted with acute intercurrent infection or following an overdose, or trauma, it is imperative that he should not

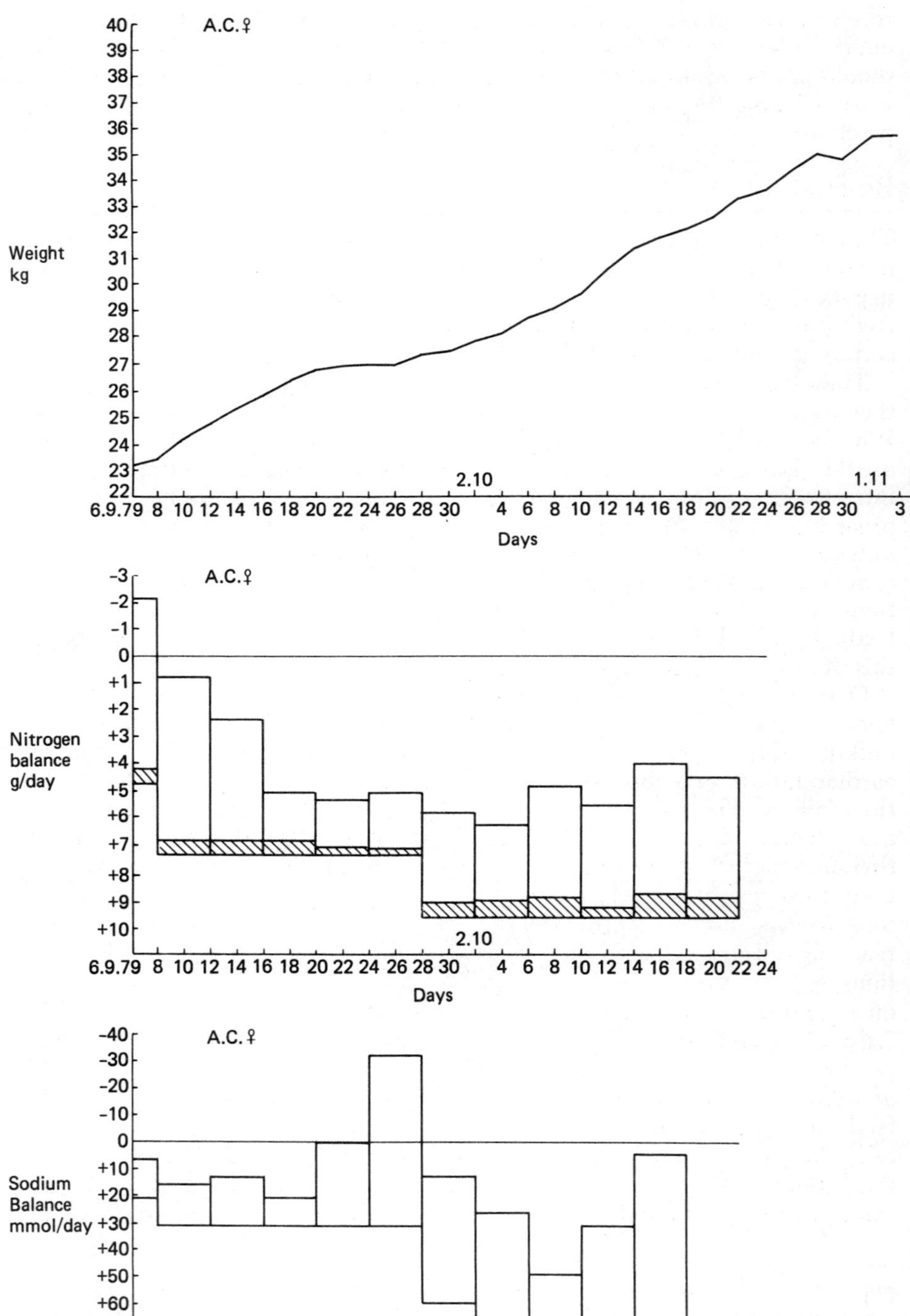
A.C.♀
Weight kg
40 39 38 37 36 35 34 33 32 31 30 29 28 27 26 25 24 23 22
2.10
1.11
6.9.79 8 10 12 14 16 18 20 22 24 26 28 30 4 6 8 10 12 14 16 18 20 22 24 26 28 30 3 5
Days
A.C.♀
Nitrogen balance g/day
-3 -2 -1 0 +1 +2 +3 +4 +5 +6 +7 +8 +9 +10
2.10
6.9.79 8 10 12 14 16 18 20 22 24 26 28 30 4 6 8 10 12 14 16 18 20 22 24
Days
A.C.♀
Sodium Balance mmol/day
-40 -30 -20 -10 0 +10 +20 +30 +40 +50 +60 +70 +80
2.10
6.9.79 8 10 12 14 16 18 20 22 24 26 28 30 4 6 8 10 12 14 16 18 20 22

receive excess intravenous electrolyte loading during resuscitation. It is also our considered view that any patient at or below 50 per cent ideal body weight should not be admitted to a psychiatric ward but rather to an acute medical ward. Clearly, the risks of demise at this stage are obviously more medical than psychiatric.

## Re-feeding

The calorie and protein content of the diet is not too important if the patient is not severely malnourished (Forbes *et al.*, 1984). There is a high mortality rate in patients with anorexia nervosa who are 50 per cent below ideal body weight (Baker and Lyen, 1982). In these patients it is most important to be absolutely certain of fluid, nutritional and the electrolyte contents of their diet.

These patients usually have normal gastrointestinal tract function unless they have been laxative abusers (Crisp, 1965; Silverstone and Russell, 1967). Whenever possible, and this applies to the vast majority, it is always safer to use the gastrointestinal tract for nutritional rehabilitation rather than resort to intravenous feeding. Total parenteral nutrition is a potentially dangerous procedure in anorexia nervosa patients (Pertschuk *et al.*, 1983). Parenteral nutrition is very rarely necessary for these patients but when it is the sodium content must be carefully noted; it is often high in the basic amino acid solutions. Acute dilatation of the stomach has been reported in patients during re-feeding (Russell, 1966) but fortunately this is a very rare complication and in this situation the patient will have to be fed parenterally.

Over recent years, we have re-fed a number of patients with severe anorexia nervosa using a fine-bore enteral feeding tube and a commercially prepared milk-based feed (Jackson *et al.*, 1981; Jackson *et al.*, in press). The danger of cardiac failure and fluid overload in these patients is well recognized and therefore especial care is required in keeping their sodium intake to a minimum. These patients have all previously adapted to low nitrogen intakes and therefore there is no indication for giving high nitrogen and caloric intakes initially to them. In severely malnourished patients with anorexia nervosa the tube feeds should be started very slowly, initially at quarter strength and reaching full strength over approximately 8 days unless there are contraindications, e.g., diarrhoea, fluid overload. The rest of such patients must be started on a quarter strength tube feed and will slowly build up to full strength. Only 7 g of nitrogen (800 kcals) are required to put most patients into positive nitrogen balance (See Fig. 7.2). Some patients will require potassium supplements *ab initio*, particularly if they have been laxative or diuretic abusers. The tube feed concentration quantity should be increased steadily over the first 2 weeks of feeding and in most patients by the end of 2 weeks it should be possible for the patient to be on at least 2 litres of full strength feed daily given by a continuous infusion. Diarrhoea rarely occurs in those patients who are given

---

Fig. 7.2 Severely malnourished female with anorexia nervosa. Weight gain, nitrogen balance and sodium balance of patient. Cross hatched areas faecal nitrogen. (Patient started on 30 g protein enteral feed which was then increased to put patient into positive nitrogen balance. Sodium balance – the patient developed fluid retention during the second week which required diuretics.)

continuous tube feeds and many of them may actually be constipated at such time requiring laxatives or suppositories. By starting with low volumes of diluted tube feed, their sodium content can be kept to a minimum during initial treatment.

These patients rarely have vitamin deficiencies but they become anabolic as the re-feeding starts and vitamins should be given at the same time. If Parentrovite Forte 1 and 2 (Bencard) is given for the first 3 days intravenously and subsequently a water soluble vitamin preparation orally, vitamin deficiency should be prevented from occurring at any time during the re-feeding phase. Zinc deficiency is best avoided by giving zinc sulphate 220 mg three times a day.

While the patient is being refed, she/he should be weighed daily to ensure there is no loss of weight and they should be encouraged to keep their own charts. By using a tube feed the total amount of nitrogen being given to a patient can be accurately assessed and if a patient's weight is not rising as quickly as calculations indicate, then by checking the urinary urea excretion it can be easily assessed whether the patient is managing to cheat even with a fine-bore tube *in situ*.

As these patients gain weight they will usually develop an appetite to start eating of their own accord with the fine-bore tube still *in situ*. It is not our policy to insist that patients eat. Most severely malnourished patients have a minimal oral intake for about 2–3 weeks. They are allowed to eat anything they want from the hospital menu, but they must still persist with their total tube feed. When the patients reach their ideal weight the nasogastric tube feed should be cut back. This initially should be done by withdrawing the feed for at least the first 6 hours during the day, then 12 hours during the day, then finally just feeding overnight. In this way, normal oral feeding can be easily re-instituted. Feeding is a social habit and it is very important that the patient starts to feed with other individuals. It may take weeks to wean the patient on to a full oral diet. Patients with anorexia nervosa usually tolerate fine-bore nasogastric tubes extremely well and co-operate by feeding themselves this way both in and out of hospital. They rarely find the tube feed a threat and in most cases do not regard the enteral feeding as a form of nutrition to concern them nor do they resist it. By using initially a 24 hour continuous feeding regimen, there are very rarely complaints from the patients of abdominal distension or discomfort which they tend to complain of when taking food orally. Some patients, however, may become very dependent on the tube for re-feeding and become frightened lest they lose weight when the tube is removed. During the period of re-feeding the patient should receive psychiatric as well as dietetic advice but they are very often happily managed on general medical wards. Anti-depressants and sedatives may be given when deemed appropriate.

In the past, anorexia nervosa patients have been heavily sedated and kept in bed whilst being re-fed but this has not been our policy. Exercise improves protein anabolism and should not be withheld from these patients. Our policy is to initially arrange for patients who are too weak to go to the gymnasium to be shown exercises to do whilst lying on their beds to increase muscle tone. As the patients' condition improves, so does the degree of their activities. It is necessary to ensure that some of the patients do not indulge in too much exercise too early in an attempt to keep their weight down. For this reason it is very important that the exercises are carefully monitored by physiotherapists.

So far with this nutritional approach and psychiatric assistance, when required, we have not lost a patient during the initial nutritional rehabilitation. This experience covers over 30 patients many of whom were below 50 per cent of ideal body weight and many of whom had already been considered psychiatric failures. We consider that patients who are properly renourished are better able to proceed and accept psychiatric guidance and treatment with hopefully better results in the majority of such cases. Our long-term success (at one year) has been 75 per cent.

## Conclusion

The traditional ways of treating severely malnourished patients with anorexia nervosa would now seem to be outdated and inappropriate. These patients can be safely and accurately returned to normal nutritional status by the use of chemically defined milk based commercially prepared feeds delivered by a fine-bore enteral feeding tube. Previous methods of treating these patients with prolonged bed-rest and often high carbohydrate diets are now extremely questionable. Our results showing that the free plasma essential amino acid concentrations were significantly lower in our anorexia nervosa patients would imply there is a marked total body depletion of these amino acids. Since these amino acids are the building blocks for protein synthesis, it may be that such depletion inhibits protein synthesis and the nutritional rehabilitation of these patients unless specific steps are taken as referred to above. It would, therefore, seem appropriate that anorexia nervosa patients should be given a properly formulated protein diet, that the exact intake is shown at any specific time and that the patient is on a fully balanced dietary intake. By this method we have shown it is possible to return such patients to full nutritional status safely in the shortest possible time with minimal complications either medically or psychiatrically.

## References


Baker, L., Lyen, K.R. (1982). Anorexia nervosa. *Current Concepts Nutr.*, **11**, 139–49.

Beaumont, P.J.V., Chambers, T.L., Rouse, L. and Abraham, S.F. (1981). The diet composition and nutritional knowledge of patients with anorexia nervosa. *J. Hum. Nutr.*, **35**, 265–73.

Boag, F., Weerakoon, J., Ginsburg, J., Havard, C.W.H., Dandona, P. (1985). Diminished creatinine clearance in anorexia nervosa: reversal with weight gain. *J. Clin. Pathol.*, **38**, 60–63.

Bowers, T.K. and Eckert, E. (1978). Leukopenia in anorexia nervosa. *Arch Intern. Med.*, **138**, 1520–23.

Crisp, A.H. (1965). The significance of some behavioural correlates of weight and carbohydrate intake. *J. Psychosom. Res.*, **11**, 117–31.

Crisp, A.H. (1970). Anorexia nervosa: 'feeding disorder' 'nervous malnutrition', or 'weight phobia'. *Wld Rev. Nutr. Diet.*, **12**, 452–504.

Dinsmore, W.W., Alderdice, J.T., McMaster, D, Adams, C.E.A. and Love, A.H.G. (1985). Zinc absorption in anorexia nervosa. *Lancet.*

Fohlin, L. (1977). Body composition, cardiovascular and renal function in adolescent patients with anorexia nervosa. *Acta Pediatr. Scand.* (Suppl) **268**, 1–20.

Forbes, G.B. (1984). Body composition changes during recovery from anorexia ner-

vosa. Comparison of two dietary regimes. *Am. J. Clin. Nutr.*, **40**, 1137–45.
Isner, J.M., Roberts W.C., Heymsfield, S.B. and Yager, J. (1985). *Ann. Intern. Med.*
Jackson, M.A., Jackson J., Talbot, S.L. and Lee, H.A. (1981) Safe effective enteral nutrition for anorexia nervosa and critically ill patients. *Recent Advances in Clinical Nutrition.*, **1**, 155–7.
Jackson, M.A. Talbot, S. and Lee, H.A. (1987). Plasma amino acid concentrations in anorexia nervosa patients. (1986) (In preparation).
Jackson, M.A., Jackson, J., Talbot, S. and Lee, H.A. (1987). Safe effective enteral refeeding in patients with anorexia nervosa. (In press).
Lefebvre, J. (1980) *Actas Psychiatr. Belg.* 551–6.
Palossy, B., Oo ME: (1977). ECG alterations in anorexia nervosa. *Adv. Cardiol.*, **19**, 280–82.
Pertschuk, M.D., Crosby, L.O. Barot L. and Mullen J.L. (1982) *Am. J. Clin. Nutr.*, 968–72.
Pertschuk, M.D., Crosby, L.O., Mullen, J.L. (1983) Total parenteral nutrition in anorexia nervosa. *Curr. Psych. Ther.*, 207–14.
Pertschuk, M.D., Forster, J., Buzby, G.P. and Mullen, J.L. The treatment of anorexia nervosa with total parenteral nutrition. *Bio. Psychiat.* (In press).
Powers, P.S. Heart failure during treatment of anorexia nervosa (1982). *Am. J. Psychiatry.* 1167–71.
Richards, P. (1975). *Lancet*, **ii**, 207–9.
Reiger, W., Brady, J.P., Weisberg, E. (1978). Haematologic changes in anorexia nervosa. *Am. J. Psychiatr.* **138**, 984–5.
Russell, G.F.M. (1966). Acute dilatation of the stomach in a patient with anorexia nervosa. *Br. J. Psychiat.*, **112**, 203–7.
Russell, G.F.M. (1967) The nutritional disorder in anorexia nervosa. *J. Psychosom. Res.*, **11**, 141–9.
Silverstone, J.T. and Russell, G.F.M. (1967). Gastric 'hunger' contractions in anorexia nervosa. *Br. J. Psychiat.*, **113**, 257–63.
Thurston, J. and Marks, P. (1974) Electrocardiographic abnormalities in patients with anorexia nervosa. *Br. Heart J.*, **36**, 719–23.
Warren, S.E. and Steinberg, S.M. (1979). Acid-base and electrolyte disturbances in anorexia nervosa. *Am. J. Psychiat.*, **135**, 415–18.
Wyatt, R.J., Fareli, M., Berry, P.L. Forristal, J., Maloney, M.J. and West, C.D. (1982). Reduced alternative complement pathway control protein levels in anorexia nervosa: response to parenteral alimentation. *Am. J. Clin. Nutr.* 973–80.
Zalin, A.M. and Lant, A.F. (1984) Anorexia nervosa presenting as reversible hypoglycaemic coma. *J. R. Soc. Med.* 193–5.

# 8 Diabetes mellitus

Harry Keen and Briony Thomas



## Introduction

Diabetes mellitus is one of the oldest diseases known to man and diet has always played a prominent part in its treatment. Before the discovery of insulin, diet represented the only hope for survival for the severe diabetic although ignorance as to how this could be achieved led to a plethora of different remedies being tried, all of which were doomed to ultimate failure. But even in the post-insulin era, dietary treatment of the diabetic has left much to be desired; development of dietary understanding has lagged far behind advances in other aspects of clinical management of the disease. Guided more by unsupported, sometimes erroneous, beliefs rather than by scientific evidence, it is hardly surprising that many of the basic tenets of diabetic philosophy for the last 60 years – in particular the need for carbohydrate restriction – have now been modified, almost reversed.

An attempt has recently been made in Britain to re-evaluate the role that diet can play in the management of diabetes and the way in which dietary principles can best be put into dietary practice. This culminated in the publication of the document 'Dietary Recommendations for Diabetics in the 1980s'

(Nutrition Sub-Committee of the British Diabetic Association, 1982) which it is hoped will lead to better, and more effective, dietary care.

## Aims of dietary treatment

The goals of dietary treatment in diabetes are undisputed. The first aim with diet, as part of the overall therapeutic approach to diabetes, is to procure the relief of symptoms – the excessive thirst, polyuria, lassitude, visual changes, the cramps, neuropathic limb pains, and irritation of the genito-urinary mucocutaneous surfaces so characteristic of untreated diabetes. Even in the absence of overt symptoms, it is now a widely accepted objective that the diabetic diet should assist in the normalization of the metabolic disorder of the disease. Though primarily the reduction of the raised blood sugar, this also includes the normalization of plasma lipids and perhaps also the control of other circulating metabolites and hormones. A further aim, of increasing importance as the life expectation of the diabetic continues to increase, is to try by dietary means to delay the appearance and to minimize the frequency of the 'long-term complications' of diabetes, a rubric which includes major arterial occlusive disease, disruption and obstruction of the microvascular circulation of the retina, kidneys and other tissues, premature and accelerated opacification of the lens of the eye, and demyelination and axonopathy in the peripheral nerves. It is these complications which have come to be the main problem for the clinician.

## Historical perspectives

In order to understand the rationale behind the new dietary recommendations it is helpful to consider the historical evolution of the diabetic diet.

Although diabetes has been recognized for such a long time, it is only comparatively recently that its pathophysiology has been understood and its multiple causation is only now becoming apparent. In particular, the clear clinical differences between the potentially lethal insulin-dependent (ID) form of diabetes and the less immediately threatening non insulin-dependent (NID) form have only comparatively recently come to be recognized as aetiologically distinct entities. Misunderstanding of the nature of the disease inevitably led to erroneous treatment. For centuries it was believed that glycosuria was not just a symptom but the fundamental lesion of diabetes causing the 'melting down of flesh and bones into urine' (Wood and Bierman, 1972). Since urinary glucose loss could not be arrested, it seemed a logical assumption that the best therapeutic measure was to replace the sugars lost to the body with a high carbohydrate diet. The earliest diabetic diets thus comprised foods such as 'honey, autumn fruits and sweet wines' (Wood and Bierman, 1972).

Not until the 18th Century was there any marked deviation from this policy. John Rollo, a surgeon in the British Navy, was the first to advocate carbohydrate avoidance with his diet based almost exclusively on meat and animal fats, preferably of a rotten or rancid nature since in this form they were believed to have anti-diabetic properties (Rollo, 1798).

Rollo's diet, either by dint of ineffectiveness or unpalatability, eventually went out of fashion and the 19th Century saw an abundance of 'diet cures' which ranged from high carbohydrate diets based on skimmed milk or oatmeal (Card, 1937) to low carbohydrate regimen containing 'vegetable thrice boiled to dissolve out their sugar' (Stowers, 1963).

In 1875 a French physician, Bouchardat, made an important discovery although its significance was not fully appreciated at the time. Bouchardat noticed that the mortality of his diabetic patients fell dramatically during the near-starvation conditions caused by the siege of Paris. Subsequently, Bouchardat found that deliberate periods of fasting significantly improved the condition of his patients.

This idea was more scientifically developed by Frederick Allen. In a series of experiments on partially depancreatized dogs, Allen clearly established the survival benefits of fasting. He also showed that dietary carbohydrate loading was specifically detrimental to remaining beta-cell function (Allen *et al.*, 1919). His 'Starvation diet' which he devised for his human diabetics of the severe ID type therefore comprised periods of fasting interspersed at intervals with a very low carbohydrate maintenance diet. This strategy was widely adopted, it was not easy or pleasant to follow but its effectiveness undoubtedly increased the longevity of many diabetics.

The discovery of insulin in 1921 revolutionized the management of diabetes but at the same time the role of diet became confused and uncertain. Compared with the dramatic effects of insulin, the importance of diet appeared to pale into insignificance. The idea that dietary consideration might be very different in the pre- and post-insulin eras was largely overlooked and its use was never properly re-evaluated. Instead Allen's warnings about carbohydrate remained uppermost in people's minds with the result that carbohydrate restriction was to remain the mainstay of dietary treatment for the next half century.

For a while, diabetic diets continued to be extremely low in carbohydrate (10–20 per cent dietary energy) but this soon led to problems of hypoglycaemia and fat-induced ketosis (Allen, 1923). Very gradually, carbohydrate was titrated back into the diet with parsimonious additions for each supplementary unit of insulin. This attitude to dietary carbohydrate was particularly devastating for growth in children and so-called 'diabetic dwarfism' – probably quite distinct from, though often grouped with, the Mauriac syndrome – was the result. As the more robust approach of R.D. Lawrence (1936) 'plenty of carbohydrate, plenty of insulin' gained acceptance, inadequate growth in children became less common and is now more likely to stem from poor diabetic control. This liberal policy was taken to unintended extremes in children by some clinicians who practiced the 'free-diet' philosophy (Lichtenstein, 1938; Guest, 1947) resulting in chaos for the parents and totally unsatisfactory management for the child. In time it was agreed that insulin-treated diabetics should be given 'reasonable' amounts of carbohydrate as part of a balanced dietary regimen, but clinical opinion on both sides of the Atlantic was reluctant to increase its proportion to more than 40 per cent of the daily total food energy, and in some hands it was significantly less (Truswell *et al.*, 1975).

The figure of 40 per cent arose mainly out of convenience; knocking off the zero from the end of the food energy allowance is an easy way of calculating the daily carbohydrate prescription in grams (eg. 1800 calories becomes 180 g carbohydrate; the latter providing 180 × 4 = 720 calories which is 40 per cent of 1800). Over the years it came to be firmly believed that more carbohydrate than this would 'exhaust' the pancreas, be detrimental to glucose tolerance and cause hypertriglyceridaemia (Albrink *et al.*, 1963). No scientific evidence for these views has ever been produced and they have become clinical axioms.

## Re-evaluation

During the 1960s facts began to emerge which gradually eroded the foundations of these traditional dietary beliefs and led eventually to a re-appraisal of the role of diet in diabetic treatment. The necessity for carbohydrate restriction began to be questioned when epidemiologists showed that diabetics living in Asia and Africa, consume a diet containing between 65–85 per cent carbohydrate without apparent harm (Patel *et al.*, 1969; Hirata *et al.*, 1970). Experimental studies confirmed that diabetics of both clinical types can be well controlled on a diet containing a high proportion of its energy in the form of carbohydrate. It was also shown that such diets do not necessarily increase the requirement for injected insulin or the endogenous insulin secretion in those with some residual beta cell function (Stone and Connor, 1963; Brunzell *et al.*, 1971; Simpson *et al.*, 1979a; Simpson *et al.*, 1979b). The body appears to adapt to a raised intake of carbohydrate through enhanced peripheral sensitivity to insulin (Lerner *et al.*, 1971) and increased activity of the glycolytic pathways (Bierman and Nelson, 1975; Wigand *et al.*, 1977). These adaptive mechanisms cannot operate in the absence of insulin, hence the well-documented adverse effect of carbohydrate in the untreated state which gave rise to the belief that carbohydrate was 'bad' for diabetics. When treatment is adequate, carbohydrate metabolism is restored towards that of normal subjects (Brunzell *et al.*, 1974).

Rather than carbohydrate, the dietary factor which appears to be of fundamental relevance to diabetic control is total energy intake. Nutrients are not metabolized in isolation but through a complex network of interrelated and often interdependent pathways where the activity of one may be greatly influenced by the activity in another. Glucose entering the circulation does not emanate solely from carbohydrate consumed. While dietary carbohydrate has a direct effect on the post-prandial glycaemic rise, all calorific nutrients have an influence on gluconeogenic and other mechanisms which determine the fasting and pre-prandial 'background' levels of circulating glucose. It was this effect which accounted for the limited successes of the starvation regime of the pre-insulin era.

The relevance of energy intake to control can most easily be demonstrated in the obese, non-insulin dependent diabetic in whom a reduction in energy intake is followed promptly by a dramatic fall in blood glucose level, the complete 'profile' of background post-prandial levels dropping long before weight reduction with its concomitant decrease in insulin resistance occurs (Weinsier *et al.*, 1974). This effect, often attributed to carbohydrate restriction (Wall *et al.*, 1973) can, in fact, be achieved by restriction of any or all of the calorific nutrients (Ernest *et al.*, 1962).

Until recently, only when obesity is present has much account been taken of dietary energy content (although a nominal recommendation about caloric intake is often made). The normal weight insulin dependent diabetic does not need caloric restriction but it may be no less important that this type of patient consumes an energy intake which matches and does not systematically exceed energy requirement.

It now seems likely that the traditional low carbohydrate diet owed its success or failure as much to the resetting of energy balance as to carbohydrate restriction *per se*. The deterioration in control which accompanies excessive carbohydrate consumption, although in part mediated by post-absorptive hyperglycaemia is also likely to be a non-specific consequence of dietary energy excess. Provided that energy intake and expenditure are in balance, it probably makes little difference to short-term diabetic control whether a diabetic diet contains a low or a high proportion of its energy as carbohydrate though other considerations may be involved (e.g. fats and arterial disease). The type of carbohydrate remains a vital consideration and is discussed below. It is the long-term impressions of high and low carbohydrate intake which have prompted the suggested change in dietary composition.

## Diet and large vessel disease (atherosclerosis)

The major long-term hazard to the Western diabetic is disease of the coronary, cerebral, and peripheral arteries – atherosclerosis. Morbidity and mortality is greatly increased in all types of diabetics whether treated with insulin, oral antidiabetic agents, or 'diet' alone. In the 16-year follow-up of the citizens of Framingham, USA, mortality from arterial disease was two- to four-fold greater in diabetics than in the population as a whole (Garcia *et al.*, 1974). In the careful 10-year follow-up study of male diabetics working for the Du Pont company, Pell and D'Alonzo (1970) found three times more deaths attributable to coronary artery and allied diseases among diabetics than among a matched non-diabetic population in the same firm. Of particular concern is the early age at which death may occur; diabetic men under the age of 34 have a cardiovascular mortality rate 12 times greater than comparable non-diabetics while in women the difference may be as much as 20-fold (Garcia *et al.*, 1974).

Arterial disease is not, however, an inevitable consequence of the diabetic state. In Japan where diabetes is at least as common as in the West, the rate of diabetic deaths ascribed to coronary disease is only one-tenth of that in the US (Goto and Fukuhara, 1968). Among East African black diabetics, Shaper and his colleagues (1962) could not find a single death from coronary disease and were only able to find one fairly certain example of cardiac ischaemia after screening and electrocardiography in over 150 diabetic patients.

These differences cannot be explained in genetic terms alone; the black diabetic living in Africa has much less vascular disease than black diabetics in the United States of America (Shaper *et al.*, 1962). Japanese diabetics who leave Japan for a more Westernized style of life in Hawaii rapidly lose their relative freedom from arterial disease (Kawate *et al.*, 1978). Many environmental changes occur on migration to a Western society but of the three major risk factors for large vessel disease (cigarette smoking, hypertension and serum cholesterol level: Kannel *et al.*, 1971) the biggest difference between Westernized and non-Westernized subjects is in their level of serum cholesterol (Keys *et al.*, 1958). Total serum cholesterol concentration carries strong predictive power for development of cardiovascular disease in normal, glucose intolerant and diabetic subjects (Kannel *et al.*, 1971); Carlson and Bottiger, 1972; Gordon *et al.*, 1974; Keys, 1970; Wilhelmsen *et al.*, 1973; Westlund and Nicolaysen, 1972) independently of the powerful inverse association between serum high density lipoprotein (HDL) cholesterol levels and cardiovascular risk (Gordon *et al.*, 1977). A large part of the Western diabetic's high susceptibility for arterial disease is due to factors which he shares with the Western non-diabetic but there is also a direct relationship between the total serum cholesterol level and the blood glucose level. Strict normoglycaemia is rarely achieved in the diabetic and their average concentrations of serum cholesterol are higher compared with non-diabetics (Hayes, 1972; Lewis, 1976) in part explaining the enhanced susceptibility to atherosclerosis. Dietary measures to minimize or counteract this tendency would therefore be of benefit. The lower serum cholesterol levels and reduced cardiovascular risk of non-Westernized diabetics (and non-diabetics) is probably related to their habitually low fat intake (Kato *et al.*, 1973). Until recently, diabetics in Western countries were given a diet which, by virtue of its carbohydrate restriction, was rich in fat and which was unlikely to lower plasma lipids and could have contributed to their elevation. Now that carbohydrate restriction is no longer seen to be an essential prerequisite for good diabetic control, such a policy can no longer be justified. The new dietary recommendations therefore suggest that diabetics should ideally consume a diet which contains at least 50 per cent of its energy from carbohydrate and no more than 35 per cent of its energy from fat.

## Diet and microvascular disease

Like large vessel disease, microvascular complications contribute heavily to the morbidity and premature mortality of the diabetic. In vessels of capillary proportions, generalized thickening of the basement membrane and progressive diminution in calibre is the characteristic abnormality and is widespread in most organs and tissues of long standing diabetics. In certain organs – the eyes, kidneys, and nerves for example – additional characteristic abnormalities of the microvasculature may develop leading to abnormalities of structure and serious disturbance of function of the areas concerned. Thus in the retinal microcirculation, capillary closure and microaneurysm formation, abnormal vascular permeability to blood constituents, and intraretinal and intravitreal neovascularization lead to gross abnormalities of retinal structure and are a major cause of blindness (Kohner and Dollery, 1975). In the kidney, glomerular capillary changes lead to urinary loss of plasma proteins and to progressive diminution in renal function.

Microvascular disease appears to be primarily associated with the duration and average control of the diabetes (Pirart, 1977) and, by implication, the length and degree of exposure to hyperglycaemia.

The role of diet in reducing the risk of these complications therefore focuses on the attainment and maintenance of near-normoglycaemia. The relevance of total energy intake rather than dietary composition *per se* to basal glycaemia has already been discussed and ensuring that a diabetic diet contains an adequate but not excessive energy content is one important aspect of treatment. The direct effect of dietary carbohydrate on the post-prandial rise in glycaemia is obviously important. Traditionally this has been tackled by the elimination of sucrose and other simple sugars from the diet on the grounds that they are absorbed more rapidly than complex carbohydrates such as starch, and thus produce undesirable peaks of glycaemia. However, experiments have shown that there is little difference between the rate of absorption and glycaemic effect of starch and glucose when given in aqueous solution (Wahlqvist *et al.*, 1978); owing to its fructose moiety, sucrose actually has a less acutely hyperglycaemic effect than either glucose or starch (Thompson *et al.*, 1978). A simple versus complex carbohydrate difference is only seen when the comparisons are made in the form of foods, for example, the effect of a sugar-containing drink with a starchy food such as bread or potato (Wishnofsky and Kane, 1935; Swan *et al.*, 1966). The difference is caused not so much by the effect of the sugar or starch *per se* but by the presence or absence of associated dietary fibre. Dietary fibre is the collective term applied to the non-digested carbohydrates of plant foods. Although a heterogeneous group of substances, dietary fibre has the general effect of delaying the absorption of carbohydrate and flattening the post-prandial glycaemic curve. A mixture of carbohydrate and fibre thus generates a smaller rise in glycaemia than the same type and amount of carbohydrate consumed alone (Jenkins *et al.*, 1976; Haber *et al.*, 1977).

The practical implications of the effects of fibre on glycaemia are considerable. Whether or not a particular carbohydrate food is suitable for a diabetic depends more on its fibre than on its sucrose content. Furthermore, different types of fibre have different effects. It is no longer realistic to propose that equal amounts of carbohydrate from different foods have the same effect on blood sugar (Crapo *et al.*, 1976; Crapo *et al.*, 1977; Jenkins *et al.*, 1980a). Beans in particular appear to have a much smaller glycaemic effect than would be expected on the basis of their carbohydrate content (Jenkins *et al.*, 1980b).

The traditional distinction between sugary and starchy foods still applies to the extent that 'starch' frequently is accompanied by some fibre whereas 'sugars' are often found in a fibre-free form. Avoidance of rapidly absorbed carbohydrate remains an important part of diabetic management. However, the over-zealous preoccupation with sucrose gave rise to many anomalies in dietary advice. Patients were told not to add sugar to drinks yet were encouraged to consume fruit juice, a fibre-free mixture of sugars and water. Desserts containing added sucrose were forbidden but those based on cornflour and milk considered suitable, despite the fact that they comprised mainly rapidly absorbed carbohydrate. Conversely, emerging evidence about the role of fibre suggests that small amounts of sucrose consumed with fibre-rich products such as wholegrain breakfast cereals or wholemeal bread may have no more (or even less) glycaemic effect than their low-fibre, sugar-free equivalents (Bantle *et al.*, 1983; Lean *et al.*, 1985).

Clearly the relationship between diet and post-prandial glycaemia is far more complex than has previously been supposed. Accompanying nutrients may also affect post-prandial glycaemia; some amino acids induce increased insulin release in patients with some remaining beta cell function (Fajans *et al.*, 1967) while the presence of fat or protein may delay the rate of gastric emptying and carbohydrate absorption (Estrich *et al.*, 1967). Much remains to be learnt about the best dietary formulation to achieve optimal glycaemic levels. Nevertheless it has become clear that a general increase in the fibre content of the diabetic diet is beneficial (Jenkins *et al.*, 1978; Miranda and

Horwitz, 1977; Anderson and Ward, 1978), and trying to ensure that every meal or snack contains at least some fibre is a useful therapeutic objective.

## General dietary considerations

However beneficial a diabetic diet may appear to be in theory, it will be of no practical value if it is not followed. Many studies have shown that compliance with traditional dietary advice is often poor. In a London diabetic clinic, Bloom (1967) found that 15 per cent of 111 diabetics followed their diet 'meticulously', 54 per cent in a general way while 31 per cent observed no dietary restrictions at all. Tunbridge and Wetherill (1970) carried out a more detailed 7-day weighed dietary assessment in 63 diabetics and found that less than one-third had a carbohydrate intake within 10 per cent of that prescribed while a further third deviated from their prescribed regime by more than 30 per cent.

A more recent survey of 218 British diabetics (Thomas, 1981) found a similarly discouraging picture (Table 8.1) and also attempted to uncover some of the reasons for poor compliance. No differences in the level of compliance were found between insulin and non-insulin dependent diabetics or between the sexes. Neither age nor duration of diabetes had any discernible effect. There was no evidence to suggest that cost was relevant; the poor compliers spent significantly more on their diet than those who followed their diet closely.

Inadequate dietary education appeared to be a likely factor in some. Dietary knowledge was unimpressive. The majority of patients knew how much carbohydrate they had been prescribed in total for each day, but few could account for how it should be distributed through the day or could be translated in terms of food. There was a clear association between lack of knowledge and lack of compliance, but this relationship may to some extent be consequential rather than causal – a person who does not bother to follow the recommended diet may forget what it should be. But even among patients who appeared to believe that they followed their diet closely, 10 per cent did not possess sufficient correct knowledge to be able to do so (other than by chance) and a further 30 per cent were making significant errors in its interpretation.

Table 8.1 Dietary compliance of 218 British diabetic adults (Thomas, 1981)

| Level of compliance | Insulin treated diabetics | Non-insulin dependent diabetics On oral hypoglycaemic drugs | On diet alone |
|---|---|---|---|
| | n = 145 | n = 55 | n = 18 |
| 'Close' (±15 % prescribed diet) | 29 % | 38 % | 28 % |
| 'Moderate' (±16–30 % prescribed diet) | 27 % | 18 % | 28 % |
| 'Poor' (>30 % prescribed diet) | 44 % | 44 % | 44 % |

None of the differences between the groups was statistically significant

Etzwiler (1972) has emphasized the ineffectiveness of a dietary prescription given out of context of a sound educational programme. Yet dietary 'education' often consists of no more than a single counselling session between patient and dietitian (and in clinics without a dietitian, between patient and a clinic nurse), usually conducted at the first visit to a diabetic clinic and hence at a time when the patient is likely to be anxious, confused and least receptive. Systematic dietary follow-up of patients does not occur in all diabetic clinics (Truswell *et al.*, 1975). Sometimes only patients with obvious dietary problems or who have failed to respond to treatment may see a dietitian on a subsequent occasion. Structured programmes of dietary education appear to be rare. Few, if any, clinics attempt to check the patient's understanding and interpretation of the principles of the diet by, for example, direct assessment of what the patient has been eating (Truswell *et al.*, 1975). Better counselling and more regular contact between the patient and his advisers is badly needed.

Lack of motivation can be a factor in non-compliance by some patients. In the above survey, 10 per cent of insulin dependent and 18 per cent of non-insulin dependent patients admitted with little show of concern that they did not bother to follow the prescribed diet. They appeared unconvinced of its importance. It is essential that all patients are told *why* they need to follow a diet as well as *how*. In diabetes where the consequences of non-compliance may be largely asymptomatic and delayed (unlike food allergy for example), explaining and re-emphasizing the reasons for the dietary manipulations are as important as the details of the advice itself.

For the majority of patients, however, inadequate education and insufficient motivation are not wholly responsible for unsatisfactory compliance. Most diabetics know something about their diet and make some effort to follow it. However, they have often been given a diet which is difficult to put into practice. The difficulties involved in changing established eating practices are often under-estimated. Food habits are highly resistant to change because each individual develops a unique eating pattern which is influenced throughout childhood by cultural, social and economic circumstances and in adulthood by occupation and lifestyle (Hinkle, 1962; Yudkin and McKenzie, 1964). To stand any chance of long-term success a prescribed diet must work with, rather than against, established eating habits. Yet in practice this rarely happens (Thomas *et al.*, 1974). In many diabetic clinics, dietary advice consists mainly of a standardized menu presented to all patients and which may reflect a lifestyle totally at variance with that of a particular individual. Such standard diet sheets usually assume that a cooked breakfast, 2 cooked main meals and afternoon tea are the norm whereas in fact this style of eating is nowadays unusual and unrealistic for most people. Little attention may be paid to the different dietary patterns of, for example, the shift worker, the travelling businessman, the working mother or those on a limited income, or the different types of foods or meals which may be consumed – canteen or restaurant meals, packed lunches or convenience foods.

Diet sheets may be accompanied by unimaginative exchange lists which offer little scope for variation. Many adopt a negative approach to the advice given with a long list of 'forbidden' foods which appears to encompass almost everything and a 'permitted' list limited to items such as salt, pepper, vinegar and diabetic squash. To compound the problem, the diet sheet itself may be badly presented and poorly reproduced so that it is uninteresting to read, difficult to understand, and perhaps also inconvenient to carry around.

Constructing individualized advice for every patient is of course a time-consuming exercise. A diet history is needed so that customary eating habits can be ascertained and then adapted into a regimen compatible with both the patient and the diabetic treatment. Adequate follow-up is essential in the early stages; it may take months to find a diet which is both effective and acceptable. Diabetic clinics must have adequate numbers of trained dietitians to do this and, moreover, to ensure that their skills are fully utilized. Dietitians should be closely involved with individualized diabetic diet formulation rather just interpreting an arbitrarily determined often standard dietary prescription.

Individualized advice initially requires a greater investment in time and manpower but will ultimately yield greater dividends in terms of better compliance and patient care. Giving advice which is not followed wastes everyone's time.

## Diabetic diet construction

### Energy intake

The first step in constructing a diabetic diet is to assess the dietary energy requirement (in either kilocalories or kilojoules). In the past this has been done by reference to tables of average energy needs according to age, sex and occupation. But this approach can no longer be considered adequate. Individual energy needs vary widely from the 'average' (Widdowson, 1962) and some individual assessment is essential. This can most easily be done by means of dietary enquiry. In a person of stable weight, habitual energy intake will equal energy output and therefore give a good guide to energy requirement. The overweight patient will of course need an energy prescription which is less than requirement.

Ideally then, a diabetic should spend time with a dietitian to assess the appropriate level of energy for the physician to prescribe. At the same time, the dietitian will gather valuable information about the patient's normal eating habits, the basis for prescriptive dietary modification.

### Fat intake

With the aim of reducing arterial disease risk, the proportion of fat in the diet should be reduced. Ideally, fat should comprise no more than 35 per cent of the total energy intake but this target will not be achieved by everyone and individual judgement is required in setting a realistic target.

Fat intake should be reduced primarily at the expense of foods rich in saturated fatty acids; suggestions for this are summarized in Table 8.2.

Supplementation with polyunsaturated fatty acids is not specifically recommended. Reduction in total fat intake is more effective in lowering serum cholesterol (Keys *et al.*, 1965). Diets rich in polyunsaturates can increase the incidence of cholelithiasis and gallstones (Sturdevant *et al.*, 1973) and a link between consumption of trans-isomers (present in some polyunsaturated

Table 8.2 Ways in which fat intake can be reduced

| *Reduce consumption of:* | *Replace with:* |
|---|---|
| Full-cream milk | Semi-skimmed or skimmed milk |
| Butter, hard and soft margarines, dripping, suet, lard | Low-fat spread (e.g. St Ivel 'Gold') |
| Full-fat dairy produce (such as most cheeses and cream) | Low-fat dairy produce (such as yogurt, cottage or curd cheese) |
| Beef, lamb, pork and avoid obvious meat fat | Chicken, turkey, fish, eggs, liver and kidneys |
| Fried food | Grilled, baked, boiled, or braised food instead. Alternatively, fry in a non-stick pan without added fat |
| 'Hidden' sources of in manufactured meat products e.g. meat pies, sausages, beefburgers, Scotch eggs | More fresh foods or home-made dishes |

margarines) and some forms of cancer has been suggested (Enig *et al.*, 1978). However, a moderate inclusion of polyunsaturated fats and oils is a better alternative than a return to more saturated alternatives.

## Carbohydrate

If fat intake is reduced, then increased carbohydrate intake can replace it to meet energy needs. At least half of the dietary energy content should be consumed in the form of carbohydrate.

Most should be eaten in the form of polysaccharides (i.e. starch) in foods rich in fibre. Isolated sources of rapidly-absorbed mono- and disaccharides (sweets, chocolate, sugar-containing drinks etc.) should be excluded from the diet except in cases of illness or hypoglycaemic emergency. Refined (i.e. fibre-free) starch-based foods should be used sparingly.

Strategies to achieve these objectives are summarized in Table 8.3.

Dietary carbohydrate must clearly be in balance with the hypoglycaemic effect of a patient's prescribed insulin or, to a lesser extent, oral drugs. The timing and quantity of carbohydrate intake are therefore important aspects of treatment for such patients. In practice, this means that some sort of carbohydrate exchange list will be required.

## Protein

Protein intake must obviously be adequate to sustain growth and replacement needs but there is no evidence to suggest that, under conditions of reasonable metabolic control, the diabetic's needs are either greater or less than those of non-diabetics. There may be a case for an increased protein intake for a short period following commencement of insulin treatment in newly diagnosed diabetics if tissue losses have been severe during the pre-diagnostic period. Severe diabetic ketoacidosis will also be accompanied by marked nitrogen losses (as much as 100 g protein per hour, Pollack, 1953) and protein supplementation may be needed during the recovery phase.

Specific consideration of protein quantity and quality may be required as a

Table 8.3 Improving the type of carbohydrate in the diabetic diet

| | Most suitable carbohydrate | Intermediate carbohydrate | Least suitable carbohydrate |
|---|---|---|---|
| *Breakfast cereals* | All-bran, Weetabix, Puffed Wheat, Shredded Wheat, Unsweetened muesli. | Porridge, cornflakes, Rice Krispies, Special K, Grapenuts, Sweetened muesli. | Sugar-coated cereals, (e.g. Sugar Ricicles). |
| *Flour, bread* | Wholemeal flour, wholemeal bread, pastry made with wholemeal flour, rye crispbread. | White flour, white or brown bread, pastry made with white flour. | Cornflour, custard powder, arrowroot. |
| *Rice, pasta* | Brown rice, brown spaghetti, brown macaroni. | White rice, white spaghetti, white macaroni. | Semolina, sago, tapioca. |
| *Fruit* | All raw fruit, all dried fruit, all cooked fruit if sweetened with an artificial sweetener, all fruit canned in natural juices. | Unsweetened fruit juices. | Sweetened fruit juices, fruit cooked with sugar, fruit pie fillings, fruit canned in syrup. |
| *Vegetables* | All vegetables and especially beans. | | |
| *Milk products* | Semi-skimmed or skimmed milk, natural yogurt. | Full-cream milk, flavoured yogurt, evaporated milk. | Condensed milk. |
| *Cakes, biscuits, snack foods* | Wholemeal or bran-biscuits, digestive biscuits. | Plain biscuits, cakes made with wholemeal flour, fruit cakes, crisps, peanuts. | Sweet biscuits, sugary cakes. |
| *Sugar and sweet foods* | | | Sugar, jams, marmalades, honey, treacle, syrup, sugar-containing drinks, sweets, chocolate. |

consequence of impaired renal function to which the long-term diabetic is especially susceptible. A more recent consideration has been the question of protein restriction in diabetics early in the phase of renal failure which may occur in up to one in three youthful onset patients. There is increasing evidence that the rate at which renal function declines, measured by progressive fall in glomerular filtration rate, can be slowed by dietary protein (and phosphorus) restriction. This is not to be confused with the treatment given to relieve symptoms in near-end stage renal failure; indeed, now that it appears possible to identify the 'subset' of insulin-dependent diabetics more susceptible to long-term diabetic renal failure by the presence of microalbuminuria (Viberti *et al.*, 1982), some thought (and experimental effort) should be directed to prophylactic lowered protein diets in such cases. However, this is as yet unestablished and requires verification before systematic application in practice.

## Alcohol

In general, there is no reason why diabetics should not consume modest amounts of alcohol if they so wish. There are, however, a few safeguards which should be observed.

Alcohol is a rich source of energy (providing 7 kilocalories per gram) and one small measure of spirits will provide 70–100 kcals. Beers and lagers provide significant quantities of carbohydrate as well. Frequent or heavy drinking upsets the energy and carbohydrate balance of the diet and hence diabetic control. The so-called diabetic beers and lagers have a reduced carbohydrate content but may have an excessively high alcohol and hence calorie content. Products reduced in both alcohol and carbohydrate (designed primarily for slimmers) may, however, be useful.

The insulin dependent diabetic has special problems with alcohol. It has a hypoglycaemic effect and can potentiate the action of insulin. They should beware of alcohol in the fasting state (the dangerous cocktail hour) and should safeguard themselves against nocturnal hypoglycaemia with an extra carbohydrate snack at bedtime after an alcoholic evening. Insulin-taking diabetics should never be tempted to drink and drive even if they are within the safe legal limit to do so; should a hypoglycaemic attack occur while the breath smells of alcohol, a diabetic may mistakenly be arrested for drunken driving instead of receiving the necessary medical help.

Chlorpropamide, the oral antidiabetic agent widely used to treat non-insulin dependent diabetes may interact with alcohol to produce an antabuse-like effect with flushing, palpitations and chest tightness (Podgainy and Bressler, 1968). These symptoms are harmless but unpleasant and the only remedy is a change of tablets or avoidance of alcohol.

Diabetics trying to lose weight should avoid alcohol because it is such a rich source of calories. Sugar-free or low-calorie soft or fizzy drinks (eg. 'Slimline' tonic water) are better and socially acceptable alternatives. There is some evidence that regular fairly heavy drinking may contribute to hypertension in non-diabetics and no reason to suppose the diabetic to be immune.

## Non-calorific nutrients

### Vitamins

Vitamin requirements in stable diabetics differ little from those of non-diabetic subjects.

Deficiencies of the water-soluble vitamins (B group, and C) can arise in a poorly controlled patient with excessive or prolonged polyuria especially if associated with an inadequate diet. During the recovery phase from ketoacidosis the abrupt change in metabolic fuel from fat and protein to glucose as insulin takes effect provokes an increased requirement for B vitamins (particularly thiamin, riboflavin and nicotinic acid) and suitable supplements, either oral or parenteral, should be provided.

## Minerals, electrolytes and trace elements

In cases of poor control and prolonged ketoacidosis, urinary losses of cations such as sodium, potassium, calcium, magnesium and zinc can be severe and require remedial treatment replacement but in general the diabetic has no special requirement.

Attention should be given to the possibility that a habitually high intake of sodium may contribute to the development of raised arterial blood pressure in genetically predisposed individuals (Prior *et al.*, 1968; Page *et al.*, 1974; Borst and Borst, 1963). A typical Western diet contains sodium far in excess of physiological need (Dahl, 1972); diabetics as a group are particularly at risk from the development of hypertension and might with prudence avoid a high sodium intake. The traditional low carbohydrate diabetic diet tended to result in a higher than average sodium intake by virtue of its reliance on salt-rich foods such as ham, cheese and other dairy produce (Thomas, 1982). This should be less likely to happen with the types of foods which the diabetic on a higher carbohydrate diet is encouraged to consume though sodium will increase with increased intake of bread.

## Substitute sweeteners

There are two distinct groups of sweeteners which can be used as substitutes for sugar by diabetics.

*Artificial sweeteners* such as saccharin or aspartame are non-toxic chemical compounds which happen to have a very sweet taste. They are many hundred times more sweet than sugar and so are only required in minute quantities. They contain no calories or carbohydrate and can be consumed freely by diabetics.

Until recently, saccharin was the only artificial sweetener permitted in this country and is the one most widely used. It is available in either tablet or liquid form, the latter being convenient for sweetening semi-solid foods such as breakfast cereals, custards or milk puddings. Saccharin has the disadvantage of producing a bitter after-taste which becomes particularly pronounced if heated. It must never therefore be added to boiling liquids or to foods before they are cooked.

Aspartame (sold under the name of Canderel) is a newcomer to the market and may in time supplant saccharine since it appears to be without a bitter after-taste.

Several other potential artificial sweeteners are currently undergoing safety evaluation and may in time increase the choice available.

*Sugar substitutes* such as sorbitol and fructose are the second type of sweeteners. Sorbitol is a 6-carbon polyalcohol which has a slow rate of passive absorption from the gut and is oxidized by the liver to fructose. Fructose is a monosaccharide, 80–90 per cent of which is actively absorbed and the remainder converted to glucose in the gut wall. Of the two, fructose is probably more useful than sorbitol. It has a more acceptable taste and, because it is one and a half times sweeter than sugar (sorbitol is only half as sweet as sugar), so less fructose is needed.

Their usefulness lies in the fact that they can supply many of the properties of sugar in addition to sweetness. Unlike saccharin and other artificial sweeteners, sorbitol and fructose can add structure and texture to baked products (such as cakes) and have preserving properties (such as in jams).

Large quantities of sorbitol and fructose can cause nausea and diarrhoea so that their intake should be limited to a maximum of 50 grams per day (including amounts consumed via diabetic foods). They should never be used 'neat', for example for sweetening drinks or sprinkled on breakfast cereals.

Sorbitol and fructose can enter tissues and be metabolized as far as trioses by the glycolytic pathway independently of insulin so they do not directly affect post-prandial glycaemia and insulinaemia. They do, however, provide energy (4 calories per gram, the same as sugar) and hence may affect long-term diabetic control if their intake is substantial. Their energy content also makes them unsuitable for diabetics who are trying to lose weight.

Large amounts of sorbitol or fructose can have undersirable effects on plasma lipids (Pelkonen *et al.*, 1972) and on serum lactate and uric acid levels (Talbot and Fisher, 1978). They can also make diabetic control worse if the diabetes is unstable or temporarily poorly controlled (e.g. during illness) and in these circumstances should be avoided.

Diabetics should be wary of the many so-called 'slimmer's sugars' on the market. A few of these 'sugars' which contain maltodextrin or lactose could be used by diabetics although they are only designed to be used for sweetening drinks such as tea and coffee and so have no real advantage over saccharine or aspartame. Many of these preparations consist of a mixture of sucrose and saccharine and hence are not suitable for diabetics.

## Diabetic foods

Many diabetics are under the misapprehension that diabetic foods are a *necessary* part of their diet; some believe they have a specific anti-diabetic effect and most assume them to contain less energy than the conventional product and thus to be useful for slimming purposes (Thomas, 1982). This defective appreciation of their nature and value is perhaps one of the most serious objections to their existence.

Diabetic products which contain sorbitol or fructose tend to be expensive, are not always well-liked and although reduced in carbohydrate will usually contain as much energy as the product they replace and sometimes even more! They also have all the attendant disadvantages of sorbitol or fructose intake (see previous section).

Diabetic foods which only contain a non-calorific sweetener such as saccharine (e.g. squash) and those lacking any added sweetener (e.g. fruit canned in natural juices) can be useful. An increasing number of 'low-calorie' foods and drinks are now available, designed primarily for slimmers but which can safely be used by diabetics as well.

A summary of the types of diabetic products available, and their usefulness, is shown in Table 8.4.

Table 8.4 Diabetic speciality foods

| Diabetic food | Sweetening agent | Suitable for diabetic slimmers | Acceptability | General comments |
|---|---|---|---|---|
| Jams, marmalades, preserves | Sorbitol or fructose | No | High | A reasonable substitute |
| Chocolate | Sorbitol or fructose | No | Debatable | May be very high in saturated fat and calories |
| Sweets | Sorbitol, fructose and/ or saccharine | Usually no | Low | Controlled ordinary 'sweets' better, sugar-free gum can be useful |
| Jellies | Sorbitol | No | Moderate | Very dense in consistency |
| Cakes | Sorbitol or fructose | No | High | Not carbohydrate-free, merely CHO reduced (by about 50%) comparatively very expensive |
| Biscuits | Sorbitol or fructose | No | Moderate | Not carbohydrate-free, merely CHO reduced (about 50%). Not always liked |
| Tinned fruit | | | | |
| in water, | — | Yes | Moderate | Useful |
| natural juice or syrup | Sorbitol or fructose | No | High | Expensive |
| Beer | — | No | High | Can have a very high alcohol content – drivers beware! Tend to be expensive |
| Squashes, pops, etc. | Saccharin Aspartame | Yes | High | Generally equivalent in cost and taste to standard product. Useful |
| Proprietary 'slimming' foods | | | | |
| 1. Slimmer's meal substitutes e.g. Limmits biscuits. | | No | | Not suitable for diabetics |
| 2. 'Low calorie' foods | | Yes | Often high | Check label carefully to ensure sugar free |

## Special dietary considerations

### Children

Children with diabetes will, almost without exception, require treatment with insulin. Most are admitted to hospital for initial stabilization and instruction on how to manage their diabetes. Dramatic changes in eating style are undesirable and unnecessary and as far as possible the meal pattern of the diabetic child should resemble, both in composition and timing, the way the child used to eat. The quantity will depend on the age, sex, activity of the child, its precise timing on the type of insulin regimen prescribed and the family dietetic practice. For the first few days of treatment the diet arrangement should be regarded as provisional, checking that the child is neither subject to periods of hunger nor confronted with meals too large to cope with. When a pattern of eating evolves which suits the child, the diabetes, and family life at home, then dietetic instruction can be consolidated. This must primarily involve the mother, but some instruction should be extended to both parents and to the child whose understanding should be as clear as possible. Undue dependence upon parental decision damages growth of independence, a quality to be promoted. Parents should be equipped with a standard carbohydrate exchange list, a proprietary foods exchange list, and diabetic recipe books so that variety can be offered. Sweets, candies, and sugar are better dropped from the diet, but emotional reasons may justify controlled inclusion in the daily schedule. A few sections of chocolate or a small candy bar may be a suitable way for the child to meet the additional carbohydrate needs of periods of greatly increased exertion – e.g. a game of football or hockey – and is a sensible precaution before energetic swimming. The child should recognize early hypoglycaemic symptoms and be instructed to carry and eat sugar lumps or compressed glucose tablets.

School meals may provide problems because few schools will have more than one or two diabetic pupils. The kitchens may co-operate in providing alternatives but the most suitable solution is for the child to take a packed lunch to school containing the correct carbohydrate and calorie content as sandwiches and fresh fruit. Visits by qualified persons to the home can solve many dietary problems and parents should have easy access to a dietitian for advice when necessary.

Children's diets need frequent review to allow for growth. Developing obesity should be checked at least annually; weight reduction is difficult and distressing in children. It is wise to avoid making an issue of food fads to which all children are prone. Adequate substitute foods can usually be found, even glucose drinks, and the phase will pass. More serious is the use of refusal to eat as a weapon in an emotional conflict. This type of behaviour disturbance usually indicates severe emotional stress in the child and should be discussed promptly with suitable experts.

A few paediatricians in this country still believe that any form of dietary restriction for a child is undesirable and advocate the so-called 'free diet'. In practice, this rarely turns out to be so, as disastrous fluctuations in glycaemia usually occur – undesirable for both the child and its parents – and a crude and little understood regime of diet and insulin is often evolved simply to keep the child out of trouble. Further difficulties arise at adolescence when the children switch from paediatrician to adult physician and find it hard to cope with even minimal dietary disciplines necessary to enable them to tackle the business of independent existence, work, and leisure.

Most children will come to accept the disciplines of a diabetic diet if time, patience, and ingenuity are expended in explaining its importance. Much depends upon parental attitudes; parents must tread the difficult path between, on the one hand, anxious, obsessional preoccupation with detail which will provoke guilt and rejection in the child, and carefree *laissez-faire* on the other. Supervised group discussions among parents of diabetic children, organized often by national Diabetic Associations, are a valuable means for achieving this balanced approach.

## Adolescents

Insulin and food requirements often change rapidly at puberty and it may take a long time before stable control is again obtained. Active adolescent boys during their peak growing period may need from 3000 to 4000 kcal/day, and girls 2000 to 3000 kcal/day. Children previously controlled on a single dose of long-acting insulin will almost always now be better managed by two injections a day of short acting preparations to which small quantities of longer acting insulins have been added. It is also a time for emotional problems with rebellion against the restrictions imposed by the diabetes often expressed by rejection of dietary regulation. Sympathetic but firm handling and perceptive advice from doctor and dietitian will usually see the youngster through this period without major catastrophes.

## The 'diet only' diabetic

Diabetics who need neither insulin nor oral hypoglycaemic agents are almost exclusively overweight. Unlike diabetics in the other two categories the timing of carbohydrate intake is irrelevant as there is no risk of drug-induced hypoglycaemia. The total amount of carbohydrate consumed is only of importance as part of the total food energy eaten (except in those individuals with Type IV hyperlipoproteinaemia who may need carbohydrate restricted to as low as 30 per cent calories). The prime aim is food energy restriction and weight reduction. Whether this is achieved by a traditional low carbohydrate diet, or 'Calorie Counting', or any other slimming regimen does not matter as long as it works. All weight reducers need intensive support and advice to achieve their desired objective and few hospital dietetic departments are able (although would like to) supply this attention. Many patients benefit from the group therapy and advice given by slimming clubs.

## Illness

Infections, trauma, and severe emotional stress will usually aggravate the metabolic disturbance of diabetes. The diabetic – even the doctor – may mistakenly think that confinement to bed and reduction in food intake will require less or no insulin. In fact, insulin requirements are often increased in such circumstances. In the absence of normal meals, carbohydrate can be taken by sipping drinks containing 20–30 g of glucose every 3–4 hours. Diet sheets should have instructions to this effect. Prolonged illness, particularly with vomiting and where there is persistent ketonuria, is more safely treated in hospital. Other disorders in diabetics involving specific dietetic measures require joint attention from physician and dietitian.

Planned surgery presents few problems, operations usually being performed with intravenous glucose infusion and short-acting insulin injections based on blood glucose control. Similarly, the postoperative course is managed most safely, until food can be taken, by intravenous glucose infusion and frequent small doses of soluble insulin or even continuous insulin infusion. Eating should restart as soon as possible following recovery from the emergency treatment of diabetic ketoacidosis.

## Pregnancy

The pregnant diabetic like her non-diabetic sister will require adequate protein, vitamins, and minerals together with an appropriate food energy intake. The nausea of early pregnancy may complicate diabetic control but a regimen of small, frequent meals rather than infrequent large ones may help. The fall in renal threshold for glucose may cause considerable urinary glucose losses, up to 70 or 80 g/day, and the ensuing carbohydrate deprivation induces a 'starvation ketonuria'. This misleading combination of glycosuria and ketonuria should clearly not be treated by raising the insulin dose but by increasing carbohydrate intake, conveniently and acceptably taken as an additional 15 g of sucrose three times a day. As pregnancy advances the insulin regimen is often changed to multiple-dose, short-acting preparations and carbohydrate distribution may require a matching adjustment. Redoubled care with dietetic and insulin control, particularly in the last trimester of a diabetic pregnancy, has greatly improved the prospect of a successful outcome.

## Travel

Travelling abroad may present difficulties for the diabetic, especially the newly diagnosed tiro. Air travel time-changes disturb the rhythm of injections and meals, and 'jet lag' may itself add control problems. Some pre-planning of diet and insulin regimen before a flight is very helpful, and frequent urine testing with small supplemental doses of soluble insulin will iron out temporary problems. National Diabetic Associations can usually provide advice and information about unusual foods.

## Immigrant groups

In the mobile world of the late twentieth century, many diabetic clinics have increasing numbers of immigrant diabetics. Their two major problems are unfamiliarity with cultural dietary and medical care patterns, and difficulties in communication. The help of an interpreter is vital. A child in the family may speak English and understand the principles of diet. Asians usually eat carbohydrate far in excess of the traditional British diet, diabetic and otherwise, and it is usually unacceptable to the patient to do more than reduce it to 55–65 per cent of food energy, by replacing some of the daily rice with more suitable vegetables. Limiting ghee (or oil) and fried meals may be required for the obese. High protein intake, though desirable, is expensive and difficult in Hindus who are often completely vegetarian. Muslim diabetics may refuse meat if they suspect that animal slaughter departs from ritual. Dietary instructions should be simple and, for the literates, written in the native language – Hindi, Urdu, Gujerati, Punjabi, or Bengali. Asian and English food equivalents should be listed, e.g. baingan (aubergine), Keke ka phate (green plantain), and moonphali (groundnuts). West Indian immigrants usually have westernized eating habits and but for native foods such as yams and green bananas, may need little special advice. A love of sugar, e.g. five or six teaspoons in tea, is a national characteristic.

## Conclusion

The new dietary recommendations are believed to be a considerable advance in diabetic management in this country. Scientific proof of their benefit based on long-term controlled clinical trials does not, and indeed may never, exist but they have more laboratory evidence and short-term and medium-term clinical trials to support them than any of their predecessors. Nor are they completely untested in practice; the majority of the world's diabetics have managed well on a more extreme version of this diet for decades. It should also be remembered that the new proposals are much in line with the principles of healthy eating, especially for the reduction of atherosclerosis risk, advocated for the whole population. If any sector of the population needs any protection from cardiovascular disease which diet can offer, then it is the atherogenically-at-risk diabetic in whom substantial improvement in prospects for health and longevity can be expected.

Details of the British Diabetic Association's 'Dietary Advice for Diabetics in the 1980s' can be obtained from the British Diabetic Association, 10 Queen Anne Gate, London W1M OBD from whom other dietary information and a list of suitable books on diabetic diet and cooking can also be obtained.

## References

Albrink, M.J., Lavietes, P.H. and Man, E.B. (1963). Vascular disease and serum lipids in diabetes mellitus. *Ann. Intern. Med.*, **58**, 305–23.

Allen, F.M. (1923). Clinical observations with insulin. *J. Metab. Res.*, **3**, 61–176.

Allen, F.M., Stillman, E. and Fitz, R. (1919). *Total Dietary Regulation in the Treatment of Diabetes*. Rockefeller Institute for Medical Research, Monograph no. 11.

Anderson, J.W. and Ward, K. (1978). Long-term effects of high carbohydrate high fibre diets on glucose and lipid metabolism: a preliminary report on patients with diabetes. *Diab. Care.*, **1**, 77–82.

Bantle, J.P., Laine, D.C., Castle, G.W., Thomas, J.W., Hoogwerf, B.J. and Goetz, F.C. (1983). Postprandial glucose and insulin responses to meals containing different carbohydrates in normal and diabetic subjects. *New Engl. J. Med.*, **309**, 7–12.

Bierman, E.L. and Nelson, R. (1975). Carbohydrates, diabetes and blood lipids. *Wld. Rev. Nutr. Diet.*, **22**, 280–87.

Bloom, A. (1967). Relation of the complications of diabetes to the clinical state. *Proc. Roy. Soc. Med.*, **60**, 149–52.

Borst, J.G. and Borst, D.G.A. (1963). Hypertension explained by Starling's theory of circulatory homeostasis. *Lancet*, **i**, 677–82.

Bouchardat, A. (1875). In: *De la Glycosurie ou Diabète Sucré: Son Traitement Hygiénique*, p. 189, Librairie Germer Billiere: Paris.

Brunzell, J.D., Lerner, R.L., Hazzard, W.R., Porte, D. Jr. and Bierman, E.L. (1971). Improved glucose tolerance with high carbohydrate feeding in mild diabetes. *New Engl. J. Med.*, **284**, 521–4.

Brunzell, J.D., Lerner, R.L., Porte, D. and Bierman, E.L. (1974). Effect of a fat-free, high carbohydrate diet on diabetic subjects with fasting hyperglycaemia. *Diabetes*, **23**, 138–42.

Card, W.I., (1937). The effect of different diets on the insulin sensitivity of diabetics. *Clin. Sci.*, **3**, 105–17.

Carlson, L.A. and Bottiger, L.E. (1972). Ischaemic heart disease in relation to fasting values of plasma triglyceride and cholesterol. *Lancet*, **i**, 865–8.

Crapo, P.A., Reaven G. and Olefsky, J. (1976). Plasma glucose and insulin responses to orally administered simple and complex carbohydrates. *Diabetes*, **25**, 741–7.

Crapo, P.A., Reaven, G. and Olefsky, J. (1977). Postprandial plasma glucose-insulin responses to different complex carbohydrates. *Diabetes*, **26**, 1178–83.

Dahl, L.K. (1972). Salt and hypertension. *Am. J. Clin. Nutr.*, **25**, 231–44.

Enig, M.A, Munn, R.J. and Keeney, M. (1978). Dietary fat and cancer trends – a critique. *Fed. Proc.*, **37**, 2215–20.

Ernest, I., Hallgren, B. and Svanborg, A. (1962). Short-term study of different isocaloric diets in diabetes. *Metabolism*, **11**, 912–19.

Estrich, D., Ravnik, A., Schlierf, G., Fukayama, C. and Kinsell, L. (1967). Effects of co-ingestion of fat and protein upon carbohydrate-induced hyperglycaemia. *Diabetes*, **16**, 232–7.

Etzwiler, D.D. (1972). The patient is a member of the medical team. *J. Am. Dietet. Ass.*, **61**, 421–3.

Fajans, S.S., Floyd, J.C. Jr., Knopf, R.F. and Conn, J.W. (1967). Effects of amino acids and proteins on insulin secretion in man. *Rec. Prog. Horm. Res.*, **23**, 617–62.

Garcia, M., McNamara, P., Gordon, T. and Kannel, W.B. (1974). Morbidity and mortality in diabetics in the Framingham population. Sixteen year follow-up study. *Diabetes*, **23**, 105–11.

Gordon, T., Castelli, W.P., Hjortland, M.C., Kannel, W.B. and Dawber, T.R. (1977). High density lipoprotein as a protective factor against coronary heart disease. The Framingham Study. *Am. J. Med.*, **62**, 707–714.

Gordon, T., Kannel, W.B., McGee, D. and Dawber, T.R. (1974). Deaths and coronary attacks in men after giving up cigarette smoking. A report from the Framingham study. *Lancet*, **ii**, 1345–8.

Goto, Y. and Fukuhara, N. (1968). Cause of death in 933 autopsy cases. *J. Jap. Diab. Soc.*, **11**, 197–206.

Guest, G.M. (1947). 'Unrestricted diet' in the treatment of juvenile diabetes. *J. Am. Dietet. Ass.*, **23**, 299–303.

Haber, G.B., Heaton, K.W., Murphy, D. and Burroughs, L.F. (1977). Depletion and disruption of dietary fibre. *Lancet*, **ii**, 679–82.

Hayes, T.M. (1972). Plasma lipoproteins in adult diabetes. *Clin. Endocrin*, **i**, 247–51.

Hinkle, L.E. Jr. (1962). Customs, emotions and behaviour in the dietary treatment of diabetes. *J. Am. Dietet, Ass.*, **41**, 341–4.

Hirata, Y., Nakamura, Y. and Kaku, M. (1970). Characteristics of the treatment of diabetics in Japan. In *Diabetes Mellitus in Asia*, pp. 216–20. Eds. Tsuji, S. and Wada, M. Excerpta Medica: Amsterdam.

Jenkins, D.J.A., Goff, D.V., Leeds, A.R., Alberti, K.G.M.M., Wolever, T.M.S.,

Garsull, M.A. and Hockaday, T.D.R. (1976). Unabsorbable carbohydrates and diabetes: decreased postprandial hyperglycaemia. *Lancet*, **ii**, 172–4.

Jenkins D.J.A., Wolever, T.M.S., Taylor, R.H., Barker, H.M., and Fielden, H. (1980b). Exceptionally low blood glucose response to dried beans: comparison with other foods. *Br. Med. J.*, **281**, 578–81.

Jenkins, D.J.A., Wolever, T.M.S., Nineham, R., Taylor, R., Metz, G.L., Bacon, S. and Hockaday, T.D.R. (1978). Guar crispbread in the diabetic diet. *Br. Med. J.*, **2**, 1744–6.

Jenkins, D.J.A, Wolever, T.M.S., Taylor, R.H., Ghafari, H., Jenkins, A.L., Barker, H. and Jenkins, M.J.A. (1980a). Rate of digestion of foods and postprandial glycaemia in normal and diabetic subjects. *Br. Med. J.*, **281**, 14–17.

Kannel, W.B., Castelli, W.P., Gordon, T., and McNamara, P.M. (1971). Serum cholesterol, lipoproteins and risk of coronary heart disease: the Framingham Study. *Ann. Intern. Med.*, **74**, 1–12.

Kato, H., Tillotson, J., Nichaman, M.Z., Rhoads, G.G. and Hamilton, H.B. (1973). Epidemiologic studies of coronary heart disease and stroke in Japanese men living in Japan, Hawaii and California: Serum lipids and diet. *Am. J. Epidemiol.*, **97**, 372–85.

Kawate, R., Miyanishi, M., Yamakido, M. and Nishimoto, Y. (1978). Preliminary studies of the prevalence and mortality of diabetes mellitus in Japanese in Japan and on the island of Hawaii. *Adv. Metab. Dis.*, **9**, 201–24.

Keys, A. (1970). *Coronary Heart Disease in Seven Countries*. American Heart Association Monograph no 29. New York.

Keys, A., Anderson, J.T. and Grande, F. (1965). Serum cholesterol response to changes in diet. I. lodine value of dietary fat versus 2S-P. *Metabolism*, **14**, 747–58.

Keys, A., Kimura, N., Kusukawa, A., Bronte-Stewart, B., Larsen, N. and Keys, M.H. (1958). Lessons from serum cholesterol studies in Japan, Hawaii and Los Angeles. *Ann. Intern. Med.*, **48**, 83–94.

Kohner, E.M. and Dollery, C.T. (1975). Diabetic retinopathy. In: *Complications of Diabetes*, pp. 7–98. Ed. Keen, H. and Jarrett, R.J. Edward Arnold: London.

Lawrence, R.D. (1936). In *The Diabetic Life*, 9th ed. Churchill Livingstone: London.

Lean, M.E.J., Tennison, B.R. and Williams, D.R.R. (1985). Glycaemic effect of bread and marmalade in insulin dependent diabetes. *Diabetic Med.*, **2**, 117–20.

Lerner, R.L., Brunzell, J.D., Hazzard, W.R., Porte, D. Jr. and Bierman, E.L. (1971). Mechanism of improved glucose tolerance on high carbohydrate diets in normals and diabetics (abstract). *Diabetes*, **20**, 342–3.

Lewis, B. (1976). In *The Hyperlipidaemias: Clinical and Laboratory Practice*, p. 294. Blackwells: Oxford.

Lichtenstein, A. (1938). Free diet in children with diabetes. *J. Paediatr.*, **12**, 183–7.

Miranda, P.M. and Horwitz, D.L. (1977). The effect of dietary fibre content on plasma glucose levels in diabetes. *Diabetes*, **26**, (Suppl. 1), 356.

Nutrition Sub-Committee of the British Diabetic Association. (1982). Dietary recommendations for diabetics for the 1980s. Reprinted in: *Human Nutrition: Applied Nutrition*, **36A**, 378–94.

Page, L.B., Danion, A. and Moellering, R.L. Jr. (1974). Antecedants of cardiovascular disease in six Solomon Island societies. *Circulation*, **49**, 1132–46.

Patel, J.C., Metha, A.B., Dhirawani, M.K., Juthani, V.J. and Aiyer, L. (1969). High carbohydrate diet in the treatment of diabetes mellitus. *Diabetologia*, **5**, 243–7.

Pelkonen, R., Aro, A. and Nikkila, E.A. (1972). Metabolism effects of dietary fructose in insulin dependent diabetes of adults. *Acta Med. Scand. Suppl.*, **542**, 187–93.

Pell, S. and D' Alonzo, C.A. (1970). Factors associated with long-term survival of diabetics. *J. Am. Med. Ass.*, **214**, 1833–40.

Pirart, J. (1977). Diabete et complications dégéneratives presentation d'une étude prospective portant sur 4400 cas observés entre 1947 et 1973. *Diab. Metab.*, **3**, 97–107.

Podgainy, H. and Bressler, R. (1968). Biochemical basis of the sulphonylurea-induced antabuse syndrome. *Diabetes*, **17**, 679–83.

Pollack, H. (1953). Treatment of diabetic coma. *Diabetes*, **2**, 177–9.

Prior, I.A.M., Evans, J.G., Harvey, H.P.B., Davidson, F. and Lindsey, M. (1968). Sodium intake and blood pressure in two Polynesian populations. *New Engl. J. Med.*, **279**, 515–20.

Rollo, J. (1798). *Cases of the diabetes mellitus*. 2nd ed. Dilly: London.

Shaper, A.G., Lee, K.T., Scott, R.F., Goodale, F. and Thomas, W.A. (1962). Chemico-anatomic studies in the geographic pathology of arteriosclerosis: Comparison of adipose tissue fatty acids and plasma lipids in diabetics from East Africa and the USA with different frequencies of myocardial infarction. *Am. J. Cardiol.*, **10**, 390–99.

Simpson, R.W., Mann, J.I., Eaton, J., Carter, R.D. and Hockaday, T.D.R. (1979b). High-carbohydrate diets and insulin dependent diabetes. *Br. Med. J.*, **2**, 523–5.

Simpson, R.W., Mann, J.I., Eaton, J., Moore, R.A., Carter, R. and Hockaday, T.D.R. (1979a). Improved glucose control in maturity-onset diabetes treated with high-carbohydrate, modified-fat diet. *Br. Med. J.*, **1**, 1753–6.

Stone, D.B. and Connor, W.E. (1963). The prolonged effects of a low-cholesterol high-carbohydrate diet upon the serum lipids in diabetic patients. *Diabetes*, **12**, 127–32.

Stowers, J.M. (1963). Nutrition in diabetes. *Nutr. Abst. Revs.*, **33**, 1–15.

Sturdevant, R.A.L., Pearce, M.L. and Dayton, S. (1973). Increased prevalence of cholelithiasis in men ingesting a serum-cholesterol lowering diet. *New Engl. J. Med.*, **288**, 24–7.

Swan, D.C., Davidson, P. and Albrink, M.J. (1966). Effect of simple and complex carbohydrates on plasma non-esterified fatty acids, plasma sugar and plasma insulin during oral carbohydrate tolerance tests. *Lancet*, **1**, 60–63.

Talbot, J.M. and Fisher, K.D. (1978). The need for special foods and sugar substitutes by individuals with diabetes mellitus. *Diabetes Care*, **1**, 231–40.

Thomas, B.J. (1981). How successful are we at persuading diabetics to follow their diet – and why do we sometimes fail? In *Nutrition and Diabetes*. Eds. Turner, M. and Thomas, B. London: John Libbey.

Thomas, B.J. (1982). Patterns of nutritional intake in diabetics and non-diabetics: relationships with vascular disease and its pathogenesis. PhD thesis, London University.

Thomas, B.J., Truswell, A.S. and Brown, A.M. (1974). Diabetic diet sheets used in Great Britain. *Nutrition*, Lond. **28**, 297–312.

Thompson, R.G., Hayford, J.T. and Danney, M.M. (1978). Glucose and insulin responses to diet. *Diabetes*, **27**, 1020–26.

Truswell, A.S., Thomas, B.J. and Brown, A.M. (1975). Survey of dietary policy and management in British diabetic clinics. *Br. Med. J.* **2**, 7–11.

Tunbridge, R. and Wetherill, J.H. (1970). Reliability and cost of diabetic diets. *Br. Med. J.* **2**, 78–80.

Viberti, G-C. Hill, R.D., Jarrett, R.J., Argyropoulos, A., Mahmud, V. and Keen, H. (1982). Microalbuminuria as a predictor of clinical nephropathy in insulin dependent diabetes mellitus. *Lancet*, **2**, 1430–32.

Wahlqvist, M.L., Wilmshurst, E.G., Murton, C.R. and Richardson, E.N. (1978). The effect of chain length on glucose absorption and the related metabolic response. *Am. J. Clin. Nutr.*, **31**, 1998–2001.

Wall, J.R., Pyke, D.A. and Oakley, W.G. (1977). Effect of carbohydrate restriction in obese diabetics: relationship of control to weight loss. *Br. Med. J.*, **1**, 577–8.

Weinsier, R.L., Seeman, A., Herrera, M.G., Assal, J-P., Soeldner, J.S. and Gleason, R.E. (1974). High and low carbohydrate diets in diabetes mellitus – study of effects on diabetic control, insulin secretion and blood lipids. *Ann. Intern. Med.*, **80**, 332–41.

Westlund, K. and Nicolaysen, K. (1972). Ten-year mortality and morbidity related to serum cholesterol. *Scand. J. Lab. Invest.*, **30** (Suppl 127), 1–54.

Widdowson, E.M. (1962). Nutritional individuality. *Proc. Nutr. Soc.*, **21**, 121–8.
Wigand, J.P., Anderson, J.W., Jennings, S.S. and Blackard, W.G. (1977). Effect of dietary composition on insulin receptors in normal subjects. *Am. J. Clin. Nutr.*, **32**, 6–9.
Wilhemsen, L., Wedd, H. and Tibblin, G. (1973). Multivariate analysis of risk factors for coronary heart disease. *Circulation*, **43**, 950–58.
Wishnofsky, M. and Kane, A.P. (1935). The effect of equivalent amounts of dextrose and starch on glycaemia and glycosuria in diabetics. *Am. J. Med. Sci.*, **189**, 545–50.
Wood, F.C. Jr. and Bierman, E.L. (1972). New concepts in diabetic dietetics. *Nutr. Today*, May/June, 4–12.
Yudkin, J. and McZenize, J.C. (1964). In *Changing Food Habits*, Macgibbon and Kee: London.

# 9 Diet in the management of cardiovascular disease

Harry A. Lee and John W.T. Dickerson



## Introduction

Cardiovascular disease (CVD) is the commonest cause of death in men aged 35–55 years of age. In 1970–71 CVD accounted for 9.1 per cent of in-patient days in the National Health Service (NHS) a proportion that was exceeded only by psychiatric disease (Black and Pole, 1975).

A number of factors are thought to be involved in the aetiology of vascular disease. Although this chapter will concentrate on diet as a risk factor and in particular as a risk factor in coronary heart disease (CHD) it is recognized that cardiovascular disease is undoubtedly multifactorial in its aetiology. It is only by recognition of this and the inclusion of any other known factors that any programme aimed to prevent, arrest or cause regression of the disease will stand any chance of success. Such programmes should therefore be incorporated in a pattern of healthy living (Morris *et al.*, 1977). CVD includes the lesions of coronary and cerebral arteries and also those of leg arteries and veins, whereas CHD includes three distinct but overlapping syndromes in middle age: myocardial infarction, angina pectoris and sudden death. Virtually all CHD results from severe atherosclerosis, but all individuals with atherosclerosis do not develop CHD.

Atherosclerosis is characterized histologically by the deposition on the intima of the vessel wall of a plaque which has a complex structure. An outer fibrous cap consisting of muscle cells, collagen and lipids, overlies a necrotic core containing cell debris, cholesterol and calcium. Regression of atherosclerosis involves dismantling this structure and the exact sequence of events leading to regression is not known. Deposition of the plaque results in narrowing of the lumen and myocardial infarction (MI) involving death of heart muscle, occurs when blood flow to the muscle is prevented by a thrombus blocking the coronary arteries. A similar process can occur in the peripheral and intestinal circulation and result in intermittent claudication and gangrene. Since the first sign of coronary disease may be infarction and sudden death before any effective therapeutic measures can be administered, it is clear that primary prevention is the only way in which the disease can be conquered.

## The lipids of atherosclerotic plaques

Cholesterol, and particularly its ester, is the predominant lipid that accumulates during plaque formation (Smith, 1965). The proportion of ester in the plaque increases during the development of the lesion (Smith *et al.*, 1967) and so, too, does that of phospholipids, but triglycerides are always present in only small amounts.

The lipids are derived primarily from the circulation, but there is also some local synthesis within the arterial wall. Active glycolysis occurs, generating $\alpha$-glycerophosphate for the synthesis of glycerides from fatty acids (Opie, 1973). High activity of the pentose pathway in arterial tissue also provides intermediates necessary for the *de novo* synthesis of glycerides. There is little evidence of cholesterol synthesis in arterial tissue and the major proportion comes from the plasma (Zilversmit, 1968; Lofland and Clarkson, 1970).

Perhaps the most important cause of cholesterol accumulation in arterial wall is the inability of the tissue to significantly metabolize the sterol, apart from some minor degradation and the formation of esters. All these compounds, because of their hydrophobic nature, induce sclerosis. Only about 20 per cent of the cholesterol ester in atheroma is produced by local synthesis, but the ester principally produced, cholesterol oleate (Bowyer *et al.*, 1968), is strongly sclerogenic (Abdulla *et al.*, 1967).

Ischaemia of the arterial wall may play a role in the deposition of lipids. Normally, the inner two-thirds of large human vessels is nourished directly from the lumen while the outer third is nourished by the vasa vasorum in the tunica adventitia (Kirk and Laursen, 1955). Thickening of the tunica intima in the aorta results in ischaemia of the tunica media and the effect of this is to impede the outflow of cholesterol from the endothelium through the tunica media and so promote accumulation of cholesterol in the tunica intima, as is seen in atherosclerosis.

## Diet as a risk factor in cardiovascular disease

There is now considerable epidemiological evidence that a number of dietary characteristics may be risk factors for CHD and that others may also be relevant to the condition (DHSS, 1974). There has been considerable discussion as to whether CHD is solely due to lipid changes and lipids in the diet, or whether it is related to sucrose, hard water, other facets of the diet, stress factors, genetics, or indeed smoking. Our aim in this chapter is not to try and define one factor that is pre-eminent but to define factors which can be modified by altered dietary intakes. Epidemiological studies have resulted in the identification of three major CHD risk factors – hyperlipidaemia (particularly hypercholesterolaemia) and hyperlipoproteinaemia, hypertension and cigarette smoking, which are amenable to preventative measures. The present discussion will be restricted largely to these topics.

## The role of dietary management in atherosclerosis

Evidence of benefit to be derived from the control of dietary factors in respect of atherosclerosis can be derived from experimental studies in animals, epidemiological studies, and primary prevention trials. Further evidence can be derived from the so-called secondary prevention trials that occur in the management of hyperlipidaemia.

### Relationships between lipid and carbohydrate metabolism

In diabetes mellitus, hyperglycaemia and hyperlipidaemia often coexist and the susceptibility of diabetic patients to vascular changes has long been recognized. This has been true even of so-called mild diabetics. Recent population studies, such as the Framingham and the Du Pont Company ones, have shown that there is a two- to three-fold increase in cardiovascular morbidity and mortality in diabetics as compared with non-diabetics. Looking at this metabolic association in a different way, others have found a relationship between raised blood sugar levels and arterial disease when analysing non-diabetic people presenting with coronary artery disease or intermittent claudication. In these studies, a greatly increased frequency of varying degrees of glucose intolerance in arteriosclerotic subjects has been found as compared with suitable controls. In a population study in Bedford (Keen, 1972), the relationship between blood sugar and arterial disease was examined and it was found that there was approximately a two-fold increase of arterial disease in the clearly diabetic group. In this study the groups with different blood sugar levels were reassessed five years later and the relative frequency of new clinical arterial events was four to five times greater in the diabetic group than in the normoglycaemic group. Epidemiological studies such as these show a definite relationship between glucose intolerance and arterial disease and may lead to the conclusion that glucose intolerance is a quantitative risk factor in relation to arterial disease. This does not imply, of course, that the glucose intolerance is the only factor.

It is not yet clear how glucose metabolism and atherogenesis are related, but it may be through the intermediary of a disorder of lipid metabolism. Hyperlipidaemia is a common accompaniment of diabetes. Several of the genetic types of hyperlipoproteinaemia, e.g. Fredrickson types 3 and 4, have an associated impairment of glucose intolerance. In other epidemiological studies the relationship between glucose tolerance and plasma lipid levels has been examined in a normal population sample. A good correlation was noticed in men and women over the age of 45 years between fasting triglycerides and glucose tolerance. This led to the conclusion that across the normal range of glucose tolerance, the higher the fasting triglyceride concentration the greater the area under the glucose tolerance curve, and therefore the greater the degree of glucose intolerance.

A causal relationship between hyperglyceridaemia and atherosclerosis was first suggested by Allbrink and Mann (1959), and more recently Carlson and Bottiger (1972) have clearly shown in a prospective ten-year study that an excess of morbidity and mortality is present in patients with raised triglyceride concentrations. They made the important observation that raised serum triglyceride concentrations had an equally predictive value with a raised blood cholesterol level.

The way in which hyperlipidaemia and glucose intolerance are related is not yet clearly understood. The role of insulin is at present purely speculative. It seems unlikely that the high triglyceride level is an antiinsulin effect, and glucose intolerance is not a feature of chronic fat-induced hyperlipidaemia. However, it has been clearly shown that both hypertriglyceridaemia and hyperglycaemia respond quite rapidly to dietary carbohydrate restriction, and this is the basis of the management of the Fredrickson types 3 and 4 hyperlipidaemias. The changes in triglyceride and glucose levels occur even without associated weight loss though this normally occurs.

To any generalization an exception will occur. It is interesting to note that Japanese diabetics have a remarkably rare incidence of diabetic gangrene and clinical coronary disease. Post-mortem surveys have further supported this observation by showing a marked diminution in the representation of coronary disease as a cause of death in Japanese diabetics e.g. 5 per cent in Japan as compared with 54 per cent in America. As Keen has pointed out, in assessing these observations, the diabetic is not necessarily doomed to severe atherosclerotic disease, but it may be that his disease in the Western environment makes him more susceptible to some particular atherogenic factor which may not yet be defined.

The role of dietary carbohydrate in producing both hyperglycaemia and hypertriglyceridaemia is not disputed. It should be noted, however, that not only the quantity but also the type of dietary carbohydrate is important when describing induced effects or trying to reverse them. Much has been said, particularly by Yudkin and his colleagues, about the relationship of sucrose to cardiovascular disease. In one of their studies the normal dietary intakes of young men were measured and 200 g of sucrose were exchanged isocalorically with starch. After two weeks of such feeding, significant increases in the concentration of plasma triglycerides were found in all subjects. In about 30 per cent of the subjects there was an increase in body weight, an increase in platelet adhesiveness, and an increase in the plasma concentration of insulin and 11-hydroxycorticosteroids. The persons in whom sucrose produces 'hyperinsulinism' may be those who are susceptible to the action of sucrose in producing CHD (Szanto and Yudkin, 1969). A high concentration of insulin has been shown to stimulate lipogenesis in arterial tissue where it is also known to inhibit lipoprotein-lipase (Stout, 1968), thus increasing deposition of lipid and inhibiting its removal. Similar changes may account for the occurrence of atherosclerosis in diabetes mellitus (Stout, 1968; Opie, 1973) in which there may be further aggravation by osmotic damage in the arterial wall due to conversion of glucose to sorbitol.

Animal experiments give some support to the view that hyperinsulinism in response to sucrose makes the individual susceptible to CHD though there are species differences. For example, in rats sucrose given for 10 weeks produces a fall in serum insulin concentration, whereas in pigs it produces a rise. Again, in rats a rise in plasma triglyceride, and occasionally of cholesterol, concentration occurs, whereas in pigs there is only a transitory rise in these constituents, and in cockerels there is a considerable rise in cholesterol only. Further differences occur inasmuch as sucrose produces hepatomegaly and this may be excessive in cockerels. Sucrose causes some enzyme changes; for example in the rat an increase in fatty acid synthetase, glucose-6-phosphate dehydrogenase and pyruvate kinase occurs in the liver at the same time as there is a decrease in fatty acid synthetase in adipose tissue. These enzyme changes may be induced quite quickly, for example 18 hours after high sucrose feeding, but there is an equally rapid fall in fatty acid synthetase activity and triglyceride levels when sucrose is withdrawn. Sucrose has been shown to produce disease in the arterial wall in rats in which it is associated with an increase in platelet aggregation. Yudkin and his colleagues have shown that sucrose produces an increase in the concentration of lipid in the aortic wall of the rat. They have also shown in cockerels that sucrose can induce aortic atheroma and that the area of atheroma is directly proportional to the level of plasma cholesterol.

Peptic ulceration may be related to CHD and Yudkin has suggested that sucrose is related to peptic ulceration. Some confirmation of this suggestion is derived from the fact that patients with peptic ulcers have improved when put on a low carbohydrate diet, and conversely that a high sucrose diet after two weeks can induce a 20 per cent increase in gastric acidity and a 200 per cent rise in peptic activity.

## Relationships between dietary lipids and plasma lipids

It seems reasonable to suppose that the concentration of lipids, and particularly cholesterol, in the plasma will be related to the deposition of lipid on the vascular intima since, as we have seen, the lipids are mainly derived from the circulation. A number of epidemiological studies have shown a relationship between hypercholesterolaemia and CHD. However, it is critical to establish the level of plasma cholesterol at which persons may be considered to be 'at risk'. The Pooling Project (1978) involved 8274 white men aged 40–64 years and results were stratified according to cholesterol concentration into five categories: < 194, 194–218, 219–240, 241–268 and > 268 mg/d*l*. A total of 647 events were recorded with an excess risk of cholesterol level at cholesterol levels of 219–240 mg/d*l*. It is clear that these are well within 'the normal' limits recorded by clinical biochemistry laboratories which often quote an upper limit of 300 mg/d*l* or more. Thus these levels have no relationship to risk of premature coronary disease (Berkson and Stamler, 1981). The optimal cholesterol level for 30 year olds is probably below 200 mg/d*l*.

Epidemiological studies have also shown a strong relationship between dietary lipid, serum cholesterol and coronary atherosclerosis at autopsy (see

Stamler, 1979). These relationships have been confirmed in prospective studies on living populations. The best known of these is the seven countries study reported by Ancel Keys and his co-workers (Keys, 1970; 1980). Data from population samples in Finland, United States and the Netherlands were compared with those from Japan and the Mediterranean countries (Greece, Yugoslavia and Italy) and showed that fat intake correlated significantly with serum cholesterol levels and with five and ten year incidence and mortality rates from CHD.

Additional evidence for a relationship between diet, blood lipids and mortality rates has come from studies of migrants from low incidence to high incidence countries. In the Ni-hon-San study of Japanese in Japan, Hawaii and California (Kagan *et al.*, 1974), CHD prevalence per one thousand of the population was found to be 25.4, 34.7 and 44.6 respectively. These differences were associated with energy intakes of 2164, 2175 and 2162 kcals per person per day respectively with total fat contributing 15.1 per cent, 33.3 per cent and 37.5 per cent of the energy, and saturated fat contributing less than 6.7 per cent, 11.8 per cent and 13.8 per cent. Intakes of simple carbohydrates were less in Japan with complex carbohydrates and total carbohydrates greater. Similar differences in foods consumed are shown by comparison of the United States and Japan with Italy in Table 9.1. Clearly, compared with America the people in Italy like those in Japan derive most of their energy from the consumption of vegetable foods, fruits, grains and legumes and eat less animal products and refined and processed sweets (Berkson and Stamler, 1981). There has been much emphasis on the protective effects of consuming large amounts of polyunsaturated fatty acids (PUFA) and this is discussed below.

Fractionation of plasma cholesterol into high, low and very low density lipoprotein (termed HDL, LDL and VLDL respectively) adds precision to the prediction of coronary events. Evidence from the Framingham study (Gordon *et al.*, 1977) as well as others (Miller and Miller 1975; Miller *et al.*, 1977;

Table 9.1 Food sources, calories and nutrients available for consumption per person per day in the United States, Italy and Japan 1954–1965 (Modified from Berkson and Stamler, 1981)

| | United States | | Italy | | Japan | |
|---|---|---|---|---|---|---|
| | kcal | % | kcal | % | kcal | % |
| Total energy | 3127 | 100.0 | 2697 | 100.0 | 2226 | 100.0 |
| Dairy, eggs, meats, poultry | | 36.1 | | 14.2 | | 3.7 |
| Fish, shellfish | | 0.7 | | 0.8 | | 3.6 |
| Fruits, vegetables, grains, legumes | | 31.3 | | 62.2 | | 80.1 |
| Oils, nuts | | 5.4 | | 11.9 | | 4.4 |
| Sugar, syrup | | 16.1 | | 8.2 | | 7.2 |
| Total protein | | 12.0 | | 11.7 | | 12.2 |
| Animal protein | | 8.7 | | 4.0 | | 2.9 |
| Total carbohydrate | | 47.6 | | 62.7 | | 76.4 |
| Total fat | | 38.9 | | 25.7 | | 10.1 |
| Saturated fat | | 14.1 | | 7.0 | | 2.0 |
| Polyunsaturated fat | | 4.6 | | 4.3 | | 2.8 |

Avogaro *et al.*, 1979) suggests that a low level of HDL may be predictive of CHD whereas a high level of HDL protects against CHD. These findings have caused a shift in the design of protective measures to an examination of those factors which raise or are associated with high HDL levels. These include female sex (Gordon *et al.*, 1977) exercise (Wood and Heskell, 1979) moderate alcohol drinking (Castelli *et al.*, 1977) and a high intake of ascorbic acid (Horsey *et al.*, 1981). Obesity and high carbohydrate diets have been found to be negatively correlated with HDL levels.

A strong positive correlation has been reported between heart attacks in young men and hypertriglyceridaemia (Carlson and Böttiger, 1972), and this might suggest that triglycerides are strongly atherogenic. However, it has been suggested (Gorringe, 1984) that they are merely the source of free fatty acids (FFA) which have been incriminated in the pathogenesis of acute heart attacks and sudden deaths (Oliver *et al.*, 1968).

## The role of other dietary factors

In a number of different parts of the world the hardness of drinking water has been correlated with cardiovascular mortality (Crawford, 1972; Neri *et al.*, 1972); the softer the water, the higher the death rate. In the UK there is a good correlation between mortality rates and the concentration of calcium in the water. It is possible that the calcium in the water prevents the absorption of toxic elements from pipes and the soil and also that by supplementing dietary calcium it prevents changes in magnesium metabolism. Tissue magnesium concentrations have been found to differ in hard and soft water areas. There is evidence (Seelig and Heggtveit, 1974) that magnesium interrelationships may play a key role in heart disease and therapeutic use of magnesium in acute CHD may be justified.

Serum and tissue cholesterol concentrations in animals are modified by altering the level of dietary ascorbic acid (Ginter *et al.*, 1971). Dietary deficiency of ascorbic acid has been found to produce atheromatous arterial lesions in guinea pigs (Willis, 1953; Willis *et al.*, 1954).

In the guinea pig, ascorbic acid deficiency reduces the conversion of cholesterol to bile salts (Ginter, 1973), the main route of excretion of the sterol.

In addition to the effects on HDL cholesterol already mentioned, extra dietary ascorbic acid reduces serum cholesterol levels in normal people under 25 years (Spittle, 1971) and in hypercholesterolaemic subjects whose initial ascorbic acid status is low (Ginter *et al.*, 1970) but not if the status is normal (Peterson *et al.*, 1975).

Much may well remain to be elucidated about the interaction of various dietary components in changing blood lipid levels and it is essential that the total diet be examined (Kritchevsky, 1976). Data summarized by Kritchevsky suggested that changes in the death rate from CHD parallel changes in the ratio of animal to vegetable protein. Persons who do not consume any food of animal origin (i.e. vegans) have lower serum cholesterol and triglyceride concentrations than age-sex-matched omnivores (Sanders *et al.*, 1978). Vegans also have less adipose tissue and this contains lower concentrations of saturated fatty acids. In the US, Seventh Day Adventists, many of whom are vegetarians, have a lower mortality from CHD than the remainder of the US population.

However, it is not possible to relate the difference in mortality solely to diet since most of them are non-smokers and are somewhat health conscious.

Another feature of a vegetarian, and particularly a vegan diet, is that it contains more 'dietary fibre' and Trowell (1972) suggested that the risk of CHD is inversely related to the amount of vegetable fibre consumed. Dietary fibre consists of a complex mixture of celluloses, hemicelluloses and pectins, and information is only now beginning to emerge on how each of these components affects metabolic processes. However, there is undoubtedly some epidemiological support for Trowell's hypothesis.

Thus, in India, Malhotra (1967) studied paired railroad workers from different parts of the country in which the risk of CHD differed by a factor of 15. This difference did not correlate with the amount of saturated fat in the diet, for workers in Udaipur, the area of lower risk, ate more saturated fat than those in the area of higher risk, Madras. Furthermore, there was no difference in the serum cholesterol concentration in the two areas. The best correlation was with the amount of vegetable fibres in the faeces. Bread can be an important source of dietary fibre, and Morris *et al.*, (1963) reported that bread consumption was related negatively to plasma cholesterol level in bank employees. Morris and his colleagues (Morris *et al.*, 1977) suggested a high intake of complex unrefined carbohydrate as part of their pattern of healthy living. However, attention has been focused on the hypocholesterolaemic effects of fruit and vegetable gels, rather than on wheat fibre (Jenkins *et al.*, 1975; Kay and Truswell 1977).

## Immunological causes

There is little doubt that at least three factors – thrombosis, lipid imbibition, and arteritis – are involved in the pathogenesis of atherosclerosis. Stated another way it is suggested that increase of endothelial permeability due to inflammation may lead to increased lipid entry. A number of experimental findings suggest that immunological mechanisms may be involved in the inflammatory process (Poston and Davies, 1974; Mathews *et al.*, 1974). Thus in the rabbit, atherosclerosis can be inhibited by antiinflammatory and immunosuppressive drugs. Ingestion of antigenic foreign protein exacerbates the atherogenic potential of high lipid diets (Minick *et al.*, 1966; Levy, 1967; Van Winkle and Levy, 1970). An increased incidence of positive skin tests to tobacco leaf protein has been found in patients with CHD who smoked (Harkavy, 1963). This appeared to be an independent risk factor, for the positive groups had a lower incidence of hypertension and hypercholesterolaemia. Absorption of intact protein from the gut is known to occur in normal infants of 1–13 months (Gruskay and Cooke, 1965). Increased levels of circulating milk protein antibodies have been found in patients with CHD (Davies *et al.*, 1969; Davies *et al.*, 1974) and there is epidemiological evidence that denatured or altered milk protein may be atherogenic (Annand, 1967, 1972). Mathews *et al.*, (1974) have postulated an immune-complex mechanism whereby circulating immune complexes could set up a vicious circle of damage to the vessel walls.

## Other factors

Cigarette smoking, heavy alcohol consumption and lack of exercise, all so much characteristic of Western societies, enhance the risk of CHD. All these factors interact with and modify the effects of dietary factors. Another factor, often overlooked and possibly independent of diet, is an individual's behavioural characteristics (Friedman and Rosenman, 1974) which have been described as 'Type A Behaviour'. This behaviour 'can be observed in any person who is aggressively involved in a chronic, incessant struggle to achieve more and more in less and less time, and if necessary against the opposing efforts of other things and other people'.

## The diet of children and atherosclerosis

Early signs of atherosclerosis – fatty streaks – have been reported in the aortas of children and the coronary arteries of most persons aged 20–29 years (Strong and McGill, 1969), and on the basis of these findings it would seem that preventative measures, to be effective, must be started within the first two to three years of life (Lloyd and Wolff, 1969). There is evidence that children, (Glueck *et al.*, 1981) like adults, who consume more saturated fat and less polyunsaturated fat have higher blood levels of cholesterol and lipoproteins. Genetically determined lipid abnormalities should be identified and treated. In their report on the prevention of coronary heart disease the joint working party of the Royal College of Physicians in London and the British Cardiac Society (1976) state that children should not be regarded in isolation from their families and that risk factors that operate in adults may equally operate in children, and similar measures for their control are indicated. It seems that bottle feeding of infants may predispose towards CHD for abnormal coronary arteries are more common in children who have been predominantly bottle fed than in those who have been breast fed. In childhood and adolescence the prevention and control of obesity is important as, too, are the overconsumption of sucrose and prevention of smoking.

# Diet and hypertension

A rise in blood pressure with age is characteristic of Western society and there are prospective epidemiological studies which lead to the conclusion that hypertension is a major risk factor in the development of both heart disease and cerebral vascular disease. There is evidence that a reduction of two to three mm in mean blood pressure as a result of antihypertensive therapy or through weight reduction has a significant effect on mortality (Marmot, 1982). Populations in the world that do not have hypertension are characterized by a lack of obesity, high levels of physical activity, diets low in animal fat, a high dietary intake of potassium and a low intake of sodium. In those at risk of rising blood pressure the tendency begins to appear early in childhood and reaches full expression in middle life.

Of the characteristics of hypertensive populations mentioned above, two seem to be causative. Thus, though the mechanism is not known, body weight and other measures of body mass are strongly correlated with blood pressure in all populations. However, once body weight has risen, and with it blood pressure above the desirable level, it is very difficult to demonstrate a consistent relationship between reduction in body weight and a lowering of blood pressure. This is probably due to the difficulty of maintaining a consistently lower weight. Considerable attention has been given to the sodium intake and more recently the importance of potassium intake in modifying the effect of excess sodium. A reduction in blood pressure on a low salt diet has been demonstrated (Morgan *et al.*, 1978; Skrabal *et al.*, 1981; MacGregor *et al.*, 1982). The estimated average salt intake in Britain is about 12 grammes per day. It seems desirable that this should be reduced to 6 grammes per day or less. A considerable reduction in the present value can be achieved simply by not adding salt in cooking or at the table. Useful discussion of the aspects of more severe reduction in dietary sodium is given by Nelson (1981).

## Diet and thrombogenesis

We have so far considered diet in relation to blood lipids and atherosclerosis. Mild myocardial infarction and sudden death involve the formation of a thrombus and any consideration of diet in relation to CHD must involve factors that may be involved in thrombus formation. Platelet sensitivity can be modified by changing dietary lipids, and dietary supplementation with linoleic acid results in a specific antithrombotic effect (Hornstra *et al.*, 1973). The importance of these effects lies in their relationship to prostaglandin and thromboxane biosynthesis and the relationship of the balance of these to haemostasis (Samuelsson *et al.*, 1976).

Linoleic acid (18:2$\omega$6) and $\alpha$-linolenic acid (18.3$\omega$3) are the most common dietary fatty acids which give rise to the three series of prostaglandins ($PG_1$, $PG_2$, $PG_3$). Linoleic is converted to di-homo-gamma-linolenic acid (DHGLA) which is further converted to arachidonic acid. In platelets, this fatty acid can be converted to thromboxane $A_2$, a powerful promotor of platelet aggregation. Arachidonic acid can also be derived from membrane phospholipids by the action of phospholipases $A_2$. In the vessel wall the major product of metabolism of prostaglandin endoperoxides is the potent anti-aggregant prostaglandin, prostacyclin (Moncada *et al.*, 1976).

Eskimos have a high fat intake and yet have a low incidence of CHD. The reason for this exception to the fat hypothesis for the genesis of CHD is now thought to lie in their consumption as a constituent of fish of a derivitive of $\alpha$-linolenic acid mainly eicosapentaenoic acid. This latter fatty acid is not found in the blood lipids of persons not consuming fish. Eicosapentaenoic acid has anti-aggregatory activity and it has been postulated that it can be converted in the vessel walls to the prostaglandin ($PGi_3$, which has anti-aggregatory properties (Dyerberg *et al.*,1978). The importance of these observations arises in the possibility that the balance between thromboxane synthesis and prostacyclin synthesis can be modified by dietary fatty acids. Another interesting connection with diet is that the activity of the enzyme prostacyclin synthetase which is involved in the conversion of prostaglandin endoperoxides to prostacyclin seems to be stimulated by vitamin E.

## The dietary treatment of hyperlipidaemia

In our discussion of the relationship of diet to CVD we have so far seen that high lipid levels, particularly those of cholesterol and LDL correlate with increased risk of CHD. Moreover, these high blood lipid levels correlate with a high intake of saturated fat, a low intake of polyunsaturated fat and possibly also with a high intake of proteins of animal origin. Furthermore, there is some evidence that elevated plasma levels of HDL diminish the risk of CHD. It is therefore pertinent to enquire whether diet may, whilst causing desirable changes in blood lipid levels, impart some protection against CHD, remembering that this may cause sudden death and therefore not be a treatable disorder. Our emphasis must clearly be on prevention.

It is possible to predict the likely magnitude of blood lipid changes that may follow changes in lipid intakes (Table 9.2). The total decrease in the plasma cholesterol that may reasonably be expected to be achieved by these dietary modifications is about 0.8 mmol/litre, less than half the difference between the values in vegans and omnivores reported by Sanders *et al.*, (1978). Two kinds of prevention trials have been done. 'Primary' prevention trials in which persons who have not had CHD change their diets (or have them changed for them!) and 'secondary' prevention trials in which the dietary changes are made following a myocardial infarct. A number of trials of each sort have been done and some of the important ones are summarized in Tables 9.3 and 9.4. The primary dietary trials involved 3283 men aged 30–64 years over periods of 5 to 8 years. A primary prevention trial using the cholesterol lowering drug, clofibrate, involved 10 627 men aged 30–59 years over a period of 5 years. The results of these trials are not very impressive. Indeed those from the Los Angeles trial give cause for concern in that a reduction in mortality from CHD

Table 9.2 Predicted effects of changes in dietary fat and cholesterol in plasma total cholesterol (Adapted from Oliver, 1981)

| | Average diet | Decrease in intake of total fat | Increase in P/S ratio | Decrease in total fat and in cholesterol increase in P/S ratio |
|---|---|---|---|---|
| Energy (kcal) | 2600 | 2600 | 2600 | 2600 |
| Calories from total fat (%) | 40 | 20 | 40 | 30 |
| Calories from saturated fat | 16 | 8 | 11 | 9 |
| Calories from PUFA (%) | 6 | 3 | 11 | 9 |
| P/S ratio | 0.4 | 0.4 | 1.0 | 1.0 |
| Dietary cholesterol (g) | 0.5 | 0.5 | 0.5 | 0.2 |
| Predicted change in plasma cholesterol concentrations (mmol/litre) due to: | | | | |
| Saturated fatty acids | – | −0.49 | −0.31 | −0.44 |
| PUFA | – | +0.1 | −0.15 | −0.1 |
| Dietary cholesterol | – | – | – | −0.21 |

Table 9.3 Summary of results of primary prevention trials (modified from Brisson, 1981)

| Source | Diet | Dietary Chol (mg 1000 kcal$^{-1}$) | P/S ratio | Duration (years) | No. of men (age in years) | Change in serum Chol as % control | Effect on mortality |
|---|---|---|---|---|---|---|---|
| New York[1] | Low SFA<br>High PUFA<br>Low CHOL | ? | 1.25–1.50 | 7 | 1242<br>(40–59) | −8 | Inconclusive |
| Los Angeles[2] | Low SFA<br>High PUFA<br>Low CHOL | 146 | 1.75 *vs.* 0.24 | 8 | 846<br>(30–59) | −13 | No effect on mortality. Cancer deaths increased |
| Chicago[3] | Low SFA<br>Low CHOL<br>Low energy | ? | ? | 5 | 519<br>(40–59) | −15 | Inconclusive |
| Helsinki[4] | Low SFA<br>High PUFA<br>Low CHOL | 100 | 1.42–1.78 *vs.* 0.22–0.29 | 6 | 676<br>(34–64) | −15 | Total mortality same in both groups |
| Edinburgh<br>Budapest<br>Prague[5] | Clofibrate<br>(1.6 g/day) | – | – | 5 | 10 627<br>(30–59) | −9 | No effect on mortality; cancers and gall-stones increased in treated groups |

1. Christakis *et al.*, (1966)
2. Dayton *et al.*, (1969)
3. Stamler (1971)
4. Miettinen *et al.*, (1972)
   Turpeinen *et al.*, (1979)
5. Oliver *et al.*, (1978)

SFA Saturated fatty acids
PUFA Polyunsaturated fatty acids
CHOL Cholesterol

was outweighed by an increase in mortality from cancer. The finding that clofibrate also produced no change in overall mortality with an increase in the incidence of cancers and gall-stones has led to the whole issue of the use of cholesteral-lowering drugs being questioned. A WHO trial has shown that over 10 years there have been 25 per cent more deaths in a group taking clofibrate than in a comparable high serum cholesterol control group (Oliver, 1981).

The results of secondary prevention trials involving some 1400 men also give little cause for encouragement. Indeed it would seem that there is little basis from these results for encouraging apparently normal subjects or, indeed, patients to radically change the fat content of their diets. This does not necessarily mean, however, that dietary change is not desirable or may not prove beneficial. It may mean that other components of the diet should be carefully

Table 9.4 Summary of results of secondary prevential trials (Adapted from Brisson, 1981)

| Source | Diet | Dietary Chol (mg 1000 kcal$^{-1}$) | P/S ratio | Duration (years) | No. of men (age in years) | Change in serum Chol as % control | Effect on deaths from CVD |
|---|---|---|---|---|---|---|---|
| London[1] | Corn oil (44 g/day) | ? | ? | 2 | 80 | −17 | None |
| London[2] | Soybean oil (80 g/day) | 108 | 2.0 | 2–7 | 393 | −10 | None |
| Oslo[3] | Low SFA High PUFA Low CHOL | 110 | 2.4 | 5 | 412 (30–64) | −14 | None, but number of relapses reduced for some cardiovascular troubles |
| New Jersey[4] | Low SFA High PUFA Low CHOL | 130 | 2.6 | 10 | 100 (30–50) | −8 | None |
| Sydney[5] | Low SFA (300 mg or less/day) High PUFA Low CHOL | | 1.7 | 2–7 | 458 (30–39) | −5 | No. of deaths slightly higher in high PUFA group |

1. Rose *et al.*, (1965)
2. Morris and Ball (1968)
3. Leren (1966)
4. Bierenbaum *et al.*, (1973)
5. Woodhill *et al.*, (1977)

considered. Dietary components interact and a therapeutic or preventive diet should include all those factors which are thought to promote the regression of atherosclerosis and the prevention of thrombosis. The effects of the different dietary components are probably additive (Lewis *et al.*, 1981). A suggested programme (Table 9.5) includes changes of life style and habit, where appropriate, and may be useful for patients with peripheral arterial disease (e.g. intermittent claudication), as well as those with coronary arterial disease (Dickerson, 1985).

Clearly, dietary recommendations (DHSS, 1984) can, and should, be at different levels (Table 9.6). We need, for instance, to consider those that can be made to the general public, which need to be gradual and economically possible in order to gain voluntary acceptance. Other recommendations can be made to medical practitioners. A report along similar lines but aimed rather more at health education was produced by James (1983) in the form of a discussion document.

Table 9.5 Programme for the prevention, or management, of vascular disease

1. Correct overweight or obesity
2. Decrease total fat, especially saturated fats. An increase in P/S ratio may be beneficial. This change will reduce energy intake
3. Reduce animal protein consumption and increase that of vegetable protein, particularly legumes
4. Include oily fish regularly, e.g. mackerel, herrings (supplies eicosapentaenoic acid)
5. Avoid 'simple' sugars but increase the intake of fibre-rich complex carbohydrate rich foods, e.g. fruit, vegetables, whole grain, cereals

*In addition to the dietary changes the following may prove worthwhile:*
Vitamin C (1g/day)
Vitamin E 300 IU/day)
Stop smoking
Take regular moderate exercise
Alcohol should be discouraged

Table 9.6 Levels of recommendations for modifications of diet in relation to cardiovascular disease (DHSS 1984)

1. *The general public*: The consumption of saturated fatty acids and of fat should be decreased; the ratio of polyunsaturated fatty acids to saturated fatty acids (P/S) should be increased to approximately 0.45. Saturated fat to provide 15 % and total fat 35 % of total energy
2. *Medical practitioners*: Special advice to be given to persons with a clinical problem; the advice to extend to close relatives of individuals with familial conditions
3. *Health education*: Inform general public of recommendations
4. *Producers, manufacturers and distributors of food and drink and caterers*: Products should be labelled with saturated and polyunsaturated fat contents
5. *Further review*: There is a need to have machinery for ongoing review
6. *Government*: Means should be found to educate the general population in the UK

## Diet and peripheral vascular disease

### Varicose veins

This condition has been reported to be virtually unknown amongst the indigenous peoples of Africa, whereas the European population of that continent has a similar incidence to that in Western nations (Dodd, 1964; Burkitt, 1970; Cleave, 1974). On the basis of these findings, they suggest that there is an association between the consumption of refined carbohydrates and the higher incidence of the condition. Cleave (1974) has suggested that varicose veins could result from venous obstruction due to unnatural loading of the colon, and lengthened transit times as the result of the consumption of a refined, Westernized diet.

## Pulmonary embolism and deep venous thrombosis

The incidence of pulmonary embolism, most of which is due to deep-leg thrombosis, has been rising in the UK during recent years. Thus, Morrell *et al.*, (1963) reported that in Oxford Hospitals, the incidence increased approximately five-fold in the decade 1952–61. The increased incidence of this condition in surgical patients seems to coincide with a decrease in the practice of pre-operative purgatives and enemas. More extensive trials are necessary before any definite advice can be given on the prevention of deep-vein thrombosis, but Latto (1972) has reported good results after instituting a routine of three tablespoonfuls of bran per day in milk, soup, or water. Excellent nursing co-operation is obviously necessary if such preventive measures are to succeed.

## Intermittent claudication

There is at present no evidence to support dietary manipulation as a treatment of this condition, but large doses of a single nutrient, vitamin E ($\alpha$-tocopherol), may prove beneficial. Studies in the 1940s by Boyd and his colleagues in Manchester suggested that clinical results in patients given 400 mg/day were better than those obtained with any other treatment then available. Haeger (1974) has reported a further trial in patients with a substantial reduction of arterial flow to the lower leg. In patients who received 300 mg of $d$-$\alpha$-tocopherol per day, the arterial flow to the lower leg increased in 20 to 25 months from 7.6 to 10.2 ml/100 g of tissue per min, whereas in patients treated with vasodilating agents, or with anticoagulants (dicoumarin), the corresponding mean values were 7.7 and 5.7 ml/100 g of tissue per min. A beneficial effect of $\alpha$-tocopherol on walking distance became evident after 3–4 months of treatment.

# Conclusion

Cardiovascular disease, and particularly coronary heart disease, often manifests itself suddenly and unexpectedly and the patient may die before therapy can be instituted. It follows, therefore, that the emphasis must move from therapy to prevention. Inasmuch as CHD is the end result of a chronic process, which may well be initiated in infancy and develop under dietary influence, there would seem to be a need for much more serious attention to life-time dietary patterns. Even in middle life, the recognition that dietary changes can influence some of the recognizable biochemical factors associated with increased susceptibility makes the changes desirable. They should be used in preference to long-term treatment with drugs whose ill-effects may be unknown or little understood.

It is clear, however, that no single dietary factor plays a dominant role, and further research is necessary to elucidate the effects of nutrient interactions and particularly the role of some of the micronutrients – the vitamins and trace elements. In addition, the influence of other factors such as behaviour (Friedman and Rosenman, 1974), smoking, and exercise cannot be ignored.

## References


Abdulla, Y.H., Adams, C.W.M. and Morgan, R.S. (1967). Connective-tissue reactions to implantation of purified sterol, sterol esters, phosphoglycerides, glyderides and free fatty acids. *J. Path. Bact.*, **94**, 63–71.

Allbrink, M.J. and Mann, E.B. (1959). Serum triglycerides in coronary artery disease. *Archs. Intern. Med.*, **103**, 4–8.

Annand, J.C. (1967). Hypothesis: heated milk protein and thrombosis. *J. Atheroscler. Res.*, **7**, 797–801.

Annand, J.C. (1972). Further evidence in the case against heated milk protein. *Atherosclerosis*, **15**, 129–33.

Avogaro, P., Bon, G.B., Cozzolato, G. and Quinci, G.B. (1979). Are apolipoproteins better discriminators than lipids for atherosclerosis. *Lancet*, **i**, 901–3.

Berkson, D.M. and Stamler, J. (1981). Epidemiology of the killer chronic diseases. In *Nutrition and the Killer Diseases*, pp. 17–55. Ed. Winick, M. John Wiley: Chichester.

Bierenbaum, M.L., Fleischman, A.I., Raichelson, R.I., Hayton, T. and Watson, P.B. (1973). Ten year experience of modified-fat diets on younger men with coronary heart-disease. *Lancet*, **1**, 1404–7.

Black, D.A.K. and Pole, J.D. (1975). Priorities in biomedical research: indices of burden. *Br. J. Prev. Soc. Med.*, **29**, 222–7.

Bowyer, D.E., Howard, A.N., Gresham, G.A., Bates, D. and Palmer, D.V. (1968). Aortic perfusion in experimental animals: a system for the study of lipid synthesis and accumulations. *Prog. Biochem. Pharmacol.*, **4**, 235–43.

Brisson, G.J. (1981). *Lipids in Human Nutrition*. MTP Press: Lancaster.

Burkitt, D.P. (1970). Relationship as a clue to causation. *Lancet*, **ii**, 1237–40.

Burkitt, D.P. (1972). Varicose veins, deep vein thrombosis, and haemorrhoids: epidemiology and suggested aetiology. *Br. Med. J.*, **ii**, 556–61.

Carlson, L.A. and Bottiger, L.E. (1972). Ischaemic heart disease in relation to fasting values of triglycerides and cholesterol. *Lancet*, **i**, 865–70.

Castelli, W.P., Doyle, J.T., Gordon, T., Hames, C.G., Hjortland, M.C., Hulley, S.B., Kagan, A., Zukel, W.J. (1977). HDL cholesterol and other lipids in coronary heart disease. The cooperative lipoprotein phenotyping study. *Circulation*, **55**, 767–72.

Christakis, G., Rinzler, S.H., Archer, M. and Krauss, A. (1966). Effect of the anti-coronary club program on coronary heart disease risk-factor states. *J.A.M.A.*, **198**, 597–604.

Cleave, T.L. (1974). *The Saccharin Disease*. Wright: Bristol.

Crawford, M.D. (1972). Hardness of drinking-water and cardiovascular disease. *Proc. Nutr. Soc.*, **31**, 347–53.

Davies, D.F., Davies, J.R. and Richards, M.A. (1969). Antibodies to reconstituted dried cow's milk protein in coronary heart disease. *J. Atheroscler. Res.*, **9**, 103–7.

Davies, D.F., Johnson, A.P., Rees, B.W.G., Elwood, P.C. and Abenethy, M. (1974). Food antibodies and myocardial infarction. *Lancet*, **i**, 1012–14.

Dayton, S., Pearce, M.L., Hashimoto, S., Dixon, W.J. and Tomiyasu, U. (1969). A controlled clinical trial of a diet high in unsaturated fat preventing complications of atherosclerosis. *Circulation*, **40**, Suppl. 2.

DHSS (1974). Diet and coronary heart disease. *Report on Health and Social Subjects*, 7. HMSO: London.

DHSS (1984). Diet and Cardiovascular Disease Committee on Medical Aspects of Food Policy. *Report on Health and Social Subjects*. 28. HMSO: London.

Dickerson, J.W.T. (1985). Diet and the regression of atherosclerosis. In *Advances in Diet and Nutrition*, pp. 19–22. Ed. Horwitz, C. Libbey: London.

Dodd, H. (1964). Cause, prevention and arrest of varicose veins. *Lancet*, **ii**, 809–11.

Dyerberg, J., Bang, H.O., Stoffersen, E., Moncada, S. and Vane, J.R. (1978). Eicosapentaenoic acid and prevention of thrombosis and atherosclerosis. *Lancet*, **ii**, 117–19.

Friedman, M. and Rosenman, R.H. (1974). *Type A Behavior and Your Heart*. Fawcett Publishers: Greenwich, Connecticut.

Garo, P., Cazzolato, G., Bittolo Bon G. and Quinci, G.B. (1979). Are apolipoproteins better discriminators than lipids for atherosclerosis? *Lancet*, **1**, 901–3.

Ginter, E., Kajaba, I. and Nizner, O. (1970). The effect of ascorbic acid on cholesterolaemia in healthy subjects with seasonal deficiency of vitamin C. *Nutr. Metab.*, **12**, 76–86.

Ginter, E., Cerven, J., Nemec, R. and Mikus, L. (1971). Lowered cholesterol catabolism in guinea pigs with chronic ascorbic acid deficiency. *Am. J. Clin. Nutr.*, **24**, 1238–45.

Ginter, E. (1973). Cholesterol: vitamin C controls its transformation to bile salts. *Science*, **179**, 702–4.

Glueck, C.J., Larsen, R., Glatfelter, L., Boggs, D., Burton, K., Smith, C., Kelly, K., Mellies, M.J., Khoury, P. and Morrison, J.A. (1981). Early feeding patterns and atherosclerosis. In *Nutrition and the Killer Diseases*, pp. 89–97. Ed. Winick, M. John Wiley: Chichester.

Gordon, T., Castelli, W.P., Hjortland, M.C., Kannel, W.B. and Dawber, T.R. (1977). High density lipoprotein as a protective factor against coronary heart disease. The Framingham study. *Am. J. Med.*, **62**, 707–14.

Gorringe, J.A.L. (1984). A fresh look at what everybody knows about ischaemic heart disease: discussion paper. *J. Roy. Soc. Med.*, **77**, 390–98.

Gruskay, F.L. and Cooke, R.E. (1965). The gastrointestinal absorption of unaltered protein in normal infants recovering from diarrhoea. *Pediatrics*, **16**, 763.

Haeger, K. (1974). Long-time treatment of intermittent claudication with vitamin E. *Am. J. Clin. Nutr.*, **27**, 1179–81.

Harkavy, J. (1963). Vascular Allergy and its Systemic Manifestations. Butterworths: Washington. Quoted by Poston and Davies (1974).

Hornstra, G., Lewis, B., Chait, A., Turpeinen, B., Karvonen, M.J. and Vergroesen, A.J. (1973). Influence of dietary fat on platelet function in men. *Lancet*, **i**, 1155–7.

Horsey, J., Livesley, B. and Dickerson, J.W.T. (1981). Ischaemic heart disease and aged patients: effects of ascorbic acid on lipoproteins. *J. Hum. Nutr.*, **35**, 53–8.

James, W.P.T. (1983). *A discussion paper on proposals for nutritional guidelines for health education in Britain*. Prepared for the National Advisory Committee on Nutrition Education (NACNE). The Health Education Council: London.

Jenkins, D.J.A., Leeds, A.R., Newton, C. and Cummings, J.H. (1975). Effect of pectin, guar gum, and wheat fibre on serum-cholesterol. *Lancet*, **i**, 1116.

Kagan, A., Harris, B.R., Winkelstein, W., Johnson, K.G., Kato, H., Syme, S.L., Rhoads, G.G., Gay, M.L., Nichaman, M.Z., Hamilton, H.B. and Tillotson, J. (1974). Epidemiologie studies of coronary heart disease and stroke in Japanese men living in Japan, Hawaii and California: demographic, physical, dietary and biochemical characteristics. *J. Chron. Dis.*, **27**, 345–64.

Kay, R.M., and Truswell, A.S. (1977). Effect of citrus pectin on blood lipids and faecal steroid excretion in men. *Am. J. Clin. Nutr.* **30**, 171.

Keen, H. (1972). Glucose tolerance, plasma lipids and atherosclerosis. *Proc. Nutr. Soc.*, **31**, 339–45.

Keys, A. (1970). Coronary heart disease in seven countries. *Circulation* **41/42**, (Suppl), 1.

Keys, A. (ed.) (1980). *Seven Countries – Diet and Coronary Heart Disease in Ten Years*. Harvard University Press: Cambridge, Massachusetts.

Kirk, J.E. and Laursen, T.J.S (1955). Diffusion coefficients of various solutes for human aortic tissue. *J. Gerontol.*, **10**, 288–302.

Kritchevsky, D. (1976). Diet and atherosclerosis. *Fedn. Proc.*

Latto, C. (1972). Effects of dietary fibre. *Br. Med. J.*, **iii**, 705.

Leren, P. (1966). The effect of plasma cholesterol lowering diet in male survivors of myocardial infarction. A controlled clinical trial. *Acta Med. Scand.*, **466**, (Suppl.), 5–92.

Levy, L. (1967). A form of immunological atherosclerosis. *Adv. Exp. Med. Biol.*, **1**, 426.

Lewis, B., Hammett, F., Katan, M., Kay, R.M., Merkx, I., Nobels, A., Miller, N.E. and Swan, A.V. (1981). Towards an improved lipid-lowering diet: additive effects of changes in nutrient intake. *Lancet*, **2**, 1310–13.

Lloyd, J. and Wolff, O.H. (1969). A paediatric approach to the prevention of atherosclerosis. *J. Atheroscler. Res.*, **10**, 135–8.

Lofland, H.B., Jr., and Clarkson, T.B. (1970). The bi-directional transfer of cholesterol in normal aorta, fatty streaks and atheromatous plaques. *Proc. Soc. Exp. Biol. Med.*, **133**, 1–8.

MacGregor, G.A., Markandu, N., Best, F. Elder, D., Cam, J. Sagnella, G.A. and Squiries, M. (1982). Double-blind randomised cross-over trial of moderate sodium restriction in essential hypertension. *Lancet*, **i**, 351–5.

Malhotra, S.L. (1967). Serum lipids, dietary factors and ischaemic heart disease. *Am. J. Clin. Nutr.*, **20**, 462–79.

Marmot, M.G. (1982). Diet, hypertension and stroke. In *Nutrition and Health*. Ed. Turner M.R. MTP Press: Lancaster.

Mathews, J.D., Whittingham, S. and Mackay, I.R. (1974). Autoimmune mechanism in human vascular disease. *Lancet*, **ii**, 1423–7.

Miettinen, M., Turpeinen, B., Karvonen, M.J., Elosuo, R. and Paavilainen, E. (1972). Effect of cholesterol-lowering diet on mortality from coronary heart-disease and other causes. A twelve-year clinical trial in men and women. *Lancet*, **ii**, 835–8.

Miller, G.J. and Miller, N.E. (1975). Plasma-high-density-lipoprotein concentration and development of ischaemic heart disease. *Lancet*, **i**, 16–19.

Miller, N.E., Thelle, D.S., Forde, O.H. and Mjøs, O.D. (1977). The Tromsø heart study. High density lipoprotein and coronary heart disease: a prospective case-control study. *Lancet*, **i**, 965–70.

Minick, C.R, Murphy, G.E. and Campbell, W.G. (1966). Experimental induction of athero-arteriosclerosis by the synergy of allergic damage to arteries and a lipid rich diet. *J. Exp. Med.*, **124**, 635–52.

Moncada, S., Gryglewski, R., Bunting, S. and Vane, J.R. (1976). An enzyme isolated from arteries transforms prostaglandin endoperoxides to an unstable substance that inhibits platelet aggregation. *Nature*, **263**, 663–5.

Morgan, T., Gillies, A., Morgan, G., Adam, W., Wilson, M. and Carney, S. (1978). Hypertension treated by salt restriction. *Lancet*, **i**, 227–30.

Morrell, M.T., Truelove, S.C. and Barr, R.A. (1963). Pulmonary embolism. *Br. Med. J.*, **ii**, 830–5.

Morris, J.N., Marr, J.W., Heady, J.A., Mills, G.L. and Pilkington, T.R.E. (1963). Diet and plasma cholesterol in 99 bank men. *Br. Med. J.*, **i**, 571–6.

Morris, J.N. and Ball, K.P. (1968). Controlled trial of soya-bean oil in myocardial infarction. Report of a Committee of the Medical Research Council. *Lancet*, **ii**, 693–9.

Morris, J.N., Mann, J.W. and Clayton, D.G. (1977). Diet and heart. *Br. Med. J.*, **ii**, 1307–14.

Nelson, M. (1981). Preparation of low salt diets. In *Nutrition and the Killer Diseases*, pp. 131–42. Ed. Winick, M. John Wiley: Chichester.

Neri, L.C., Mandel, J.S. and Hewitt, D. (1972). Relation between mortality and water hardness in Canada. *Lancet*, **i**, 931–4.

Oliver, M.F. (1981). Serum cholesterol – the knave of hearts and the joker. *Lancet*, **ii**, 1090–95.
Oliver, M.F., Heady, J.A., Morris, J.N. and Cooper, J. (1978). A co-operative trial in the primary prevention of ischaemic heart disease using clofibrate. Report from the Committee of Principal Investigators. *Br. Heart J.*, **40**, 1069–1103.
Oliver, M.F, Kurien, V.A. and Greenwood, T.W. (1968). Relation between serum-free-fatty acids and arrhythmias and death of acute myocardial infarction. *Lancet*, **i**, 710–15.
Opie, L.H. (1973). Lipid metabolism of the heart and arteries in relation to ischaemic heart disease. *Lancet*, **i**, 192–5.
Peterson, V.E., Crapo, P.A., Weininger, J. Ginsberg, H. and Olefsky, J. (1975). Quantification of plasma cholesterol and triglyceride levels in hypercholesterolaemic subjects receiving ascorbic acid supplements. *Am. J. Clin. Nutr.*, **28**, 584–7.
Pooling Project Research Group (1978). Relationship of blood pressure, serum cholesterol, smoking habit, relative weight and ECG abnormalities to incidence of major coronary events. Final report of the Pooling Project. *J. Chron. Dis.*, **31**, 201–306.
Poston, R.N. and Davies, D.F. (1974). Immunity and inflammation in the pathogenesis of atherosclerosis. *J. Atheroscler. Res.*, **19**, 353.
Rose, G.A., Thomson, W.B. and Williams, R.T. (1965). Corn oil in treatment of ischaemic heart disease. *Br. Med. J.*, **1**, 1531–33.
Royal College of Physicians of London and the British Cardiac Society (1976). Prevention of coronary heart disease. *J. R. Coll. Phys.*, **10**, 1–63.
Samuelsson, B., Hamberg, M., Malmsten, C. and Svensson, J. (1976). The role of prostaglandin endoperoxides and thromboxanes in platelet aggregation. *Adv. in Prostaglandin Thromboxane Res.*, **1**, 737–46.
Sanders, T.A.B, Ellis, F.R. and Dickerson, J.W.T. (1978). Studies of vegans: the fatty acid composition of plasma choline phosphoglycerides, erythrocytes, adipose tissue and breast milk and some indication of susceptibility to ischaemic heart disease in vegans and omnivore controls. *Am. J. Clin. Nutr.*, **31**, 805–13.
Seelig, M.S. and Heggtveit, H.A. (1974). Magnesium interrelationships in ischaemic heart disease: a review. *Am. J. Clin. Nutr.*, **27**, 59–79.
Skrabal, F., Aubock, J. and Hortnagl, H. (1981). Low sodium/high potassium diet for prevention of hypertension: probable mechanism of action. *Lancet*, **ii**, 895–900.
Smith, E.B. (1965). The influence of age and atherosclerosis on the chemistry of aortic intima. Parts I and II. *J. Atheroscler. Res.*, **5**, 224–48.
Smith, E.B., Evans, P.H. and Downham, M.D. (1967). Lipid in the aortic intima: the correlation of morphological and chemical characteristics. *J. Atheroscler. Res.*, **7**, 171–86.
Spittle, C.R. (1971). Atherosclerosis and vitamin C. *Lancet*, **ii**, 1280–81.
Stamler, J. (1971). Acute myocardial infarction – progress in primary prevention. *Br. Heart. J.*, **33** (Suppl.) 145–64.
Stamler, J. (1979). Population studies. In *Nutrition Lipids and Coronary Heart Disease*, pp. 25–88. Eds. Levy, R., Rifkind, B. Dennis, B. and Ernst, N. Raven Press: New York.
Stout, R.W. (1968). Insulin-stimulated lipogenesis in arterial tissue in relation to diabetes and atheroma. *Lancet*, **ii**, 702–5.
Strong, J.P. and McGill, H.C. (1969). The pediatric aspects of atherosclerosis. *J. Atheroscler. Res.*, **9**, 251–65.
Szanto, S. and Yudkin, J. (1969). The effect of dietary sucrose on blood lipids, serum insulin, platelet adhesiveness and body weight in human volunteers. *Post-grad. Med. J.*, **45**, 602–7.
Trowell, H. (1972). Ischaemic heart disease and dietary fibre. *Am. J. Clin. Nutr.*, **25**, 926–32.

Turpeinen, O., Karvonen, M.J., Pekkarinen, M., Miettinen, M., Elosuo, R. and Paavilainen, E. (1979). Dietary prevention of coronary heart disease: the Finnish mental hospital study. *Int. J. Epidemiol.*, **8**, 99–118.

Van Winkle, M. and Levy, L. (1970). Further studies on the reversibility of serum sickness cholesterol induced atherosclerosis. *J. Exp. Med.*, **132**, 858–67.

Willis, G.C. (1953). An experimental study of the intimal ground substance in atherosclerosis. *Can. Med. Ass. J.*, **69**, 17–22.

Willis, G.C., Light, A.W. and Gow, W.S. (1954). Serial arteriography in atherosclerosis. *Can. Med. Ass. J.*, **71**, 562.

Wood, P.D. and Haskell, W.L. (1979). The effect of exercise on plasma high density lipoproteins. *Lipids*, **14**, 417–27.

Woodhill, J.M., Palmer, A.J., Leelarthalpin, B., McGilchrist, C. and Blacket, R.B. (1977). Low fat, low cholesterol diet in secondary prevention of coronary heart disease. In *Drugs, Lipids and Atherosclerosis*, pp. 317–30. Eds. Kritchevsky D., Padletti, R. and Holmes, W.L., Plenum Press: New York.

Zilversmit, D.B. (1968). Cholesterol flux in the atherosclerotic plaque. *Ann. N.Y. Acad. Sci.*, **149**, 710–24.

# 10 Diseases of the alimentary tract

John W.T. Dickerson and Harry A. Lee



## Introduction

The alimentary tract is the normal route of entry of nutrients into the body and diseases of the tract have particular relevance and importance to nutritional status. Furthermore, treatment of the various diseases of the tract, whether by surgery, radiotherapy, or drugs, can have a profound effect on the digestion and absorption of foodstuffs. Appetite is affected by the nature, and mode of presentation of food, and disease affects the nature of the food that can be eaten.

The identification of deficiencies of individual nutrients involves clinical, dietary, and biochemical assessment, and detailed descriptions of these methods are beyond the scope of this book. Sometimes, however, and particularly in relation to diseases of the alimentary tract, it is desirable to assess the general state of nutrition of the patient and to follow this through a period of recovery. The methods that can be used in the assessment of nutritional status are discussed in Chapter 21.

## The mouth

### Vitamin deficiencies

Lesions of the mouth occur in blood disorders of nutritional origin. Thus, in iron-deficiency anaemia there is usually a loss of filiform papillae around the edges, and usually over the dorsum, so that the whole appearance is of a smooth, glazed tongue. In pernicious anaemia the tongue is often sore and the filiform papillae reduced. This is the commonest early sign of cyanocobalamin (vitamin $B_{12}$) deficiency in vegans.

Deficiencies of practically all the vitamins of the B group have an effect on the soft tissues of the mouth, but the clinical picture caused by deficiencies of individual vitamins is often obscured by the concomitant anorexia and resulting multiple deficiencies. A dietary deficiency of thiamine may give rise to increased sensitivity of the mouth and to small herpetic-like lesions, but not to glossitis. Intravenous solutions of dextrose can precipitate, or aggravate, thiamine deficiency, and thiamine should always be given with them.

Angular stomatitis is a somewhat non-specific sign, but often responds to large doses of riboflavin, and sometimes to pyridoxine. It also occurs in iron-deficiency anaemia and other debilitating diseases. Lack of riboflavin causes cheilosis and a painful superficial glossitis. The tongue may have a characteristic magenta or bright red appearance. Glossitis also occurs in pellagra and responds dramatically to niacin. The glossitis of sprue and coeliac disease responds to folic acid.

A deficiency of ascorbic acid causes premature cessation of dentine formation with secondary overcalcification. The periodontal fibres are weakened and the teeth may become loose and fall out. The gums become hyperaemic and cyanotic and bleed easily and these are amongst the earliest signs of ascorbic acid deficiency. In his classical study of scurvy, Lind described varicose veins under the tongue as a sign of the disease, and it has been suggested that 'sublingual petechiae' may be due to ascorbic acid deficiency (Taylor, 1976). This view appears to be supported by the observation that these lesions are associated with low leucocyte levels of the vitamin (Andrews and Brook, 1966), but it has yet to be proved whether there is a causal relationship.

A deficiency of vitamin A may cause hypoplasia in the enamel and dentine of teeth. Tooth formation is not affected, after the age of 6 years, because by that age the crowns are complete. In adults, a deficiency of vitamin A may cause hyperkeratosis of the oral mucosa.

Defective calcification of the dentine of the teeth occurs in rickets; a deficiency of vitamin D has been thought by some to be involved in caries susceptibility.

### Dental caries

Dental caries is extremely prevalent in most civilized societies. The aetiology is almost certainly connected with diet (Hartles and Leach, 1975), for African natives and Eskimos are immune to it until they become 'Westernized' in their feeding habits.

Hypoplasia and a low intake of fluoride are predisposing factors, but the principal cause is undoubtedly a high intake of refined carbohydrate, and particularly of sucrose. The most likely immediate cause of caries is the exposure of enamel to acids (lactic, acetic, or formic) at about pH5. Such concentrations of acid are produced in the mouth by the action of commensal bacteria (*Streptococcus* species) on carbohydrates which have become trapped in the plaque formed by bacteria from polymers of glucose and fructose. The importance of the physical form of sugary foods was demonstrated in a long-term experiment in Sweden (Gustafsson *et al.*, 1954). Eating sticky toffees and caramels between meals caused a sharp increase in dental caries whereas sucrose solutions taken with meals had little effect. The administration of vitamin supplements and other sweetened solutions in dummies and reservoir feeders is to be deprecated for it is associated with a high incidence of dental caries in 3 to 4-year-old children (Committee on Medical Aspects of Food Policy, 1969).

An important preventive measure, in addition to reducing the consumption of sweets between meals, is the consumption of drinking water containing 2 p.p.m. of fluoride (Royal College of Physicians, 1976). Alternatively, topical application of fluorides has been shown to reduce caries (Holloway *et al.*, 1963). It has also been suggested that fluoride might be added to milk or table salt.

## Cancer of the mouth and pharynx

Carcinoma of the hypopharynx may be more common in women than in men. The explanation appears to be that the mucosal atrophy that occurs in the dysphagia of chronic iron-deficiency anaemia, the Patterson–Kelly or Plummer–Vinson syndrome, is itself a pre-malignant condition, as far as the post-cricoid region is concerned (Owen, 1950).

These tumours are treated by surgical excision or radiotherapy, or by a combination of these methods. Cytotoxic drugs are also sometimes used. Each of these methods creates nutritional problems. Where surgery is used this may necessitate extensive reconstruction of the mouth, and during the early stages of rehabilitation tube feeding will be necessary. After extensive surgery and reconstruction the patient may be severely disfigured, and it is important that interest in the diet of such patients be seen as part of their rehabilitation. Radiotherapy to the mouth may damage the taste buds and have profound psychological, physiological, and nutritional after-effects. The nutritional problems associated with cancer are discussed in Chapter 16.

# The oesophagus

## Benign diseases with nutritional involvement

### Dysphagia

A number of benign conditions may make the swallowing of food difficult or painful. Thus, in achalasia weak oesophageal peristalsis and the inability of the internal cardio-oesophageal sphincter to relax causes the collection of food in the oesophagus. Here it causes first discomfort and then, after fermentation, oesophagitis and pain. Modifications in the nature and mode of consumption of food may give relief. A bland semi-fluid diet is often helpful. If a milk-based diet is found to be the most suitable it is essential that particular attention is given to the provision of ample quantities of water-soluble vitamins. The patient may also find that standing up several times through a meal, drinking a glass of water, or taking a deep breath and exhaling hard forces food into the stomach (Truelove and Reynell, 1972).

Benign stricture of the oesophagus causes dysphagia with resulting weight loss, but appetite is usually readily regained after treatment. However, if the stricture is extensive and has to be removed surgically, the patients benefit from some dietary advice. Frequent small meals, with added carbohydrate in the form of Caloreen to increase the energy density may be useful in helping the patient to regain weight.

Dysphagia can occur in patients with long-standing iron-deficiency anaemia (the Patterson–Kelly or Plummer–Vinson syndrome). This is principally a disease of middle-aged women, and has now become rare in this country.

**Perforation, caustic burns**

If the oesophagus becomes perforated as a result of trauma, the continued taking of food by mouth results in a chylothorax which has to be drained by suction. The injury may heal spontaneously or require surgical repair. Regardless of the course to be adopted, an alternative means of feeding must be instituted, and this can be parenterally, or via a jejunostomy. Suitable feeds are described in Chapters 22 and 23, respectively. A tube-feed through a jejunostomy is perhaps preferable, for with skilled administration it causes less discomfort to the patient, is attended by less risk of complications, and is considerably cheaper.

Caustic soda is sometimes ingested accidentally by children or intentionally in attempted suicide by adults. This destroys the oesophageal mucosa and may penetrate the muscular coats. Again, it is essential that the damaged area is 'rested' as much as possible, particularly if, as with other kinds of trauma, there is risk of perforation. The patient is fed through a gastrostomy with a tube-feed.

**Hiatus hernia, gastro-oesophageal reflux, and chronic peptic ulcer (Barrett's ulcer)**

Hiatus hernia often occurs in obese individuals due to the bulk of the abdominal contents exerting pressure on the hiatus. Pregnancy and chronic cough act in a similar way. On the basis of epidemiological data it has been suggested that a low roughage diet may also be an aetiological factor because of the often concomitant constipation (Burkitt and James, 1973; Burkitt, 1978) although this view has been challenged (Cleave, 1974). The heartburn that occurs in a patient with a hiatus hernia may be accompanied by regurgitation of acid fluid into the mouth after meals. It is usually associated with a change of posture, and may occur on lying down at night. The pain may be severe, and the patient may complain of food sticking in the throat. Bleeding may occur and the patient may thus have iron-deficiency anaemia.

The disorder is more common in women than in men. Women should be advised not to wear corsets or tight garments, and to avoid stooping. An obese patient should be put on a strict programme of weight reduction as by this treatment the symptoms often disappear and the condition is alleviated. The patient is advised to take a bland diet, with no solid food for three hours before going to bed. Meals should be small and frequent. Spirits, hot drinks, and hard, hastily chewed food should be avoided. Antacids are used until the oesophagitis subsides. Anaemia is treated with oral iron, or, if severe, with blood transfusions. Patients should stop smoking, as many of them admit that they get more heartburn after smoking (Dennish and Castell, 1971; Stanciu and Bennett, 1972), due to its effect in decreasing the lower oesophageal sphincter pressure.

An association between heartburn and the ingestion of specific kinds of foods in different individuals is well known. It seems that the lower oesophageal sphincter pressure is important in preventing reflux symptoms after food ingestion (Castell, 1975). Release of gastrin and other gastrointestinal hormones may play a role in changing lower oesophageal sphincter pressure. The release of cholecystokinin in response to a fatty meal may be the mechanism by which fat induces reflux in a large number of patients with fatty food intolerance. Chocolate, coffee, and caffeine also cause a lowering of lower oesophageal sphincter pressure and reflux and this is probably due to their content of methylxanthines. A lowering of sphincter pressure with resulting acid reflux is also likely to occur after the ingestion of alcohol (Hogan *et al.*, 1972). Spicy foods, tomato juice and citrus juices also cause reflux in some individuals.

Chronic peptic ulcer of the oesophagus is treated, as elsewhere, by rest, posture, alkalis, and a non-irritant diet.

## Malignant disease

Cancer of the oesophagus is more common in males than in females, and also occurs more commonly in alcoholics, associated with coeliac disease, and also with achalasia. The patient usually complains of pain and dysphagia on swallowing solid foods, and of a loss of body weight. The extent of weight loss is related to the chronicity of the dysphagia. If the weight loss is considerable with accompanying anaemia, the patient may be a poor operative risk.

Though the value of pre-operative nutritional rehabilitation of patients with cancer of the oesophagus may still be a matter of debate, some surgeons provide full parenteral regimes for those who cannot swallow (Watson, 1982; McKeown, 1985). It remains to be shown whether a comparatively short period of intravenous nutrition improves operative outcome. It seems that most attention should be paid to problems of anaemia and dehydration. Feedings via a gastrostomy or jejunostomy may be contraindicated as the tubes interfere with subsequent surgical procedures and increase the risk of sepsis. The presence of anaemia may be masked by dehydration but when present it should be corrected by blood transfusion well before the operation. Survival times following operations for oesophageal cancer are disappointing and expectation of a cure therefore remote. Restoration of the ability to swallow is the primary objective. In severe cases removal of the tumour may not be possible, even as a palliative measure. This is particularly true for elderly frail patients and those with cardiovascular disease. In these patients it may be necessary to resort to feeding through a permanent gastrostomy, or through a fine-bore nasogastric tube (Nazari *et al.*, 1984). The nutritional status of patients with unresectable disease has been found to improve following endoscopic intubation (Fellows *et al.*, 1984). Nutritional rehabilitation after oesophagectomy or oesophagogastrectomy often presents a considerable problem. Parenteral feeding may be necessary or a tube feed may be given with a nasogastric tube remaining *in situ* for some time following the operation. However, there is some risk of ulceration at the lower end if the tube remains in for a long time. Alternatively, it may be necessary to feed the patient through a jejunostomy. Whichever route is chosen, feeding should be started as soon as possible, and up to 3000 kcal (12.6 MJ) and 100 g protein (16 g nitrogen) should be given per day together with appropriate supplements of iron, trace elements and water-soluble vitamins. The composition of suitable tube-feeds is discussed in Chapter 22.

More work is necessary to ascertain the level of the various nutrients that should be given to obtain an optimum rate of recovery. A deficiency of essential fatty acids has been reported in the serum of patients with cancer of the oesophagus (Wapnick *et al.*, 1974), but the significance of this finding is not at present known.

After surgery, some patients have persistent diarrhoea, poor appetite, and difficulty in regaining weight. Continuing dietary advice and encouragement is necessary. The patients should be advised to take frequent small meals after leaving hospital and the psychological benefit of repeated consultation should not be underrated. These factors are obviously more important when there has been extensive resection, for this increases the risk of metabolic problems. Steatorrhoea has been reported (Shils and Gilat, 1966; Shils, 1971), and is thought to be due to the sacrifice of the vagus nerves at operation, but it is not an invariable consequence of vagotomy (Johnston *et al.*, 1972). Be this at it may, it is unwise to increase the fat content of the diet in order to increase the calorie density of the food, for dietary fat will retard gastric emptying in those patients with a remaining stomach. Under these circumstances medium-chain triglycerides (see p. 222) have proved useful. Additional energy can also be given as Caloreen. In patients who fail to respond to these measures, it may be beneficial to attempt to stimulate appetite by giving an anabolic steroid such as Durabolin.

In the more favourable of McKeown's (1985) patients 37 per cent had died by the end of the first year and 55 per cent at the end of the second. The reasons for this high wastage are not clear. It is tempting to suggest that malnutrition could contribute to the risk of fatal anastomic leaks. However, with patients with cancer of the oesophagus, as with those with tumours at other sites, perhaps too much emphasis has been placed on crude survival rates. There is undoubtedly a need to assess the effect of treatment on quality of life and therefore the ability to swallow and the maintenance of nutritional status make an important contribution to this.

## The stomach

The stomach functions as a reservoir for ingested food and plays a role in the digestion and absorption of nutrients. It follows, therefore, that disease may result from the exposure of the mucosa to ingested irritant or toxic materials, and to the results of deranged digestive and absorptive function. Surgical treatment of gastric disease is likely to have considerable nutritional consequences.

## Benign diseases with nutritional involvement

### Gastritis

Diet may be involved in the aetiology of acute gastritis. Alcohol, allergic reactions to specific foods, drugs such as aspirin, or the ingestion of foods infected with staphylococci may be involved. Chronic gastritis may follow repeated attacks of acute gastritis, and is commoner in those who smoke or drink heavily, in the lower income groups, than in other people. Reflux of duodenal contents, together with a reduced resistance of mucosal cells due to the irritant effect of bile salts is another cause. Faulty diet, malnutrition, and autoimmune reactions are other possible causes.

Iron-deficiency anaemia is common, and this is due to inadequate iron intake, poor absorption and recurrent bleeding from minor gastric erosions. There may be decreased production of intrinsic factor with subsequent development of $B_{12}$ deficiency. This may not progress to pernicious anaemia, but the associated clinical manifestations including weakness, loss of memory, and mental depression frequently respond to treatment with $B_{12}$.

### Peptic ulcer disease

The view that peptic ulcer disease reflects an abnormality of gastric secretion, or a failure of a physiological mechanism to check excessive secretion (Dragstedt, 1969) is now generally accepted. However, the geographical distribution of gastric and duodenal ulcers is different and they are now considered as separate diseases and have been reviewed (Jones, 1957; Sircus, 1973). Gastric ulcer differs from duodenal ulcer in its lower output of acid both in the resting state and on maximum stimulation. Duodenal ulcer is believed to be due to vagal hyperactivity. Claims that dietary factors might cause gastric ulcers are based on the finding that in Great Britain between the two world wars it was between two and five times more prevalent in the lower than in the upper social classes. People in the poorest social class were, at that time, consuming diets which were well below physiological standards both in quality and quantity. It seems likely, however, that better methods of treatment, rather than improvement of the diet could well account for the fall in deaths from gastric ulcer in recent years.

The aims of medical treatment are threefold – relief of symptoms, healing of the ulcer, and the prevention of recurrence. The principles of treatment (Davidson *et al.*, 1979) are: (1) rest, both physical and psychological; (2) a bland diet, given in small amounts at frequent intervals to provide 'physiological rest' for the stomach; (3) drugs – sedatives, antacids, antispasmodics, and carbenoxolone; (4) the cessation of smoking.

Strict diets used to be prescribed for patients with gastric ulcers. The Sippy regimen of hourly milk combinations was interspersed with antacid powders. Strict diets are now not necessary (Ingelfinger, 1966), and indeed may be positively harmful because they may result in patients becoming undernourished. Such diets may, however, be self-prescribed, and attention must be paid to the water-soluble vitamins, and especially to ascorbic acid, the intake of which is often low. If antacids are used extensively, it may be necessary also to take supplements of thiamine, as antacids are known to destroy this vitamin or prevent its absorption.

Patients, should generally be encouraged to eat ordinary foods, avoiding large meals and taking three or four snacks per day between meals. In this way, the risk of further attack by acid on the gastric mucosa is minimized. Individual differences are found in the foods that can be tolerated, and these must be found by trial and error. There is no evidence that a dietary regime accelerates healing of an ulcer; its main purpose is to reduce the dyspepsia. It is important therefore to omit from the diet substances that are known to stimulate acid secretion such as alcohol and caffeine-containing beverages, or those that are direct mucosal irritants such as black pepper, chili, vinegar, mustard, pickles, and irritating spices. Such foods should probably be avoided for at least two years. Aspirin should also be avoided.

If the symptoms are severe, or if there has been a haemorrhage, seven small meals should be given each day, and the main ingredient of these should be milk, eggs, and fruit juice. Blood transfusions may be necessary in very debilitated anaemic subjects.

The use of vitamin E in the treatment of gastric ulcers may warrant further investigation. Following a report by Solar (1959) that patients with ulcers improved on vitamin E, Kangas *et al.*, (1972) reported a substantial increase in the rate of healing of gastric ulcers produced experimentally in the rat. Deficiencies of vitamin E have also been found to cause peptic ulceration in human volunteers (Horwitt, 1959).

## Gastric carcinoma

Carcinoma of the stomach accounts for the death of about 14 000 people each year in England and Wales. The disease chiefly affects middle-aged and elderly persons and the sex ratio is 3:2, with men being affected more commonly than women.

The influence of environmental factors has been discussed by Doll (1956). There are considerable geographical variations in its distribution and deaths due to the disease are four times higher in Japan than amongst the white population of the United States and twice as high as in England. Observations made on Japanese immigrants to the United States are strongly in favour of environmental factors, probably dietary, being of major importance. In patients in whom the disease is too advanced for surgery, treatment must be palliative. Such patients should be encouraged to eat what they like and any anaemia present should be treated appropriately. Those patients treated surgically by partial gastrectomy, total gastrectomy or, in the case of carcinoma of the cardia, by oesophagogastrectomy, require careful nutritional management, either orally, by tube-feeding, or occasionally parenterally.

## Nutrition after gastric surgery

Gastric resection and reconstruction can be performed in a variety of ways. Alternatively, gastric ulcers may be treated by vagotomy and pyloroplasty.

Table 10.1 Changes in function following gastric resection and reconstruction (Celestin, 1974)

| |
|---|
| Rapid emptying of the stomach remnant |
| Reduced secretion of hydrochloric acid and pepsin |
| Reduced secretion of intrinsic factor |
| Reduced secretion of pancreatic enzymes |
| Inadequate mixing of food with enzymes and bile |
| Reduced absorption of certain food substances, especially protein and fat. Glucose is absorbed very rapidly |
| Abolition of normal pH gradient in the alimentary canal |
| Increased intestinal mobility |
| Altered bacteriological state of intestine occasionally |
| Effects related to the creation of the afferent loop |

Each of the possible procedures is followed, to a greater or lesser degree, by disturbances in gastric function (Table 10.1). Some of these follow soon after taking food and can be described as the early or post-cibal syndromes (Table 10.2); others develop later due to the long-term effects of disturbed functions. These are described as the 'late symptoms'. These complications have been reviewed a number of times (Stammers and Williams, 1963; Wright and Tilson, 1973). Problems following vagotomy have been discussed by Williams and Cox (1969).

**Early symptoms**

The 'dumping' syndrome was a term given by Mix (1922) to a group of sensations coming on after food and thought to be due to rapid emptying from the stomach of food which is 'dumped' in the small intestine. Knowledge of the pathophysiology of the condition stems from the demonstration by Machella (1950) that the syndrome could be reproducibly initiated 5 minutes after the infusion of 10 per cent dextrose solution into the jejunum. The entry of a hypertonic solution into the intestine causes a movement of extracellular fluid into the lumen of the bowel, with a consequent reduction of plasma volume. It may be felt quite soon or after 2 to 4 hours, and occurs more frequently in women than in men, and usually lasts about 30 minutes.

The aim of medical treatment is the relief of symptoms by reducing the osmolarity of the solution entering the intestine and by prolonging the emptying of the gastric remnant. Dietary modifications that are helpful in achieving this aim are as follows: meals should be small, frequent, and dry. Soups, milk, and sweets should be avoided; the diet should contain little carbohydrate and particularly sugar, but it should have a high content of protein and fat; drinks should be taken separately from the main meals; and it may be of advantage to lie down for a short period after meals. This regime together with the use, if necessary, of anticholinergic drugs, helps most patients and only about 1 per cent require remedial surgery (Wright and Tilson, 1973). Those patients who have late symptoms such as reactive hypoglycaemia may be helped by tolbutamide taken at the time of eating (Drapanas, 1967).

The vomiting of bile occurs intermittently and is thought to be due to transient obstruction of the afferent loop which holds up the bile and pancreatic

Table 10.2 Post-gastrectomy syndromes (Celestin, 1974)

A Early post-cibal, symptoms:
1. The 'dumping syndrome'
2. The 'hyperglycaemic syndrome'
3. Bile vomiting

B Late symptoms – nutritional disturbances
1. Weight loss and steatorrhoea
2. Iron deficiency anaemia
3. Megaloblastic anaemia
4. Vitamin $B_{12}$ deficiency
5. Severe malnutrition

juice. Prevention is surgical, rather than dietary, by reducing the size of the afferent loop.

**Late symptoms – nutritional disturbances**

Weight loss is a well-known consequence of gastric surgery, occurring more frequently in women than in men, and is a consequence of a reduced food intake. A similar finding has been reported after vagotomy and gastroenterostomy (Wheldon *et al.*, 1970). It may be accompanied by malabsorption – particularly of fat, and sometimes also of protein. Persistent encouragement of the patient is often necessary for him to regain weight, and this is particularly so after the more extensive total gastrectomy or oesophagogastrectomy. Co-operation from the patient is of the utmost importance, and, as mentioned above in relation to oesophagectomy, patients should be seen by a nutritionist in the early weeks following the operation so that a satisfactory regime can be worked out. There is a tendency to revert to an inadequate food intake when the patients leave hospital (Bradley *et al.*, 1975). Meals must be small and frequent. A small amount of alcohol, about 30 minutes before a meal, is sometimes useful in increasing appetite. Occasionally anabolic steroids have been given with advantage to patients recovering from oesophagogastrectomy.

Malabsorption is discussed more fully on p. 222 but it should be noted here that some malabsorption of fat is common after gastrectomy (MacKay, 1970), and it also occurs after vagotomy and gastroenterostomy (Shils, 1971). The osteomalacia that occurs in about 25 per cent of patients after gastrectomy (Eddy, 1971) is statistically correlated with faecal fat excretion and this suggests that malabsorption could be the dominant factor in its aetiology.

There is a gradual fall in the concentration of haemoglobin in the blood after partial gastrectomy, and this fall is faster in females than in males (Baird, 1967). Iron deficiency is by far the commonest cause of anaemia in these patients. It seems that there is a defect in the mechanism by which increased absorption of dietary iron occurs in response to anaemia. It seems almost certain, however, that a reduction in iron intake, accompanying the usually occurring reduction in energy intake, could be a contributing factor since there is normally a linear relationship between these in the diet. This form of anaemia responds well to iron supplements (Baird, 1967). It is well known that ascorbic acid facilitates the absorption of iron, and this potentiation occurs in post-gastrectomy patients (Baird *et al.*, 1974). The absorption of ascorbic acid itself has been reported to be reduced in patients undergoing vagotomy for peptic ulcer, probably as a consequence of reduced gastric acid (Macdonald and Cohen, 1972).

In a study of about 300 patients, Hoffbrand (1967) found uncomplicated megaloblastic anaemia, due to $B_{12}$ deficiency, in only 4 per cent of patients and a mild megaloblastic anaemia, due to folate deficiency, in a further 2 per cent. Serum $B_{12}$ levels have been found to be subnormal in approximately 10–20 per cent of patients. The $B_{12}$ level does not change appreciably during the first two years, but falls rapidly after about six years. The time lag is due to the time taken to exhaust liver stores. The fall in $B_{12}$ values is much more severe in patients who survive five years after total gastrectomy.

Folate deficiency is a much less important cause of anaemia than $B_{12}$ deficiency, in spite of the fact that Hoffbrand found subnormal serum folate concentrations in about 40 per cent of his patients. Impaired absorption of folate occurs in some gastrectomy patients (Elsborg, 1974). Serum folate is a poor index of folic acid status, however, and it could be argued that it is not necessary merely to correct a biochemical deficiency. However, since a number of drugs, including alcohol, interfere with folic acid metabolism it would seem wise to correct an identified deficiency.

Severe protein–energy malnutrition has been described after polyapartial gastrectomy (Neale *et al.*, 1967).

## Miscellaneous diseases of the stomach and duodenum

Crohn's disease has been described in the stomach and duodenum. There is no special dietary regimen for the condition other than that used for the basic disease, that is a diet which is nutritionally adequate in every respect and which is easily tolerated without producing further gastrointestinal irritation and pain. The response of patients to food is variable and for some it is necessary to have a bland low-residue diet.

Menetrier's disease is characterized by large, prominent, gastric folds found diffusely throughout the stomach or localized in the antrum, and is a protein-losing gastropathy. Treatment is symptomatic with antacids to reduce dyspepsia and a high protein diet when hypoalbuminaemia is present.

## The small intestine

The digestion and absorption of carbohydrates, proteins, and fats is completed in the small intestine and the absorption of vitamins and minerals is almost restricted to this part of the digestive tract. The mucosal cells themselves play an important role in these processes and at the same time act as a barrier to the entry of non-nutrient material. Inflammation by micro-organisms, chemical irritants, immunological reactions, or genetic defects may damage one or both functions in a specific or non-specific manner with nutritional consequences.

## The malabsorption syndrome

The most frequent clinical signs of disease of the small intestine are diarrhoea, steatorrhoea and the consequent weight loss and nutritional deficiencies. The treatment of diarrhoea can be one of the most challenging therapeutic problems in medicine. Whatever the cause, be it cholera, other acute bacterial infections, or massive resection of the gut, the general principles of management apply. These are the replacement of fluid, electrolytes, minerals, and vitamins and the restoration and maintenance of adequate nutrition of the patient. In acute diarrhoea, the loss of water and electrolytes is greater than in the chronic condition. In inflammatory states, the fluid that is lost tends to resemble plasma and the loss of protein as well as electrolytes occurs. Quantitative aspects of replacement will vary according to the severity of the condition. In the more chronic forms, such as gluten enteropathy, transit time is longer and consequently there is time for the more readily absorbed nutrients to pass from the lumen and the chief manifestation of the disease is steatorrhoea. This term is often used synonymously with the 'malabsorption syndrome' whereas it strictly applies to the passage of excess fat in the stools, and the malabsorption syndrome is a condition in which there is multiple malabsorption of nutrients (fats, protein, minerals, and vitamins) from the intestine (Escovitz and Rubin, 1973).

There are many different causes of steatorrhoea (Losowsky *et al.*, 1974). Thus, it may be due to intestinal mucosal lesions (e.g. gluten-sensitive enteropathy, tropical sprue), structural lesions of the intestine (Crohn's disease, radiotherapy), drugs (alcohol), infection within the gut (acute enteritis, especially in children, small bowel stasis), maldigestion (bile salt deficiency, pancreatic enzyme deficiency), surgery (gut resection, gastric surgery), bio-chemical abnormalities (alactasia, lipoprotein deficiency, the Zollinger–Ellison syndrome), or disease elsewhere (tumours, ulcerative colitis, Paget's disease, malnutrition).

When considered in relation to the nutritional consequences of the disease and nutrient needs, the specific nature of the pathological process responsible for the malabsorption may be of little relevance. However, treatment must be based on clear understanding of the site, aetiology, and extent of the gut disorder. For example, diarrhoea caused by bacterial overgrowth requires treatment with antibiotics, whereas diarrhoea caused by a deficiency of gut enzymes requires the elimination of the non-utilizable substrate.

In conditions in which steatorrhoea is a serious problem, the maintenance of the energy intake on a low-fat diet may present a problem. In such conditions medium-chain triglycerides (Senior, 1968) may be substituted in the diet in place of normal fat containing long-chain triglycerides. Medium-chain triglycerides are those with a chain length of 6–10 carbon atoms, in contrast to the long-chain triglycerides of food which have a chain length of 12–18 carbon atoms. The studies of Hashim *et al.*, (1960) are amongst those which pioneered the use of medium-chain triglycerides in the human. These lipids are hydrolysed more rapidly than those of normal fat (Greenberger *et al.*, 1966) and the fatty acids are absorbed directly into the portal system. Moreover, in the absence of pancreatic lipase, the triglycerides are absorbed directly without hydrolysis, thus permitting their use in patients with pancreatic insufficiency. It is clear also that the mode of absorption bypasses the necessity of the complex resynthesis of triglyceride in the mucosal cell and subsequent formation of chylomicrons necessary for the absorption of long-chain fatty acids. Medium-chain triglycerides are therefore of use in the management of children with abetalipoproteinaemia.

**Gluten-sensitive enteropathy**

Sometimes known as coeliac disease, or non-tropical sprue, gluten-sensitive enteropathy is usually a disease which manifests itself in early childhood. There are no accurate figures for its incidence in Great Britain, but it is said to occur in 1 in 2000 to 1 in 8000 of the population. Its incidence may be increasing, however, due to the early inclusion of wheat products in infant feeds (Arneil *et al.*, 1973). The disease also occurs in adults as an acquired condition. It is characterized by diffuse involvement of the entire small bowel with atrophy of the villi, and hypoplasia of the crypts, with consequent prevention of proper absorption of nutrients. The intestinal mucosa also becomes permeable to substances which have a deleterious effect upon the health of the patient and cause some of the symptoms of the disease. The causative agent is the gliadin fraction of wheat gluten. Four gliadin fractions can be separated electrophoretically and each is toxic (Ciclitira *et al.*, 1984). However, sensitivity to gluten occurs in other diseases and in dermatitis herpetiformis results in intestinal changes similar to those in coeliac disease (Anderson *et al.*, 1984). However, the mechanism of its action is not really known. One theory links coeliac disease to the absence of a critical enzyme in the jejunum, and the other suggests that the jejunum in coeliac disease is more susceptible to antigenic reaction to gliadin thus causing submucosal lesions.

As soon as the diagnosis is made, the patient should be put on to a gluten-free diet. It may take several weeks to obtain a satisfactory response to the diet, but after this time, failure to respond should raise a suspicion that there has been an error in diagnosis, and that the steatorrhoea is secondary to some other organic disease. The response of the patient is shown by rapid gain in weight and height (Young and Pringle, 1971) and parallel with this there is biochemical evidence of the restoration of normal jejunal mucosa. This can be checked by doing a mucosal biopsy, but usually a faecal fat determination is sufficient. A recurrence of fatty stools should raise the question as to the strict adherence of the patient to the diet, and failure here may result from the kindness of relatives and friends who offer the child biscuits, bread, or cake. Different patterns of response to the diet are, however, found, and these are summarized in Fig. 10.1. Life-long adherence to the diet is necessary. Fetal abnormalities (Mortimer *et al.*, 1968), and infertility that was improved by diet (Morris *et al.*, 1970) have been reported in women with coeliac disease. Furthermore, irreversible deterioration may be precipitated in a patient who has been maintained in good health for a number of years on a gluten-free diet (Booth, 1970).

Only wheat and rye gluten are harmful; barley may also be harmful but definite evidence of this is at present lacking. Maize flour, rice, and potatoes are harmless, and so too is gluten-free flour made from wheat and rye. Except in the early stages, the diet need not be restricted in fat. However, great care must be taken in selecting other items of the diet as many of these, for instance

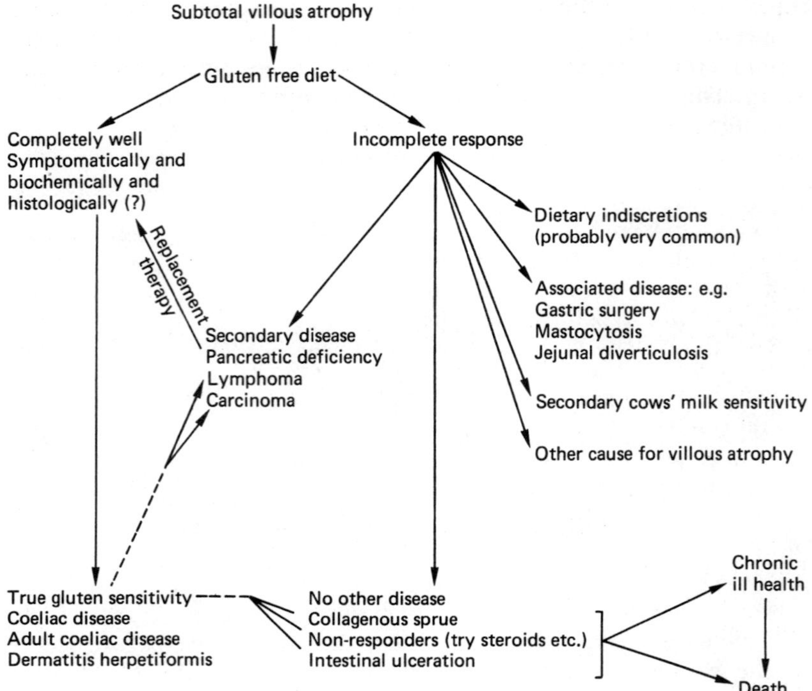


Fig. 10.1 Varying response of patients with subtotal villous atrophy to a gluten diet (from Losowsky *et al.*, 1974). --- indicates that the course is followed by only a minority of subjects. Reproduced by permission of Churchill Livingstone, Edinburgh.

some brands of ice cream and sweets, may contain flour. A sample gluten-free diet is shown in the Appendix (Table 1). A thoroughly practical book of gluten-free recipes is available (Hills, 1977) and can be strongly recommended. It should be noted that gluten-free products based on wheat starch contain gliadin which exacerbates coeliac disease (Ciclitira *et al.*, 1985).

Hypoalbuminaemia occurs in about 50 per cent of patients with coeliac disease, and depending on the severity of the disease, the patient may require supplements of vitamins and minerals. Clinical deficiency of vitamin A has not been reported and the assessment of vitamin E status is made difficult by the absence in the human of a specific disease due to its deficiency. Vitamin K deficiency occurs in over 70 per cent of patients with coeliac disease (Bossak *et al.*, 1957). It appears that restoration of a normal mucosa is necessary before vitamin D can enhance calcium absorption (Nassim *et al.*, 1959). A deficiency of magnesium has been reported in various forms of steatorrhoea, and the degree of depletion may be related to the amount of fat excreted (Booth *et al.*, 1963). Malabsorption of folic acid is almost invariable in coeliac disease and that of $B_{12}$ occurs in about 40 per cent of cases and is related to the severity of the disease. Unequivocal evidence for deficiencies of other water-soluble vitamins appears to be lacking, although a proportion of patients show impaired absorption of vitamin $B_6$ (Brain and Booth, 1964), and it is probable that ascorbic acid supplements should be given. Low plasma zinc concentrations, and a reduction in taste acuity which is associated with zinc deficiency (Hambidge *et al.*, 1972), have been reported in adults with coeliac disease (Solomons *et al.*, 1976). The patients also had low plasma albumen concentrations due to the concomitant protein-losing enteropathy. However, there was a poor correlation between the plasma levels of zinc and albumen suggesting that they were not causally related. The authors suggested that malabsorption of zinc may have occurred due to intestinal chelation with fatty acids.

**Tropical sprue**

This is a disease of unknown aetiology which in many respects closely resembles coeliac disease in both its clinical manifestation, and the changes that occur in the physiology of the small intestine. There are, however, important differences between gluten-induced enteropathy and tropical sprue, for whereas the former responds to a gluten-free diet and not to folic acid, the latter responds to folic acid and not to a gluten-free diet (Jeejeebhoy *et al.*, 1966). There is impaired glucose, fat, vitamin $B_{12}$, and folic acid absorption, and there may be a consequent megaloblastic anaemia. The general mode of treatment is to give vitamin $B_{12}$ by injection and folic acid by mouth. Multivitamin tablets should also be administered, and if there is a sign of bony changes then effervescent calcium tablets should also be given. Sometimes an iron preparation is necessary.

**Crohn's disease**

The cause of Crohn's disease is still unknown and its management remains unsatisfactory. The disease is uncommon in the upper part of the small intestine but may well occur in the lower part and in such patients malabsorption may be severe. It is not surprising that malnutrition is common in this condition (Harries *et al.*, 1982) and is probably multifactorial (Grand, 1980). Folic acid (Hoffbrand *et al.*, 1968) and ascorbic acid (Gerson and Fabry, 1974) deficiencies are probably due to malnutrition caused by nutritionally poor low-residue diets. Malnutrition is also associated with iron deficiency anaemia (Harries *et al.*, 1984). Symptoms of zinc deficiency are frequent complications in patients with low serum zinc levels (McClain *et al.*, 1980). In some but not all Crohn's patients who have small-bowel resection the low serum zinc concentrations correlate with low muscle zinc concentrations (Hessov *et al.*, 1983). It is clear that deficiencies of vitamins and minerals should be identified and rectified. It is particularly important to exclude $B_{12}$ deficiency before folic acid supplements are given. Some patients benefit from a low fat diet which results in a decrease in the diarrhoea and faecal electrolyte loss. In patients who have small bowel resections a low fat diet increases zinc absorption (Hessov *et al.*, 1983). Feeding patients parenterally to achieve total bowel rest has been advocated in the management of patients with Crohn's disease, but this seems not to be necessary (Lochs *et al.*, 1983). Elemental diets such as Vivonex (p. 489) have been used over long periods in severely malnourished patients with satisfactory results (Goode *et al.*, 1976). More recently, attention has been directed to the possibility that specific food intolerance may play an important role in Crohn's disease. Of 29 patients having food intolerances, 21 remained in remission on diets alone for a mean period of 15 months

(Workman *et al.*, 1984). The most important foods provoking symptoms were wheat and dairy products.

**Radiotherapy**

The epithelium of the small intestine is second only to the bone marrow in its sensitivity to radiation. Altered intestinal function may occur during therapy and usually disappears. However, patients with persistent and recurring damage are often difficult to manage. The measures outlined above are usually helpful. The fat content of the diet should be reduced or the fat replaced with medium-chain triglycerides and appropriate vitamin and mineral supplements given parenterally if necessary.

**Drugs**

The effects of drugs on the digestion and absorption of nutrients is discussed in Chapter 18.

**Blind loop syndrome**

Small bowel stasis gives rise to the 'blind loop syndrome' and this may develop in patients with blind loops, fistulas, strictures, and diverticulae. The causes of the malabsorption that occurs in this condition are not well understood (Goldstein, 1971), but it has been established that bacteria colonize the loop and use vitamin $B_{12}$ and other essential nutrients for their own metabolism. The steatorrhoea that occurs is caused by bacterial deconjugation of bile salts which then become less efficient in forming micelles necessary for the absorption of fat. In some patients anorexia and general malaise may result from the absorption of toxic metabolites produced by bacterial action in the lumen of the intestine. Chenodeoxycholate has been suspected as one possible metabolite causing fever and liver abnormalities. Treatment is usually by surgery, but vitamin $B_{12}$ in large doses is often required.

Maldigestion may occur as a result of a deficiency of bile salts or pancreatic enzymes. Replacement of bile salts is not practicable because they cause irritation in the colon, but pancreatic enzymes can be given orally. In the absence of bile salts, dietary fat should be replaced by medium-chain glycerides.

Protein insufficiency may develop in those patients with oedema and hypoalbuminaemia as the only symptom, but occasionally a more serious condition resembling kwashiorkor may develop. There may be interference with the absorption of some amino acids by bile salts. Low concentrations of essential amino acids have been found in the serum of patients with the blind loop syndrome, and this suggests that bacteria may metabolize amino acids to a form in which they are unavailable to the host. These changes are completely reversed by antibiotics. A few patients may show evidence of malabsorption of carbohydrates.

**Short bowel syndrome**

The availability of methods of nutritional maintenance which necessitate a minimal absorption capacity (elemental diets) or none at all (parenteral hyperalimentation) now tempts surgeons to perform resections that would have been rejected previously because of high initial mortality and morbidity rates. Whilst it is reasonably easy to provide adequate nutrition parenterally during the initial period following such operations, and in some cases this has been extended to periods exceeding a year (Shils, 1975), it is necessary to consider more carefully the potential for long-term rehabilitation of these nutritional cripples. In addition to those resections that are carried out for disease of the small bowel, the short gut syndrome may be produced iatrogenically by reversible bypass procedures in the treatment of the morbidly obese. The absorptive defects resulting from gut resection depend upon the degree of resection, the area resected, the presence or absence of the ileocaecal valve, and the state of the remaining bowel (Zamchek and Broitman, 1973). Gastric hypersecretion, diminished absorption of bile salts, and complicating pancreatic insufficiency contribute to the problem.

Three clinical stages have been described in patients after resection of the small intestine (Pullan, 1959). In the first stage, immediately after surgery, the survival of the patient is threatened by fluid and electrolyte losses due to vomiting and diarrhoea and by bowel complications such as fistula and intra-abdominal sepsis. Nothing is gained by premature oral feeding, and all essential fluid, electrolyte and nutrient requirements should be met parenterally (Wright and Tilson, 1973). These authors recommend that nothing be given by mouth while diarrhoea exceeds 2 litres/day, or seven or eight bowel movements. This diarrhoea may not start for several days, or it may be delayed for 2 to 3 weeks. It is important not to be deceived by the apparent early good progress.

Normal water and electrolyte needs should be met daily. Hypokalaemia commonly occurs unless the replacement of potassium is quantitative. Losses of 150–200 mmol of potassium per day may occur in these patients. Clinically significant deficiencies of calcium, phosphate, and magnesium take some weeks to develop (Ladefoged *et al.*, 1980).

Parenteral nutrition is discussed in Chapter 23 and there are now a number of extensive reviews of the subject. It is important to recognize that the aim of parenteral nutrition is to maintain the ideal lean body mass, and that this cannot be done by giving 5 per cent dextrose solutions (Table 10.3).

Oral or tube-feeding should be started as soon as possible but the restoration of enteral nutrition must be done cautiously in those patients in whom a considerable proportion of the small intestine has been removed (Wright and Tilson, 1973). Suitable diets for administration by tube are presented elsewhere (Chapter 22). It is often advantageous to give these feeds as a slow continuous 24-hour drip which allows for more complete absorption and diminishes the diarrhoea. If there is evidence of gastric hypersecretion, or the diarrhoea is uncontrollable, further surgery may be necessary. Experiments with dogs

Table 10.3 Energy value of different volumes of 5 % dextrose solution

| Volume (ml) | Total dextrose content (g) | Energy yield (kcal) |
|---|---|---|
| 1 000 | 50 | 200 |
| 5 000 | 250 | 1000 |
| 10 000 | 500 | 2000 |
| 12 500 | 625 | 2500 |

suggest that adequate parenteral nutrition during this stage may play an important role in the adaptation of the small intestine to resection, and hence to the progress of the patient to the second stage (Wilmore *et al.*, 1971).

Stage two is characterized by a subsidence of the diarrhoea and the accompanying fluid and electrolyte problems. There is a return of appetite, and bowel function becomes quite normal in the absence of eating. The emphasis moves to the restoration of normal and adequate nutrition by the use of normal foods. This move must again be made cautiously. At first the feeds must be small and repeated every 2 hours during the course of the day. Skimmed milk should be used because of its lower fat content. If the milk potentiates the diarrhoea (particularly in the black races) the patient should be investigated for lactase deficiency (Wapnick, 1972). The primary problem is the delivery of hypertonic solutions of high calorie value to a deficient gut without potentiating diarrhoea. Solutions should at first be isotonic and usually cannot be raised much above 400–450 mosmol/kg body weight for several weeks (Wright and Tilson, 1973). Such solutions are often unpalatable and poorly consumed.

The diet can only be enriched by trial and error and Wright and Tilson (1973) recommended that carbohydrate be added first and no further additions made until the gut can absorb 50 to 100 g/day. Protein should then be added as lean meat. Fibrous foods should be avoided. Ordinary foods may be supplemented by the use of elemental diets (so-called 'space-diets') containing L-amino acids, glucose, vitamins, minerals, and ethyl linoleate.

These nutrients are rapidly absorbed from the upper gastrointestinal tract and leave a minimum of residue in the lower gastrointestinal tract. They are believed not to stimulate intestinal secretion and therefore tend to reduce the output from gastrointestinal fistulas. It is important, however, to remember that they are very hypertonic with an osmolarity of about 1200 mosmol/litre. It is probably best for the patient to sip these diets throughout the day. The addition of fat to the diet is desirable because it makes the diet more interesting and increases its energy content. However, an increase in steatorrhoea must be avoided and considerable trial and error may be necessary on the part of dietitian, cook, and patient to produce an acceptable formula. Medium-chain triglycerides have been used with success in patients with massive gut resection (French, 1968; Bochenek *et al.*, 1970), but diarrhoea may not be reduced for several days after their incorporation into the diet. The reason for this delay is not known, but it is clear that the triglycerides must be given a fair trial before being rejected. Many patients do not accept the oil well, and Wright and Tilson (1973) comment that they have not been able to induce patients to take much more than 40–50 g daily. It has been suggested that one contributing cause of the diarrhoea in patients who have had partial enterectomy is the failure of the enterohepatic circulation of bile salts so that abnormal amounts of bile salts pass into the colon where they inhibit the absorption of water (Hofmann, 1967). In support of this suggestion, it has been found that patients with resections of less than 100 cm, but not more, responded favourably to the administration of cholestyramine (Hofmann and Poley, 1972).

Patterns of unsaturated fatty acids suggesting essential fatty acid deficiency have been found in the serum of patients who have had gut resections and in those with carcinoma of the oesophagus (Wapnick *et al.*, 1974). In the former group, the degree of deficiency was not related to the magnitude of the resection. Press *et al.*, (1974) found that patients who had no more than 90 cm of small bowel remaining, and who had been on a low fat diet, had a dry scaly skin rash and a serum lecithin fatty acid pattern indicative of essential fatty acid deficiency. The deficiency in these patients was reversed by the cutaneous application of sunflower seed oil. The cutaneous absorption of essential fatty acids has been confirmed in experimental essential fatty acid deficiency (Böhles *et al.*, 1976). About 75 per cent of patients with ileal resection develop hyperoxaluria, and 10–20 per cent of these develop nephrolithiasis (Sickinger, 1975). This complication is related to the deconjugation of bile acids in the small intestine, and to an increase in the ratio of glycine to taurine conjugates. The most likely immediate cause of the complication is an increased absorption of oxalic acid in the small intestine. There are three possible ways of preventing the hyperoxaluria and hence preventing also the more serious nephrolithiasis. Cholestyramine may be given to bind bile acids and thus reduce the amounts of conjugates formed. Alternatively, taurine, in a dose of 9 g per day, may be given orally to replenish the taurine pool and thus reduce the endogenous synthesis of glycine. Finally, tetracycline may be used to reduce the amounts of deconjugation due to bacterial flora and thus reduce the amount of oxalic acid formed in this way.

Supplements of calcium, magnesium, and vitamins as suggested in Table 10.4 should be given as necessary.

Those patients who survive to stage 3 reach a final period in which maximum weight is achieved, and this is usually within 20 per cent of the ideal value. They are usually those patients with less extensive resections, and those who can take a more or less normal diet divided into a number of small meals rather than the usual three. Diarrhoea may continue to be a problem, but with time the colon adapts.

Bypass operations offer the opportunity for weight loss in the extremely obese without recourse to drastic diets, diuretics, appetite suppressants, and stimulants. Patients must clearly be well-motivated to undergo such procedures, but the general conclusion from the literature seems to be that the advantages outweigh the comparatively minor inconveniences. Three types of bypass have been performed: jejunocolic and jejuno-ileo (Payne *et al.*, 1973), and gastric (Printen and Mason, 1973). Jejuno-ileal bypass tends to be associated with an increased fat deposition in the liver during the period of rapid weight loss (Payne *et al.*, 1973; Bendezu *et al.*, 1976). In a study of 29 patients 21 months after bypass, the last authors reported a significant fall in serum cholesterol, serum triglycerides, blood sugar after a glucose load, and fasting plasma insulin levels. They also noted occasional increased secretion of oxalate and hypomagnesaemia. Hypomagnesaemia may also be found pre-operatively because obese patients are often given diuretics (Swenson *et al.*, 1974).

**Sugar malabsorption**

Defective digestion and absorption of dietary carbohydrate is common in infants and children (Holzel *et al.*, 1959) and occurs also in adults. It may result from a primary inherited enzyme defect and thus be permanent, or be a secondary phenomenon of temporary duration following mucosal damage or bacterial colonization of the intestine. Disaccharidase deficiency may be

**Table 10.4** Suggested doses for repletion of vitamins and minerals (adapted from Losowsky *et al.*, 1974)

| | |
|---|---|
| Vitamin A | Deficiency, 30 000 μg (100 000 units) retinol per day initially. Maintenance 9000 μg (30 000 units) retinol per day. |
| Vitamin D | Biochemical deficiency, 1250 μg (50 000 units) per day with twice weekly monitoring of serum Ca, reducing dose rapidly as necessary.<br>Severe deficiency 2500 μg (100 000 units) intramuscularly weekly initially.<br>In severe steatorrhoea 2500 μg (100 000 units) intramuscularly monthly with occasional checks on serum Ca. |
| Vitamin E | If deficiency suggested by biochemical and haematological findings, give 50 to 100 mg per day. No clear-cut syndrome except in infants. |
| Vitamin K | Haemorrhage, 10 mg intramuscularly (or intravenously), repeated after several hours if necessary. |
| Riboflavin | Suspected deficiency, up to 50 mg per day orally. Parenteral preparation available. |
| Nicotinic acid | Suspected deficiency, up to 500 mg per day orally. Intravenous injection of up to 100 mg in encephalopathy. |
| Pyridoxine | Up to 50 mg per day, or more, may be used. |
| Folic acid | 5 mg three times per day by mouth. Intramuscular preparation available. |
| Vitamin $B_{12}$ | 1000 μg hydroxocobalamin daily for 7 days then every 2 months. |
| Ascorbic acid | 200 to 1000 mg per day orally in deficiency. |
| Iron | Many oral preparations. Intramuscular and intravenous preparations available. |
| Calcium | Milk and milk products are a good source. Calcium Sandoz chocolate tablets, four 3 times daily. Intravenous calcium gluconate can be given in an emergency. If there is difficulty in raising serum Ca levels, consider Mg replacement. |
| Magnesium | 15 to 125 mmol of chloride or hyroxide per day orally as necessary.<br>Intravenous or intramuscular preparations are available.<br>Magnesium sulphate or chloride can be given intravenously in saline to replace calculated extracellular deficit during 24 hours. There is danger in too-rapid injection. |

specific or general and in either case diarrhoea is the principal symptom. The diarrhoea results when the offending carbohydrate(s) is present in the diet and is more severe in infants and children than in adults. The diarrhoea is osmotic in origin and is caused by the presence of undigested disaccharides in the lumen of the intestine.

It is necessary to distinguish between 'sugar intolerance' which is a treatable disorder in which diarrhoea and/or vomiting is caused when a particular sugar or sugars are ingested, and 'sugar malabsorption' which may be diagnosed when there is laboratory evidence of disordered sugar absorption (Walker-Smith, 1975). A diagnosis of sugar malabsorption does not necessarily imply that there is a clinically important degree of sugar intolerance.

Table 10.5 Varieties of sugar malabsorption and their dietary management (modified from Walker–Smith, 1975)

| | |
|---|---|
| *Disorders of disaccharide absorption* | |
| 1. Primary | |
| congenital alactasia. Permanent | Lactose-free diet. |
| sucrose–isomaltase deficiency. Probably permanent | Sucrose-free diet. |
| 2. Secondary: | |
| caused by a number of conditions including gastroenteritis, coeliac disease, giardiasis, protein–energy malnutrition, following neonatal surgery, cows' milk protein intolerance, cystic fibrosis, immunodeficiency syndromes, massive resection of the small intestine. Transient | Lactose-free diet. |
| 3. Later onset or 'racial' lactose intolerance: common in Africans, Greek Cypriots, Indians, Chinese, American Negroes, New Guinea natives and Australian Aborigines. Rare in Caucasians. May be transient | Variable degree of lactose intolerance. |
| *Disorders of monosaccharide absorption* | |
| 1. Primary: | |
| congenital glucose-galactose malabsorption. Permanent | Child able to include some milk and sugar in the diet in later years but unrestricted leads to recurrence of symptoms. |
| 2. Secondary: | |
| can occur following neonatal surgery and in protein-energy malnutrition. Transient | Carbohydrate-free formula for short time to which glucose and/or fructose may be added in increments of 1 %. |

The varieties of sugar malabsorption that have been described, together with indications for their dietary management, are shown in Table 10.5. Clinical assessment combined with laboratory investigations are necessary for the diagnosis of sugar intolerance in children and a scheme for the investigation of post-operative diarrhoea in a neonate is shown in Fig 10.2. The carbohydrate content of various milks and milk formulas is shown in Table 10.6.

It is important to note the wide range of diseases and conditions which may give rise to secondary lactose intolerance. Those listed in the table are largely those that occur in infants and children. Adults with diarrhoea due to inflammatory bowel disease or gastrectomy occasionally improve when milk and milk products are omitted from the diet.

The rare inherited disorder acrodermatitis enteropathica becomes manifest at weaning or before weaning in bottle-fed babies and is characterized by lactose intolerance. The skin lesions and the bowel functions return rapidly to normal when the child is given supplements of zinc sulphate (Moynahan,

Table 10.6 Carbohydrate content of various milks and milk formulas (g/100 ml) (adapted from Walker–Smith, 1975)

| | Lactose | Sucrose | Glucose | Starch | Others |
|---|---|---|---|---|---|
| Breast milk | 7 | – | – | – | – |
| Cows' milk | 4.5 | – | – | – | – |
| Cow & Gate Half Cream Babymilk 1 | 7.1 | – | – | – | – |
| Cow & Gate Full Cream Babymilk 2 | 4.2 | 3.3 | – | – | – |
| Cow & Gate V formula | 7.0 | – | – | – | – |
| Ostermilk 1. Half Cream | 7.0 | – | – | – | – |
| Ostermilk 2. Full Cream | 4.7 | 2.0 | – | – | – |
| Lactogen | 5.3 | 1.4 | – | – | – |
| Sweetened condensed milk diluted 1 in 8 | 1.8 | 6.7 | – | – | – |
| SMA | 7.0 | – | – | – | – |
| S 26 | 7.0 | – | – | – | – |
| Enfamil | 7.0 | – | – | – | – |
| Nutramigen (Australia) | – | – | 5.8 | 2.6 | – |
| Nutramigen (UK) | – | 6.1 | – | 2.7 | – |
| Sobee | – | 1.2 | – | 2.6 | 3.6* |
| Pro-Sobee | – | 3.8 | – | – | 3.0† |
| Galactomin 17 | – | – | 1.25 | – | 5.0** |
| Galactomin 19 | – | – | – | – | 7.3†† |
| Pregestemil | – | – | 6.3 | 2.3 | – |
| Al 110 | – | – | 7.1 | – | – |

* Dextrimaltose. † Corn sugars. ** Maltose, dextrins, and higher sugars. †† Fructose.

1974). The optimum dose appears to be 150 mg of zinc sulphate per day in divided doses. An acrodermatitis-like rash has been reported in two infants fed parenterally for diarrhoea (Arakawa *et al.*, 1976). This condition was characterized by low plasma zinc concentrations and responded dramatically to oral zinc sulphate (35 mg/day).

Vitamin K deficiency may occur in infants with chronic diarrhoea (Thomas *et al.*, 1972) and be a cause of subdural haematoma.

### Abetalipoproteinaemia

Lipoprotein deficiency occurs as a genetic disorder, abetalipoproteinaemia, which is characterized by an inability to absorb normal fat due to the lack of the specific lipoprotein required to coat the chylomicrons in the mucosal cell and so permit their passage into the lymph. These patients can, however, absorb medium-chain triglycerides and these should be used instead of ordinary fat.

### Tumours

Intestinal obstructions due to tumours cause loss of fluid and electrolytes which must be made good by appropriate infusions and intravenous feeding if necessary.

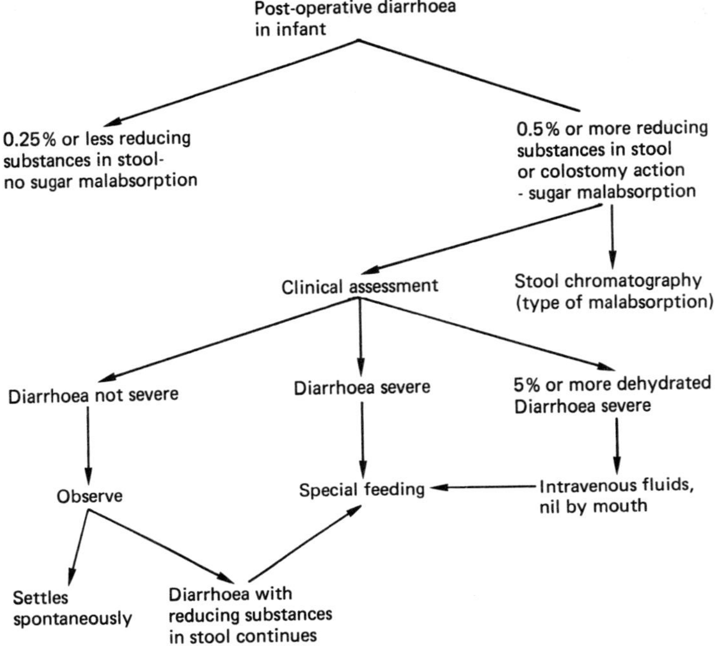


Fig. 10.2 Scheme for investigation of post-operative diarrhoea in a neonate, for sugar malabsorption (from Walker–Smith, 1975). Reproduced by permission of Pitman Medical Publishing Co. Ltd, Tunbridge Wells.

**Fistulas**

Gastrojejunocolic fistulas produce diarrhoea and steatorrhoea in which bacterial overgrowth in the small intestine plays a role. Fistulas may also occur between the small intestine, large intestine, bladder, and abdominal wall in Crohn's disease. Wherever they occur, fistulas result in abnormal losses of intestinal contents and malnutrition and hypoproteinaemia is not uncommon. The nutrition of the patient plays an important role in deciding whether surgery is necessary or not, and should be provided by the use of low residue tube-feeds as a continuous drip or parenterally. Delay in instituting adequate nutrition may be life-threatening and the patient may succumb to infection.

## Protein-losing enteropathies

This is a term used for a group of abnormal conditions in which there is excessive loss of plasma protein into the gastrointestinal tract with resulting oedema and hypoproteinaemia (Waldmann, 1966; Schussheim, 1972). Diseases showing protein-losing enteropathy (PLE) have no single common aetiology. Excessive protein loss into the bowel may result from obstructed outflow of the gastrointestinal lymphatics (e.g. lymphangiectasia, and carcinoma), exudation through an inflamed and ulcerated mucosa (e.g. regional enteritis, ulcerative colitis, coeliac disease), excessive secretion of mucus (e.g. atrophic gastritis, gastrointestinal cancer), or excessive loss in other disorders (e.g.

nephrosis, defective gamma globulin synthesis). Losses of iron, copper, calcium, and lipid may accompany the loss of protein. The latter may amount to 30–60 per cent of the circulating protein pool, or 1–2 g protein per kg body weight per day. Treatment must be directed to the primary cause of the condition, but management with gluten-free diet or medium-chain triglycerides has been found useful. It is also necessary to give intravenous infusions of albumin and fluids.

## The large intestine and rectum

### Irritable bowel syndrome

This disorder may affect up to a quarter of the population, the majority of whom suffer in silence. Nevertheless, the minority of the afflicted population constitute a major part of a gastroenterologist's workload (Fielding, 1977). The symptoms of IBS are variable. They include abdominal pain, flatulence, dyspepsia and irregular bowel habits. It has been suggested that a fibre-depleted Western diet is responsible for the condition and many gastroenterologists recommend bran or other bulk additives in its management, in spite of conflicting evidence of their value (Heaton, 1985). The suggestion (Alun-Jones *et al.*, 1982) that food intolerance plays a major role in its pathogenesis is largely unsubstantiated.

Chaudhary and Truelove (1962) identified two sub-groups of patients; those with 'spastic colon' who complained of pain associated with variable bowel habits, and those with painless diarrhoea. Read (1984) has suggested that for the purpose of clinical trials the following symptomatic definition should be used for what he calls the irritable 'colon' rather than the irritable bowel syndrome: abdominal pain together with a disturbance of bowel habit, which may be either diarrhoea or constipation or both and often encompasses urgency, frequent calls to stool and feelings of incomplete evacuation. The definition should also include the statement that these symptoms cannot be explained by specific pathology of the colon.

IBS appears to be a predominantly female complaint commonly presenting in the third or fourth decade. Thus the majority of sufferers are pre-menopausal women and it is therefore possible that changes in hormonal status may be an aetiological factor. This suggestion is supported by the finding (Wald *et al.*, 1981) that the luteal phase of the menstrual cycle is associated with increased progesterone levels and prolongation of gastrointestinal transit time. Studies by Christofides *et al.*, (1982) in relation to pregnancy suggest that progesterone causes the inhibition of the gut-stimulatory hormone motilin, which has powerful effects on the smooth muscle of the gastric antrum, duodenum and colon (Christofides, 1978). The passing of loose motions at the beginning of menstruation (Rees and Rhodes, 1976; Wald *et al.*, 1981; Leeds *et al.*, 1982; Davies *et al.*, 1986) has been attributed to the release of prostaglandins E2 and F2d by endometrial tissue (Gonzalez, 1980). These observations may, in some women, seriously question the validity of a diagnosis of IBS if emphasis is placed upon alterations in bowel function (Drossman *et al.*, 1982).

The treatment of IBS is largely symptomatic. Increasing the fibre content of the diet may paradoxically reduce constipation and ease diarrhoea. The possibility that the condition is caused or exacerbated by adverse reactions to specific dietary constituents should be investigated. In this connection, it is important to take a full dietary and symptom history. Foods which seem to be associated with symptoms can then be eliminated from the diet for a trial period without the necessity for going through a full elimination programme.

## Ulcerative colitis

This is the commonest cause of chronic diarrhoea in temperate climates. Its aetiology is unknown although a number of theories have been put forward. One of these is that the disorder is an allergic disease, and it is of interest that a high incidence of known allergic diseases such as hay fever and eczema has been found in patients with ulcerative colitis and also in their relatives. In about 20 per cent of patients there seems to be some allergy to cows' milk protein (Wright and Truelove, 1965), and these patients benefit from a milk-free diet. Another contributing reason for the beneficial effect of such a diet is that a minority of patients are deficient in lactase and the diet results in exclusion of lactose.

The disease in often associated with psychological disturbances and this is one reason for not imposing an unreasonably restricting diet. However, in the acutely ill patient a diet consisting of toast, butter, soft boiled eggs, meat, potatoes, clear broth, tea, rice, jelly, and custards has been recommended (Zamchek and Broitman, 1973). Further liberalizations by the addition of cooked vegetables and canned fruits can occur when the stools are consistently formed and free of blood. Frequent small meals, attractively presented to help the appetite, are generally better tolerated than three regular ones. Zamchek and Broitman suggest that a diet containing 2400 to 3600 kilocalories (10.1 to 15.1 MJ) and 125 to 150 g protein may be necessary to restore nitrogen balance.

## Cancer

In western countries, cancer of the colon is second only to that of the lung as a killing neoplasm, and these tumours have the same epidemiology as diverticular disease. It remains to be shown, however, whether individuals such as vegans and vegetarians who normally consume more fibre have a lower incidence of the disease. It is interesting in this connection that the gut flora of Americans and Britons degrade bile to form potential carcinogens. There is a tendency for the disease to relapse spontaneously, but for others surgery is often required. A diet rich in protein and carbohydrate with vitamin supplements is required. Faecal loss of fluid, electrolytes, and blood must be made good and every attempt made to maintain the patient in nitrogen balance. Considerable loss of protein amounting to up to 50 g per day in the stools occurs in some patients with carcinoma of the colon and benign papillomas of the colon and rectum and this complicates the management.

The principal function of the colon is the absorption of water and electrolytes which escape reabsorption in the small bowel. Surgery of the large bowel generally results in diarrhoea though a few patients after colostomy complain of constipation. This condition usually results from a change of dietary habits to produce a very high residue stool. It is customary to advise colostomy patients to take a low residue diet, but this may produce a high volume stool which is unacceptable because of its demands on colostomy care. Reversal to a high residue diet then produces constipation. Dietary adjustment must be made by trial and error. In a survery of members of the Ileostomy Association of Great Britain and Ireland, questionnaires from 952 people were analysed with special reference to the production of watery flow, upset of timing of filling of the bag, flatulence, pain, and odour (Thomson *et al.*, 1970). It was concluded that patients should not omit any particular item from their diets unless it repeatedly caused dyspepsia.

## Diverticular disease

Epidemiological evidence suggests that the incidence of diverticular disease has increased during the last century or so and that it is a disease of western civilization (Painter, 1975). The percentage of individuals presenting with diverticuli in the colon increases with age and some reports put the incidence as high as 35 per cent of individuals over the age of 60. The aetiology of the disorder is unknown, but it is strongly suspected that a dietary deficiency of fibre in the diet may play a role (Painter and Burkitt, 1971). This deduction is based upon the epidemiology of the disease, and the fact that increasing the fibre content of the diet of patients with diverticular disease results in an improvement of the condition (Painter *et al.*, 1972). The diet contains a high proportion of vegetable fibre and in addition crude bran is given at the rate of 2 to 6 dessertspoonfuls per day. Bran tablets (Fybranta) containing 2 g bran per tablet given at the rate of 9 tablets per day have given relief which is superior to that obtained with a high roughage diet (Taylor and Duthie, 1976). Dietary fibre is a complex mixture of indigestible material and the role of its individual components in the possible aetiology of this, or any other condition, is at present unknown.

## Constipation

Constipation may be secondary to other pathological conditions and to psychiatric states, but simple constipation does occur as a troubling disorder in many people and particularly during pregnancy and in the elderly. According to Jones (1972) it can result from lack of roughage in the diet, ignoring the call to evacuate the rectum, emotional disturbances, and travelling. Dietetic treatment would seem to be preferable to the use of laxatives. Increasing the fibre content of the diet has been found to reduce the problem of constipation during pregnancy (Anderson and Whichelow, 1985) and in geriatric hospitals. Whole wheat bread, the use of All-Bran, Shredded Wheat, or Weetabix as a breakfast cereal, and generous portions of green vegetables and salads all help to decrease the transit time of the food through the gut. Fat intake should be generous, but not excessive and the intake of starchy foods, particularly cakes and biscuits, and also sugar, sweets, and chocolates should be reduced. It is also advisable to reduce consumption of milk because milk and milk dishes in some people are prone to give rise to excessive wind. Milk in tea or coffee is allowed, but extra fluid should be taken as water, fruit juice, lager, beer, or stout. In addition to the above dietary changes, the individuals should be encouraged to take a regular walk morning or evening.

## The pancreas

The syndrome of pancreatic insufficiency characterized by weight loss, and steatorrhoea, with or without diabetes mellitus, occurs as the result of chronic pancreatitis or, less commonly, carcinoma of the pancreas. A special diet is not essential in uncomplicated cases of pancreatic insufficiency. Defects in the digestion of carbohydrate and protein, as well as that of fat, are usually present. In order to maintain a high caloric content, however, fat must be included in the diet. Its tolerance varies from case to case and can be between 50 and 150 g per day. Visible fat should be replaced in part, or in its entirety, by medium-chain triglycerides. Only skimmed milk should be used, but chicken, lean meat, or white fish can be taken with any vegetables (except fried potatoes). Fruits, jams, jelly, and sugar should be taken liberally, and extra protein can be obtained from Casilan or Lonalac, preparations of dried milk proteins. Regular parenteral administration of fat-soluble vitamins, and possibly also of $B_{12}$, should be given at intervals of 1–4 weeks. Actual deficiency of $B_{12}$ is rare. It appears that the vitamin is not absorbed well by patients with chronic pancreatitis in the fasting state, but absorption is normal when food is given (Henderson *et al.*, 1972). Most patients improve clinically and benefit from pancreatin (5–10 g) given with meals. The most suitable form of pancreatic replacement therapy seems to be with Cotazym, the contents of 2–3 capsules which are sprinkled over each main meal (Naish and Read, 1974).

Pancreatic insufficiency is a common consequence of cystic fibrosis, and is responsible for the nutritional abnormalities found in patients with the disease. In some cases the condition is complicated by small bowel malabsorption and hepatic abnormalities. The condition is often helped by a high protein, low fat diet with adequate supplements of fat-soluble vitamins and enzyme preparations (Dhar *et al.*, 1973). A relatively high dose of pancreatic enzymes (0.1 to 0.3 g pancreatin per kg body weight per day) is required. Disaccharidase deficiency may necessitate the elimination of milk products from the diet. Medium-chain triglycerides may be used with advantage (Huang, 1968).

## Conclusion

Almost all diseases of the alimentary tract affect the digestion and absorption of food. In some diseases, dietary modification is an important part of treatment. In others, adequate nutrition contributes greatly to the success of other forms of treatment, be it surgery, radiation, or drugs, and plays an important role in the rehabilitation of the patient and the protection against infection. The elucidation of nutritional deficiencies in individual cases may necessitate close collaboration between clinician, biochemist and nutritionist and implementation by informed nursing staff.

## References


Alun Jones, V., Shorthouse, M., McLaughlan, P., Workman, E.M. and Hunter, J.O. (1982). Food intolerance: a major factor in the pathogenesis of Irritable Bowel Syndrome. *Lancet*, **ii**, 1115–17.

Anderson, A.S. and Whichelow, M.J. (1985). Constipation during pregnancy: dietary fibre intake and the effect of fibre supplementation. *Hum. Nutr. Appl. Nutr.*, **39A**, 202–207.

Anderson, H., Björkman, A.C., Gillberg, R., Kastrup, W., Mobacken, H. and Stockbrügger, R. (1984). Influence of the amount of dietary gluten on gastro-intestinal morphology and function in dermatitis herpetiformis. *Hum. Nutr.: Clin. Nutr.*, **38C**, 279–85.

Andrews, J. and Brook, M. (1966). Leucocytes – vitamin C content and clinical signs in the elderly. *Lancet*, **i**, 1350–1.

Arakawa, T., Tamura, T., Igarashi, Y., Suzuki, H. and Sandstead, H.H. (1976). Zinc deficiency in two infants during total parenteral alimentation for diarrhoea. *Am. J. Clin. Nutr.*, **29**, 197–204.

Arneil, G.C., Hutchinson, J.H. and Shanks, R.A. (1973). Personal communication. Referred to in Present-day practice in infant feeding (1975). *DHSS Report on Health and Social Subjects*, No. 9, p. 15. HMSO: London.

Baird, I.M. (1967). Iron deficiency. In *Post-Gastrectomy Nutrition*, pp. 43–53. Ed. Krikler, D.M. Lloyd-Luke: London.

Baird, I.M., Walters, R.L. and Sutton, D.R. (1974). Absorption of slow-release iron and effects of ascorbic acid in normal subjects and after partial gastrectomy. *Br. Med. J.*, **iv**, 505–8.

Bendezu, R., Wieland, R.G., Green, S.G., Hallberg, M.C. and Marsters, R.W. (1976). Certain metabolic consequences of jejunoileal bypass. *Am. J. Clin. Nutr.*, **29**, 366–70.

Bochenek, W., Rodgers, J.B. and Balint, J.A. (1970). Effects of changes in dietary lipids on intestinal fluid loss in the short bowel syndrome. *Ann. Intern. Med.*, **72**, 205–13.

Böhles, H., Bieber, M.A. and Heird, W.C. (1976). Reversal of experimental fatty acid deficiency by cutaneous administration of sunflower oil. *Am. J. Clin. Nutr.*, **29**, 398–401.

Booth, C.C. (1970). The enterocyte in coeliac disease. *Br. Med. J.*, **iv**, 14–17.

Booth, C.C., Hanna, S., Babouris, N. and MacIntyre, I. (1963). Incidence of hypomagnesaemia in intestinal malabsorption. *Br. Med. J.*, **ii**, 141–4.

Bossak, E.T., Wang, C.I. and Aldersberg, D. (1957). Clinical aspects of the malabsorption syndrome (idiopathic sprue). *J. Mt. Sinai Hosp.*, **24**, 286–303.

Bradley, E.L., Isaacs, J., Hersh, T., Davidson, E.D. and Millikan, W. (1975). Nutritional consequences of total gastrectomy. *Ann. Surg.*, **182**, 415–29.

Brain, M.C. and Booth, C.C. (1964). The absorption of tritium-labelled pyridoxine HCl in control subjects and in patients with intestinal malabsorption. *Gut*, **5**, 241–7.

Burkitt, D.P. and James, P.A. (1973). Low-residue diets and hiatus hernia. *Lancet*, **ii**, 128–30.

Burkitt, D.P. (1978). Mechanical effects of fibre with reference to appendicitis, hiatus hernia, haemorrhoids and varicose veins. In *Dietary Fibre: Current Developments of Importance to Health*, pp. 35–40. Ed. Heaton, K.W. Libbey: London.

Castell, D.O. (1975). Diet and the lower oesophageal sphincter. *Am. J. Clin. Nutr.*, **28**, 1296–8.

Celestin, L.R. (1974). Postgastrectomy and postvagotomy problems. In *Basic Gastroenterology*, p. 94. Eds. Naish, J.M. and Read, A.E. Wright: Bristol.

Chaudhary, N.A. and Truelove, S.C. (1962). The irritable colon syndrome. A study of the clinical features, predisposing causes and prognosis in 130 cases. *Q. J. Med.*, **31**, 307–22.

Christofides, N.D. (1978). Importance of the jejunal hormone motilin. In *Gastrointestinal and related hormones*, pp. 51–57. Eds. Walters G. and Bloom, S.R., (Suppl.) *J. Clin. Path.* London: British Medical Association.

Christofides, N.D., Ghatei, M.A., Bloom, S.R., Borberg, C. and Gillmer, M.D.G. (1982). Decreased plasma motilin concentrations in pregnancy. *Br. Med. J.*, **285**, 1453–4.

Ciclitira, P.J., Ellis, H.J. and Fagg, N.L.K. (1984). Evaluation of a gluten-free product containing wheat gliadin in patients with coeliac disease. *Br. Med. J.*, **289**, 83.

Ciclitira, P.J., Cerio, R., Ellis, H.J., Maxton, D., Nelufer, J.M. and Macartney, J.M. (1985). Evaluation of a gliadin-containing gluten free product in coeliac patients. *Hum. Nutr.: Clin. Nutr.*, **39C**, 303–308.

Cleave, T.L. (1974). *The Saccharine Disease*. Wright: Bristol.

Committee on Medical Aspects of Food Policy (1969). Panel on cariogenic foods. First Report. *Br. Dent. J.*, **126**, 273–80.

Davidson, S., Passmore, R., Brock, J.F. and Truswell, A.S. (1979). *Human Nutrition and Dietetics*, 7th ed. Churchill Livingstone: Edinburgh.

Davies, G.J., Crowder, M., Reid, B. and Dickerson, J.W.T. (1986). Bowel function measurements of individuals with different eating patterns. *Gut*, **27**, 164–9.

Dennish, G.W. and Castell, D.O. (1971). Inhibitory effect of smoking on the lower bowel sphincter. *N. Engl. J. Med.*, **284**, 1136–7.

Dhar, P., Zamcheck, N. and Broitman, S.A. (1973). Nutrition in diseases of the pancreas. In *Modern Nutrition in Health and Disease*, 6th ed. Ch. 28, Section C, pp. 819–28. Eds. Goodhart, R.S. and Shils, M.E. Lea and Febiger: Philadelphia.

Doll, R. (1956). Environmental factors in the aetiology of cancer of the stomach. *Gastroenterologia, Basel*, **86**, 320–28.

Dragstedt, L. (1969). Peptic ulcer: an abnormality of gastric secretion. *Am. J. Surg.*, **117**, 143–56.

Drapanas, T. (1967). Discussion following W.H. Gerwig. Gerwig, W.H., Easley, G.W. and Mendoza, C.B. Results following remedial operation for severe dumping syndrome. *Archs Surg.*, **95**, 631–5.

Drossman, D.A., Sandler, R.S., McKee, D.C. and Lovitz, A.J. (1982). Bowel patterns among subjects not seeking health care. *Gastroenterology*, **83**, 529–34.

Durnin, J.G.V.A., and Womersley, J. (1974). Body fat assessed from total body density and its estimation from skinfold thickness: measurements on 481 men and women aged 16 to 72 years. *Br. J. Nutr.*, **32**, 77–97.

Eddy, R.L. (1971). Metabolic bone disease after gastrectomy. *Am. J. Med.*, **50**, 442–9.

Elsborg. L. (1974). Malabsorption of folic acid following partial gastrectomy. *J. Gastroent.*, **9**, 271–4.

Escovitz, G.H. and Rubin, W. (1973). The malabsorption syndrome. *Med. Clins N. Am.*, **57**, 907–23.

Fellows, I.W., Greensmith, J. and Atkinson, M. (1984). The nutritional effects of endoscopic intubation for carcinoma of the oesophagus and cardia. *Clin. Nutr.* **2**, 167–8.

Fielding, J.F. (1977). New aspects of the irritable bowel syndrome. *Ir. Med. J.*, **70**, 304–306.

French, A.B. (1968). Effect of graded increment of medium chain triglycerides on nutrient balance in subjects with intestinal resection. In *Medium-Chain Triglycerides*, pp. 109–19. Ed. Senior, J.R. Univ. of Pennsylvania Press: Philadelphia.

Gerson, C.D. and Fabry, E.M. (1974). Ascorbic acid and fistula formation in regional enteritis. *Gastroenterology*, **67**, 428–33.

Goldstein, F. (1971). Mechanisms of malabsorption and malnutrition in the blind loop syndrome. *Gastroenterology*, **61**, 780–84.

González, E.R. (1980). New era in treatment of dysmenorrhea. *J.A.M.A.*, **244**, 1885–6.

Goode, A., Hawkins, T., Feggetter, J.G.W. and Johnston, I.D.A. (1976). Use of an elemental diet for long-term nutritional support in Crohn's disease. *Lancet*, **i**, 122–4.

Grand, R.J. (1980). Malnutrition and inflammatory bowel disease. In *Nutrition and Gastroenterology*. pp. 125–40. Ed. Winick, M. Chichester: Wiley.

Greenberger, N.J., Rodger, J.B. and Isselbacher, K.J. (1966). Absorption of medium and long chain triglycerides: Factors influencing their hydrolysis and transport. *J. Clin. Invest.*, **45**, 217–27.

Gustafsson, B.E. (1954). Vipeholm dental caries study: survey of literature on carbohydrates and dental caries. *Acta Odont. Scand.*, **11**, 207–31.

Hambidge, K.M., Hambidge, C., Jacobs, M. *et al.*, (1972). Low levels of zinc in hair anorexia, poor growth, and hypogeusia in children. *Pediatr. Res.*, **6**, 868–74.

Harries, A.D., Fitzsimons, E., Dew, M.J., Heatley, R.V. and Rhodes, J. (1984). Association between iron deficiency anaemia and mid-arm circumference in Crohn's disease. *Hum. Nutr.: Clin. Nutr.*, **38C**, 47–53.

Harries, A.D., Jones, L., Heatley, R.V. and Rhodes, J. (1982). Malnutrition in the inflammatory bowel disease: an anthropometric study. *Hum. Nutr.: Clin. Nutr.*, **36C**, 307–313.

Hartles, R.L. and Leach, S.A. (1975). Effect of diet on dental caries. *Br. Med. Bull.*, **31**, 137–41.

Hashim, S.A., Arteaga, A. and Van Itallie, T.B. (1960). Effect of saturated medium-chain triglyceride on serum lipids in man. *Lancet*, **i**, 1105–108.

Heaton, K.W. (1985). Functional diarrhoea: the acid test. *Br. Med. J.*, **290**, 1298–9.

Henderson. J.T., Simpson, J.D., Warwick, R.R.G. and Shearman, D.J.C. (1972). Does malabsorption of Vitamin $B_{12}$ occur in chronic pancreatitis. *Lancet*, **ii**, 241–3.

Hessov, I., Hasselblad, C., Fasth, S. and Hultén, L. (1983). Zinc depletion after small-bowel resections for Crohn's disease. *Hum. Nutr.: Clin. Nutr.*, **37C**, 353–9.

Hills, H.C. (1977). *Good Food*: Grain-free, Milk-free. Roberts Publications: London.

Hoffband, A.V. (1967). Vitamin $B_{12}$ and folic acid. In *Post-Gastrectomy Nutrition*, pp. 1–15. Ed. Krikler, D.M. Lloyd-Luke: London.

Hoffbrand, A.V., Stewart, J.S., Booth, C.C. and Mollin, D.L. (1968). Folate deficiency in Crohn's disease: incidence, pathogenesis and treatment. *Br. Med. J.*, **ii**, 71–5.

Hofmann, A.F. (1967). The syndrome of ileal disease and the broken enterohepatic circulation: cholerheic enteropathy. *Gastroenterology*, **52**, 752–7.

Hofmann, A.F. and Poley, J.R. (1972). Role of bile salt malabsorption in pathogenesis of diarrhoea and steatorrhoea in patients with ileal resection. 1. Response to cholestyramine or replacement of dietary long-chain triglyceride with medium-chain triglyceride. *Gastroenterology*, **62**, 918–34.

Hogan, W.J., Viegas De Andrade, S.R. and Winship, D.H. (1972). Ethanol-induced acute esophageal motor dysfunction. *J. App. Physiol.*, **32**, 755–60.

Holloway, P.J., James, P.M.C. and Slack, G.L. (1963). Dental disease in Tristan da Cunha. *Br. Dent. J.*, **115**, 19–25.

Holzel, A., Schwarz, V. and Sutcliffe, K.W. (1959). Defective lactose absorption causing malnutrition in infancy. *Lancet*, **i**, 1126–8.

Horwitt, M.K. (1959). Tocopherol requirements of man. *Fedn Proc.*, **18**, 530 (abstract).

Huang, N.N. (1968). Medium-chain triglycerides in cystic fibrosis. In *Medium-Chain Triglycerides*, pp. 207–17. Ed. Senior, J.R. Univ. Pennsylvania Press: Philadelphia.

Ingelfinger, F.J. (1966). Let the ulcer patient enjoy his food. In *Controversy in Internal Medicine*. Saunders: Philadelphia.

Jeejeebhoy, K.N., Desai, H.G., Noronha, J.M., Antia, F.P. and Parek, H.D.V. (1966). Idiopathic tropical diarrhoea with or without steatorrhoea (tropical malabsorption syndrome). *Gastroenterology*, **51**, 333–4.

Johnston, D., Humphrey, C.S., Walker, B.E., Pulvertaft, C.N. and Goligher, J.C. (1972). Vagotomy without diarrhoea. *Br. Med. J.*, **iii**, 788–90.

Jones, F.A. (1957). Clinical and social problems of peptic ulcer. *Br. Med. J.*, **i**, 719–23; 786–93.

Jones, F.A. (1972). Management of constipation in adults. In *Management of Constipation*, Ch. 4, pp. 97–131. Eds. Jones, F.A. and Godding, E.W. Blackwell: Oxford.

Kangas, J.A., Schmidt, K.M. and Solomon, G.F. (1972). Effect of vitamin E on the development of stress-produced gastric ulceration in the rat. *Am. J. Clin. Nutr.*, **25**, 864–6.

Ladefoged, K., Nicolaidau, P. and Harnum, S. (1980). Calcium, phosphorus, magnesium, zinc and nitrogen balance in patients with severe short bowel syndrome. *Am. J. Clin. Nutr.*, **33**, 2137–44.

Leeds, A.R., Khumalo, T.D., Ndaba, N.G. and Lincoln, D. (1982). Haricot beans, transit time and stool weight. *J. Pl. Fds.*, **4**, 33–41.

Lochs, H., Meryn, S., Marosi, L., Ferenci, P. and Hörtnagl, H. (1983). Has total bowel rest a beneficial effect in the treatment of Crohn's disease? *Clin. Nutr.*, **2**, 61–4.

Losowsky, M.S., Walker, B.E. and Kelleher, J. (1974). *Malabsorption in Clinical Practice*. Churchill Livingstone: Edinburgh.

MacCarthy-Leventhal, E.M. (1959). Post-radiation mouth blindness. *Lancet*, **ii**, 1138–9.

Macdonald, J.A.E. and Cohen, M.M. (1972). Effect of vagotomy on ascorbic acid, nutrition in patients with peptic ulcer. *Br. Med. J.*, **ii**, 738–40.

Machella, T.E. (1950). Mechanisms of the postgastrectomy dumping syndrome. *Gastroenterology*, **14**, 237.

MacKay, C. (1970). Postgastrectomy steatorrhoea. *Am. J. Surg.*, **120**, 324–8.

McClain, N., Soutor, C. and Zieve, L. (1980). Zinc deficiency: a complication of Crohn's disease. *Gastroenterology*, **78**, 272–9.

McKeown, K.C. (1985). The surgical treatment of carcinoma of the oesophagus. *J. R. Coll. Surg.*, **30**, 1–14.

Mix, C.L. (1922). 'Dumping stomach' following gastrojejunostomy. *Surg. Clin. N. Am.*, **2**, 617.

Morris, J.S., Adjukiewicz, A.B. and Read, A.E. (1970). Coeliac infertility: An indication for dietary gluten restriction? *Lancet*, **i**, 213–14.

Mortimer, P.E., Stewart, J.S., Norman, A.P. and Booth, C.C. (1968). Follow-up study of coeliac disease. *Br. Med. J.*, **iii**, 7–9.

Moynahan, E.J. (1974). Acrodermatitis enteropathica: a lethal inherited human zinc-deficiency disorder. *Lancet*, **ii**, 399–400.

Naish, J.M. and Read, A.E. (1974). *Basic Gastro-enterology*. Wright: Bristol.

Nassim, J.R., Saville, P.D, Cook, P.B. and Mulligan, L. (1959). The effects of vitamin D and gluten-free diet in idiopathic steatorrhoea. *Q. Jl Med.*, **28**, 141.

Nazari, S., Dionigi, P. and Dionigi, R. (1984). Nasogastric tube substitution for nutritional support in patients with oesophageal cancer: a simple method. *Clin. Nutr.*, **3**, 59–60.

Neale, G., Antcliff, A.C., Welbourn, R.B., Mollin D.L. and Booth, C.C. (1967). Protein malnutrition after partial gastrectomy. *Q. Jl Med.*, New Series **xxxvi**, 469–94.

Owen, R.D. (1950). The problem of hypopharyngeal carcinoma. *Proc. Roy. Soc. Med.*, **43**, 157–68.

Painter, N.S. (1975). *Diverticular Disease of the Colon*. Heinemann Medical: London.

Painter, N.S., Almeida, A.Z. and Colebourne, K.W. (1972). Unprocessed bran in

treatment of diverticular disease of the colon. *Br. Med. J.*, **ii**, 137–40.
Painter, N.S. and Burkitt, D.P. (1971). Diverticular disease of the colon: A deficiency disease of Western civilizations. *Br. Med. J.*, **ii**, 450–54.
Payne, J.H., Dewind, L., Schwab, C.E. and Kern, W.H. (1973). Surgical treatment of morbid obesity. *Archs Surg.*, **106**, 432–7.
Press, M., Hartop, P.J. and Prottey, C. (1974). Correction of essential fatty acid deficiency in man by the cutaneous application of sunflower-seed oil. *Lancet*, **i**, 597–8.
Printen, K.J. and Mason, E.E. (1973). Gastric surgery for relief of morbid obesity. *Archs Surg.*, **106**, 428–31.
Pullan, J.M. (1959). Massive intestinal resection. *Proc. Soc. Med.*, **52**, 31–7.
Read, N.W. (1984). Bowel transit time of food in man: measurement, regulation and possible importance. *Scand. J. Gastroenterol.*, **19** (Suppl. 96), 77.
Rees, W.D.W. and Rhodes, J. (1976). Altered bowel habit and menstruation. *Lancet*, **ii**, 475.
Royal College of Physicians of London (1976). *Fluoride, Teeth and Health.* London: Pitman.
Schussheim, A. (1972). Protein-losing enteropathies. *Am. J. Gastroenterol*, **58**, 124–32.
Senior, J.R. (1968) (Ed.). *Medium-Chain Triglycerides.* Univ. Pennsylvania Press: Philadelphia.
Shils, M.E. (1971). The esophagus, the vagi and fat absorption. *Surgery Gynec. Obstet.*, **132**, 709–15.
Shils, M.E. (1975). A program for total parenteral nutrition at home. *Am. J. Clin. Nutr.*, **28**, 1429–35.
Shils, M.E. and Gilat, T. (1966). The effects of esophagectomy on absorption in man: clinical and metabolic observations. *Gastroenterology*, **50**, 347–57.
Sickinger, K. (1975). Clinical aspects and therapy of fat malassimilation with particular reference to the use of medium-chain triglycerides. In *The Role of Fats in Human Nutrition*, pp. 116–209. Ed. Vergroessen, A.J. Academic Press: London.
Sircus, W. (Ed.) (1973). *Clins Gastroenterology*, **2**, 217.
Solar, C.J. (1959). Vitamin E and ulcers. *Revta esp. Enferm. Apar. dig. Nutr.*, **18**, 745.
Solomons, N.W., Rosenberg, I.H. and Sandstead, H.H. (1976). Zinc nutrition in coeliac sprue. *Am. J. Clin. Nutr.*, **29**, 371–5.
Stammers, F.A.R. and Williams, J.A. (1963). *Partial Gastrectomy.* Butterworths: London.
Stanciu, C. and Bennett, J.R. (1972). Smoking and gastro-oesophageal reflux. *Br. Med. J.*, **iii**, 793–5.
Swenson, S.A., Lewis, J.W. and Sebby, K.R. (1974). Magnesium metabolism in man with special reference to jejunoileal bypass for obesity. *Am. J. Surg.*, **127**, 250–5.
Taylor, G. (1976). Vitamin C and stroke. *Lancet*, **i**, 247.
Taylor, I. and Duthie, H.L. (1976). Bran tablets and diverticular disease. *Br. Med. J.*, **i**, 988–90.
Thomas, J., Collipp, P.J., Schussheim, A. and Pochedly, C. (1972). Vitamin K deficiency in infants with chronic diarrhoea. *Clin. Med.*, **79**, 25–8.
Thomson, T.J., Runcie, J. and Khan, A. (1970). The effect of diet on ileostomy function. *Gut*, **11**, 482–5.
Truelove, S.C. and Reynell, P.C. (1972). *Diseases of the Digestive System*, 2nd ed. Blackwell: Oxford.
Wald, A., Van Thiel, D.H., Hoechstetter, L., Gavaler, J.S., Egler, K.M., Verm, R., Scott, L. and Lester, R. (1981). Gastrointestinal transit: the effect of the menstrual cycle. *Gastroenterology*, **80**, 1497–1500.
Waldmann, T.A. (1966). Protein-losing enteropathy. *Gastroenterology*, **50**, 422–43.
Walker-Smith, J. (1975). *Diseases of the Small Intestine in Childhood.* Pitman Medical: Tunbridge Wells.

Wapnick, S. (1972). Milk and lactose intolerance following distal small bowel resection. *Am. J. Clin. Nutr.*, **25**, 655–60.

Wapnick, S., Norden, D.A. and Venturas, D.J. (1974). Essential fatty acid deficiency in patients with lesions of the gastrointestinal tract. *Gut*, **15**, 367–70.

Watson, A. (1982). A study of the quality and duration of survival following resection, endoscopic intubation and surgical intubation in oesophageal carcinoma. *Br. J. Surg.*, **69**, 585–8.

Wheldon, E.J., Venables, C.W. and Johnston, I.D.A. (1970). Late metabolic sequence of vagotomy and gastrojejunostomy. *Lancet*, **i**, 437–40.

Williams, J.A. and Cox, A.G. (1969). *After Vagotomy*. Butterworths: London.

Wilmore, D.W., Dudrick, S.J., Daly, J.M. and Vars, H.M. (1971). The role of nutrition in the adaptation of the small intestine after massive resection. *Surgery Gynec. Obstet.*, **132**, 673–80.

Workman, E.M., Alun Jones, V., Wilson, A.J. and Hunter, J.O. (1984). Diet in the management of Crohn's disease. *Hum. Nutr.: Appl. Nutr.*, **38A**, 469–73.

Wright, H.K. and Tilson, M.D. (1973). *Postoperative Disorders of the Gastrointestinal Tract*. Grune and Stratton: New York.

Wright, R. and Truelove, S.C. (1965). Circulating antibodies to dietary protein in ulcerative colitis. *Br. Med. J.*, **ii**, 142–4.

Young, W.F. and Pringle, E.M. (1971). 110 children with coeliac disease, 1950–1969. *Archs Dis. Child.*, **46**, 421–36.

Zamchek, N. and Broitman, S.A. (1973). Nutrition in diseases of the intestines. In *Modern Nutrition in Health and Disease*, Ch. 28, Section B, pp. 785–818. Eds. Goodhart, R.S. and Shils, M.E. Lea and Febiger: Philadelphia.

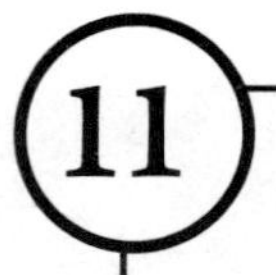

# Disorders of the liver and gall bladder

Neil McIntyre and Carol Bateman



## Introduction

The liver plays a central role in the metabolism of many dietary constituents. It receives portal blood directly from the intestine and removes many water-soluble foodstuffs; it handles lipids and lipid-soluble substances which enter the systemic circulation via the thoracic duct; and by secreting bile into the intestinal lumen plays a major part in the digestion and absorption of fat.

The relationship between food and the liver has been recognized for centuries; as diseases of the liver are often accompanied by anorexia, nausea, vomiting and food intolerance it is hardly surprising that dietary measures have been advocated in their management. These include the use of mineral waters, the avoidance of coffee and spices (because they were thought to cause hyperaemia of the liver), and the administration of liver or liver extracts; even Hippocrates is thought to have used raw liver as treatment. Little or no evidence has been presented to support most of these dietary regimens. A low fat diet is often advocated for hepatitis and cirrhosis. It is bad treatment (except for a small number of patients) but it is still widely used.

This situation reflects a widespread lack of knowledge amongst doctors about the nutritional aspects of liver disease. This is unfortunate. Bad dietary habits may cause hepatobiliary disease and good dietary advice may be invaluable in the management of a number of diseases of the liver.

## Dietary factors in the pathogenesis of liver disease

Some liver diseases are due to excessive ingestion of normal dietary constituents; others have been attributed to dietary deficiency.

### Alcoholic liver disease (Brunt, 1971; Orrego *et al.*, 1981)

This is the most important liver disease induced by dietary indiscretion, at least in western communities. Matthew Baillie linked excessive alcohol intake and a nodular liver in 1793 and the evidence incriminating ethanol as a cause of liver disease is now overwhelming. The mechanism by which it produces liver damage remains obscure. Fatty liver is produced quite rapidly by the ingestion of ethanol but there is little evidence to suggest that fat *per se* causes serious liver damage. Fatty liver resolves with cessation of alcoholic intake.

A proportion of those who drink excessively develop liver cell necrosis and infiltration with inflammatory cells. This alcoholic 'hepatitis' is a precursor of cirrhosis. Only 8–15 per cent of alcoholics are found to have cirrhosis but the risk of developing it is related both to the amount of alcohol ingested and the length of alcohol history. Women may develop cirrhosis more quickly than men. It used to be thought that an excessive alcohol intake would only cause cirrhosis if it was associated with a poor diet. The studies of Lieber and his colleagues have shown that this is not true. Alcohol can produce cirrhosis even when the diet is adequate (Lieber, 1975). All types of alcoholic drinks seem to be capable of damaging the liver and ethanol itself appears to be the common factor. With cessation of alcohol ingestion cirrhosis does not revert to normal and the patient may die of the complications of cirrhosis; despite abstinence, hepatitis may continue to progress to cirrhosis. Even so, the prognosis of alcoholic liver disease is greatly improved by abstinence and every effort should be made to stop alcoholics drinking (Brunt *et al.*, 1974). The short-term effects of abstinence are not impressive: acute exacerbations of alcoholic hepatitis may persist for weeks or months after stopping drinking and large amounts of alcohol can be given to patients with acute alcoholic hepatitis without apparent influence on the rate of recovery (Reynolds *et al.*, 1965).

### Malnutrition (Conn, 1982)

Malnutrition has been considered to be an important factor in the pathogenesis of cirrhosis. In experimental animals cirrhosis can be produced by diets deficient in protein, choline, and vitamins. But in man there is no convincing evidence that cirrhosis is caused by malnutrition *per se*. The liver is certainly affected by undernutrition. Kwashiorkor, a disease of children, occurs when there is protein malnutrition but an adequate caloric intake from carbohydrate. There is a large fatty liver but cirrhosis is a rare consequence.

## Fatty liver (Alpers and Sabesin, 1982)

Fatty liver occurs not only with an excess of alcohol and with protein malnutrition; it may be found when an excessive caloric intake leads to obesity and it sometimes results from parenteral hyperalimentation. The hepatomegaly of obesity is rarely accompanied by significant impairment of liver function and improves rapidly with weight reduction. The hepatomegaly of parenteral hyperalimentation may be associated with elevated serum aspartate aminotransferase and alkaline phosphatase. It has been attributed to a relative excess of carbohydrate over protein and if continued intravenous feeding is essential the proportion of carbohydrate should be reduced.

## Inborn errors of metabolism

Even the constituents of a normal diet may cause disease in some patients; an inborn error of metabolism may interfere with the metabolism of substances such as tyrosine, galactose, fructose, copper and iron, and liver damage can result. The treatment of several of these conditions, e.g. tyrosinosis, galactosaemia, and hereditary fructose intolerance, is critically dependent on early diagnosis and on the exclusion of the offending substance from the diet. But they are all rare diseases and those interested in their dietary management should refer to appropriate chapters in Stanbury *et al.*, (1983).

For Wilson's disease (hepatolenticular degeneration) in which excessive amounts of copper are deposited in the tissues, dietary control is less important than the prompt and prolonged administration of D-penicillamine; this is given to chelate excess tissue copper and to remove it via the urine. But it is sensible to reduce the intake of copper-rich foods and patients should be advised to avoid shellfish, dried fruit, nuts, chocolate, mushrooms and liver.

For genetically determined haemochromatosis, in which tissue iron is excessive, the keystone of treatment is the removal, by venesection, of body iron in the form of haemoglobin. In this condition it is not necessary to recommend a low iron diet, which is unpalatable, as the amount of iron normally absorbed is negligible compared to the amount removed by venesection.

In black Africans marked siderosis can occur in association with the chronic ingestion of a diet high in iron; this comes from iron cooking pots and from iron drums in which alcoholic beverages are prepared. Again, venesection is used to get rid of the iron but in this situation it is sensible to change the cooking utensils and to avoid the ingestion of iron-rich beverages.

## Dangerous foods and dietary contaminants (McIntyre and Morgan, 1979)

Some liver diseases occur from the ingestion of certain foods. The food itself may be toxic, e.g. the mushroom *Amanita phalloides* can cause fatal hepatitis; plants of the genera *Crotalaria* and *Senecio*, which are used to make bush tea, can cause an obstruction of centrilobular hepatic veins due to their content of pyrrolizidine alkaloids. Other foods are dangerous because they are contaminated by noxious agents. Fascioliasis of the liver results from eating water cress contaminated with the metacercariae of *Fasciolia hepatica*. Epidemics of viral hepatitis have been traced to the ingestion of infected clams and oysters.

## Effect of liver disease on nutritional status

### Effect of cirrhosis and other diseases

Many patients with acute or chronic liver disease show no evidence either of general nutritional deficiency or of deficiency of a single substance. Those who are ill commonly lose weight; other clinical signs of malnutrition are rare but detailed biochemical studies frequently reveal a covert nutritional disturbance.

In alcoholics these disturbances are common and are usually attributable to an inadequate diet. Morgan *et al.*, (1976) described a variety of nutritional disturbances in non-alcoholic patients with cryptogenic cirrhosis and chronic aggressive hepatitis. The incidence of these disturbances was lower than in alcoholics. Some (40 per cent) showed evidence of fat-soluble vitamin deficiency (vitamins A, E and carotene) but less than 10 per cent of the patients had deficiencies of vitamin $B_{12}$, nicotinic acid, thiamine or riboflavin; 17 per cent had evidence of folate deficiency. The observed disturbances did not appear to be due to dietary inadequacy, age, or interference with fat absorption.

A small number of patients with liver diseases show florid nutritional deficiency. Those with beriberi, scurvy, folate deficiency, and/or peripheral neuropathy, etc., tend to be alcoholics. Although they have a deficient dietary intake related to poverty, drunkenness and/or anorexia, other factors may play a part. When ethanol intake is high it can provide a large number of calories which render other foods unnecessary simply as a source of energy. Consequently, the vitamins which they contain are lost. A heavy alcohol intake may also increase requirements for thiamine and there may be malabsorption of vitamins, due to mucosal damage or to chronic alcoholic pancreatitis.

Drug therapy may interfere with nutritional status. In a large series of patients with various liver diseases, leucocyte ascorbic acid levels were reduced only in alcoholics and in patients with primary biliary cirrhosis (Beattie and Sherlock, 1976). In the latter group dietary histories did not suggest poor intake but the low ascorbate levels were associated with cholestyramine therapy. In children on cholestyramine, low folate levels have been found (West and Lloyd, 1975). These findings suggest that ascorbate and folate polyglutamates may bind to cholestyramine within the intestinal lumen.

It is important to recognize diseases such as beriberi and scurvy. If they are treated early they will respond rapidly and well to treatment, but severe neurological damage due to thiamine deficiency may persist despite therapy.

The presence of liver disease may interfere with the response to vitamin therapy, as the absorption of vitamins and their conversion into metabolically active compounds may be impaired (Danford and Munro, 1982). Reduced thiamine absorption and deficient thiamine phosphorylation have been reported in liver disease. Low activity of red cell transketolase, a thiamine dependent enzyme, may not respond to thiamine, suggesting a defect in the enzyme apoprotein. Plasma levels of pyridoxal-5-phosphate may be low in liver disease, possibly due to increased clearance, and there is not the usual increase following the administration of pyridoxine.

Vitamin A (retinol) absorption is impaired when bile secretion is reduced (Glickman, 1983). But parenchymal liver disease may impair synthesis of retinol binding protein (RBP), and thus the release of vitamin A from hepatic stores, and synthesis of prealbumin which binds RBP in plasma. Zinc deficiency is found in cirrhosis; as the enzyme converting retinol to retinal is a zinc dependent enzyme, further impairment of vitamin A metabolism may occur in liver disease.

A low plasma vitamin $B_{12}$ concentration is uncommon in patients with non-alcoholic liver disease, and absorption and transport of the vitamin are usually normal. In contrast, high circulating vitamin $B_{12}$ levels are found in patients with viral hepatitis, liver abscess, metastatic carcinoma and active cirrhosis. In hepatitis free vitamin increases and which is assumed to come from damaged hepatocytes, while the bound form is increased in cirrhosis (Danford and Munro, 1982).

In acute viral hepatitis serum iron and serum ferritin concentrations are often raised; maximum values are not seen until bilirubin and transaminase levels have reached their peak. The increased ferritin presumably comes from damaged liver cells but this could only account for a small part of the rise in serum iron. Transferrin iron must also be raised but the mechanism is unclear. Diminished utilization of iron for haemoglobin synthesis, impaired reticulo-endothelial uptake, and impaired hepatic storage of iron may all play a part.

In patients with non-alcoholic chronic liver disease iron deficiency is uncommon in the absence of malabsorption, gastrointestinal bleeding or a bleeding diathesis. Nevertheless, evidence of iron deficiency with or without anaemia has been found in up to 25 per cent of patients with cryptogenic cirrhosis or chronic hepatitis; it was attributed to occult gastrointestinal blood loss, or possibly to poor dietary intake (Morgan *et al.*, 1976).

Plasma albumin levels are often low in liver disease and in the absence of fluid retention it reflects a decrease in albumin synthesis as albumin catabolism tends to be reduced when serum albumin levels are low. But when oedema and ascites are present a low serum albumin may be misleading as high albumin synthetic rates may be present; under these circumstances the low albumin is due to its distribution into a much larger extravascular volume (Rothschild *et al.*, 1983).

Changes in plasma amino acids in liver disease relate to the severity, activity and aetiology of the liver disease (Morgan *et al.*, 1982). In fulminant hepatic failure the levels of most plasma amino acids are high, but those of the branched chain amino acids (BCAA) are normal or low. This reflects peripheral release of amino acids and reduced hepatic uptake; BCAA, however, are mainly removed by muscle. In chronic liver disease, with or without encephalopathy, plasma BCAA are low while the aromatic amino acids, phenylalanine, tyrosine, and methionine are increased. These changes appear to result from poor hepatic function, portal systemic shunting and high insulin and glucagon levels.

In patients with severe protein deficiency total plasma amino acid levels may be reduced. One might expect amino acid levels to fall in patients with hepatic encephalopathy whose protein intake is restricted (see later), but usually levels are well maintained on the protein intake used therapeutically. The pattern of individual plasma amino acids in patients with chronic liver disease is abnormal. Fischer and his colleagues (1975) found that in patients with severe parenchymal liver disease and those with hepatic encephalopathy (see later), there was a reduction in the plasma concentration of valine, leucine and isoleucine and an increase in phenylalanine and tyrosine. The altered ratio of these amino acids in patients with severe hepatocellular failure was thought to be important in causing the observed alterations in cerebral function. But similar changes occur in patients with parenchymal liver disease even when liver damage is minimal and encephalopathy absent.

The nutritional disturbances in patients with liver disease may have no obvious clinical consequences. Even so, it is useful to know about them so that abnormal laboratory results may be correctly interpreted when they are observed. It would also seem sensible to correct reversible deficiencies when this is possible. They may have deleterious effects on hepatic function which, although unrecognized, may affect prognosis. For example, patients with liver disease and ascorbic acid deficiency have a significantly longer antipyrine half-life than patients with liver disease alone (Beattie and Sherlock, 1976). Supplementation with ascorbic acid might improve hepatic drug handling.

## The effects of obstructive jaundice

When the biliary tree is obstructed there is a reduction in the secretion of bile salts and other substances. The severity of the resulting nutritional disturbance depends on the completeness of the obstruction and on the reduction of food intake, either from anorexia or by deliberate changes of the diet. Its clinical significance, however, depends on the prognosis of the obstructing lesion and on the extent to which induced metabolic changes can be reversed by treatment.

Steatorrhoea is common. It is rarely gross because fat can be absorbed from the intestine even when a luminal deficiency of bile salts reduces the size of the micellar phase. But reduced micelle formation has serious consequences for the absorption of fat-soluble vitamins. Phylloquinones and menaquinones (the naturally occurring vitamins $K_1$ and $K_2$) are adequately absorbed from the intestine only in the presence of bile salts (Friedman, 1982). Vitamin K is initially concentrated in the liver but the concentration declines rapidly when absorption is impaired. Vitamin K is a cofactor for the gamma carboxylation of glutamic acid residues during the synthesis of several coagulation factors including prothrombin. Without this post-translational modification the factors are inactive. The stores of vitamin K are small and with biliary obstruction impaired coagulation appears within weeks. When it is severe spontaneous bleeding occurs. With straightforward biliary obstruction the bleeding disturbance is rapidly corrected by the administration of vitamin K parenterally and its administration prior to surgery is mandatory. If there is hepatocellular damage the response to vitamin K may be poor as the liver may be unable to synthesize adequate amounts of prothrombin and factors VII, IX and X; large amounts of vitamin K may even depress prothrombin levels.

Vitamin D absorption is impaired with biliary obstruction but the clinical effects of this absorptive defect are not seen as quickly as in the case of vitamin

K (Smith, 1982). Not only are there large body stores of vitamin D (which would last approximately one year) but much of the daily requirement for this vitamin is supplied by synthesis in the skin (although in the jaundiced patient the bilirubin in the skin may interfere with vitamin $D_3$ synthesis by absorbing ultraviolet rays). With biliary obstruction of short duration, as with most surgically remediable lesions, the consequences of vitamin D deficiency do not become apparent and no treatment is necessary. Only with long-standing biliary obstruction, e.g. due to biliary stricture or primary biliary cirrhosis, do problems arise: failure to give parenteral vitamin D may then cause osteomalacia to appear in a small number of patients. Reduced vitamin D absorption and osteomalacia may also occur in a small number of patients with severe and chronic parenchymal liver disease who show disturbances of fat absorption.

Vitamin D is converted within the body to 25-hydroxyvitamin D and then to 1,25 dihydroxyvitamin D. The latter metabolite is probably the major functional form of vitamin D and is the most potent metabolite identified yet. The initial hydroxylation at the 25-position takes place in the liver; 1-hydroxylation occurs in the kidney. As one might expect levels of 25-hydroxyvitamin D tend to be reduced in patients with cirrhosis and in patients with obstructive jaundice but they correlate poorly with the degree of osteomalacia (which probably depends on levels of 1,25 dihydroxyvitamin D).

Factors other than vitamin D deficiency may affect calcium absorption in patients with liver disease. There may be a deficient dietary intake of calcium. When triglyceride absorption is impaired excessive amounts of long-chain fatty acids may be present in the intestinal lumen; these may form insoluble soaps with intraluminal calcium ions and so depress calcium uptake. The latter effect is not seen with medium-chain triglycerides which promote calcium uptake in experimental animals.

One should avoid symptomatic steatorrhoea in patients with obstructive jaundice by reducing the intake of dietary fat to a tolerable level. Theoretically medium-chain triglyceride would be a useful substitute but in practice it is rarely necessary. The effect of vitamin D on calcium absorption is so dominant that calcium absorption returns to normal when vitamin D metabolism is corrected. When vitamin D therapy is commenced in patients who have been vitamin D deficient (and therefore calcium deficient) it is obviously sensible to give dietary calcium supplements.

Some patients with liver disease develop osteoporosis. The cause is not clear. It may be due to a generalized nutritional disturbance, to chronic protein deficiency, or to other interference with protein metabolism. Osteoporosis is particularly common in 'liver patients' treated with steroids; they may develop collapsed vertebrae and other clinical manifestations of the condition.

A small number of patients with primary biliary cirrhosis develop severe bone pain despite long-term treatment with vitamin D. The cause of this bone pain is not certain; it may respond to intravenous infusion of calcium, with remission of the pain for several months (Ajdukiewicz *et al.*, 1974). The pain does not appear to respond to oral calcium and there is no evidence that it is nutritional in origin.

The absorption of the fat-soluble vitamins A and E may be impaired in patients with either obstructive jaundice or parenchymal liver disease. The resulting deficiency of vitamin E has no obvious consequences in adults but may cause neurological problems in children (Elias *et al.*, 1980). Vitamin A deficiency does produce clinical manifestations although they are often overlooked. Evidence of impaired dark adaptation can be found with special tests but only occasional patients, with severe depletion, complain of night blindness. Vitamin A deficiency is also associated with keratinization of epithelia, especially of the conjunctiva and cornea; in addition there may be an impairment of taste and smell which probably results from the keratinizing effect. Retinol (vitamin A) is released from the liver into plasma bound to a retinol binding protein; plasma vitamin A concentrations tend to be reduced with liver disease presumably because of a defect in release from the liver (Glickman, 1983).

## Diet in the treatment of liver diseases

Dietary advice is often important in the management of liver disease and its complications. Unfortunately many patients receive advice of doubtful value. Even if asymptomatic they may be given a low fat diet or asked to abstain from alcohol; more rigorous restrictions may be suggested in some cases. There is no good evidence to support dietary restriction for patients with few symptoms (except for those with alcoholic liver disease who should abstain from alcohol!). If nausea, vomiting, and/or abdominal pain occur after meals the patient should obviously avoid foods which are regularly associated with the symptoms. Similarly, when anorexia is present, the patient should not be given unattractive dishes; he should be allowed to select meals which appeal to him. These simple recommendations are all that is necessary for most patients.

When nutritional deficiency is severe and the patient is unable to eat adequate amounts of food, it may be necessary to supplement the diet with food given via a nasogastric tube or even by the use of intravenous nutrition. There has been concern about the use of i.v. nutrition in liver disease, particularly with lipid preparations, but it is clear that many patients tolerate modern intravenous sources of protein and fat without complications.

### Viral or drug-induced hepatitis

Patients with hepatitis who have few symptoms need no restrictive dietary advice; they should be encouraged to eat normally. Even when a patient has severe anorexia, nausea, and vomiting he can usually take small amounts of food by mouth and drink enough to prevent significant dehydration. He should be encouraged to do both and should be tempted with attractive food and drink. It is rarely necessary to feed through a nasogastric tube or to use intravenous supplementation.

There should be no attempt to restrict fat in patients with hepatitis. Low fat diets are bulky; they are generally unappetizing and may exacerbate anorexia. Hoagland and his colleagues showed in 1946 that patients allowed a high fat, high protein diet consumed more calories than those allowed only a low fat diet. They gained more weight and appeared to recover more quickly from the disease. Chalmers *et al.*, (1955) force-fed servicemen with viral hepatitis (using a stomach tube in a small number!) to ensure a diet containing at least

3000 kcal (and upwards of 150 g of both protein and fat). The illness in these patients was shorter, by about 6 days, than that of patients eating *ad lib.*, whose caloric intake was considerably lower. This benefit is relatively small and the authors did not advocate force-feeding of civilians! Even so, it seems sensible to advise patients with hepatitis to take as high a calorie intake as they can tolerate.

Patients with acute hepatitis are often advised to abstain from alcohol during the attack and for six months to a year afterwards. It is harmless advice which focuses attention on the potential hepatotoxicity of alcohol at a time when the patient is introspective about his liver. But it must be confessed that there is no good evidence that alcohol in moderation has a deleterious effect on the liver either during an acute attack or during convalescence. However, excessive amounts of alcohol may be hepatotoxic in their own right and a relapse of hepatitis associated with alcohol abuse has been noted in a number of patients (Damodaran and Hartfall, 1944).

## Cirrhosis of the liver

The preceding remarks about the dietary management of viral and drug-induced hepatitis are generally applicable to the care of patients with uncomplicated cirrhosis of the liver. Dietary restriction is unnecessary and patients should avoid only foods which upset them. A small number of cirrhotic patients have symptomatic steatorrhoea and require dietary fat restriction. In this case fats rich in polyunsaturated fatty acids should be used as they supply essential fatty acids such as linoleic and linolenic. For patients with certain complications of cirrhosis, dietary control may be critically important.

Patients with cirrhosis frequently have dilated veins in the oesophageal wall; they are relatively thin walled and may rupture and bleed profusely into the lumen. Although there is no evidence that the texture of food influences bleeding it seems sensible to warn patients about the possible risk of ingesting fragments of bone or other hard, sharp-edged foods. Patients who are confused, or who cannot chew their food properly, should be given soft, pulpy foods which cannot cause mucosal damage.

### Hepatic encephalopathy (Sherlock 1982; Jones, 1983)

Patients with severe parenchymal liver disease or shunting of blood from the portal to the systemic circulation may show evidence of cerebral dysfunction. The cause(s) of 'hepatic encephalopathy', which may be of more than one type, is not yet certain, but dietary protein is clearly an important precipitating factor. In some patients with cirrhosis and stupor or coma, and/or other neurological manifestations, products of protein catabolism (which may have been produced within the body, i.e. after absorption), are presumably acted upon by intestinal bacteria to produce substances toxic to the brain. These may be produced in normal subjects, but it is assumed that they are cleared by healthy liver cells, and that this process is enhanced because intestinal blood passes through the liver before entering the systemic circulation.

No protein (or less than 20 g a day) should be given at the start of an episode of encephalopathy. The protein of existing intestinal contents should be removed by the use of purgatives and enemata. These are particularly useful following gastrointestinal haemorrhage which presents a large protein load to the gut and often precipitates hepatic coma. Complete protein restriction can only be a short-term measure. On recovery or after a day or so of such treatment, protein should be given to minimize negative nitrogen balance. Unfortunately, oral protein cannot be replaced by intravenous infusion of conventional amino acid mixtures as these may also exacerbate encephalopathy (Webster and Davidson, 1957; Fischer *et al.*, 1974). The infusion of amino acid mixtures containing high concentrations of branched-chain acids (valine, leucine, and isoleucine) may be of value in hepatic coma (Fischer *et al.*, 1975).

Protein should be reintroduced gradually into the diet in increments of 10 to 20 g per day. The aim is to give just enough protein to prevent negative nitrogen balance, as its encephalopathic effect is thought to be related to the amount of protein administered. If one used first-class protein rich in essential amino acids 30 g of protein per day might be adequate. In practice it is difficult to prepare a palatable diet using only protein of high biological value. There are studies which suggest that protein of vegetable origin is better tolerated than animal protein in patients with encephalopathy (Greenberger *et al.*, 1977) but in practice it is difficult to persuade seriously ill patients to take sufficient protein if they are only provided with the bulky vegetable regimen. Fortunately, patients with encephalopathy can usually be stabilized on 50 g or more of protein daily. This protein should be distributed fairly evenly throughout the day as a sudden load may make the encephalopathy worse: following an oral load of protein the electroencephalographic pattern deteriorates within about 2 hours. The low protein diets used at the Royal Free Hospital are presented in the Appendix (Table 2).

The ability to tolerate dietary protein can be enhanced by the administration of a non-absorbable antibiotic such as neomycin, which presumably reduces the production of the cerebral toxin, or of the synthetic disaccharide lactulose which may reduce its absorption. Using such compounds patients may be able to take 80 g of protein daily: larger amounts of protein are not necessary. With progression of the liver disease the tolerance to dietary protein gradually decreases despite treatment with neomycin or lactulose.

When protein is restricted carbohydrate must be given to reduce endogenous protein catabolism and to promote the anabolic use of administered protein. A daily carbohydrate load of 1600 calories has been recommended and this has often been given intravenously either as glucose or fructose. Walker *et al.*, (1974) gave oral glucose supplements to cirrhotics on a diet containing 40–60 g protein. They used oral glucose to boost plasma insulin levels and to reduce plasma glucagon, as oral glucose gives higher insulin levels than fructose or intravenous glucose. In each case blood ammonia, which has been incriminated in encephalopathy, fell significantly. This suggests that we should, whenever possible, give oral glucose rather than fructose or intravenous glucose to patients with encephalopathy. Glucose is preferable to fructose, particularly in acute hepatic failure, as hypoglycaemia itself causes an encephalopathy in this condition and fructose may precipitate lactic acidosis.

Bleeding from oesophageal varices is sometimes treated by the construction of a portacaval shunt. These patients have a high incidence of chronic hepatic encephalopathy within 3 years of the operation. They may also have transient encephalopathy in the immediate post-operative period when liver cell function may be depressed due to the surgery. For this reason we restrict protein immediately after surgery; we work up to normal protein intake over a week or so increasing the protein in the diet by about 20 g at a time.

**Fluid retention**

Many patients with cirrhosis of the liver have disturbances of renal functioning which lead to the retention of salt and water. This excess fluid may cause swelling of the ankles and/or abdominal distension (ascites); both may be uncomfortable and inconvenient for the patient.

The reasons for the fluid retention are poorly understood and this limits our ability to treat it effectively. On an empirical basis it has been established that the manipulation of dietary salt and water may be of therapeutic benefit.

The degree of renal functional disturbance may be assessed arbitrarily by the ability of the kidneys to excrete salt and to clear free water. Some patients with fluid retention pass relatively large amounts of urinary sodium and are able to generate free water (i.e. are 'water tolerant'). Such patients will usually lose fluid with moderate restriction of dietary sodium. If there is avid sodium retention more severe sodium restriction is necessary. Although it is possible to reduce dietary sodium to less than 10 mmol/day this cannot be done without an unacceptably low protein intake or the use of artificial protein preparations which are very unpalatable. By using unsalted bread and no salt in cooking, and with protein restricted to only 60 to 70 g daily, it is possible to reduce sodium intake to around 20 mmol/day. Fortunately most patients respond adequately to a daily intake of around 40 mmol; this is still severe sodium restriction in dietary terms but it is a more practicable goal for therapy. The low sodium diet used at the Royal Free Hospital is presented in the Appendix (Table 3).

The patient and his doctors must be on the look-out for foodstuffs which have an unacceptably high salt content. The patient must also avoid alkali preparations such as Mist. Mag. Trisil which contain a lot of sodium; sodium-free preparations should be prescribed.

Some patients with a low urinary sodium output are 'water tolerant'. They respond to diuretics and a low salt diet. The most difficult group to treat are patients with a low urinary sodium who are water intolerant. Often their inability to excrete free water is reflected in hyponatraemia. They are usually treated with a low salt diet, diuretics and by restriction of dietary water intake to around 1 litre a day. The results of treatment are generally poor and the life expectancy of these patients is short, as they also tend to develop functional renal failure. There is evidence that water intolerance and renal failure are due to reduced renal production of prostaglandins, which in turn may be secondary to diminished availability of their precursor, arachidonic acid (Perez-Ayuso *et al.*, 1984). Whether these complications can be delayed by administration of arachidonate, or its precursor, linoleic acid, is not yet known.

Salt restriction is unpleasant for the patient and treatment with diuretics may also be associated with a number of untoward consequences. It is probably wise not to treat patients with fluid retention unless oedema and/or ascites are causing troublesome symptoms which distress the patient; it is certainly unwise to treat too vigorously. When diuretics are used salt intake is usually restricted, but some doctors believe that the restriction of salt need not be too rigorous providing the patient goes into negative sodium balance (Reynolds *et al.*, 1978). Further studies are needed to determine optimal sodium intake when diuretic therapy is used in patients with cirrhosis.

**Carbohydrate intolerance**
Impaired glucose tolerance is commonly seen in patients with cirrhosis of the liver. It is not usually associated with insulin deficiency. Plasma insulin levels tend to be high in cirrhosis and there is a resistance to the action of exogenous insulin. Symptomatic diabetes is less common and when polyuria does occur it can usually be treated by simple dietary restriction of carbohydrates. A small number of patients with cirrhosis are insulin dependent and it seems likely that their diabetes mellitus is different from the glucose intolerance usually seen with cirrhosis.

## The diet and hyperbilirubinaemia

Gilbert's syndrome is a chronic, benign, non-haemolytic, unconjugated hyperbilirubinaemia. Fasting increases plasma bilirubin levels in subjects with this condition. The effect may be an extrahepatic one or a direct effect on the liver cell; although the exact mechanism is not known it seems to be related not to the caloric intake but to the presence or absence of fat in the diet whether this is given orally or intravenously (Gollan *et al.*, 1976).

The diet-induced increase in hyperbilirubinaemia is relatively unimportant in terms of the patient's well-being but it is worthy of recognition. Gilbert's syndrome is common, occurring in up to 6 per cent of the population. It is usually unrecognized but unconjugated hyperbilirubinaemia may be detected when patients in hospital are starved or fed only with intravenous glucose or amino acids. Gilbert's syndrome should be considered as a diagnosis before there is a vigorous search for other more sinister causes of jaundice. An injection of Intralipid should lower the plasma bilirubin level in patients with this benign condition.

Gollan and his colleagues speculated that the low lipid content of some feeding regimes used for premature infants might exacerbate neonatal hyperbilirubinaemia; they suggested on this basis that lipid should be included in the diets given to jaundiced neonates.

## Dietary management of biliary obstruction

Patients with an obstruction to the flow of bile into the duodenum have a number of nutritional disturbances which were described earlier. When the obstruction is surgically remediable there is little indication for specific dietary measures as reversible metabolic disturbances will correct themselves rapidly following relief of the obstruction. Vitamin K deficiency should be corrected preoperatively by the intramuscular injection of phytomenadione in a dose of 10 mg daily. Steatorrhoea, and possibly pain of biliary origin, may improve with fat restriction. (It is, of course, essential that dehydration and other obvious metabolic disturbances should be corrected as far as possible before surgery.)

In patients with chronic biliary obstruction due to primary biliary cirrhosis, biliary stricture, biliary atresia, etc., more active dietary measures may be necessary. If steatorrhoea disturbs the patient then the intake of long-chain fatty acids should be reduced to a tolerable level. Usually the caloric intake will still be adequate but if it is necessary to boost caloric intake, or if it is necessary to provide a large caloric intake for the purposes of growth, as in young children with biliary atresia, then this can be accomplished by the administration of medium-chain triglycerides which do not require bile salts for their absorption (see Appendix, Table 4).

Fat soluble vitamins do require bile salts for their absorption and patients with chronic biliary obstruction require supplementation with vitamins A, D and K on a long-term basis. This may be conveniently provided by the monthly intramuscular injection of 10 mg of phytomenadione and 100 000 units each of vitamins A and D (which can be given in one injection if a special preparation is made). There is now evidence that vitamin E deficiency is common in chronic obstructive jaundice. The significance of this deficiency in adults is not clear but it appears to cause serious neurological abnormalities in children with conditions such as biliary atresia (Elias *et al.*, 1980). Vitamin E should clearly be given to such children.

For reasons which were given earlier it is also sensible to give calcium supplements to patients with chronic biliary obstruction, particularly when they are first treated with vitamin D as their requirements for calcium at this time will be high. Calcium can be given conveniently in a variety of forms in a dose of about 1 g (25 mmol) of elemental calcium daily. Effervescent tablets, such as Calcium Sandoz (which contains calcium lactate gluconate), are more palatable than other preparations. It should be noted that effervescent calcium preparations contain relatively large amounts of sodium. Recently it has been claimed that oral administration of a microcrystalline hydroxyapatite compound, Ossopan, gives improved calcium absorption in patients with biliary obstruction (Epstein *et al.*, 1982).

## Diet and gall bladder diseases

In this section we will confine our remarks to dietary agents in the pathogenesis of gallstones and in the treatment of some of their 'non-obstructive' complications. The nutritional implications of biliary obstruction, whether due to gallstones or other biliary tract diseases such as stricture, sclerosing cholangitis, or atresia, have been discussed earlier.

### The pathogenesis of gallstones (Bennion and Grundy, 1978)

It is hardly surprising that dietary factors have been incriminated in the production of cholesterol gallstones. Gallstone disease is a disease of civilized communities and is strongly associated with disorders such as obesity, diabetes mellitus and hypertriglyceridaemia. Each of these may be 'cured' by treatment with a low calorie diet and they are often considered as diseases of overnutrition. In general the 'western' diets associated with these conditions are characterized by a high intake of refined carbohydrates and a relatively low intake of dietary fibre. Refined carbohydrates may be a causal factor in terms of excessive caloric intake because they provide concentrated calories without the appetite satisfying properties of bulky, unrefined foods or of fats.

Gallstones are usually formed in the gall bladder and presumably their genesis and growth must be affected not only by the volume and composition of the bile reaching the gall bladder from the hepatic ducts but also by various aspects of functioning of the gall bladder. The lithogenicity (or stone-forming tendency) of hepatic bile will be increased if there is an increase in its cholesterol content or a reduction in its content of bile salt or phospholipid, while the tendency of stones to grow in the gall bladder will presumably be enhanced if the lithogenicity of the bile increases within it or if there is prolonged stasis of bile in the gall bladder due to infrequent or sluggish emptying.

Gallstone formation can undoubtedly be induced by dietary means in experimental animals. It is of interest that it appears to be necessary to use diets rich in refined carbohydrate. The mechanism may not be related simply to overnutrition as such diets cause a suppression of bile salt production and consequently a small bile acid pool.

The relative proportions of different bile salts may also be important in gallstone production. There is evidence to suggest that the lithogenicity of bile may be proportional to its content of deoxycholic acid, a secondary bile acid produced in the colon by the dehydroxylation (at position 7) of cholic acid. There is epidemiological evidence to suggest that some African populations with a low incidence of gallstones have a low concentration of deoxycholate in bile and faeces. They eat a diet high in fibre. The addition of bran to a diet rich in refined sugars reduces the deoxycholate content of bile which becomes less lithogenic.

If dietary factors increased biliary cholesterol output one would expect an increased incidence of gallstones. It has been claimed that cholesterol feeding has this effect but the evidence to date is far from convincing. Some workers believe that a reduction in the dietary content of animal fat causes a mobilization of plasma and tissue cholesterol with increased excretion in bile; indeed this may be the mechanism for the lowering of plasma cholesterol with a low animal fat diet. Some support for this hypothesis comes from the studies of Sturdevant *et al.*, (1973) who found a greater prevalence of gallstones in subjects eating a diet low in saturated fat and cholesterol but high in unsaturated fat and plant sterol.

The type of food eaten may not be the only dietary factor involved in the pathogenesis of gallstones. It has been shown that fasting causes bile to become lithogenic and that nocturnal bile is more lithogenic than bile produced during the day. Furthermore without food intake there will be no release of cholecystokinin and the bile will remain stagnant in the gall bladder. For both reasons one might expect a greater incidence of gallstones in subjects who miss breakfast and who eat only one or two meals a day (Capron *et al.*, 1981).

The evidence connecting dietary factors and gallstone production does not as yet justify widespread dietary modification purely to reduce the incidence of gallstones. But the advice which one might give for this purpose is also sensible on other grounds. Reduction of dietary intake of refined carbohydrate would help to control obesity and dental decay and to reduce the incidence of diabetes mellitus. Increasing bran intake would improve constipation and reduce the incidence of diverticular disease (and possibly of haemorrhoids and varicose veins!). Reduction of cholesterol intake would do no harm and might reduce the risks of atheroma. The only dilemma is whether we should reduce the intake of animal fats and use polyunsaturated fats in their place. If this diet proves to be effective in reducing coronary heart disease then clearly it should be recommended even if the risk of gallstones is thereby increased. This issue is still controversial but the balance of evidence suggests that reduction in animal fat intake is a sensible precaution.

## Diet in the treatment of cholelithiasis

Patients with gallstones which are producing no symptoms pose a problem for their doctors. There is no evidence that dietary treatment can disperse the gallstones. They may disappear with treatment with chenodeoxycholic or ursodeoxycholic acids but if this is stopped they tend to return and the place of chemical dissolution in the long-term treatment of gallstones is not yet clear. Many doctors advocate elective surgery for silent gallstones (Editorial, 1975) but although the mortality in good hands is small it is not negligible.

Dyspepsia is often attributed to the presence of stones in the gall bladder but several studies have suggested that symptoms such as flatulent dyspepsia, abdominal pain, specific food intolerance and heartburn are equally common in patients with and without gallstones (Morris, 1973). This casts doubt upon the concept of 'gall bladder dyspepsia'.

There is also doubt about the pathophysiological significance of fat intolerance. This complaint is common in patients with gastrointestinal symptoms but, on average, the same foods are incriminated by all patients with digestive complaints, whether caused by hepatobiliary diseases or by functional disorders, peptic ulcer, or by ulcerative and inflammatory disease of the small and large intestines. Patients with gallstones have no greater incidence of fat intolerance (Koch and Donaldston, 1964). Taggart and Billington (1966) fed fat in a disguised form to twelve patients who complained of fat intolerance. Dyspeptic symptoms occurred with only 8 per cent of challenges; the authors concluded that dyspepsia after 'fatty' foods was not related to the fat ingested but to prejudice about fat or to domestic or personal disturbances at the time of eating.

There is only one widely accepted indication for dietary fat restriction in the treatment of gallstone disease (although there is, as far as we know, no 'hard' evidence to support it!). When patients are suffering from acute cholecystitis or from an obstructed gall bladder, fat intake should be restricted, or calories should be given intravenously, in order to reduce the secretion of cholecystokinin. This hormone is released from the small intestine by fat and the products of lipolysis, and to a lesser extent by amino acids and small peptides.

Cholecystokinin contracts the gall bladder and simultaneously relaxes the sphincter of Oddi. When there is no obstruction to the biliary tree one would expect a higher pressure to result from contraction of the gall bladder; this might cause more severe pain or perforation of the gall bladder.

When the patient is very ill intravenous fluids and calories should be given. If the patient can take food by mouth and surgery is not imminent then dietary fat should be reduced to 25 per cent of calories or less; it may, however, be necessary to reduce the fat content to less than 10 per cent (Council on Foods and Nutrition of AMA, 1962).

## Conclusion

Dietary factors may be important in the pathogenesis and the management of hepatobiliary diseases. In many instances our understanding of the physiological and biochemical mechanisms concerned is poor and this limits the way in which we can use dietary modifications to minimize symptoms and to improve prognosis. But when dietary changes are necessary it is usually essential that the dietary composition should be strictly controlled. This is not an easy matter for the practising doctor who would be wise to seek help from a dietitian when this is available. If such help is not to hand then he must do his best using referencce sources such as the Appendix to this book, or the books by Francis (1974) and Davidson *et al.*, (1979). Tables of diets relating to this Chapter are given in the Appendix, p. 512.

## References

Ajdukiewicz, A.B., Agnew, J.E., Byers, P.D., Wills, M.R. and Sherlock, S. (1974). The relief of bone pain in primary biliary cirrhosis with calcium infusions. *Gut*, **15**, 788–93.

Alpers, D.H. and Sabesin, S.M. (1982). Fatty liver: biochemical and clinical aspects. In *Diseases of the Liver*, pp. 813–45. Eds. Schiff, L. and Schiff, E.R. Lippincott: Philadelphia.

Bailey, A., Robinson, D. and Dawson, A.M. (1977). Does Gilbert's disease exist. *Lancet*, **i**, 931–8.

Beattie, A.D. and Sherlock, S. (1976). Ascorbic acid deficiency in liver disease. *Gut*, **17**, 571–5.

Bennion, L.J. and Grundy, S.M. (1978). Risk factors for the development of cholelithiasis in man. *N. Engl. J. Med.*, **299**, 1161–7, 1221–7.

Brunt, P.W. (1971). Alcohol and the liver. *Gut*, **12**, 222–9.

Brunt, P.W., Kew, M.C., Scheuer, P.S. and Sherlock, S. (1974). Studies in alcoholic liver disease in Britain: clinical and pathological patterns related to natural history. *Gut*, **15**, 52–8.

Capron, J.P., Delamarre, J., Herve, M.A., Dupas, J.L., Poulain, P. and Descombes, P. (1981). Meal frequency and duration of overnight fast: a role in gallstone formation? *Br. Med. J.*, **283**, 1435.

Chalmers, T.C., Eckhardt, R.D., Reynolds, W.E., Cigarroa, J.G., Deane, N., Reifenstein, R.W. and Smith, C.W. (1955). The treatment of acute infectious hepatitis: studies of the effects of diets, rest, and physical reconditioning on the acute course of the disease and on the incidence of relapse and residual abnormalities. *J. Clin. Invest.*, **34**, 1163–235.

Conn, H.O. (1982). Cirrhosis. In *Diseases of the Liver*. Eds. Schiff, L. and Schiff, E.R., pp. 847–977. Lippincott: Philadelphia.

Council on Foods and Nutrition of the American Medical Association (1962). The regulation of dietary fat. *J. Am. Med. Ass.*, **181**, 411–29.

Damodaran, K. and Hartfall, S.J. (1944). Infective hepatitis in the garrison of Malta. *Br. Med. J.*, **ii**, 587–90.

Danford, D.E. and Munro, H.N. (1982). The liver in relation to the B vitamins. In *The Liver: Biology and Pathobiology*. Eds. Arias, I.M., Popper, H., Schachler, D. and Shafritz, D.A. pp. 367–84. Raven Press: New York.

Davidson, S., Passmore, R., Brock, J.F. and Truswell, A.S. (1979). *Human Nutrition and Dietetics*, 7th ed., pp.412–21. Churchill Livingstone: Edinburgh.

Editorial. (1975). Dangers of silent gall stones. *Br. Med. J.*, **i**, 415.

Elias, E., Muller, D.P.R. and Scott, J. (1980). Association of spinocerebellar disorders with cystic fibrosis in chronic childhood cholestasis and a very low vitamin E. *Lancet*, **ii**, 1319–21.

Epstein, O., Kato, Y., Dick, R. and Sherlock, S. (1982). Vitamin D, hydroxyapatite and calcium gluconate in treatment of cortical thinning in post-menopausal women with primary biliary cirrhosis *Am. J. Clin. Nutr.*, **36**, 426–30.

Farivar, M., Bucher, N.L.R., Wands, J. and Isselbacher, K.J. (1976). Beneficial effect of insulin and glucagon on fulminant murine hepatitis. *Gastroenterology*, **70**, 981.

Fischer, J.E., Yoshimura, N., Aguirre, A., James, J.H., Cummings, M.G., Abel, R.M. and Deindoerfer, F. (1974). Plasma aminoacids in patients with hepatic encephalopathy: effects of aminoacid infusions. *Am. J. Surg.* **127**, 40–47.

Fischer, J.E., Yoshimura, N., Aguirre, A., James, J.H., Keane, J.M., Wesdorp, R.I.C., Yoshimura, N. and Westman, T. (1975). The role of plasma amino acids in hepatic encephalopathy. *Surgery*, **78**, 276–88.

Francis, D.E.M. (1974). *Diets for Sick Children*, 3rd ed. Blackwell: Oxford. (4th ed. in press.)

Friedman, P.A. (1982) Vitamin K. In *The Liver: Biology and Pathobiology*, pp. 357–65. Eds. Arias, I., Popper, H., Schachter, D., and Schafritz, D. Raven Press: New York.

Glickman, R.M. (1983). Vitamin A and the liver. Chapter 42 in *Liver in Metabolic Diseases*. Eds. Bianchi, L., Gerok, W., Landmann, L., Sickinger, K. and Stalder, G.A. M.T.P Press: Lancaster.

Gollan, J.L., Bateman, C. and Billing, B.H. (1976). Effect of dietary composition on the unconjugated hyperbilirubinaemia of Gilbert's syndrome. *Gut*, **17**, 335–40.

Greenberger, N.J., Carley, J., Schenker, S., Bettinger, I., Stamnes, C. and Beyer, P. (1977). Effect of vegetable and animal protein diets in chronic hepatic encephalopathy. *Am. J. Digest. Dis.*, **22**, 845–55.

Hoagland, C.L., Labby, D.H., Kunkel, H.G. and Shank, R.E. (1946). An analysis of the effect of fat in the diet on recovery in infectious hepatitis. *Am. J. Pub. Hlth.*, **36**, 1287–92.

Jones, E.A. (1983). The enigma of hepatic encephalopathy. *Postgrad. Med. J.*, **59**, (Suppl. 4), 42–54.

Koch, J.P. and Donaldson, R.M. (1964). A survey of food intolerances in hospitalised patients. *N. Engl. J. Med.*, **271**, 657–60.

Leevy, C.M. and Kiernan, T. (1975). Nutritional factors and liver disease. In: *Modern Trends in Gastroenterology*, Vol. 5, pp. 250–61. Ed. Read, A.E. Butterworths: London.

Lieber, C.S. (1975). Liver disease and alcohol: fatty liver, alcoholic hepatitis, cirrhosis and their interrelationships. *Ann. N. Y. Acad. Sci.*, **252**, 63–84.

Morgan, M.Y. and McIntyre, N. (1985). Nutritional aspects of liver disease. In: *Liver and Biliary Disease*, 2nd ed., pp. 119–160. Eds. Wright, R., Millward-Sadler, G.H., Alberti, K.G.M.M. and Karran, S. W.B. Saunders Company: London.

Morgan, A.G., Kelleher, J., Walker, B.E. and Losowsky, M.S. (1976). Nutrition in cryptogenic cirrhosis and chronic aggressive hepatitis. *Gut*, **17**, 113–18.

Morgan, M.Y., Marshall, A.W., Milson, J.P. and Sherlock, S. (1982). Plasma amino acid patterns in liver disease. *Gut*, **23**, 362–70.

Morris, J.S. (1973). Dyspepsia and its investigation. *Br. J. Hosp. Med.*, **10**, 144–7.

Orrego, H., Israel, Y. and Blendis, L.M. (1981). Alcoholic liver disease: information in search of knowledge. *Hepatology*, **1**, 267–83.

Perez-Ayuso, R.M., Arroyo, V., Camps, J., Rimola, A., Gaya, J., Costa, J., Rivera, F.

and Rodes, J. (1984). Evidence that renal prostaglandins are involved in renal water metabolism in cirrhosis. *Kidney Int.*, **26**, 72–80.

Reynolds, T., Lieberman, F.L. and Goodman, A.R. (1978). Advantages of treatment of ascites without dietary sodium restriction and without complete removal of excess fluid. *Gut*, **19**, 549–53.

Reynolds, T.B., Redeker, A.G. and Kuzma, O.T. (1965). Role of alcohol in pathogenesis of alcoholic cirrhosis. In *Therapeutic Agents and the Liver*, pp. 131–42. Eds. McIntyre, N. and Sherlock, S. Blackwell: Oxford.

Rosenthal, W.S. and Glass, J. (1970). Vitamin $B_{12}$ and the liver. *Prog. Liver Dis.*, **3**, 118–46.

Rothschild, M.A., Oratz, M. and Schrieber, S.S. (1983). Serum albumin in liver disease. Chapter 6. In *The Liver in Metabolic Diseases*, Eds. Bianchi, L., Gerok, W., Landmann, L., Sickinger, K. and Stalder, G.A. M.T.P. Press: Lancaster.

Sherlock, S. *Diseases of the Liver and Biliary system*, 6th ed. (1982). Blackwell: Oxford.

Smith, J.E. (1982). Vitamin D metabolism. In *The Liver in Metabolic Diseases*, Eds. Bianchi, L., Gerok, W., Landmann, L., Sickinger, K. and Stalder, G.A. M.T.P. Press: Lancaster.

Stanbury, J.B., Wyngaarden, J.B., Fredrickson, D.S., Goldstein, J.L. and Brown, M.S. (1983). *The Metabolic Basis of Inherited Disease*, 5th ed. McGraw Hill: New York.

Sturdevant, R.A.L., Pearce, M.D., and Dayton, S. (1973). Increased prevalence of cholelithiasis in men ingesting a serum-cholesterol-lowering diet. *N. Engl. J. Med.*, **291**, 168–71.

Taggart, D. and Billington, B.P. (1966). Fatty foods and dyspepsia. *Lancet*, **ii**, 464–6.

Walker, C., Peterson, W. and Unqar, R. (1974). Blood ammonia levels in advanced cirrhosis during therapeutic elevation of insulin–glucagon ratio. *N. Engl. J. Med.*, **291**, 168–71.

Webster, L.T. and Davidson, C.S. (1957). Cirrhosis of the liver. Impending hepatic coma and increased blood ammonium concentrations during protein hydrolysate infusion. *J. Lab. Clin. Med.*, **50**, 1–10.

West, R.J. and Lloyd, J.K. (1975). The effect of cholestyramine on intestinal absorption. *Gut*, **16**, 93–8.

# 12 The nutritional management of renal disease

Harry A. Lee



## Introduction

When considering the nutritional needs of renal failure patients certain basic concepts have to be recognized such as:

1. the influence of the uraemic environment upon the utilization of given substrates;
2. whether the substrates given orally or intravenously adversely affect the uraemic status as a whole or in part, e.g., accentuating acidosis;
3. the effects that such substrates may have upon the well-being of the uraemic individual; and
4. whether time duration effects of the uraemia or, in turn, of the nutritional programme have to be modified with either continuing uraemia or prolonged administration of the therapeutic regimen.

Correction of nutritional deficits in uraemic patients is different from that of malnutrition in individuals with normal organ function. Although many of the principles governing the nutritional management of acute and chronic renal failure are similar, they are sufficiently different to warrant their separate consideration. Many of the disturbances of intermediary metabolism are similar in acute and chronic renal failure, for example, lipid handling. However, such disturbances only have real significance in patients with chronic renal failure because of their longer duration which may result in pathological consequences, e.g. atheroma.

## Acute renal failure

### Oral nutritional management

Although many advances have been made over the past 30 years in the management of acute renal failure patients with respect to dialysis techniques and metabolic care, the mortality rate remains high around 40–50 per cent. Of course, this figure has to be considered against the background that patients now accepted for acute renal failure management would not have been 30 years ago. Patients now being referred to Acute Renal Failure Units are more severely compromised than years ago simply because dialysis techniques have improved. Nevertheless, the observations of Montgomerie *et. al.*, in 1968, remain the same–that malnutrition complicating acute renal failure is associated with a high infection rate and increased mortality. The nutritional management of acute renal failure patients has become more simplified and requires a more aggressive approach than practised hitherto.

It should also be recognized that the nutritional management of acute renal failure patients is also determined by other considerations such as:

1. the severity of the acute renal failure i.e., degree of catabolism;
2. whether there is normal gastrointestinal function;
3. whether the patient requires dialysis and what frequency and type of dialysis procedure e.g., peritoneal dialysis, haemodialysis or haemofiltration;
4. whether only intravenous nutrition can be considered; and
5. the significance of any other extra renal losses e.g., gastrointestinal fistulae, nasogastric aspiration.

Conservative treatment is still mainly that of modest protein and fluid restriction with provision of minimal amounts of electrolytes. The time honoured approach of 500 ml/day of fluid plus any fluid losses from the previous day, e.g., urine, diarrhoea, fistula losses, vomiting, increased sensible losses (e.g., pyrexia), remains appropriate. In the calculation of fluid requirements for such patients it is important to include the water of metabolism amounting to 0.4–0.5 litre/day in adults. Unless this is included in any calculation it is readily appreciated that over a 7 day period a water excess amounting to 3.5 litres may accumulate leading to serious clinical consequences, particularly in elderly patients.

The protein restricted regimens have been based on the Giovannetti principles whereby 0.3 g protein/kg body weight/day with 40–50 kcal/kg body weight/day were given. It is now appreciated that urea recycling mechanisms

Table 12.1 Suggested classification of acute renal failure (Bu = blood urea)

| | |
|---|---|
| Group 1 – 'Medical' | Daily Bu rise 4.8 mmol/litre (= 4.6–9.8 g nitrogen breakdown/day)* |
| Group 2 – 'Surgical' | Daily Bu rise 8.12 mmol/litre (= 9.3–13.8 g nitrogen breakdown/day) |
| Group 3 – 'Hyper catabolic' | Daily Bu rise > 12 mmol/litre (= 13.8 g nitrogen breakdown/day) |
| *Nutrition* | |
| Group 1 – Protein restrict, either route (i.e. oral or intravenous) | Groups 2 and 3 – Feed normally, dialyse appropriately |

* Based on 70 kg patient; water 60 % body weight = 42 litres

Table 12.2 Dialysis nutritional losses

| |
|---|
| *Peritoneal dialysis* |
| 20–30 g protein/40 litre dialysis |
| 13–15 g amino acid/40 litre dialysis |
| *Haemodialysis* |
| 2–3 g amino acid/hour dialysis |
| *Both* |
| Water-soluble vitamins |
| Essential biological elements |

have no nutritional significance in the management of acute renal failure patients. Nevertheless, as shown by Berlyne *et. al.*, 1967, protein restricted regimens in acute renal failure patients of modest catabolism, i.e., group 1 (Table 12.1) are associated with an increased sense of well-being, a diminished requirement for dialysis, fewer complications and a seemingly improved nutritional equilibrium. Such regimens provide approximately 20–30 mmol of sodium/day and keep the potassium allowance below 40 mmol/day. As shown in Table 12.2 when such patients require dialysis procedure, then it is important to make allowances for the nutritional losses necessarily incurred in such dialysis procedures. These are minimal with haemofiltration. It is important to realize that in peritoneal dialysis both proteins and amino acids are lost whereas in haemodialysis only amino acids are lost. In haemofiltration only amino acids are lost but to a lesser degree than in haemodialysis (Table 12.2). Consideration of these points, however, reminds the clinician that it is not surprising that hypoproteinaemia occurs particularly with peritoneal dialysis and protein restricted regimens in groups 2 and 3 patients. A number of studies have shown that amino acid losses across peritoneal dialysis can be compensated for by adding an amino acid solution to the peritoneal dialysate. The mean serum amino acid nitrogen concentration in renal failure patients is around 7–9 mg/100 ml and if 10 ml of Vamin N (a complete amino acid solution) are added or some other similar preparation, this gives a dialysate concentration of 9.4 mg amino acid nitrogen/litre thus obviating the obligatory losses. Occasionally, in these patients, one may have to compensate for the protein losses by giving intravenous plasma, albumin or human plasma protein faction (HPPF). Note importantly that only one-third of the total body albumin resides in the circulating vascular compartment and two-thirds is in the extra-vascular, extra-cellular fluid compartment.

For patients with hypercatabolic acute renal failure, or for that matter, moderately increased catabolism (groups 3 and 2 respectively) there is no place for severely restricted protein regimens. These patients, from a purely metabolic aspect, behave in a similar way to normal patients with respect to their response to trauma or infection. Many such patients may catabolize between 100 and 120 g of protein daily, equivalent to at least 16–19 g of nitrogen. These patients will require more frequent dialysis procedures or haemofiltration (CAVH) than their normo-catabolic counterparts which will further accentuate their tendency towards negative nitrogen balance and its sequelae unless compensated for. Negative nitrogen balance in acute renal failure patients is associated with the same sequelae, i.e., loss of body weight, decreased muscle mass, diminished serum albumin concentration, diminished immunoglobulin concentration, impaired immunocompetence (both cellular and humoral), increased incidence of infection and diminished rates of wound healing and more frequent wound dehiscence. Furthermore, hypoproteinaemia is associated with impaired efficiency of the microcirculation with attendant bed sores.

In such patients, therefore, it is reasonable to use haemodialysis and/or haemofiltration as the methods of choice of maintaining metabolic equilibrium. There can be no rationale for the attitude that one must use protein restricted regimens in these patients to reduce the frequency of haemodialysis and/or haemofiltration. The adage must be that in hypercatabolic or moderately catabolic patients, dialyse as frequently as necessary to accommodate the normal nutritional requirements and not restrict. This philosophy was established many years ago by Silva *et al.*, 1967, when they noted that frequent dialysis and a good food allowance was associated with better patient survival and diminished morbidity. As indicated in Table 12.2, it is important to make appropriate compensation for the inherent nutritional losses found with dialysis procedures.

With respect to oral management there is no need to have specifically designed enteral feeds, supplementary feeds or special, pure amino acid preparations. It is most important that the clinicians realize that providing *normal* nutritional requirements and preparations will suffice in these patients and that one may have to dialyse more frequently to accommodate the fluid and normal metabolic load.

## Intravenous nutritional management

This whole area has been simplified by the recognition that for intravenous nutrition in acute renal failure patients, there is no need for specially designed solutions. Furthermore, there is no need to use high glucose concentrations and insulin regimens to accommodate energy needs. In acute renal failure both glucose and fat metabolism are impaired by the uraemic status. However, if a patient is frequently dialysed, restoring the internal environment to near normal, then, of course, the utilization of both glucose and fat approximates to normal. There has been much debate in the past about what type of amino acid solution should be used for IV nutrition and how energy provision should be divided between glucose and fat provision. It is now recognized in the UK and, I believe, in many other countries, that one can use a nutritional regimen of a suitable full profile amino acid solution (both essential and non-essential) and an equi-energetic distribution between glucose and fat mixed in a 3 litre bag. By using a glucose/fat combination there is no longer the need to have a further potential complicating administration feature of an insulin infusion. Furthermore, with the advent of CAVH techniques there is absolutely no fluid volume constraint with respect to nutritional support regimens. Therefore, routine full profile amino acid solutions, fat emulsions and carbohydrates can be used as one would for the non-acute renal failure surgical counterparts.

A mistake often made with intravenous nutritional regimens is that they must be both phosphate and potassium deplete. With either frequent haemodialysis or CAVH there will inevitably be substantial losses of both potassium and phosphate from the patient and unless these are rectified in the nutritional regimen then nitrogen homeostasis cannot be obtained in the presence of both hypokalaemia and hypophosphataemia. Indeed, as shown in the accompanying figure (Fig. 12.1) considerable supplements of potassium and phosphate may need to be given to such patients.

It has long since been established that the infusion of intravenous fat emulsions as part energy source across a dialysis procedure does not interfere with the clearance of dialysance characteristics of artificial kidney or CAVH membranes. It is no longer necessary, in my opinion, to use insulin infusions as an automatic part of IV nutritional management of acute renal failure patients unless, of course, they are diabetic too. The old approach of using 300–400 units of insulin daily is now quite obsolete.

Although it has been the traditional American approach to use pure essential amino acid solutions in the management of acute renal failure patients, one must be mindful that their patients were carefully selected to be the least catabolic. As other investigators have shown there is absolutely no evidence to support the concept that giving essential amino acids only improves the survival rate of acute renal failure patients. Conversely, it must also be recognized that although some acute renal failure patients will lose more than 30–40 g nitrogen/day, one must never attempt to replace more than 20 g nitrogen daily otherwise the ability of the liver to cope with such amino acid loading is exceeded and simply more deamination results with the greater urea production. Similarly, one should not infuse in general more than 2500 kcal/day.

Nowadays, the management of acute renal failure patients by IV nutrition has been considerably simplified by the fact that all hospital pharmacies have the facility to prepare 3 litre bags in which suitable amino acid solutions, glucose and fat emulsions are mixed in a totally compatible manner and can be given to patients over a 24 hour period. No longer is there the need for glucose monitoring by Ames meters, constant infusion pumps to provide insulin or, indeed, complicated bottle procedures to make sure all nutrients were delivered over a 24 hour period.

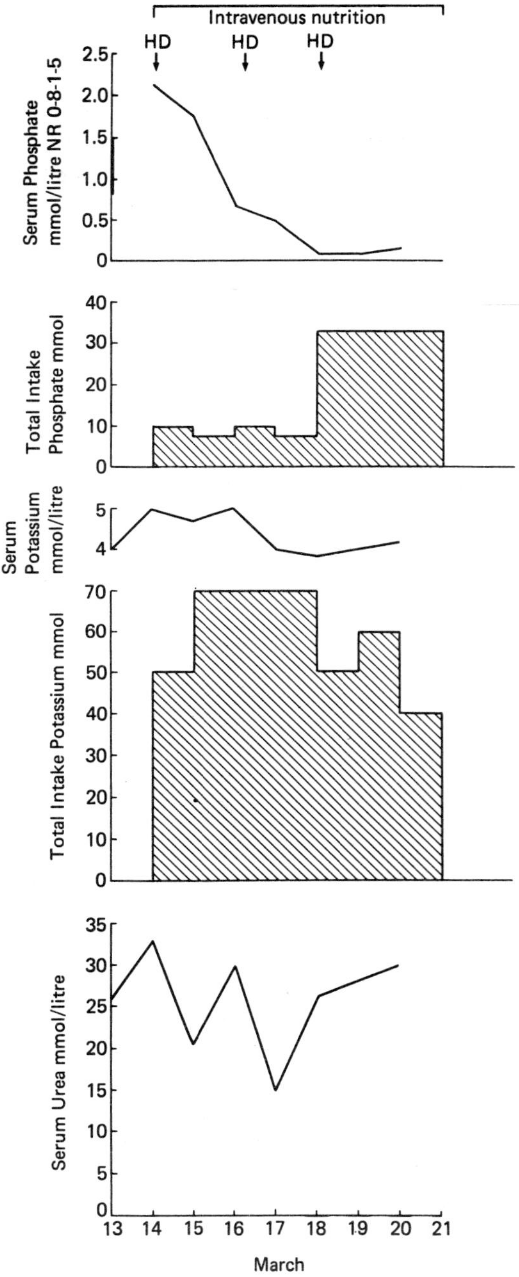


**Fig. 12.1** Patient T.M. Major gastrointestinal surgery, secondary G.I. fistula formation and acute renal failure with septicaemia. H.D. = haemodialysis. Intravenous nutrition programme provided 10 g nitrogen (Vamin-glucose) and 2500 kcals (at least 80 per cent per day as glucose-insulin) daily. Note even with high phosphorus supplementation (Boots neutral phosphate solution) profound hypophosphataemia persisted. Serum potassium concentration maintained within normal limits. Patient died of pulmonary embolism.

# Chronic renal failure (CRF), conservative management

## Low protein diet

It is intriguing to realize that since the original publications of Giovannetti and Giordano in 1964, low protein diet regimens have now two distinct areas of influence in the management of chronic renal failure. Traditionally, low protein diets (0.3 g/kg body weight) have been given to patients when their glomerular filtration rate (GFR) had fallen below 10 ml/minute. In these patients the rationale for giving low protein diets was to provide symptomatic relief from nausea, vomiting, pruritus, shortness of breath and low haemoglobin concentration etc., rather than have any curative effect on the renal disease *per se*. However, it is now recognized that if low protein (0.6 g/kg) diets with energy from fat and carbohydrate at up to 35 kcal/kg body weight are instituted much earlier in the course of chronic renal failure, e.g., GFR$\simeq$50 ml/minute (serum creatinine 150–200 $\mu$mol/litre) then there may actually be a beneficial effect upon the renal pathological processes themselves. It is interesting to reflect that in 1975 an editorial in the BMJ quoted '. . . Imposition of an unpalatable diet solely in an imperious attempt to improve the biochemical profile is neither reasonable nor kind . . .'. This is not disputed, but it must now be equally recognized that low protein diets have two distinct functions: (a) in certain patients they can decelerate the rate of renal functional deterioration; and (b) they can definitely ameliorate the symptoms of chronic renal failure. The symptoms of advanced chronic renal failure are many (Table 12.3) and any patient who can be relieved of such a profile of symptoms can only but feel better. However, the author would remind clinicians that dietary management is not a substitute for end-stage renal failure replacement therapy when that is indicated and available. On the other hand, it must equally be recognized that low protein amino acid supplemented diets can offer a very important interim therapy when dialysis procedures fail and an alternative treatment is being sought.

Previously it has been claimed that chronic renal failure is simply a variant of chronic malnutrition. This most certainly need not be the case and, indeed, one can use the usual parameters of establishing nutritional homeostasis e.g., body weight, serum albumin concentration, short half-life protein such as C-3 complement and transferrin, skinfold thickness, mid-arm muscle circumference measurement and in the more erudite atmosphere, serum amino acid profile, nitrogen balance and serum 3 methylhistidine concentrations.

Much of the disillusionment with low protein diets has arisen from their poor application. Clearly, if a patient on a low protein diet does not ingest the total prescribed then inevitably he must go into negative nitrogen balance with the attendant consequences. This is a basic point often not appreciated by the clinician.

## Low protein diets in early chronic renal failure

These form part of the overall profile of nutritional/metabolic management of such patients. It is now common practice to institute a 40 g protein (0.6 g/kg)

Table 12.3 Symptoms of chronic renal failure that can be modified by dietary management

| |
|---|
| Nausea |
| Vomiting |
| Apathy |
| Pruritus |
| Shortness of breath |
| Fatigue, lethargy |
| Oedema |
| Polyuria; polydipsia |
| Bone pain |
| Joint pain (pseudogout) |
| Red eyes |
| Paraesthesiae; weakness |
| Visual disturbances |

diet at serum creatinine concentrations of around 200 μmol/litre. It has been shown in those patients with a vaso-reactive renal parenchymal vasculature that they respond to reducing the protein load. This really is a reflection of the observation in diabetic patients that controlling the glucose intake controls hyperglycaemia and the resultant renal hyperperfusion and increased GFR which results in morphological damage to the capillaries and tubules. A number of studies have clearly shown that the institution of low protein diets early in chronic renal failure (chronic glomerulonephritis, the commonest cause of ESRF, chronic pyelonephritis, polycystic renal disease, some cases of essential hypertension) can decelerate the rate of progression of the renal failure. However, it must equally be appreciated that low protein diets in isolation are not sufficient and associated hyperphosphataemia, hyperuricaemia and hyperlipidaemia also need to be treated. Indeed, there is continuing debate amongst nephrologists whether low protein diets alone are sufficient in the early stages of chronic renal failure or whether these should be combined with;

1. phosphate restriction e.g. 600–1000 mg daily;
2. modified emphasis on fat intake particularly polyunsaturated fatty acids and;
3. better control of hyperuricaemia.

Over the past decade, there has been considerable resolution of the problems concerning whole protein, amino acid and keto acid analogue administration to chronic renal failure patients. There is no evidence in adults to suggest that giving amino acid supplements and/or keto acid analogues in any way alters the rate of progression of chronic renal failure or improves nitrogen balance. Certain investigators have indicated that using the reference of the reciprocal of the serum creatinine is a better guide of the progression of renal failure and gives early warning as to when a patient may require end-stage renal failure replacement. At the time of writing, it is by no means concluded whether low protein diets in isolation or in combination with phosphate restriction, fat intake modification and uric acid control give the best result and in which

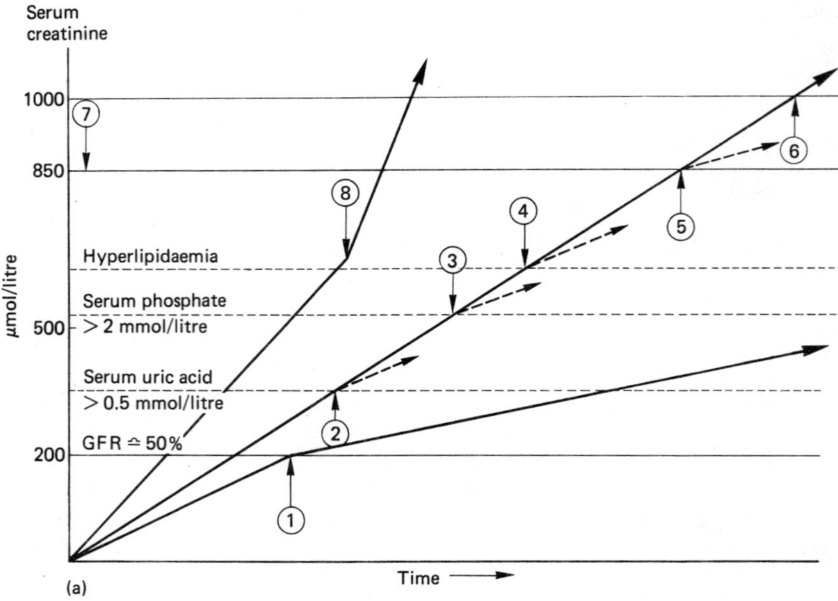


**Fig. 12.2(a)** Schematic representation of effects of dietary modifications on progression of chronic renal failure. Key: Lines indicate deceleration in rate of progression dependent upon dietary manoeuvre introduced. They do not all represent same degree of improvement. GFR = glomerular filtration rate. (1) Introduction of low protein diet e.g. 40 g/day – not likely to achieve any symptomatic relief at this level. (2) Use of allopurinol to control hyperuricaemia. (3) Use of aludrox (or similar compound) to control hyperphosphataemia – note evidence of renal osteodystrophy tends to occur earlier with renal tubular diseases. (4) Control of hyperlipidaemia (2/3 hypertriglyceridaemia 1/3 mixed cholesterol and triglyceride (type IIB)) by diet and later hypolipidaemic drugs. (5) Late introduction of low protein diet e.g. 30 g/day – now likely to achieve more symptomatic relief than 'physiological' improvement. (6) Introduction of P6 dietary formulation as a 'holding operation'. (7) Fashion angio access for haemodialysis patients or start diabetics on C.A.P.D. (8) Deleterious effect of development of accelerated hypertension – every effort must be made to control this if beneficial effects of dietary manipulations to be maintained.

types of chronic renal failure (Fig. 12.2). However, it is now generally agreed that early protein restriction in chronic renal failure will benefit a patient from a renal function and overall biochemical standpoint even if not symptomatically. Hence the extreme importance of gaining patient compliance by giving the individual accurate and practical information.

## Late chronic renal failure

All too often patients are referred late in the course of their disease when their GFR will already be below 10 ml/minute. In such patients there is no doubt that severe protein restriction (0.25 g/kg body weight) with essential amino acid supplementation can be of considerable benefit. Some years ago, both

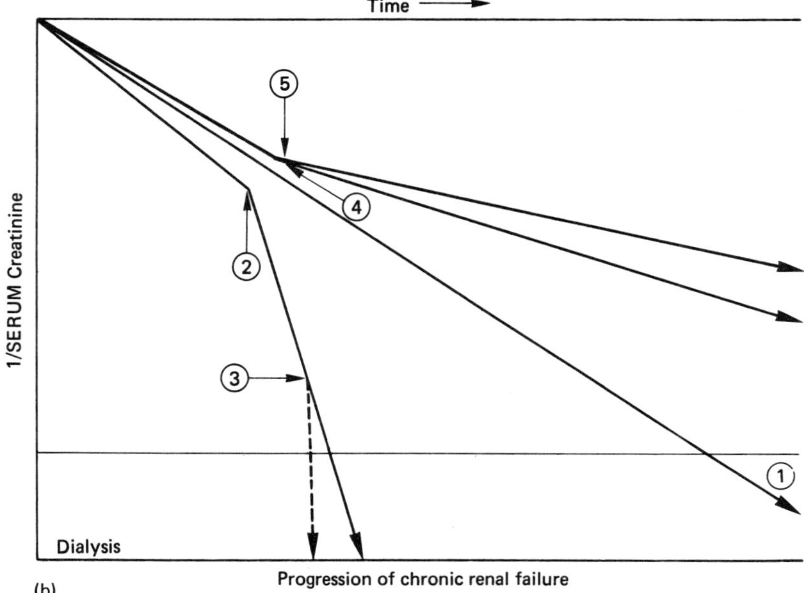


**Fig. 12.2(b)** Schematic representation of effects of dietary modifications on disease processes upon rate of progression of chronic renal failure. (1) Untreated case of chronic renal failure. (2) Deleterious effect of untreated accelerated hypertension. (3) Added deleterious effects of intercurrent infections e.g. urinary tract infection and/or surgery. (4) Improvement gained by early introduction of low protein diet. (5) Improvement achieved by combined effects of low protein diet, control of hyperphosphataemia, hypercalciuria and hyperlipidaemia.

Japanese and the UK investigators showed that the use of a P6 (protein 6 g equivalent) amino acid supplemented regimen could be of value in ameliorating the monotony of low protein diets. It has been shown that such regimens symptomatically improve patients and the need for dialysis is deferred, particularly if intercurrent problems occur with one dialysis procedure, e.g., CAPD peritonitis and patients are waiting to go on to regular haemodialysis. Low protein diets with amino acid supplementation can provide a good quality of life for the patient and delay either the need to start dialysis treatment or prolong the interval at changeover between different dialysis modalities. Furthermore, the P6 regimen has shown clearly that a patient can have both high and low biological class protein improving the palatability of such diets.

All clinicians should be aware that certain factors will influence the efficacy of low protein dietary regimens with or without amino acid supplementation (see Table 12.4). Equally, patients must be instructed about the importance of the diet and to recognize that it is essential to take the full diet and any other therapeutic regimen prescribed. A number of studies have conclusively shown that low protein diets supplemented by essential amino acid supplement can be effective.

As always, those patients with accelerated hypertension do less well with such a dietary regimen. The type of response that may be anticipated from a

Table 12.4 Factors influencing effect of dietary management of CRF

1. May need preliminary dialysis
2. Must take *whole* diet
3. Takes up to *one month* to stabilize
4. Care with salt and water balance
5. Effects of intercurrent illness

low protein dietary regimen is shown in Table 12.5. An important practical point is not to overlook the dietary compensation required for proteinuria. Although physiologically it is normal for proteinuria to decrease with a falling GFR, there are nevertheless the exceptions when, even with a GFR well below 10 ml/minute, proteinuria may exceed 10 g/day.

In adult practice, it has now been established that there is no place for the keto acid analogues of some essential amino acids as a supplement in low protein diets in the management of chronic renal failure. However, a different situation applies in paediatric practice which will not be discussed in this chapter.

## Disturbance of lipid metabolism

Hyperlipidaemia is a well recognized metabolic complication of chronic renal failure. About two-thirds of all patients will have some lipid disturbance and about two-thirds of these will have a Type IV hyperlipidaemia (hypertriglyceridaemia). Formerly, it was thought that the dietary management of such patients should be modified according to whether they had a Type IIb or Type IV disturbance of lipid metabolism. It has been decided, however, that all such patients should receive a high polyunsaturated fat dietary intake so that the P/S ratio approximates 1; this makes dietary management much easier. It is no longer necessary to insist that patients with Type IV hyperlipidaemia should have a low carbohydrate intake and those with a Type IIb a low cholesterol intake. The studies of Gokal and his colleagues have shown very conclusively that an overall low fat, low carbohydrate, dietary P/S ratio approximating 1 is sufficient for the management of hyperlipidaemic problems. It is now hoped that the traditional approach of giving extra calories to chronic renal failure patients by 'extra dollops of double cream' has now ceased.

Table 12.5 Factors influencing degree of, and response to, protein restriction in dietary management of CRF

1. GFR 10–15 ml/min – 40 g protein diet
2. GFR 5–10 ml/min – 30 g protein diet
3. GFR < 5 ml/min – strict LPD

Group (1) Blood urea returns to near normal
Group (2) Blood urea falls into 6–12 mmol/litre
Group (3) Blood urea falls into 15–20 mmol/litre

urea/creatinine ratio <27.5

## Other dietary considerations

As indicated earlier, low protein dietary management of chronic renal failure needs also to accommodate the separate problems of hyperphosphataemia, hyperuricaemia and hyperlipidaemia. I do not believe in the prescription of ultra low phosphate diet but rather the adequate prescription of phosphate binders, Alu-caps, Aludrox or sucralfate. Hyperuricaemia is adequately controlled by appropriate doses of allopurinol though in a small percentage of cases hypersensitivity reactions may occur. Renal osteodystrophy may occur in those with chronic renal failure secondary to, in particular, tubular diseases (e.g. chronic pyelonephritis, analgesic nephropathy), and for these, treatment with l-alphahydroxycholecalciferol (1αOHCC) is sufficient. Nevertheless, in a small percentage of patients, though rarely before dialysis, total parathyroidectomy may be required and long-term replacement treatment with 1αOHCC started.

## Chronic renal failure in diabetics

Chronic renal failure remains the major cause of death in juvenile onset diabetes mellitus. Surveys suggest that 50 per cent of patients will die of chronic renal failure if diabetes mellitus occurs before the age of 20 years. There is approximately 15 years between the on-set of diabetes mellitus and the occurrence of proteinuria. However, once proteinuria has occurred, as a result of diabetic nephropathy, then the time course to end-stage renal failure is 4–5 years. If a diabetic patient becomes frankly nephrotic as a result of his renal lesion, then the time course is somewhat shorter. Furthermore, once the blood urea has reached $>$ 10 mmol/litre or the serum creatinine $>$ 200 μmol/litre, it takes only 2 years to reach end-stage renal failure and death if no alternative programme is available. Fortunately, with the advent of chronic ambulatory peritoneal dialysis (CAPD) the future is much brighter for such patients and they can be transplanted from the CAPD programme.

Hitherto, there has been scant attention to the question of protein restriction in patients with early diabetic nephropathy, the emphasis always being on glycaemic control. The policy should now be that patients with evidence of diabetic nephropathy should be referred early to nephrology units who can cope best with both their diabetic and renal problems. Diabetic patients with chronic renal failure are subject to the same metabolic secondary effects as non-diabetic patients and these include not only uraemia itself, but renal osteodystrophy (particularly rare in diabetic patients), hyperuricaemia, hyperlipidaemia (more common), hyperglycaemia and hyperkalaemia. It is now recommended that diabetic patients with a serum creatinine of 300–400 μmol/litre should be put on a 40 g protein diet (modified according to body weight) and this be tailored down to a 30 g protein intake when their serum creatinine reaches 500–600 μmol/litre. Equally, it must be emphasized that the application of ultra low protein diets (e.g. P6 formulations – see above) should not be given so as to delay a diabetic patient starting CAPD treatment. The philosophy should be that a modicum of dietary protein restriction is essential but one should not delay referring patients with end-stage renal failure for management when their serum creatinine has reached 750 μmol/litre.

There is increasing evidence (Author's observations not yet published) that when the serum creatinine is below 120 μmol/litre protein restriction can effect a dramatic stabilization of GFR if this is already reduced. Of course, for the diabetic patient already subject to the glucose restrictions, the added restrictions of protein intake modification can be irksome, but it should be emphasized to such patients that strict dietary compliance can not only

1. delay the time when they will need end-stage renal replacement therapy, but also
2. diminish associated complications, e.g., hyperlipidaemia and vascular disease.

It is hoped that in the future more diabetologists will recognize the importance of starting early dietary protein restriction in the diabetic patient long before the serum biochemistry overtly indicates the onset of chronic renal failure.

## Regular haemodialysis (RDT) patients

There is now general agreement that if such patients receive 1–1.25 g protein per kg body weight/day no other specific dietary treatment is required. On average most patients receive 60 g protein/day on the assumption they have two haemodialyses of 6–9 hours per week (depending on the efficiency of the dialysis procedure used). It is no longer customary to give such patients amino acid supplements or other dietary supplements other than tab. aneurin co. forte, ascorbic acid and folic acid as deemed appropriate.

Occasionally, chronic renal failure patients on RDT require supplementary feeding because of intercurrent illness and inability to maintain a normal oral intake. For such patients a 3 litre bag IV nutritional approach can be used across dialysis time providing 9–13 g nitrogen and 2000–2500 kcals per dialysis. Although in the past much debate has taken place, particularly amongst Europeans, about how much, if any, amino acid supplementation should be given across (i.e. intravenously) each regular haemodialysis treatment, it is now generally accepted this is no longer necessary. Thus, provided adequate protein and energy intakes are given together with vitamin, iron and other requirements, no amino acid supplements are required. Of course, if a regular haemodialysis patient acquires an intercurrent illness, i.e., infection or surgical intervention, then he may be regarded as an acute renal failure patient in the immediate post-crisis period receiving more frequent dialyses and a more nearly normal nutritional intake, be that enterally or parenterally.

Perhaps a point that has previously been overlooked is not whether nutrition is adequate but whether patients comply strictly with dialysis instructions. Therefore, it is frequently noted with regular haemodialysis patients that their serum urea and creatinine concentrations are much higher than anticipated but this in turn relates to

1. not performing haemodialysis appropriately; and to
2. breaking by a considerable margin their advised dietary intake.

## Chronic ambulatory peritoneal dialysis (CAPD)

The protein requirements for patients on CAPD are 1–1.25 g/kg body weight for those having 3 or 4 exchanges/day. This applies equally to the diabetic and non-diabetic patients. Although there will clearly be a certain amount of glucose absorption during CAPD this of itself does not necessarily result in a higher degree of secondary hyperlipidaemia though there is a tendency to hypertriglyceridaemia if too many strong glucose bags are used. Many diabetic patients prefer to carry on with their routine subcutaneous insulin injections rather than add insulin to the intraperitoneal fluid. Although some studies have shown that intraperitoneal insulin results in a better glycaemic control, this should not be regarded as mandatory in diabetics. Although amino acid and protein losses are greater in peritoneal dialysis and for that matter in CAPD, there is no need to make any compensatory dietary adjustments for such losses.

In both RDT and CAPD patients hyperlipidaemic problems may occur and these can be resolved either by

1. dietary modification e.g., lowering the dietary saturated fatty acid or carbohydrate content or;
2. adding hypolipidaemic agents such as bezafibrate which have the particular advantage of lowering serum triglycerides whilst augmenting the HDL2 fraction of HDL lipoprotein.

Although it was formerly thought there were certain parallelisms between uraemic and hepatic coma, this no longer has any therapeutic significance. Therefore, there is not any particular attention that needs to be given to the branch chain amino acid content of the protein allowance for either RDT or CAPD patients.

## Other renal diseases requiring specific dietary management

### Idiopathic hypercalciuria

Firstly, it is important to ascertain the degree of hypercalciuria. If a patient has hypercalciuria of less than 12.5 mmol/day, then it is likely that he will respond to dietary management. This implies the use of a water softener and a dietary calcium intake of 20 mmol or less daily. However, if the urinary calcium excretion is greater than 12.5 mmol daily then dietary management alone will not suffice and additionally either cellulose phosphate 5 g t.d.s. and/or bendrofluazide 5–10 mg daily will be required. Many patients with hypercalciuria will have an associated degree of hyperoxaluria. This should be differentiated from primary hyperoxaluria. The prime sources of dietary oxalate intake are:

1. tea;
2. certain fruits and vegetables e.g., strawberries, tomatoes, spinach.

In general one can say that if a patient with idiopathic hypercalciuria with a urinary calcium excretion of less than 12.5 mmol daily undertakes modest calcium restriction with water softening then a greater than 60 per cent success rate with respect to:

1. stone formation,
2. symptomatic renal tract colic or;
3. operative intervention, can be achieved.

With those having a greater than 12.5 mmol daily excretion then the addition of cellulose phosphate and/or bendrofluazide can add another 20 per cent overall success rate. Certain patients do not respond to these measures and may require ultra severe dietary calcium intake. This means getting the dietary calcium intake below 8 mmol daily, an extremely tedious and boring dietary regimen. In addition to calcium restriction, cellulose phosphate and bendrofluazide, it has been shown in world-wide studies that stone formation is more common in those populations with a higher protein intake. Therefore, some authorities suggest that 100–200 mg of allopurinol should be prescribed daily.

In the final analysis whenever considering the problem of idiopathic hypercalciuria it is not simply a matter of biochemical measurement. The important factors are whether;

1. the patient feels better;
2. has less colic episodes;
3. requires less surgical interventions and;
4. whether clinically and radiologically one can prove there is a diminished incidence of stone formation.

## Cystinuria

This rare genetically determined biochemical disorder of the basic amino acids resulting in cystinuria, a highly insoluble amino acid in acid urine, is associated with the formation of cystine renal calculi. Penicillamine has proved the turning point in the management of this disorder. However, occasional patients react with a hypersensitivity reaction to this drug either by developing the nephrotic syndrome or a bone marrow suppression problem. This complication is rare but nevertheless merits consideration of alternative approaches. If a patient cannot tolerate penicillamine, then the alternatives are:

1. a high fluid intake with;
2. alkalinization of the urine or;
3. a low methionine diet.

Clearly such patients need to be instructed very carefully about their dietary and fluid management and, because they know the consequences, the compliance factor is high. The normal recommended daily methionine intake for a 70 kg man is 2.2 g, i.e., twice the absolute minimum required. Methionine is an essential amino acid and one could doubt the wisdom of a low methionine diet on a long-term basis. However, when faced with a patient who has only one kidney, who continues to develop renal calculi and for whom you know no other therapeutic approach is available (because of previous penicillamine sensitivity) a dietary approach is the only alternative. It would be assumed that such a patient was on an alkalinizing regimen (1 g sodium bicarbonate t.d.s or q.d.s.) and a high fluid intake (3–4 litres/day and 0.5 litres at 2 a.m.) and subsequently a 400 mg methionine dietary intake daily. I have repeatedly studied such a patient over 4 years without any obvious clinical, nutritional or metabolic abnormalities developing.

## Oxalosis

This rare inborn error of metabolism results in the formation of oxalate calculi. Oxalate stones also form in patients who have had ileojejunal bypass operations for obesity and are not uncommon in patients with Crohn's disease.

The dietary management of this condition is to refuse the intake of such foods that contain a high content of oxalate, e.g., rhubarb, and other fruits such as strawberries. The formation of oxalate stones in bowel disorders is related in part to altered glycine metabolism and partly to increased intestinal absorption of oxalic acid. Oral administration of 9 g taurine daily may reduce the endogenous formation of glycine.

## Gout

There is no longer the need for severe dietary regimens in the management of this condition. Clearly, one can advise the patient against a high alcohol intake, but by and large this can be accommodated by the use of allopurinol in the vast majority of cases. Allopurinol is a potent xanthine oxidase inhibitor and will decrease the serum uric acid concentrations and thereby the propensity toward renal calculus formation. This applies equally well to the acute situations where myeloproliferative disorders are treated with cytotoxic agents.

## Nephrotic syndrome

Nephrotic patients may lose vast amounts of protein in the urine, e.g., in excess of 20 g daily leading to a serum albumin concentration of less than 10 g/litre in extreme cases. It is important to recognize that at least 10 g of dietary protein are required to replace 1 g of serum albumin. Only one-third of the total body albumin resides in the circulating vascular compartment of the extra-cellular fluid volume space, the other two-thirds being in the non-vascular compartment of the ECF. Only occasionally is it necessary to feed such patients by an enteral feeding approach as most will tolerate up to 100 g of protein daily. However, the problem arises particularly in children who may well need nasogastric feeding with some proprietary preparation. Thus, the management of the nephrotic syndrome comprises:

1. high protein intake;
2. not too much attention to salt intake;
3. use of high dose diuretic regimen where indicated and;
4. being aware that resolution of the problem may take weeks or, indeed, months rather than days.

Only rarely in adult practice is it necessary to resort to intravenous HPPF to improve the circulating blood volume temporarily to improve renal perfusion and thereby the GFR to improve filtration whereby diuretic treatment might have effect. Overall, the management of nephrotic syndrome is one of patience, high protein intake and appropriate diuretic dosage.

## Renal disease in hypertension

Salt restriction is now less important than it used to be because of the potency of currently available diuretics. It is more important that patients have a palatable diet with which they can be compliant than insist upon ultra rigid regimens whereby salt intake is below 40 mmol/day which few people nowadays can tolerate. Therefore, in my view, no specific dietary management is really required.

## Starvation syndromes in regular dialysis patients (RDT and CAPD)

By and large this is a syndrome of the past. Occasionally a regular dialysis patient with non-volume dependent hypertension will become emaciated and require bilateral nephrectomy. It is more important this sort of patient gets recognized early rather than embark upon a rigid dialysis protocol, weight reduction and severe salt restriction. In my view enteral and intravenous feeding have no part to play in the management of such patients. Either their hypertension can be controlled or they should have bilateral nephrectomy. However, there are other patients on regular dialysis programmes who have intercurrent illnesses and thereby cannot take their normal oral intake. In such cases the dialysis protocol should be increased from two to three times weekly and dialysis time be used to infuse a 3 litre bag containing 9–13 g of nitrogen and 2000–2500 kcals.

## Renal transplantation patients

Athough it has been traditional to accuse such patients of being overweight because they are either on steroids or over indulgent this is not necessarily the case. There is no evidence whatsoever to prove that necessarily steroid treated patients must become obese and acquire hyperlipoproteinaemic problems. Nowadays, more than 50 per cent of patients undergoing cadaveric renal transplantation will be on cyclosporin A which has no relevance to either obesity, hyperlipidaemia or other metabolic consequences. In my view all renal transplant patients should:

1. be educated about the need to observe a sensible dietary intake;
2. be encouraged to keep to a target weight and;
3. be advised of the iniquities of being overweight.

# Conclusion

From the foregoing it can be seen that the role of diet is of paramount importance in the management of acute and chronic renal failure patients. Although there are many similarities in all patients as a result of uraemia the time duration factor is of paramount importance to separating out acute from chronic renal failure. It is also my firm view that no self respecting Renal Unit can operate without a full time dietitian in attendance to explain in detail the minutiae of dietary management to the patients involved. Over the last 30 years there has been a revolution in terms of low protein dietary management in chronic renal failure, being initially to ameliorate symptoms and now actually being therapeutic in terms of reducing the rate of renal functional deterioration. It has not yet been defined which patients may most benefit from the early introduction of low protein diet and this will depend upon the availability of more readily practised out-patient investigations.

## References

Blacklock, N.J. and Macleod M.A. (1974). The effect of cellulose phosphate on intestinal absorption and urinary excretion of calcium. *Br. J. Urol.*, **46**, 385–92.

Brenner, B.M., Meyer, T.W., and Hostetter, T.H. (1982). Dietary protein intake and the progressive nature of kidney disease. *N. Engl. J. Med.*, **307**, 652–9.

Editorial. (1982). Diet and the progression of chronic renal failure. *Lancet*, **ii**, 1314–15.

El Nahas, A.M., Masters-Thomas, A., Brady, S.A., Farrington, K., Wilkinson, J., Hilson, A.J.W., Varghese, Z. and Moorhead, J.F. (1984). Selective effect of low protein diets in chronic renal diseases. *Br. Med. J.*, **289**, 1337–41.

Giordano, C. (1982). Protein restriction in chronic renal failure. *Kidney Int.*, **22**, 401–408.

Giordano, C. and Friedman, E.A. (eds) 1981). *Uraemia: pathobiology of patients treated for 10 years or more.* Wichtig Editore: Milan.

Grant, A. and Todd, E. (1982). *Nutrition in renal failure in enteral and parenteral nutrition: A Clinical Handbook*, pp. 121–8. Eds. Grant, A. and Todd, E. Blackwell Scientific Publishers: Oxford.

Lee, H.A. (1981). Acute renal failure. In *Nutrition and the Surgical Patient*, pp. 236–52. Ed. Hill, G.L. Churchill Livingstone: Edinburgh.

Lee, H.A. (1981). *Diet and Renal Failure in Recent Advances in Clinical Nutrition*, 1, pp. 159–69. Eds. Howard, A. and McLean Baird, I. John Libbey: London.

Lee, H.A. (1981). What are the nutritional problems in renal failure? 2nd European Congress on Parenteral and Enteral Nutrition, pp. 318–26. Ed. Wright, P.D., *Acta Chir. Scand.* (Suppl. 507).

Lee, H.A. and Jackson, M.A. (1981). Keto acid therapy in chronic renal failure patients on moderately protein restricted diets in uraemia: pathobiology of patients treated for 10 years or more, pp. 9–16. Eds. Giordano, C., and Friedman, E.A. Wichtig Editore: Milan.

Lee, H.A., Talbot, S., Rowlands, A. and Jackson, M.A. (1980). Dietary management of chronic renal failure with oral amino acids. *Nutr. Metab.*, **24**, 50–63.

Mitch, W.E., Abras, E., and Walser, M. (1982). Long term effects of a new keto acid-amino acid supplement in patients with chronic renal failure. *Kidney Int.*, **22**, 48–53.

Pak, C.Y.C., Delea, C.S. and Bartter, F.C., (1974). Successful treatment of recurrent nephrolithiasis (calcium stones) with cellulose phosphate. *N. Engl. J. Med.*, **290**, 175–80.

Rose, G.A. and Harrison, A.R. (1974). The incidence, investigation and treatment of idiopathic hypercalciuria. *Br. J. Urol.*, **46**, 261–74.

# Anaemias and coagulation disorders of nutritional origin

Israel Chanarin



## Normal blood values

Normal levels of haemoglobin and red cells vary with age and sex. Adult values are shown in Table 13.1.

The newborn have relatively high haemoglobin levels and red cell counts and these values rapidly fall in the first few months to be succeeded by values below those found in adults until the age of 5 to 7 years. At puberty male values become higher than female values. The newborn is macrocytic (mean corpuscular volume, MCV, above values in healthy adults), whereas red cells for the subsequent few years are microcytic, when the MCV is smaller than in adults. Adult MCV values are attained after the age of 7 to 8 years.

## Nutritional requirements for red cell production

Anaemia appears as a major manifestation of a deficiency of some nutrients such as iron, $B_{12}$, and folate. Lack of vitamin K affects blood coagulation. Protein deficiency leads to anaemia as part of kwashiorkor in infancy or as in gross malnutrition in adults.

Vitamin $B_6$ (pyridoxine) is required for haem synthesis and anaemias

Table 13.1 Normal values in adults at sea level (mean ± 2 standard deviations)

| | Male | Female |
|---|---|---|
| Red cells ($\times 10^6/\mu l$) | 5.0 ± 0.6 | 4.6 ± 0.5 |
| Haemoglobin (g/100 ml) | 14.7 ± 1.8 | 13.5 ± 1.2 |
| PCV (%) | 42.8 ± 4.9 | 39.5 ± 3.7 |
| MCV (fl) | 85.2 ± 4.8 | 85.8 ± 3.9 |
| MCH (pg) | 29.3 ± 1.6 | 29.2 ± 1.5 |
| MCHC (%) | 34.4 ± 1.3 | 34.0 ± 1.3 |

responding to pyridoxine occur (sideroblastic anaemias). These, however, do not arise from simple nutritional deficiency but from defects in haem synthesis which are corrected in some cases by large doses of pyridoxine far in excess of the normal daily requirement of 1 – 2 mg. Lack of riboflavin can cause anaemia in animals but this is exceptionally rare in man. The role of niacin in the production of anaemia is uncertain although patients with pellagra are anaemic. Scurvy regularly produces anaemia, although whether this is due entirely to lack of ascorbic acid or to associated folate deficiency is uncertain.

Vitamin E deficiency has been thought to be a cause of anaemia in premature infants due to the premature destruction of red cells.

The role of copper in anaemia is poorly understood. Deficiency is rare, and mainly occurs in children. However, it has also been reported as a complication of total parenteral nutrition (see p. 509).

## Age, sex, race and climate

Anaemia due to malnutrition is more frequent in infancy due to high growth requirements and in old age due to incapacity and often poverty. It is also more common in women of child bearing age due to menstrual loss, and to increased iron and folate requirements in pregnancy and lactation.

Certain congenital disorders which increase folate requirements are prevalent in certain races. The most important are abnormal haemoglobins. Haemoglobin S (HbS) and/or C are present in one-third of the population of Nigeria and Ghana. Thalassaemia is widespread in Asia and along the Mediterranean coast. Hindu Indians are strict vegetarians and eat no foods of animal origin, hence nutritional $B_{12}$ deficiency is very common among them.

Climatic and hygienic conditions determine the frequency of hookworm infestation throughout the world and this is a major cause of intestinal blood loss and iron deficiency. Malaria causes red cell destruction and leads to an increased folic acid requirement. Other dietary deficiencies are often superadded to the increased iron and folate requirements in such conditions.

## Iron

A mixed western-type diet supplies an average of 14 mg of iron daily. The iron is present either as inorganic iron or as iron incorporated into haem, usually the myoglobin of meat. Inorganic iron is best absorbed when it is in the more soluble reduced ferrous state and reducing agents (e.g. ascorbic acid) as well as contact with gut mucosa favour reduction of iron. However, it is the over-all composition of the meal that determines the availability of iron for absorption. Iron is well absorbed when it is present with meat, fish, and liver and less well absorbed in the presence of eggs, cream, corn, or beans and, indeed as part of a vegetarian meal. Apart from soluble ferrous iron, complexes are formed between iron and food components (chelates) which determine absorption. Absorption of haem iron is not influenced by these factors and is unaffected by reducing agents and gastric acid which enhance inorganic iron uptake.

Iron is absorbed from the upper 40 cm of the small gut, where haem enters the mucosal cells. The iron is split from the haem intracellularly and joins other iron within the cell. Inorganic iron entering the cell becomes attached to a protein in the sap and if the cell itself requires iron some will be taken up by mitochondria. Thereafter some iron passes out of the cell to be transported by transferrin, an iron-carrying protein in body fluids and plasma. The remaining intracellular iron is taken up by apoferritin to form ferritin and is retained within the cell. The cells on the surface of the villi are renewed by cell division at the base of the villi and the older cells progress to the end of the villus and are shed into the gut lumen with the iron-ferritin complex. The amount of apoferritin in the cell thus acts as a controlling factor regulating the amount of iron absorbed. In iron deficiency the cell ferritin content is very low so that most of the absorbed iron is transferred to plasma. When the iron stores are adequate much of the iron is retained in the cell.

Normally 1–2 mg of iron are absorbed each day, the higher values occurring in women with higher iron needs due to iron losses in menstruation. In iron deficiency and in normal pregnancy absorption is augmented so that about 4 mg are absorbed daily. A greater demand for iron than this cannot be met by further improvement in absorption of food iron so that negative iron balance develops. Significant changes in red cells and in haemoglobin values occur in about 15 per cent of apparently normal healthy women when given iron and this suggests the presence of undiagnosed iron deficiency in this group.

A specific protein, transferrin, transports iron in the plasma not only from the gut but also iron derived from iron-storage cells throughout the body and from effete red cells to the marrow, where the iron is utilized for the synthesis of haemoglobin in erythroblasts. Transferrin, in terms of its iron-binding capacity is present in plasma at concentrations of 260–400 μg/100 ml. One-third is normally bound to iron so that the serum iron level is 60–160 μg/100 ml. In iron deficiency the serum iron is low and the transferrin concentration is increased.

Iron is stored in fixed macrophages as ferritin. The ferritin molecule is a protein shell within which up to 400 iron atoms are stored. Haemosiderin is degraded ferritin.

*Iron deficiency*. The anaemia leads to tiredness and shortness of breath. Lack of iron may arise from:

1. Increased iron loss due to persistent bleeding. Most of the iron in the body is present in red cells and blood loss is the commonest way in which iron is lost. Many disorders of the gastrointestinal tract ranging from gastric or duodenal ulcers and aspirin ingestion, to cancers of the large gut, piles and hookworm infestation all cause regular blood loss. Menstrual losses are of great importance in women.
2. An increased requirement for iron arises in pregnancy, which usually leads to iron deficiency if additional iron is not given. Reference has already been made to the anaemia associated with rapid growth.
3. Inadequate iron intake due to a poor diet, or less commonly to impaired absorption, as after partial gastrectomy, or to a combination of these factors, is also an important cause of iron deficiency. Iron-deficiency anaemia is found particularly in women from deprived economic circumstances taking a poor diet and who have menorrhagia. There is a significant association in pregnancy between folate and iron deficiency due to poor dietary intake of these substances, for diets providing inadequate amounts of iron also provide inadequate amounts of folate as well as other nutrients such as ascorbic acid.

*Diagnosis.* The blood film is typical with characteristic haematological indices – reduced haemoglobin concentration, low mean corpuscular volume and low mean corpuscular haemoglobin. The blood film shows red cells with thin rims of haemoglobin and the mean corpuscular haemoglobin concentration is low in the more severe cases.

The serum-iron and ferritin levels are low and the serum iron-binding capacity is raised. Tissue stores of iron are severely depleted, as demonstrated by staining marrow or liver for iron by the prussian blue method.

Once iron deficiency is diagnosed the cause must be determined by careful enquiry about excessive menstrual blood losses or gastrointestinal blood loss in both sexes. Tests for faecal occult blood losses are important. Labelling the patient's red cells with $^{51}Cr$ and noting the $^{51}Cr$ in the faeces is another valuable method of quantitating intestinal blood loss. A dietary history may also be very helpful.

*Treatment.* Prophylactic treatment is important in pregnancy where 30 mg of elemental iron daily in the form of any of the currently available preparations such as ferrous sulphate are adequate (Chanarin and Rothman, 1971).

Correction of iron deficiency consists of dealing with the cause of blood loss as well as replacement therapy. Ferrous sulphate remains the cheapest and most effective form of therapeutic iron.

## Vitamin $B_{12}$ and folate

Lack of either of these vitamins may give rise to a megaloblastic anaemia. Symptoms include tiredness, lassitude, shortness of breath and a sore mouth and/or tongue. Patients with vitamin $B_{12}$ deficiency may complain of paresthesiae in the hands and feet, loss of taste and smell and sometimes difficulty in walking, with difficulty in micturition. Most of these latter symptoms are due to degeneration of nerve tissue (i.e. subacute combined degeneration of the spinal cord).

The earliest haematological evidence of lack of these vitamins is a raised MCV on doing a blood count and macrocytic blood film followed by progressive anaemia, leucopenia and thrombocytopenia. This altered mode of blood formation is characterized by a megaloblastic marrow as compared to normal blood formation, i.e. normoblastic.

Macrocytosis with a normoblastic marrow occurs in other disorders such as alcoholism, aplastic anaemia, haemolytic anaemia, sideroblastic anaemia and liver disease.

### Cobalamin

Vitamin $B_{12}$ or cobalamin is similar in structure to haemoglobin. It is composed of four modified pyrrole groups, forming a corrin ring linked to a cobalt atom. Benzimidazole is linked to this corrin ring.

The source of vitamin $B_{12}$ is bacterial synthesis. In ruminants $B_{12}$ is synthesized by bacteria in the foregut. Man obtains pre-formed $B_{12}$ from foods of animal origin, e.g. meat, milk, eggs. Vitamin $B_{12}$ is not required by plants and is not present in vegetables and fruits. The only $B_{12}$ present in a vegetarian diet is that provided by bacterial contamination or via water contaminated by $B_{12}$ originally produced by soil bacteria.

Vitamin $B_{12}$ is stable and can withstand a wide range of pH as well as heat. A mixed diet supplies a variable but adequate amount of $B_{12}$ ranging from 1 to 8 $\mu$g in a relatively poor diet, to 4 to 85 $\mu$g daily in a so-called high-cost diet. A 'vegetarian' diet will supply less than 1 $\mu$g $B_{12}$ daily. The daily $B_{12}$ requirement is 2–4 $\mu$g and this equals the daily loss as assessed by long-term whole body counting techniques following a tracer dose of $^{60}Co$–$B_{12}$.

Most of the vitamin $B_{12}$ in food is available for absorption. In the stomach the $B_{12}$ binds to intrinsic factor, a glycoprotein secreted by the parietal cell of the gastric mucosa and the $B_{12}$-intrinsic factor complex passes down to the distal ileum where it becomes attached to specific receptor sites on the surface of the epithelial cells lining the villi.

Vitamin $B_{12}$ alone is absorbed from the ileum, maximum transfer to blood taking place after 8–12 hours. A specific transport protein, transcobalamin II, is necessary for normal $B_{12}$ transport.

Vitamin $B_{12}$ status can be assessed by measuring the serum $B_{12}$ level – almost all this $B_{12}$ is attached to transcobalamin I. The normal range is about 170–1000 pg/ml, the precise values depending upon the assay method employed.

Vitamin $B_{12}$ is required to maintain normal folate function, but the precise biochemical pathways by which this occurs remain uncertain. The failure of folate function leads to a megaloblastic anaemia. Vitamin $B_{12}$ is also required in mammals for the synthesis of methionine and for the conversion of methylmalonic acid to succinic acid.

*Deficiency of vitamin $B_{12}$.* The causes are:

1. Nutritional deficiency, e.g. due to a strict vegetarian diet.
2. Impaired absorption due to
   (a) Gastric causes – atrophy (pernicious anaemia), gastrectomy.
   (b) Intestinal causes – coeliac disease, tropical sprue, anatomical abnormalities of gut giving an abnormal small gut bacterial flora, fish tapeworm, Crohn's disease.

*Manifestations of $B_{12}$ deficiency.* These are due to a megaloblastic anaemia as described. The earliest evidence is a rise in the MCV.

In addition to erythropoiesis, $B_{12}$ is needed for normal function and integrity of nerve tissue. About one-third of patients with pernicious anaemia have evidence of peripheral neuritis and about 10 per cent involvement of the central nervous system (spinal cord and brain).

*Nutritional vitamin $B_{12}$ deficiency.* This is commonplace in communities who for religious reasons do not consume any food of animal origin. This applies to Hindu vegetarians who are found not only in India but also among Indian immigrants throughout the world. Despite low serum $B_{12}$ levels and considerably reduced body stores of $B_{12}$, the majority of these people are healthy. There were no differences in the heights and weights of Indian students taking mixed diets and those taking strictly vegetarian diets. The mean serum $B_{12}$ level among healthy vegetarians was 121 pg/ml as compared to 366 pg/ml in a group taking a mixed diet (Mehta *et al.*, 1964), and about half had $B_{12}$ levels below 100 pg/ml.

Megaloblastic anaemia due to $B_{12}$ deficiency is common. The anaemia may be mild or very severe. In younger women it may be associated with infertility. The serum vitamin $B_{12}$ level is low in such women but unlike all other patients with vitamin $B_{12}$ deficiency, they absorb vitamin $B_{12}$ in a normal manner.

The diagnosis is established by demonstrating an adequate haematological response to oral vitamin $B_{12}$ treatment in the dose they would receive from a normal diet, viz. about 5 $\mu$g $B_{12}$ daily.

Other causes of $B_{12}$ deficiency should not be overlooked in this group of patients. True pernicious anaemia is present with the same incidence as in Caucasians.

**Folate**

Folic acid is a complex molecule consisting of a bicyclic structure (a pteridine ring), *para*-aminobenzoic acid, and between 1 and 6 glutamic acid residues. The compounds with more than one glutamic acid are called folate polyglutamates. The natural folates are reduced, that is, they have four additional hydrogens in the pteridine ring to form tetrahydrofolic acid. Thus the natural compounds are very susceptible to oxidative damage even on exposure to atmospheric oxygen. Finally the folate compounds function in the transfer of single carbon units which are generally carried as formyl (—CHO) or methyl (—$CH_3$) groups.

*Dietary sources.* Folate compounds are widely distributed and almost all foodstuffs contain a variable amount. A normal mixed diet supplies between 100 and 300 $\mu$g of total folate per day. Of this about one-quarter is largely in the monoglutamate form (available for microbiological assay without further treatment) and is almost completely absorbed from the gut. The remainder is in the form of polyglutamates. These must have the glutamic acid chain removed by a conjugase enzyme in order to make them available to assay organisms as well as during the course of intestinal absorption in man. A substantial amount of polyglutamate is absorbed but the quantitative aspects are uncertain. Most natural folates have methyl or formyl substituents. Food folate is lost with storage of the food, exposure to ultraviolet light and during cooking.

The daily requirement is 100–200 $\mu$g in adults, 200–300 $\mu$g in pregnancy, and 50–100 $\mu$g in the first two years of life.

During the intestinal absorption of natural folates, the molecule is changed in the gut cells so that methyltetrahydrofolate only reaches the portal blood. In the intestinal cell, folates are reduced and methylated, and with polyglutamates the glutamic acid chain is removed. Pteroylglutamic acid itself, used in folate therapy, is not present in natural materials such as foodstuffs. It is absorbed largely unchanged and further metabolized in the body.

Folate coenzymes are concerned with the transfer of single carbon units in the synthesis of purines and pyrimidines. These two types of compounds are constituents of nucleic acids and hence are required in increased amount when there is increased cell turnover. Thus folate is essential for fetal growth, in infancy and for cell renewal as in haemolytic anaemia.

**Causes of folate deficiency**

1. Nutritional deficiency.
2. Malabsorption as in gluten sensitivity or tropical sprue.
3. Increased requirement in pregnancy, haemolytic anaemia, tumours.
4. Interference by drugs such as anticonvulsants, folate antagonists, salazopyrine.

*Manifestations of folate deficiency.* The anaemia that develops in folate deficiency is similar in all respects to that due to $B_{12}$ deficiency and once again macrocytosis is the earliest manifestation. Clinically there are few early symptoms other than lack of energy. Subsequently a sore, smooth tongue and sore mouth, pallor and shortness of breath occur.

The blood and marrow changes are identical to those described in megaloblastic anaemia due to $B_{12}$ deficiency.

Diagnosis of folate deficiency as the cause of megaloblastic anaemia depends on: (1) excluding $B_{12}$ deficiency; (2) showing abnormal results for tests for folate deficiency; and on occasion (3) showing a haematological response to treatment with 200 $\mu$g folate daily. Vitamin $B_{12}$ deficiency is excluded by showing that the patient absorbs $B_{12}$ normally, assuming that the patient is not a vegetarian, or has a normal serum $B_{12}$ level. Patients with folate deficiency usually have abnormally low serum folate levels, low red cell folate levels and increased urinary excretion of formimino-glutamic acid after an oral histidine load.

*Nutritional folate deficiency* occurs more often in old people, pregnant women and premature infants. Premature infants may be born with reduced folate stores and receive a poor folate intake from heated and reheated artificial milk feeds. Initial heating of a milk preparation is likely to destroy the ascorbate which preserves reduced folate. Reheating before feeding, in the absence of ascorbate, destroys folate. Recognition of these problems has led to folate supplementation of milk feeds. Such infants show falling serum and red cell folate concentration which may reach very low levels. A small number develop increasingly severe anaemia which does not respond to iron therapy. There is an excellent response to folate therapy (Vanier and Tyas, 1967).

Folate deficiency develops in pregnancy if the daily folate intake does not meet the increased folate need during pregnancy. This increased requirement arises from the increase of the maternal blood volume, and growth of the uterus, placenta and fetus. Not only may a megaloblastic anaemia appear in the mother but folate deficiency can lead to placental insufficiency and to the birth of a small premature infant. Low birth weight infants and prematurity due to folate deficiency are preventable by folate supplements during pregnancy (Baumslag *et al.*, 1970).

When folate deficiency occurs in pregnancy it is usually associated with iron deficiency. Both are basically due to poor nutritional intake. In the UK a usually mild megaloblastic anaemia develops in about 2 per cent of pregnant women. This is recognized in the last weeks of pregnancy or during the puerperium. This anaemia is largely prevented by oral folate supplements throughout pregnancy. In practice a combined iron and folic acid tablet is prescribed to be taken once daily throughout pregnancy.

Old people, because of poverty, lack of interest, or immobility, may take an inadequate folate intake and some 8 per cent of people over the age of 65 in the

UK have abnormally low red cell folate concentrations. Nutritional folate deficiency has been found in those living on a diet of tea and toast, in those with psychiatric disturbances and in those requiring admission to old people's homes. A raised MCV is the most sensitive index of something untoward in the blood and confirmation is sought by a marrow aspiration to demonstrate megaloblastosis. There is a low serum and red cell folate level. Measurement of serum $B_{12}$ level, $B_{12}$ absorption, and if necessary, further tests to ensure that the patient does not have $B_{12}$ deficiency should be carried out, since long-term folate therapy in patients who really have $B_{12}$ deficiency may produce neurological damage.

Nutritional folate deficiency may be associated with alcoholism and scurvy. Alcohol is itself a marrow toxin leading to a normoblastic macrocytosis which is reversible on alcohol withdrawal. In severe alcoholics further changes are found which include abnormal vacuolation of marrow cells, accumulation of iron granules in normoblasts (sideroblasts) and megaloblastic changes. When the changes are due to alcohol alone, folate levels in serum, red cells and liver are normal. In about one-third of alcoholics additional nutritional folate deficiency is present. The subjects are usually spirit rather than beer drinkers and have a very poor dietary energy and protein intake. In these both oral folate as well as alcohol withdrawal are required before the blood returns to normal. A substantial beer intake may supply fair amounts of folate (Wu *et al.*, 1975). The folate activity for *L. casei* of one brand of beer has been estimated to be 136 $\mu$g/kg (Herbert, 1963).

Deficiency of vitamin C and folic acid go hand in hand. They occur in similar foodstuffs, both are labile and ascorbate tends to preserve folate. It is not surprising that most scorbutics are also folate deficient and megaloblastic.

## Protein–energy malnutrition

Uncomplicated protein-energy malnutrition (kwashiorkor) is accompanied by a mild anaemia which is usually normocytic or slightly macrocytic. The marrow may be either of normal cellularity or hypocellular. Haemodilution partly contributes to this reduced haemoglobin level. With protein repletion there is a further initial fall in haemoglobin accompanied by a slow reticulocytosis. There is some evidence that this phase is accompanied by low levels of erythropoietin (Finch, 1975).

However, uncomplicated protein–energy malnutrition is the exception and usually there is evidence of accompanying infection and iron and folate deficiency. Iron deficiency almost invariably appears once recovery is apparent and iron supplements must be given. Occasionally megaloblastosis is present *de novo* but megaloblastosis is not a major factor in cases diagnosed early. However, in South India (Pereira and Baker, 1966), South Africa (Walt *et al.*, 1956), Egypt (Khalil *et al.*, 1973) and Colombia (Velez *et al.*, 1963), megaloblastosis may be present in about one-third of children and is due to folate deficiency. Evidence of these deficiencies may appear after protein repletion and may be accompanied by temporary failure in marrow function.

Associated infection produces a further depression of appetite and increases nitrogen loss (Scrimshaw, 1975) and causes impaired digestion and absorption of protein. The malnutrition causes an increased susceptibility to infection for it has long been recognized that malnutrition is associated with impaired immunocompetence.

## Vitamin K and blood coagulation

Vitamin K is needed for the synthesis of six apparently separate factors needed for normal blood coagulation. These factors are prothrombin (Factor II), Factor VII, Christmas factor (Factor IX), Protein C, Protein S and Stuart–Prower factor (Factor X). All these factors are synthesized in the liver.

Nutritionally, vitamin K occurs as either vitamin $K_1$ (phylloquinone) in vegetable oils and leafy plants, or as vitamin $K_2$ (menaquinones) which is produced by a wide variety of bacteria. Man probably has a dietary requirement for vitamin K. The normal gut flora does produce vitamin K but this is present in the large gut or colon, whereas normal intestinal absorption occurs from the generally sterile small gut. Vitamin K is a fat-soluble vitamin and, like vitamins A and D, its absorption is facilitated by bile salts and this is impaired in malabsorption states and in jaundiced subjects in whom secretion of bile salts into the gut in hindered. Significant body stores of vitamin K have not been demonstrated. Coumarin-type drugs (warfarin, phenindione) inhibit the action of vitamin K in the synthesis of the six coagulation factors.

### Haemorrhagic diseases of the newborn

The six vitamin K-dependent coagulation factors are present at birth in plasma at concentrations of 20–50 per cent of that found in adult life. This is due to immaturity of synthetic pathways in the infant's liver and is unrelated to availability of vitamin K. There is a further fall in the infant's plasma level of vitamin K-dependent factors in the first 2–4 days of life and this secondary fall is preventable by giving vitamin K to either mother or infant. The fall in plasma activity is more pronounced in premature infants.

Haemorrhagic disease of the newborn (HDN) is an exaggeration of this fall in vitamin K-dependent factors and it is due to a deficiency of vitamin K. The initial fall in plasma activity is exaggerated and the recovery is delayed.

Bleeding may be severe beginning on the second or third day of life. It may occur from the umbilical stump, from the gut (melaena), below the scalp (cephalhaematoma), or following a circumcision. There may be generalized bleeding in skin and limbs. Laboratory tests show a prolonged prothrombin time, and usually prolonged cephalin–kaolin time.

Treatment is by injection of 0.5 to 1 mg of vitamin $K_1$. The prothrombin time should be shortened significantly in hours and there should be rapid cessation of bleeding. In severe cases the dose can be repeated 4 hourly for three doses. Fresh plasma will replace the missing factors rapidly and if anaemia is present whole blood may be needed.

Prevention of HDN can be achieved either by giving the newborn 2 mg of vitamin $K_1$ orally or 1 mg by injection, or by giving the mother vitamin K antepartum. Mothers receiving long term anticonvulsant therapy for the treatment of epilepsy are especially liable to have infants with HDN and all infants of these mothers should receive prophylactic vitamin K.

## Nutritional vitamin K deficiency in adults

This may rarely develop in adults with nutritional deficiency who are given a broad-spectrum antibiotic. The latter presumably interferes with intestinal bacterial synthesis of vitamin K. Similarly antibiotics may increase the toxicity of anticoagulant drugs (coumarins) by altering the availability of competitive vitamin K. A dose of 10–20 mg of vitamin $K_1$ orally should reverse the coagulation abnormalities in 24 hours, but if anticoagulants are to be continued, infusion of fresh frozen plasma to supply the missing factors is preferable. Vitamin K renders the subject resistant to coumarin drugs for several weeks.

## References


Baumslag, N., Edelstein, T. and Metz, J. (1970). Reduction of incidence of prematurity by folic acid supplementation in pregnancy. *Br. Med. J.*, **i**, 16–17.

Chanarin, I. and Rothman, D. (1971). Further observations on the relation between iron and folate status in pregnancy. *Br. Med. J.*, **ii**, 81–4.

Finch, C.A. (1975). Erythropoiesis in protein–calorie malnutrition. In *Protein–Calorie Malnutrition*, pp. 247–56. Ed. Olson, R.E. Academic Press: New York.

Herbert, V. (1963). A palatable diet for producing experimental folate deficiency in man. *Am. J. Clin. Nutr.*, **12**, 17–20.

Khalil, M., Tanios, A., Moghazy, M., Aref, M.K., Mahmoud, S. and El Lozy, M. (1973). Serum and red cell folates, and serum vitamin $B_{12}$ in protein–calorie malnutrition. *Archs Dis. Child.*, **48**, 366–9.

Metha, B.M., Rege, D.V. and Satoskar, R.S. (1964). Serum vitamin $B_{12}$ and folic acid activity in lactovegetarian and non-vegetarian healthy adult Indians. *Am. J. Clin. Nutr.*, **15**, 77–84.

Pereira, S.M. and Baker, S.J. (1966). Hematologic studies in kwashiorkor. *Am. J. Clin. Nutr.*, **18**, 413–20.

Scrimshaw, N.S. (1975). Interactions of malnutrition and infection: Advances in understanding. In *Protein–Calorie Malnutrition*, pp. 353–67. Ed. Olson, R.E. Academic Press: New York.

Vanier, T.M. and Tyas, J.F. (1967). Folic acid status in premature infants. *Archs Dis. Child.*, **42**, 57–61.

Velez, H., Ghitis, J., Pradilla, A. and Vitale, J.J. (1963). Cali-Harvard nutrition project. I. Megaloblastic anemia in kwashiorkor. *Am. J. Clin. Nutr.*, **12**, 54–65.

Walt, F., Holman, S. and Hendrickse, R.G. (1956). Megaloblastic anaemia of infancy in kwashiorkor and other diseases. *Br. Med. J.*, **i**, 1199–203.

Wu, A., Chanarin, I., Slavin, G. and Levi, A.J. (1975). Folate deficiency in the alcoholic – its relationship to clinical and haematological abnormalities, liver disease and folate stores. *Br. J. Haemat.*, **29**, 469–78.

# 14 Mineral metabolism

## Trevor C.B. Stamp



## Introduction

Twenty-five of the 96 elements present on earth are indispensable to animal life. The lighter the element the more abundant it is on earth, two-thirds (22) of the 34 lightest elements being also biologically essential. Essential elements fall into three broad overlapping groups according to their general function. The first group comprises major structural elements, H, O, C, N, P and S that provide the basic building units of the organism, amino-acids, sugars, fatty acids and nucleotides. The second group maintains ionic equilibrium, electrochemical functions and membrane potential. This group includes Na, K, Mg, Ca and Cl. The third and most numerous group consists mainly of essential metals, present in trace concentrations, that participate in enzyme systems and specialized transport proteins. The six most important of these are Fe, Cu, Zn, Mn, Mo and Co. Others present in still more minute concentrations include nickel, chromium, selenium, tin and vanadium, the essential nature of some having been demonstrated only in mammals other than man. Of the four non-metals boron appears to be capable of incorporation only into plant structure. Roles for silicon and fluoride have been indicated (see below).

Metal ions participate in nearly one-third of all enzymes (Vallee and Wacker, 1970). These enzymes can be considered in two groups, metalloenzymes and metal ion-activated enzymes. In the former, a specific metal is firmly bound in a fixed molar ratio to specific sites within the molecule and does not dissociate under physiological conditions; its removal destroys all enzyme activity but this may usually be restored by replacing the original metal. The metal ion-activated enzymes show only loose binding to the metal, other ions may sometimes substitute, the enzyme may show certain activity in the absence of the metal, and full activity is always restored by its replacement. The ubiquitous alkaline earths, calcium, magnesium, sodium and potassium are also involved in many active metal-enzyme complexes. Sodium and potassium fall outside the scope of mineral metabolism, leaving calcium, phosphorus and magnesium pre-eminent.

Calcium occupies a unique position in terms of its functional significance, considered below. The need to regulate skeletal homeostasis and to maintain precise extracellular calcium homeostasis in the body fluids that bathe this vast skeletal reservoir has 'evolved' a complex set of control mechanisms including the vitamin D-endocrine and parathyroid systems, calcitonin, and phosphate itself. They appear to influence magnesium as well although the influences are less well understood. Experimentally, the non-essential alkaline earths strontium and barium may also compete with calcium in parts of the vitamin D and parathyroid systems.

The present chapter is concerned with the physiological importance of minerals and their concentrations in the human body, origins in food, daily intakes and requirements, mechanisms of absorption, excretion and internal homeostasis, their inter-relationships and the acquired and hereditary diseases associated with deficiency or excess.

## Evolutionary aspects of mineral metabolism

Mineral metabolism becomes a little clearer if its evolutionary course over a thousand million years is considered. Among much conjecture certain probabilities of natural selection have been established (Prosser and Brown, 1961). The earth's early atmosphere was rich in hydrogen, methane and ammonium and poor in oxygen. Pre-Cambrian seas where life first evolved were rich in potassium and magnesium. The earliest organic molecules and sub-cellular organelles thus developed and reproduced in this medium. As time passed and cells developed, concentrations of magnesium and potassium fell while the seas became richer in calcium and sodium. Evolving cellular forms, adapted to their internal environment of magnesium and potassium, developed membrane pumps to maintain it. But as multicellular organisms slowly developed tissues their extracellular fluid cations came to consist predominantly of sodium and calcium. Respiration was at first anaerobic, as is the tricarboxylic acid cycle, and was thus catalysed by enzymes activated mainly by magnesium ions, and membrane potential being maintained partly through magnesium-dependent adenosine triphosphatase. One evolutionary aspect of trace-metal metabolism is the similar trace concentrations of these metals in the oceans, $10^{-5}$ or $10^{-6}$, to that of the alkaline earths (Frieden, 1973). Their physiological significance partly consists of the stronger chelates they tend to form with proteins, and in the value of the resulting complexes to the organism. Increasing amounts of oxygen in the earth's atmosphere, producing hydrogen peroxide and the superoxide ion, would have been toxic to primitive life-forms. The particular oxygen-combining properties of iron and copper, with their primitive protein ligands, would at first have protected these organisms. But as adaptation to aerobic respiration evolved so did the value of iron and copper as essential metal-enzyme complexes in the link between molecular oxygen and electron transport. It has been suggested that if any one enzyme could be described as the most vital in biochemistry it might be cytochrome c oxidase, containing one atom of iron and one of copper in each molecule, which stands at the end of the electron transport chain (Frieden, 1973).

Two further evolutionary events require brief consideration, the development of a calcified endoskeleton and migration of life to the land. The variable supply of vital calcium ions in both aquatic and terrestrial environments would certainly have made a reservoir, within the bony skeleton, advantageous. Our polypeptide hormones have been conserved from evolutionary antiquity. Calcitonin is present in bacteria and its earliest functions may have concerned osmotic regulation in sea- and fresh-water as well as calcium homeostasis (Orimo *et al.*, 1972; Copp, 1972). While phosphorus is virtually a trace element in oceans and large fresh-water lakes it is abundant in a terrestrial existence. Fishes in their calcium-containing environment do not possess parathyroid glands and the development of these glands in amphibians was a further evolutionary stage, providing for precise homeostasis of plasma calcium and phosphorus.

## Calcium

It is perhaps not surprising, considering the hundreds of millions of years of evolution in a calcium-rich environment, that so much structure and function is mediated by this element. The skeleton is founded on a 'rock' of calcium and phosphorus in the solid state; amorphous calcium phosphates and carbonate account for up to 40 per cent of the total and a highly organized crystal lattice of hydroxyapatite with an overall formula of $Ca_{10}(PO_4)_6(OH)_2$, comprises the remainder (Vaughan, 1975). Solid calcium gives strength to the teeth, and is deposited as carbonate in the otolith organ for maintenance of equilibrium. Calcification is controlled to a large part by the local concentration of ionic calcium in the specialized bone-extracellular fluid (ECF), which is lower than in general ECF (Neuman and Ramp, 1971). Ionized calcium controls electrical transmission throughout the nervous system and at neuromuscular junctions; it preserves membrane potential and muscle contractility. It is important in transmission of hormonal activity too: most, if not all, hormones that express their activity through the second messenger, cyclic adenosine monophosphate (cyclic AMP) require calcium ions for this process; examples include the actions of releasing factors for growth hormone and thyrotrophin in the anterior pituitary cells, TSH on the thyroid, LH on the corpus luteum, parathyroid hormone, histamine, adrenalin on other organs, and many other effects of hormonal as well as other specific stimuli (Rasmussen, 1972). A host of enzymes are activated by calcium ions and even more are inhibited (Dixon and Webb, 1964). Blood clotting is dependent on calcium ions including both activation of Factor VIII and conversion of prothrombin to thrombin. Finally many antigen-antibody reactions are calcium-dependent (Liberti *et al.*, 1973).

The adult human body contains approximately 1 kg calcium (25 000 mmol) of which nearly 99 per cent is in the skeleton (Fig. 14.1). The new-born skeleton contains only 30 g of calcium and imposes a trivial burden on maternal stores. For comparison, the skeleton also contains 88 per cent of the body's total phosphorus, 80 per cent of its carbonate, over 60 per cent of its magnesium and 35 per cent of its sodium. Many of the essential elements are also present in trace concentrations.

Plasma contains calcium in three main forms, ionized, protein-bound and complexed as citrate, phosphate and proteinate. The ionized form, approximately 46–48 per cent of the total under normal conditions (Walser, 1961; Lingärde, 1972) is the only clinically important fraction for reasons which have been discussed. Nearly half the overall total is bound to protein (approximately 46 per cent; Walser, 1961), nearly 90 per cent to albumin

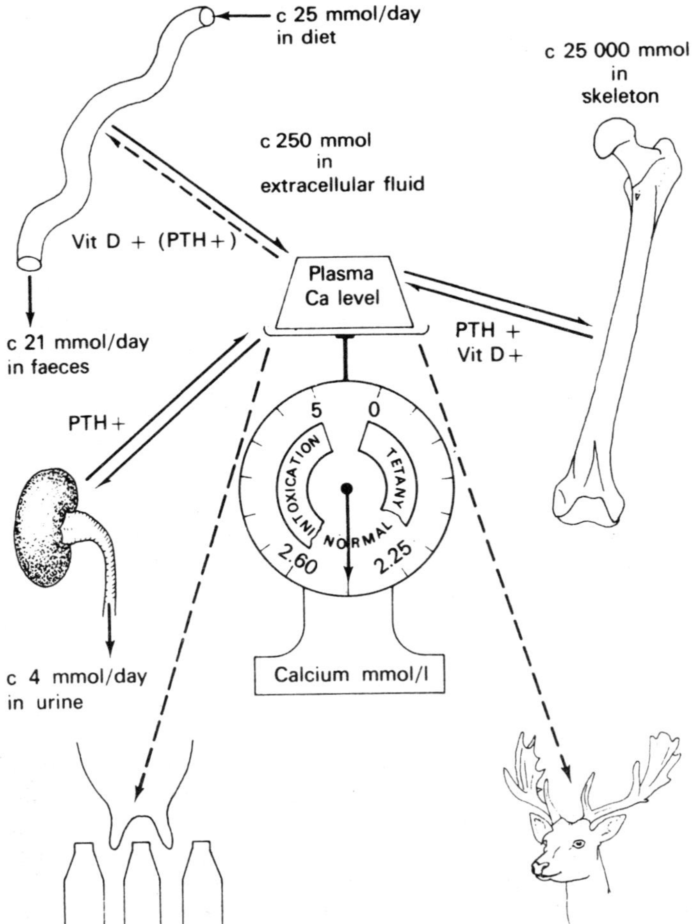


Fig. 14.1 Simplified scheme of extracellular calcium transport and homeostasis.

(Lingärde, 1973). The degree of binding is sensitive to pH and changes in the same direction, acidosis reducing the protein-bound fraction. The small proportion of complexed calcium is diffusible calcium citrate and undiffusible proteinate. Measurement of total plasma calcium is only important as an index of ionized calcium which is much harder to determine accurately. Correction factors for protein binding have increased the accuracy with which total calcium reflects ionized calcium concentration. Simultaneous measurement of plasma albumin allows adjustment of measured total calcium to a 'corrected' level. For higher values than 40–41 g/litre for albumin (each laboratory should ideally set its normal values and correction factors) a standard equivalent for calcium is subtracted, and for lower values a strict proportion of calcium is added (Dent, 1962; Peacock and Nordin, 1973; Berry *et al.*, 1973): a typical correction factor is 0.1 mmol/litre calcium for 6 g/litre albumin below or above 41 g/litre with intermediate values corrected proportionally. This simple correction allows for influences on total plasma calcium which would otherwise confuse diagnosis and treatment including haemo-concentration and dilution which varies with upright and recumbent posture and with venous stasis during blood sampling, and pathological deficiency in plasma albumin. There may be a small rise in plasma calcium after meals and a diurnal variation has also been noted with lowest levels being found at night (Peacock and Nordin, 1973).

The normal range for corrected plasma calcium is approximately 2.25–2.6 mmol/litre, depending on the analytical method. Normal corrected calcium in the fasting state lies within a range of 0.35 mmol/litre (Davies *et al.*, 1971; Purnell *et al.*, 1971).

Dairy products are the richest dietary source of calcium except for butter. Cows' milk contains up to 30 mmol/litre, nearly four times the calcium content in human milk. Hard cheese is also an excellent source but creamed cheese is much poorer. Eggs are a fair source (over 1.25 mmol/100 g), and certain green leafy vegetables such as cabbage and spinach make a more meagre contribution. The calcium content of hard water is 2.5–3.5 mmol/litre. In Britain flour is fortified with calcium carbonate although EEC regulations threaten discontinuation and bread is therefore, at present, still a good source of calcium. Meat contains little (McCance and Widdowson, 1943).

Daily calcium intakes in Britain may vary widely round a mean of 20–25 mmol. In the adult in calcium equilibrium approximately one-fifth of dietary calcium is absorbed and four-fifths are excreted in faeces (Fig. 14.1). As intake increases above 12 mmol/day there is a small progressive increase in net absorption by passive diffusion although its proportion to dietary intake declines, thus providing an increasingly effective intestinal barrier to absorption at high levels of intake. At very low levels of intake the proportion of net absorption to intake appears to decline owing to obligatory faecal loss from endogenous secretion into the gut of about 4 mmol/day: at intakes below 5–7.5 mmol/day faecal calcium may exceed intake (Brine and Johnston, 1955; Stanbury, 1976). Pooling of metabolic balance data obtained during the 1930s and 1940s showed that apparent calcium equilibrium in the adult was achieved by mean intake of 10 mg/kg/day (Irving, 1973). Distinction may be drawn between recommended minimal adult requirement, which is the mean intake required to preserve mean balance (set at 10 mmol/day: FAO/WHO,

1962), and recommended allowance which is the intake which will preserve balance in 95 per cent of the population; the latter was set at 12.5 mmol in the UK in 1969 and 20 mmol in the USA in 1974 but calculation from more recent extensive data suggests this figure might be as high as 22.5 mmol/day (Nordin *et al.*, 1979; Parfitt, 1983). Extensive longitudinal studies have been published in the past 10 years concerning prevention of age-related fractures and osteoporosis by calcium supplementation. Estimates of age-related bone loss, calcium balance, height loss and vertebral fracture rate suggest that calcium intakes of the order of 1.5 g (37.5 mmol) daily, achieved by supplementation if necessary, may protect against osteoporosis particularly in post-menopausal females (for reviews see Nordin *et al.*, 1979; Parfitt, 1983; Nagant de Deuxchaisnes, 1983). The degree of protection may be a minor one and plenty of studies have not achieved statistical significance. But osteoporosis is a problem on a national scale and every opportunity of benefit, however small, particularly if it is also cheap and harmless, is welcome. Studies have not distinguished between various forms of calcium supplementation and microcrystalline hydroxyapatite compound, soluble calcium preparations and even calcium carbonate have all been reported effective (see below).

Calcium requirements are different during growth and maternal lactation. Children retain about 5 mmol calcium daily, with maximum positive calcium balances of 8–9 mmol daily during the puberty growth spurt. Similar values can be calculated from data on total body calcium at different ages (Irving, 1973). There is one report of osteoporosis in childhood resulting from a self-chosen diet containing less than 5 mmol calcium daily, the disease being cured when the child was persuaded to increase his calcium intake (Dent, 1973). Recommendations for childhood calcium intake may be simply made by adding these values of 5–9 mmol/day for calcium retention to the adult recommendation of 10 mmol/day.

The full-term fetus contains 750 mmol calcium which could be supplied with little risk entirely by the maternal skeleton. Much more calcium is lost during lactation, however, on average 10 mmol daily over 6 months. Fortunately intestinal calcium absorption is increased during pregnancy and lactation so maternal dietary sources normally provide all the infant's calcium. Clearly maternal calcium requirements become significant during lactation. A figure for this requirement may be arrived at by adding these 10 mmol from daily lactation to the rather arbitrary 10 mmol/day suggested for healthy adults although a value in excess of this has been given (FAO/WHO, 1962).

Healthy adults in calcium equilibrium excrete calcium in the urine equivalent to their net calcium absorption, the normal range in males being approximately 5–7.5 mmol/24 hours and in females 4–6 mmol/24 hours (Fig. 14.1). Much lower urine calcium is seen in the adolescent growth spurt. Finally, calcium may be lost through the skin in sweat in amounts which can vary between 0.5–9 mmol per day (Isaksson *et al.*, 1967; Carr *et al.*, 1973). Regulation of calcium and phosphorus metabolism is discussed below.

## Phosphorus

The body contains about 26 000 mmol phosphorus as organic and inorganic phosphate of which 88 per cent is concentrated in the skeleton. Organic phosphates are present in every large structural molecule. Inorganic phosphate provides a major buffer system in the regulation of acid-base balance particularly by its renal excretion, shares in skeletal structure and helps to control mineralization; it regulates calcium directly both outside and within the cell, helps to control other aspects of cell function and it is subject, directly or indirectly, to similar endocrine influences.

Plasma inorganic phosphate is present in a number of ionized, protein-bound and complexed forms. The ionized forms are free $HPO_4^{2-}$, $NaHPO_4^-$ and $H_2PO_4^{2-}$ in that order of magnitude and comprise 82 per cent of the total (Walser, 1961). Only 12 per cent is protein-bound and the remainder is complexed with calcium and magnesium. Total plasma phoshporus levels show a wider variation than calcium but are still subject to homeostatic control. Levels rise after ingestion of dietary phosphate and fall during the night or after ingestion of carbohydrate; phosphorus levels are plainly less responsive to protein changes than those of calcium. Normal fasting plasma phosphorus levels range from 0.80–1.45 mmol/litre in adults but the range is appreciably higher in childhood and adolescence.

Dietary phosphorus deficiency is virtually impossible for humans to sustain except in experimental conditions. The intestine absorbs two-thirds to three-quarters of the normal dietary intake of 25–45 mmol by mechanisms that are less precisely controlled than those for calcium. A large amount of phosphate is thus available for urinary combination with hydrogen ion and excretion as 'titratable acid'. The effects of dietary calcium and phosphorus on mutual intestinal absorption were once controversial. While calcium may be absorbed in the absence of phosphorus, there is evidence that optimal calcium absorption requires its presence (Clark, 1969; Omdahl and De Luca, 1973). While excess calcium salts may inhibit phosphate absorption it is no longer accepted that excess inorganic phosphate may inhibit net calcium absorption by precipitating insoluble calcium phosphate in the gut (Albright and Reifenstein, 1948; Stamp, 1972; Stanbury, 1976; and see Parfitt 1983 for review). Absorbable phosphate food additives do not appear relevant to human nutrition: the Ca/P ratio of 'Western' diets is in any case higher than that in the developing world. Only when phosphate is complexed either as phytate (inositol hexaphosphate) in flours or as cellulose phosphate (e.g. in treatment of idiopathic hypercalciuria) can it bind calcium in the gut. There is no clear evidence that excess dietary phytate contributes to human illness either.

## Regulation of calcium and phosphorus

Calcium and phosphorus homeostasis is maintained by the vitamin D-endocrine system, parathyroid hormone (PTH), calcitonin (to a still-uncertain degree) and calcium and phosphate ions themselves.

Parathyroid hormone is a polypeptide containing 84 amino acid residues; it is synthesized in the parathyroid cell as an appreciably larger peptide, this initial product representing all the structural information encoded in the gene for PTH (Habener and Jacobs, 1982). PTH is secreted by the parathyroid glands at an inversely proportional rate to the level of plasma calcium (Mayer, 1975). All the calcium effects of PTH tend to raise the plasma calcium level:

PTH thus stimulates renal tubular calcium reabsorption, a major influence on plasma calcium. It mobilizes bone calcium by direct stimulation of osteoclasts and it enhances intestinal calcium absorption in man (Stanbury, 1976) by day-to-day control of 1,25-dihydroxyvitamin D synthesis in kidney (see below). PTH inhibits renal tubular phosphate reabsorption and thus lowers plasma phosphorus. Within the cell it exerts its effect via the second messenger cyclic AMP following activation of the magnesium-dependent adenyl cyclase system. The first detectable event in its action on bone cells is an increase in calcium uptake which is rapidly followed by release of calcium from bone into the ECF. It then begins to stimulate new osteoclast formation and bone turnover increases owing to a secondary rise in osteoblastic activity. Attempts to demonstrate a primary anabolic effect of synthetic human N 1–34 PTH in man (Reeve *et al.*, 1976) have failed to show any net gain in skeletal mineral.

Vitamin D exists in two forms, the natural (animal) vitamin cholecalciferol (vitamin $D_3$) and the synthetic vitamin ergocalciferol (vitamin $D_2$). Both are ultraviolet irradiation products of respective precursor sterols. The animal precursor 7-dehydrocholesterol is synthesized in liver, stored in the deeper layers of the epidermis and converted by solar ultraviolet and body heat to cholecalciferol. Ergosterol is synthesized by certain yeasts and its irradiation yields vitamin $D_2$. Vitamin $D_1$ was described many years ago and was later discovered to be merely a mixture of antiricketic sterols so the term has been discarded.

Unlike certain experimental animals such as the rat, man is utterly dependent on vitamin D for active intestinal calcium absorption and calcification of cartilage and bone matrix (osteoid); its deficiency produces the classical disease of rickets in childhood and osteomalacia in adults. Vitamin D may also be ingested in the diet but unless food is fortified artificially only oily fish (sardines, herring, mackerel, salmon, tuna) contain enough to compensate for sunshine deprivation. Only in the last decade has this relatively trivial contribution of dietary sources been appreciated and all published recommendations regarding vitamin D intake have thus been concerned with apparent dietary requirement. Traditionally established international units (IU) of vitamin D are a measure of the power of an administered test substance to cure experimental rickets by cumbersome bioassay in rats. Pure vitamin $D_2$ or $D_3$ contains 40 000 IU per mg (1 IU is therefore 0.025 $\mu$g). Dietary 'requirements' were said to be 400 IU daily for infants and children and 100 IU daily for adults (Yendt, 1970; FAO/WHO, 1970). In addition to oily fish and the liver oils of certain white fish (cod, halibut) eggs provide a reasonable source, but milk with only 2–7 IU per pint (varying in amount from winter to summer) and other dairy products are clearly rather poor sources and meat is poorer still. Fortified products include baby foods, margarine, some commercial yogurts, beverages and breakfast cereals. In the USA and most of Canada, milk is fortified to the extent of 10 $\mu$g per quart. The (more recent) Canadian experiment abolished a problem of rickets in Quebec (C.R. Scriver, personal communication).

Vitamin D has no direct action on its target organs but requires successive hydroxylations first in liver to produce 25-hydroxyvitamin D (25-OHD) and second in kidney to produce 1,25-dihydroxyvitamin D (De Luca, 1979; Norman and Ross, 1979; Fraser, 1980; see Fig. 14.2). 25-OHD is the major

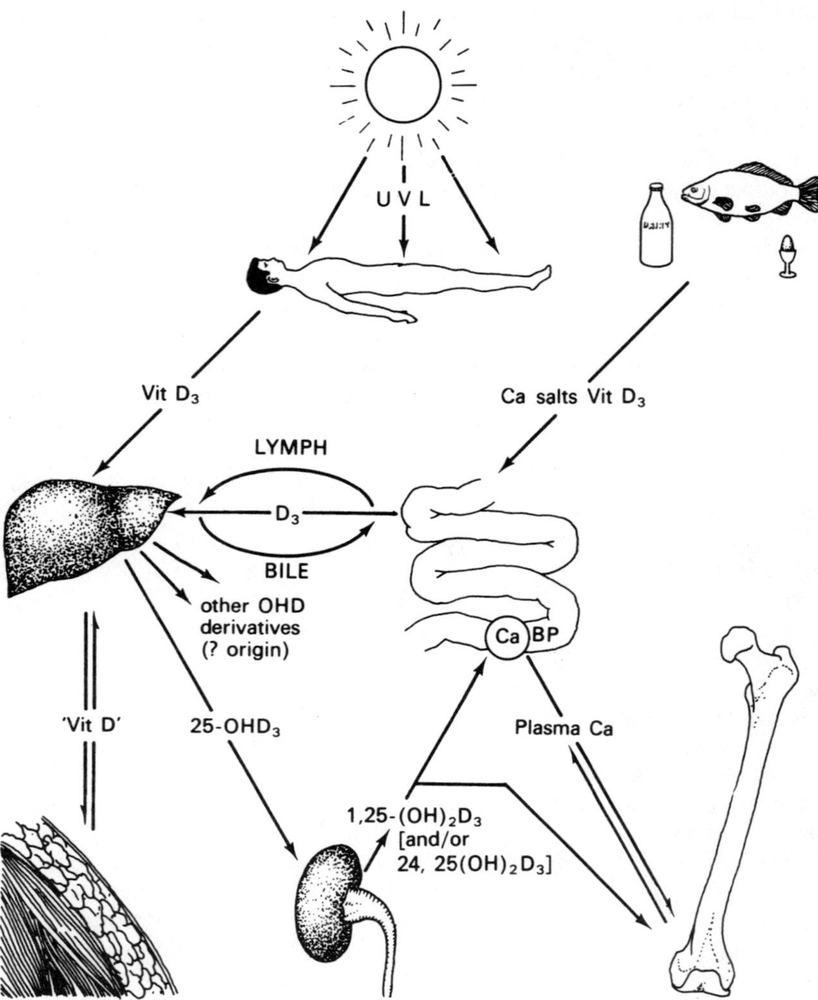


Fig. 14.2 Vitamin D metabolism; nutrition, transport and function (see text for further explanation). UVL, ultraviolet light; $25\text{-}OHD_3$, 25-hydroxycholecalciferol; $1{,}25(OH)_2D_3$, 1,25-dihydroxycholecalciferol; $24{,}25(OH)_2D_3$, 24,25-dihydroxycholecalciferol; CaBP, calcium-binding protein.

circulating form of the vitamin and shows a marked seasonal variation in Britain in both white subjects and Asians indicating the importance of summer sunshine as the major determinant of vitamin D nutrition (Stamp and Round, 1974). Mean levels in healthy white subjects are approximately 32 nmol/litre in early spring and 55 nmol/litre in late summer and early autumn but levels vary widely. In the United Kingdom deficiency occurs in the Asian community among the elderly and in the institutionalized. But rickets occurs in all societies where adults and children are screened from sunlight including desert Bedouin tribeswomen in their goatskin tents. Skin pigmentation with melanin is at worst only a minor hindrance to endogenous vitamin D synthesis (Stamp, 1975). Comparison of circulating 25-OHD levels in subjects receiving intensive solar or artificial ultraviolet irradiation with levels in patients receiving oral vitamin D suggests that maximum endogenous vitamin D synthesis may reach 8000–10 000 i.u. daily (Stamp *et al.*, 1977).

The true hormonal form of vitamin D, 1,25-dihydroxyvitamin D ($1,25(OH)_2D$, calcitriol) is normally synthesized only in renal tubules (De Luca, 1979; Norman and Ross, 1979; Fraser, 1980). It is potent in concentrations as low as $10^{-10}$M and its level in normal human plasma is approximately 0.14 nmol/litre (Haussler and McCain, 1977). A second compound, 24,25-dihydroxyvitamin D ($24,25(OH)_2D$), is synthesized in kidney in inverse proportion to the active form and circulates in higher concentrations. Its possible function in humans, if any, remains uncertain. $1,25(OH)_2D$ synthesis is stimulated experimentally by low calcium diets (Boyle *et al.*, 1971), by parathyroid hormone (Fraser and Kodicek, 1971) and by low phosphorus levels within renal cortex (Tanaka and De Luca, 1973); other possible regulatory mechanisms include the concentration of $Ca^{++}$ at some intracellular site and the concentration of $1,25(OH)_2D$ itself (MacIntyre *et al.*, 1975). The adaptation to low calcium diets may be explained by stimulation of $1,25(OH)_2D$ synthesis.

In intestinal mucosa $1,25(OH)_2D$ combines initially with a cytosol receptor protein and then localizes in nuclear chromatin where, in the manner of a true steroid hormone, it regulates DNA transcription, formation of messenger RNA and the eventual synthesis of calcium-binding protein. However, $1,25(OH)_2D$ enhances calcium transport in advance of calcium-binding protein synthesis (Wasserman *et al.*, 1974), suggesting that other as yet uncertain mechanisms may be important.

$1,25(OH)_2D$ promotes bone resorption directly, an apparently paradoxical situation since the hormone is required for adequate calcification of cartilage and osteoid. However, if normal concentrations of calcium and phosphorus are delivered to bone experimentally in the absence of vitamin D, or if calcification is promoted in human osteomalacia by treatment with phosphate alone, the resulting pattern of calcification is abnormal: it is randomly distributed instead of forming an organized calcification front which is required for normal construction of lamellar bone (Rasmussen and Bordier, 1974). Thus vitamin D functions in some way to order the correct pattern of calcification.

Calcitonin, a hormone produced in man by the C-cells of the thyroid gland (Copp, 1972) has uncertain relevance to human metabolism. It inhibits bone resorption by inhibiting osteoclastic activity and PTH-induced osteoclast proliferation. Calcitonin levels rise during pregnancy and lactation, fall after the menopause and are elevated by oestrogen therapy in post-menopausal females. These findings have suggested to some a protective effect against calcium loss from the female skeleton (MacIntyre *et al.*, 1980).

## Disorders of calcium homeostasis

The main forms of disturbed calcium metabolism are illustrated in Fig. 14.3. Full accounts are available in reference works on metabolic bone disease (see

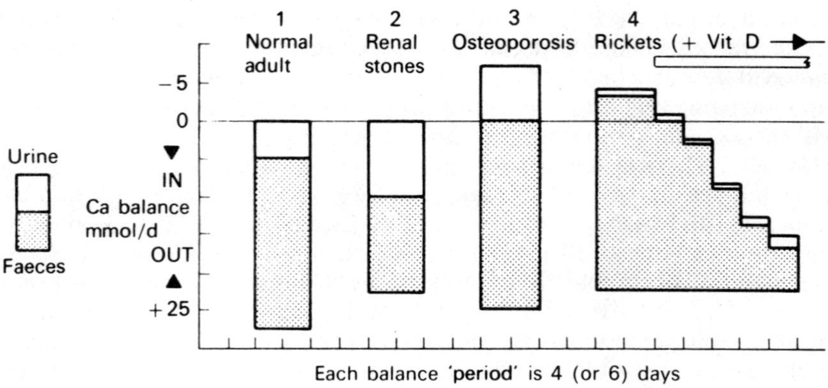


**Fig. 14.3** Patterns of normal and abnormal calcium metabolism. Data are plotted in the classical manner (Albright and Reifenstein, 1948): intake is plotted downwards, as an area, from the zero line, faecal excretion is added upwards from the intake line, urine excretion is added above faecal excretion, and the resulting difference from the zero line represents either positive balance (below the zero line), negative balance (above the zero line), or calcium equilibrium. A healthy child is normally in positive balance. 1. Healthy adult showing approximately four-fifths of the calcium intake excreted in the faeces; 2. a patient with renal stones showing as much as half the dietary calcium absorbed and excreted in the urine; 3. a patient with active osteoporosis showing that skeletal calcium is lost both in the faeces (faecal calcium approximates intake), and in the urine (mild hypercalciuria is evident); 4. a patient with rickets: faecal calcium exceeds (or approximates) intake but urine calcium is low (usually). Note the steady decrease in faecal calcium during effective vitamin D therapy, resulting in progressively positive calcium balance: urine calcium may remain low during much of the healing phase.

Avioli and Krane, 1977, 1978; Avioli and Raisz, 1980; Parsons, 1982). Certain disorders warrant further present discussion in relation to nutrition.

In addition to classicial rickets and osteomalacia from dietary or ultraviolet deprivation there are over 40 forms of metabolic rickets which need to be carefully differentiated for optimum therapy (Stamp, 1982). The curative dose of vitamin D may be up to 1000 times that required for the nutritional form. Figure 14.2 shows all the functional sites at which disturbance may give rise to metabolic rickets. Most malabsorption syndromes arising from small-intestinal disease may produce malabsorption of vitamin D. Osteomalacia following partial gastrectomy may be due to avoidance of fatty foods which contain the vitamin; self-chosen diets may thus be deficient in vitamin D and the disease may respond to physiological supplements of the vitamin (Morgan *et al.*, 1965; Morgan *et al.*, 1970). A small minority of 'food-faddists' may develop similar disease (Dent and Smith, 1969). Bile salts appear necessary for vitamin D absorption so biliary disease may produce a deficiency which can be cured by *parenteral* administration of physiological amounts of vitamin D (Dent and Stamp, 1970a). A special form of ultimate vitamin D deficiency may occur among epileptic patients receiving long-term high-dosage anti-convulsant therapy, despite an apparently adequate vitamin D intake. The rickets or osteomalacia may be related to the effect of anticonvulsant drugs which induce microsomal liver enzymes: enhanced enzyme activity may vicariously divert vitamin D from its normal functional pathway but the disease may also be multifactorial (Stamp *et al.*, 1978).

Phosphate depletion alone may rarely produce osteomalacia in humans as a result of ingesting large quantities of non-absorbable alkali (e.g. aluminium hydroxide) which bind phosphate in the gut and produce hypophosphataemia. Phosphate binders may be given to patients with chronic renal failure and phosphate retention in order to lessen the dangers of ectopic calcification and hyperparathyroid bone disease: hypophosphataemic osteomalacia has been reported in this situated (Baker *et al.*, 1974). Self-medication with enormous doses of antacids among patients with long-standing dyspepsia has also produced hypophosphataemic osteomalacia (Lotz *et al.*, 1964; Dent and Winter, 1974); this form of osteomalacia is uniquely associated with marked hypercalciuria, presumably from increased production of $1{,}25(OH)_2D$ stimulated by hypophosphataemia. Phosphate depletion by aluminium hydroxide gel ('Aludrox') may be attempted for ectopic calcification in diseases other than chronic renal failure such as calcinosis circumscripta and calcinosis universalis (Nassim and Connolly, 1970).

Aluminium is toxic, however. It is absorbed from the gastrointestinal tract and is also present in tap-water. A particular danger has recently become apparent in patients with chronic renal failure using tap-water for chronic haemodialysis and oral phosphate-binders (Wills and Savory, 1983). Features of aluminium toxicity include dialysis encephalopathy with convulsions and dementia. Aluminium deposition in bone produces vitamin D-resistant osteomalacia as a separate event from hypophosphataemia by direct interference with calcification in osteoid. Excess aluminium may also be a factor in both the anaemia and the vascular calcification of chronic renal failure.

In the short term, aluminium hydroxide has had other uses. Following surgical removal of a parathyroid tumour which has produced bone disease (osteitis fibrosa) a 'hungry bones' stage of rapid recalcification produces severe hypocalcaemia (Albright and Reifenstein, 1948) with possible convulsions and consequent pathological fracture. It may not readily respond to high doses of calcitriol or dihydrotachysterol (DHT, AT 10) despite oral or parenteral calcium supplements. In this situation Aludrox reduces available phosphate for calcification, lowers the extreme positive calcium balances and lessens the severity of hypocalcaemia until the clinical situation has stabilized (Dent, 1962; Stamp, 1972). In all these situations it may be given in a dose of 40 ml three or four times daily simultaneously with all meals (that is, at all times of phosphate ingestion).

The central role of the kidney in vitamin D metabolism has clarified the problem of renal rickets. Renal tubular disease may be hereditary or acquired. The large number of hereditary diseases ranges from cystinosis, where rickets is associated with a progressive severe destruction of all renal tubular function and ultimate glomerular failure as well, to X-linked hypophosphataemic rickets where a life-long renal tubular 'leak' of phosphate is the only detectable abnormality of renal function. Acquired disorders include obstructive uropathies, heavy metal poisoning, and the rare adult-presenting form of primary hypophosphataemia. Rickets and osteomalacia result either from loss of 1,25$(OH)_2$D production, or from the phosphate drain or from both. Phosphate supplements have been used by some in addition to vitamin D in X-linked hypophosphataemia and appear essential in the adult-presenting disease. Sodium, potassium and bicarbonate supplements may also be required depending on the nature of the disease.

Phosphate administration may also be useful in the treatment of hypercalcaemia, particularly in inoperable hyperparathyroidism and certain types of malignant disease. Its hypocalcaemic effect has been known for many years: metastatic precipitation of calcium phosphate is a risk, but phosphate is nevertheless valuable in carefully chosen situations (Lancet, 1972). Infants are particularly sensitive to the hypocalcaemic effect of phosphate. Cows' milk contains much more phosphorus than human milk, and certain synthetic infant foods may be rich in phosphorus, a significant cause of neonatal hypocalcaemic tetany.

The major importance of adequate calcium intake for growth and maternal lactation is discussed above. Calcium supplementation is also sensible during the early healing stages of severe rickets and osteomalacia, during the post-operative stage of parathyroidectomy and in the long-term treatment of hypoparathyroidism. Hypoparathyroidism is better managed, however, by vitamin D or one of its more potent and quick-acting derivatives.

The problem of calcium supplementation in osteoporosis and age-related fractures is considered above. Slow loss of bone mineral after the approximate age of 40 is almost universal. In some patients, however, this loss may accelerate and produce the syndrome of osteoporosis with pathological fractures, particularly of lumbar and thoracic vertebrae, and associated height loss. A large number of unrelated diseases are also associated with osteoporosis including cortico-steroid excess whether from treatment or Cushing's disease, alcoholism, rheumatoid arthritis and other, sero-negative, arthritides, hypopituitarism or primary hypogonadism, intestinal malabsorption syndromes (particularly chronic liver disease) and immobilization. Major reviews of pathogenesis and treatment in all these forms are available (Barzel, 1979; De Luca *et al.*, 1981; Dixon *et al.*, 1983). Among many other aspects of calcium metabolism which change with age, net intestinal calcium absorption decreases (Bullamore *et al.*, 1970) – that is, a relatively higher proportion of dietary calcium is excreted in the stools. However, faecal calcium may be raised (i.e. there is 'calcium malabsorption') in most if not all forms of skeletal rarefaction including acute idiopathic disease in children or young adults, cortico-steroid therapy, immobilization, rickets and osteomalacia, or neoplastic bone resorption (Lancet, 1976a). One must therefore guard against uncritical acceptance of 'calcium malabsorption' as such as a primary cause of rarefaction in involutional and post-menopausal osteoporosis. Certain neoplastic diseases, particularly myelomatosis and some lymphomas, may produce clinical syndromes mimicking osteoporosis and require careful differential diagnosis. All secondary forms of osteoporosis should be sought since in some the primary cause may be amenable to treatment. In post-menopausal osteoporosis good longitudinal studies have recently provided evidence for skeletal benefits from exercise, cyclical oestrogen replacement, and treatment with sodium fluoride provided that high calcium supplementation is assured (Barzel, 1979; De Luca *et al.*, 1981; Riggs *et al.*, 1982; Dixon *et al.*, 1983).

**Renal stone formation**

Attention to clinical nutrition, with mineral restriction or supplementation, is important in the management of many patients who suffer recurrent renal stones. Over 90 per cent of renal stones are composed mainly of calcium oxalate and over 90 per cent of these result from the condition of idiopathic hypercalciuria. Ninety per cent of these patients are male. The diagnosis should not imply a strict upper normal limit for urinary calcium since many healthy males excrete over 7.5 mmol/24 h. About 5 per cent of calcium stone formers, most commonly females, suffer from primary parathyroid disease and rarer causes include medullary sponge kidney, renal tubular acidosis and primary and secondary hyperoxaluria. The majority of patients who develop a calcium oxalate stone will probably never get another one but recurrent stone-formers require variably stringent control. Some limitation of calcium intake is indicated and can usually be directed at avoiding milk and hard cheese. Hard water, as in the London area, may be a problem (some mineral waters such as Perrier contain even more calcium) but only severe cases need be advised to boil water first to reduce its calcium content. Calcium restriction for intestinal calcium overabsorption does not seem to put the skeleton at risk in Britain. Sodium loading increases serum $1,25(OH)_2D$ and urine calcium and may be an additional risk factor in idiopathic hypercalciuria (Silver *et al.*, 1983). Only one-third of urinary oxalate is derived from diet and perhaps only regular consumption of high-oxalate foods, particularly all forms of nuts, needs to be discouraged unless they are also good sources of calcium such as spinach, broccoli and milk chocolate. Additional mainstays of treatment include orthophosphate supplements and thiazide derivatives (Pak, 1980). Magnesium (see below) solubilizes calcium salts and magnesium supplements have proved beneficial in primary hyperoxaluria (Dent and Stamp, 1970b). Calcium stone formation in hyperoxaluria is also reduced by pyridoxine (Watts *et al.*, 1979). All these measures may rarely deserve trial in other forms of intractable calcium oxalate lithiasis. Accurate diagnosis is of prime importance, however, since alkalinizing therapy is the only successful treatment for renal tubular acidosis and may be required along with other measures for unrelated problems of cystine or uric acid stone formation. The role of urinary infection is outside the scope of present discussion.

**Other considerations**

Certain rare inborn errors of metabolism have been treated by calcium restriction. These include idiopathic hypercalcaemia of infancy where there is hypersensitivity to vitamin D analogous to hypercalcaemic sarcoidosis in adults, the severe autosomal recessive form of 'marble-bones' disease where calcium restriction has until recently offered the only hope for developing a marrow cavity adequate for haemopoiesis, and progressive diaphyseal dysplasia (Engelmann's disease) in which bone pain associated with progressive overgrowth has been relieved by dietary calcium restriction.

Calcium and skeletal homeostasis are understandably influenced by other minerals. Magnesium shares a common control mechanism in the parathyroid gland and is required to maintain plasma calcium. Non-essential alkaline earths compete experimentally with parathyroid regulation and for calcium-binding protein. Strontium inhibits 1,25$(OH)_2$D synthesis and produces experimental rickets. Copper is required for normal synthesis of skeletal collagen. Fluoride may guard against osteoporosis as well as against dental caries. Manganese may be important for mucopolysaccharide synthesis. These properties are considered below.

## Magnesium

Magnesium is the fourth most abundant cation in the body; adults contain about 1200 mmol of the element, one half to two-thirds in the skeleton. Magnesium is not incorporated into the crystal lattice of hydroxyapatite nor does it probably penetrate into the crystal surface but remains in the hydration shell (Vaughan, 1975). Nevertheless only 2 per cent of bone magnesium is 'exchangeable'. Although total body magnesium is less than one twentieth that of calcium, outside the skeleton their molar ratios are quite similar. As considered above calcium is mainly extracellular, while magnesium is mainly intracellular, the distribution of these elements being analogous to sodium and potassium.

Just as calcium, but not magnesium, is responsible for the structural integrity of the cell membrane, so magnesium but not calcium is responsible for structural integrity of the mitochondrial membrane. Magnesium ions are required for anaerobic glycolysis and oxidative phosphorylation; they activate alkaline and acid phosphatases, pyrophosphatase and ATPase and participate in molecular phosphate transfer. Cyclic AMP synthesis is dependent on Mg-activated adenyl cyclase. In nuclei, synthesis and stability of DNA require Mg ions. Magnesium, like calcium, is involved in neuronal and neuromuscular excitability and in muscle contractility and in clinical practice its effects may be difficult to separate from those of calcium. Isolated hypomagnesaemia may rarely produce tetany identical to that produced by hypocalcaemia.

Plasma magnesium concentration normally ranges from 0.71–0.96 mmol/litre. A higher proportion is diffusible than that of calcium, approximately 70 per cent; a higher proportion than that of calcium is bound to globulin (Sunderman and Sunderman, 1967). Magnesium homeostasis is less well-understood than that of calcium but seems more loosely regulated. Plasma magnesium falls more readily than calcium by dietary restriction or gastro-intestinal loss but this apparently weaker conservation may be misleading since the main store of magnesium is intracellular where less is known about homeostasis.

The average daily adult intake of magnesium is 10.0–12.5 mmol, about half that of calcium. Plants such as green leafy vegetables are a fairly rich source of magnesium which is present in chlorophyll. Meat and offal are also good dietary sources but milk and dairy products are low in magnesium. About one-third of dietary magnesium is absorbed from the gut, a higher proportion than calcium. Metabolic balance studies (Jones *et al.*, 1967) have suggested that intakes of 8.3–12.5 mmol daily, equivalent to 0.15–0.17 mmol/kg (Wacker and Parisi, 1968), are required to maintain magnesium balance and this forms the basis of fairly loose recommendations (WHO, 1973). However, the gut may adapt well to low magnesium intake by increasing proportionate absorption (Wacker and Parisi, 1968); the statistical regression of faecal magnesium on dietary magnesium shows near-zero faecal magnesium at zero intake (King and Stanbury, 1970); very little faecal magnesium is endogenously derived; finally, the kidneys conserve magnesium well and can normally reduce excretion to less than 0.5 mmol per day. All these findings suggest that adults diets may need little magnesium. Magnesium allowances in infants and children are based on the magnesium content of human milk, about 1.7 mmol/litre (one-third the content of cows' milk). Based on a minimum intake of one litre human milk daily up to the age of one year the magnesium allowance increases steadily from 1.7 mmol daily at that age.

Urinary magnesium excretion in adults is normally in the region of 4.4 ± 1.0 mmol/day (Heaton *et al.*, 1964; Clarkson *et al.*, 1967), as expected from knowledge of dietary intake and intestinal absorption. Some workers have reported considerably higher normal values in the London area, up to 8–9 mmol/day for magnesium and 11 mmol/day for calcium (Evans *et al.*, 1967). Renal tubular magnesium reabsorption occurs mainly from the thick ascending limb of the loop of Henle and is inhibited by many diuretics (Dirks and Quamme, 1980). Approximately 0.6 mmol magnesium is lost daily in sweat, and heavy sweating may occasionally be a significant factor in magnesium loss.

There is a relationship between the concentration ratios of K:Na and Mg:Ca in a wide variety of cells and organelles (Williams and Wacker, 1967). From this a cell membrane pump may be inferred which regulates calcium and magnesium transport in opposite directions similar to the pump mechanisms for sodium and potassium transport. Among other influences, the thyroid hormones L-thyroxine and tri-iodothyronine produce a striking cellular influx of magnesium into two cell pools, lowering plasma magnesium and raising urinary magnesium excretion, probably in association with enhanced intestinal absorption and positive magnesium balance (Dimich *et al.*, 1966; Jones *et al.*, 1966). Converse changes occur in hypothyroidism.

Intestinal calcium and magnesium absorption are interrelated. Experimental dietary restriction of one element may increase intestinal absorption of the other in animals, suggesting competition for an absorptive pathway (Alcock and MacIntyre, 1962; MacIntyre, 1963), although there is less evidence in man. The effects of supplementation are also less clear-cut; while calcium supplementation may diminish magnesium absorption in man and lower plasma and urinary magnesium (Clarkson *et al.*, 1967) the converse does not seem to apply; indeed magnesium supplementation may actually decrease faecal calcium and increase urine calcium (Heaton and Parsons, 1961). Magnesium absorption bears a more similar proportion to intake than calcium over a wide range, intestinal absorption being therefore less tightly regulated than calcium. Magnesium ions do not compete for binding to intestinal calcium-binding proteins (Bruns and Avioli, 1975). Long-term magnesium supplementation appears not to affect calcium metabolism. Parathyroid hormone stimulates both calcium and magnesium absorption from the intestine, enhanced absorption of both elements being a feature of hyperparathyroidism (Heaton and Pyrah, 1963; Wacher and Parisi, 1968; King and Stanbury, 1970). However, while PTH stimulation of calcium absorption is dependent on vitamin D, magnesium absorption is not impaired in vitamin D deficiency and administration of vitamin D produces only small and inconstant changes in magnesium absorption. Finally, magnesium absorption is unimpaired in chronic renal failure (Clarkson *et al.*, 1965) indicating its independence from diminished renal tubular synthesis of $1,25(OH)_2D$.

Parathyroid hormone enhances renal tubular magnesium reabsorption just as it does with calcium (MacIntyre, 1963; Shelp *et al.*, 1966). Nevertheless, plasma magnesium is usually normal in patients with hyperparathyroidism although there is a significant negative correlation between plasma calcium and magnesium in hyperparathyroidism, a small minority showing hypomagnesaemia (Sutton, 1970). This contrasts with normal subjects who show a positive correlation between plasma calcium and magnesium (Briscoe and Ragan, 1967) and may be due to inhibition of tubular magnesium reabsorption by hypercalcaemia (Massry *et al.*, 1969; Dirks and Quamme, 1980). In chronic renal failure urinary magnesium excretion inevitably falls with declining glomerular filtration rate; plasma levels usually remain normal presumably owing to diminished intake (Clarkson *et al.*, 1965). Primary hyperaldosteronism produces hypomagnesaemia and increased urinary magnesium excretion and plasma magnesium is raised in Addison's disease (Wacker and Parisi, 1968). These effects remain poorly understood.

As with calcium, parathyroid hormone control of magnesium metabolism is subject to a feed-back mechanism, although on a molar basis magnesium is two to three times less effective than calcium in suppressing PTH secretion both *in vitro* and *in vivo* (Habener and Jacobs, 1982; Buckle *et al.*, 1968; Mayer, 1975). However, a critical magnesium level is necessary below which PTH secretion is severely inhibited. Human hypomagnesaemia may produce severe hypocalcaemia which is resistant to treatment with vitamin D and which may be worsened by calcium treatment which further depresses the plasma magnesium. Circulating PTH may be low or undetectable and rapidly rises to normal or even supranormal values following magnesium administration, restoring total and ionized calcium and increasing renal phosphate clearances (Anast *et al.*, 1972; Suh *et al.*, 1973). These findings may be due at least in part to the dependency on magnesium of parathyroid adenyl cyclase, an enzyme which mediates PTH release. There may be additional reasons for the hypocalcaemia of hypomagnesaemia including impaired end-organ response to PTH in kidney and bone (Habener and Jacobs, 1982).

Calcitonin has not been shown to affect magnesium metabolism. Magnesium ions stimulate calcitonin secretion at abnormally high perfusate concentrations (Care *et al.*, 1971; Pento *et al.*, 1974) but this finding has no known physiological significance at present.

The clinical effects of hypomagnesaemia are well-known both in adults and infants (Hanna *et al.*, 1960; Wacker and Parisi, 1968; Editorial, 1973). There may, however, be considerable difficulty in distinguishing symptoms of magnesium depletion from associated deficiencies and other abnormalities; symptoms which have responded to magnesium repletion alone include muscle weakness, ataxia, tetany, vertigo, depression and cardiac abnormalities. Any gastrointestinal disease associated with a malabsorption syndrome or prolonged diarrhoea may produce magnesium deficiency. Prolonged intravenous feeding without magnesium supplements, particularly if accompanied by naso-gastric aspiration, may also produce it. In infants excessive dietary phosphate in cows' milk may precipitate hypomagnesaemia as well as hypocalcaemia. Renal causes include prolonged diuretic therapy; alcohol produces a rapid magnesium diuresis possibly by a specific action – alcoholics are particularly prone to magnesium deficiency and additional causative factors include dietary deficiency, diarrhoea and secondary hyperaldosteronism in cirrhosis. Hyperparathyroidism is an uncommon cause, and hypoparathyroidism has also been incriminated. Diabetic ketosis may result in magnesium depletion by the same means which give rise to potassium depletion.

Idiopathic hypomagnesaemia results from a primary defect in intestinal magnesium absorption. It may represent an inborn error of metabolism and, since it has been reported in offspring of a first cousin marriage, may be transmitted as an autosomal recessive characteristic. It presents as fits in infancy between one and four months of age (Friedman *et al.*, 1967; Salet *et al.*, 1966; Nordio *et al.*, 1971; Haijamae and MacDowell, 1972). Very low magnesium levels, with near-zero magnesium balance, were associated with good positive calcium balances and on magnesium repletion calcium balance became negative (Friedman *et. al.*, 1967); the possible mechanisms responsible for these findings have already been discussed.

Oral magnesium repletion may be achieved with salts such as the glycerophosphate, 6 g daily of the salt providing 26.75 mmol Mg (Friedman *et. al.*, 1967), magnesium acetate (Heaton and Parsons, 1961) and magnesium oxide or hydroxide as Mist. Mag. Hydrox. B.P. (Dent and Stamp, 1970b). Intravenous therapy is given as a solution of magnesium sulphate ($MgSO_4.7H_2O$) and a total dose of 20–25 mmol is generally enough to achieve repletion after which subsequent losses can be balanced. The use of magnesium in treatment of renal stones is discussed above.

There is no significant metabolic cause of symptomatic hypermagnesaemia; this has usually resulted from vigorous therapy and in particular the treatment of maternal eclampsia with magnesium salts has produced magnesium intoxication in the infant (Editiorial, 1973).

## Other alkaline earths

The remaining alkaline earths strontium, barium and radium are not essential elements but all of them can exchange with and replace calcium within the hydroxyapatite crystal. Strontium follows calcium in the periodic table, shows most similarity to calcium in its overall metabolism, and has been intensively studied. $^{85}$Strontium has been used as a tracer for calcium in metabolic studies while the bone-seeking $^{90}$strontium has represented one of the main dangers of nuclear 'fall-out'. The body discriminates against strontium in favour of calcium in at least two ways: there is a stonger barrier to its intestinal absorption, relatively more strontium is excreted in the urine, and there may be a relative blood:bone barrier as well (Wasserman and Comar, 1961;

Vaughan, 1975). The adult skeleton contains 4 mmol stable strontium from a dietary intake of about 23 $\mu$mol daily. Parenteral calcium and strontium are largely excreted in the urine while injected barium and radium are largely excreted in the stools.

Strontium and to a much lesser extent barium compete with calcium for binding to intestinal calcium-binding protein (Wasserman *et. al.*, 1974; Bruns and Avioli, 1975). This competition is also seen with zinc, manganese and cadmium but, as previously mentioned, magnesium is virtually inactive in this system. In high experimental concentrations strontium inhibits PTH secretion and stimulates calcitonin secretion (Care *et al.*, 1975); it also produces experimental rickets, inhibiting intestinal calcium absorption, calcium binding protein synthesis and $1,25(OH)_2D$ synthesis in kidney. Its further study may lead to better understanding of the molecular aspects of vitamin D metabolism.

Barium sulphate has often been usefully employed, because of its insolubility, as an internal faecal marker for metabolic balance studies.

## Fluoride

The protective effects of fluoride against tooth decay are fully established (Editorial, 1972(a)) but it has more recently been found essential for optimal growth and fertility in animals (Rheinhold, 1975). It may have an additional role in maintaining skeletal strength. Fluoride is an avid bone-seeking element and readily replaces $OH^-$ in the apatite crystal lattice; resulting crystals (fluorhydroxyapatite) are both larger, stronger and less soluble in water than calcium apatite and it is these properties which have been thought to protect dentine and tooth enamel against caries.

Body fluoride increases steadily with age to about 160 mmol/kg (3 g/kg). It is mainly ingested in drinking water which varies widely in fluoride content from 2.5 $\mu$mol/litre to 1.0 mmol/litre depending on the area. Fish is a fair source of fluoride and meat also contains appreciable quantities. Fluoride is readily absorbed from the intestinal tract (Faccini, 1969). Although the anion is toxic to many enzymes its avid subsequent uptake by bone may well afford protection against adverse effects. In addition to the changes it produces is bone crystal structure and function it also stimulates osteoblastic activity (Jowsey *et al.*, 1968); however, the resulting excess osteoid in poorly mineralized (Burkhart and Jowsey, 1968) and fluoride therapy without large calcium supplements produces a histological picture similar to osteomalacia. The action of fluoride on bone may be further complicated by parathyroid hormone stimulation (Faccini and Care, 1965; Teotia and Teotia, 1973) although it is not clear whether this is the cause of the increased bone resorption which is also found, nor has it been unequivocally established in man.

Most recent argument has been concerned with the role of fluoride in the prevention and treatment of osteoporosis. There is conflicting epidemiological evidence for its prophylactic value in high and low fluoride areas (Bernstein *et al.*, 1966; Affram *et. al.*, 1969; Parfitt, 1983). The situation may be different regarding treatment of established disease. While fluoride alone is harmful, in combination with massive calcium supplementation it may increase trabecular bone volume judged micro-radiographically (Riggs *et al.*, 1973), and histomorphometrically (Briançon and Meunier, 1981). Decrease in spinal crush fracture rate in osteoporosis has been reported (Riggs *et al.*, 1982). Metabolic balance studies have, however, failed to show net calcium retention and the trabecular bone changes may therefore be accomplished at the expense of increased intracortical porosity.

For adequate prevention of dental caries fluoride concentration in drinking water should approximate 50 μmol/litre or 1 part per million (p.p.m., mg/litre) (WHO, 1970; Editorial, 1972(a)). In certain localities well water may contain excessive concentrations of fluoride; its prolonged consumption during growth eventually produces skeletal fluorosis in which the bones become excessively dense but more brittle and their histology shows the gross features described above. Periosteal activity is excessive and although the bones do not expand as in Paget's disease extraskeletal ossification occurs at tendon and ligamentous insertions.

## Zinc

Among the essential biological metals zinc is second in prevalence only to iron. The dietary requirement for zinc is the same as that for iron but unlike iron there is no functional pool of zinc (Golden and Golden, 1981); body zinc is half that of iron but ten times more than that of the next most prevalent metal, copper. Several reviews of zinc metabolism are available (Underwood, 1977; Burch *et. al.*, 1975; Burch and Sullivan, 1976; Golden and Golden, 1981).

The number of known zinc metalloenzymes has steadily increased to a recent count of 80 (Golden and Golden, 1981). They include carbonic anhydrase, alkaline phosphatase, alcohol dehydrogenase, carboxypeptidases A and B, certain collagenases and enzymes involved in vitamin A metabolism. Other metals may substitute for the same enzymes in different species. Zinc is involved in a number of metal-ion activated enzymes including several peptidases, for example arginase and aminopeptidase; and many enzymes involved in synthesis and metabolism of protein, RNA and DNA are zinc metalloproteins. Zinc also appears necessary for normal bone development (Colhoun *et. al.*, 1974). The features of zinc deficiency include defective growth and sexual maturation, poor wound healing, susceptibility to infection, skin and intestinal defects; they are common to man, livestock and experimental animals. Acrodermatitis enteropathica is a specific human zinc deficiency disease (see below).

The human body contains between 22 and 35 mmol zinc of which 98 per cent is intracellular as might be expected with an element which is chelated so strongly by its cytosol and microsomal apo-enzymes. Normal plasma zinc levels range from 11.5–17.6 μmol/litre with a mean of about 15 μmol/litre (Halstead *et. al.*, 1974). Plasma levels decline with stress, infection, pregnancy, oral contraceptive and corticosteroid therapy. Thirty to forty per cent of plasma zinc is firmly bound to a specific α2-macroglobulin and the remainder is more loosely bound to albumin (Parisi and Vallee, 1970). Over 75 per cent of whole blood zinc is contained in red cells, mainly associated with carbonic anhydrase. Skin, bone, visceral organs and the prostate gland are relatively rich in zinc; in bone it is sequestered and largely unavailable for metabolic purposes.

Dietary zinc intake is normally 0.15–0.23 mmol daily of which half to two-thirds is absorbed, all through the small intestine. However, the availability of dietary zinc, and other trace metals, for absorption is much more variable than with other minerals since it is so readily chelated by other dietary and intestinal contents such as phytate and many peptides and amino acids. Provisional dietary requirements have therefore been calculated for each of several arbitrary percentages of 'available zinc' (WHO, 1973): these authorities have also calculated that requirements are doubled in lactating women. The value given above for average intake covers the majority of requirements in all other ranges for age and sex.

Good dietary sources of zinc are meat, fish and other sea food, and legumes. The great bulk of zinc in wheat, basically a good dietary source, may be lost in highly milled flour. On the other hand, there is an uncertain danger that availability of zinc in all vegetable sources may be limited by phytate content.

Not much is known of the mechanisms which control zinc absorption. In experimental animals intestinal mucosa contains at least two zinc-binding proteins (Van Campen and Kowalski, 1971) and zinc absorption may be inversely related to intestinal mucosal zinc content (Evans *et. al.*, 1973). Zinc and copper inhibit absorption of each other, suggesting that they may share certain aspects of absorption. In man absorption of radioactive zinc is apparent 15 minutes after ingestion and peak plasma levels are reached in 4 hours. Zinc is mainly excreted in the stool. About 5–11 μmol zinc is excreted in the urine in 24 hours; urinary zinc is increased by parenteral amino acids and penicillamine. Sweat contains 15 μmol Zn/litre.

A syndrome of zinc deficiency in man has been extensively reported (Prasad, 1966; Burch and Sullivan, 1976) mainly in Iran and Egypt despite the problem of differentiating its special features from those of other dietary deficiencies and of parasitic infections; zinc deficiency was also recorded in some subjects without clinical abnormalities. Existence of the syndrome was supported by the clinical response to zinc supplementation (Sanstead *et al.*, 1967). Affected patients, usually adolescents, were dwarfed and sexually retarded; their endocrine abnormalities resembled hypopituitarism. Zinc deficiency may also retard wound healing and alter senses of taste and smell (Hambidge, 1974). It has also been implicated in human teratogenicity (Hambidge *et. al.*, 1975; Burch and Sullivan, 1976).

Acute zinc deficiency from total parenteral feeding has resulted in diarrhoea, mental depression, para-orificial dermatitis and hair loss. Plasma zinc levels only fell during a phase of sustained anabolism and weight gain (Kay *et al.*, 1976). The disease is very similar to acrodermatitis enteropathica (see below). Other states associated with zinc depletion include alcoholic cirrhosis, when urinary zinc is increased, malabsorption syndromes, pancreatitis, diabetes and sickle cell anaemia. The zinc content of hair has been used as a measure of deficiency but may show paradoxical results (Bradfield and Hambidge, 1980).

Acrodermatitis enteropathica (AE) is a primary inborn error of zinc metabolism characterized by specific intestinal malabsorption. The degree of zinc malabsorption in this disease is of the same order as that of magnesium in idiopathic hypomagnesaemia (Moynihan, 1974). AE is inherited as an autosomal recessive characteristic. The disease presents at weaning or earlier if the infant is not breast fed. Restoration of breast feeding produces remission but inevitable relapse follows re-introduction of other diets. Severe dermatitis of the extremities is associated with severe diarrhoea and without treatment death occurs in infancy. Following fortuitous improvement when zinc was given for a presumed dietary deficiency Moynihan (1974) demonstrated a unique deficiency of zinc and full regression followed zinc supplementation (Moynihan, 1975). The distribution of symptoms recalls the role of zinc in collagen metabolism and in digestive enzymes and the poor wound healing associated with other states of zinc deficiency. The cause of zinc malabsorption in AE is unknown. Jackson (1977) estimated body zinc deficit in an adult with AE and measured the increase in zinc absorption produced by Diodoquin: no changes were seen in calcium, phosphorus or magnesium balance. Treatment requires 35–100 mg elemental zinc daily, various salts being available. For a young woman during pregnancy 200–300 mg zinc sulphate daily was adequate. Zinc intoxication has been reported following domestic renal haemodialysis using water stored in a galvanized tank.

## Copper

As with other trace metals much knowledge of mammalian copper metabolism and its deficiency diseases derives from veterinary medicine. The signs of human deficiency reflect the known actions of the copper-containing enzymes and match those in domestic animals, the ataxia of grazing cattle and sheep, the anaemia of pigs and the cardiovascular and skeletal defects in poultry and other animals. Comprehensive reviews of history and biochemistry are available (Underwood, 1977; Burch *et. al.*, 1975; O'Dell, 1976). Copper plays a vital role in the metabolism of nervous tissue, in haemopoiesis, and in skeletal and connective tissue formation, revealing an importance far in excess of its concentration in the body. Interrelationships between the metabolism of most trace metals are well-illustrated with respect to copper, iron, zinc and molybdenum.

Copper and iron share a unique position in electron transport both being an integral part of cytochrome c oxidase, and the major importance of copper enzymes lies in this ability to accept electrons and transfer molecular oxygen (see *Evolutionary Aspects*). Since cytochrome c oxidase comes at the end of the electron transport chain all oxidative phosphorylation, coupled with the formation of high-energy phosphate bonds is dependent on copper. The special needs of the brain and central nervous system for energy may explain why this tissue suffers so early from copper deficiency, particularly from abnormalities in myelination (see below). Other major copper enzymes include the 'multifunctional' caeruloplasmin (also known as ferroxidase), superoxide dismutase, amino oxidase, uricase and tyrosinase. Caeruloplasmin is vital to iron transport; it oxidizes iron from the ferrous storage form to the ferric state that is required for stable complexing with the specific iron transport protein transferrin (hence, 'ferroxidase'); copper deficiency can thus produce hypochromic anaemia with low serum iron but excessive iron stores. Occasional problems in the differential diagnosis of apparent iron-deficiency anaemia are obvious. Caeruloplasmin also oxidizes catecholamines, serotonin and ascorbic acid. The toxic superoxide ion which inhibits cytochrome c oxidase is broken down by superoxide dismutases (cupreins) in red cells, brain and liver. Superoxide is generated by xanthine oxidase which contains both iron and molybdenum as essential metals. Intestinal copper absorption is also affected by molybdenum, as it is by zinc (see below). Amine oxidase participates in the formation of collagen and elastin, specifically in its oxidation of the end carbon (c-terminal) of lysine and hydroxylysine to form highly reactive aldehyde groups; these groups are the immediate precursors of cross-linkages between the collagen or elastin chains; deficiency can weaken blood vessel walls and cause skeletal deformities. Lathyrism is produced by substances known as lathyrogens such as the naturally occurring B-aminoproprionitrile in sweet-pea seeds. Lathyrogens inhibit amine oxidase and produce a connective tissue disturbance that mimics copper deficiency. Tyrosinase is required in melanin production and pigmentary abnormalities might therefore be expected in states of copper deficiency.

The adult human body normally contains between 1.3 and 1.9 mmol copper; half is in bone and muscle but liver and brain have the highest tissue concentrations. Copper concentration in the new-born is three times greater than in the adult but rapidly falls between 1 and 3 months of age as liver reserves fall, at which time the infant is most susceptible to the anaemia of copper deficiency. Premature infants have lower concentrations and are also at risk from deficiency. Plasma copper levels are normally 24 μmol/litre; they rise in situations where zinc and iron levels fall i.e. in periods of stress, infection, pregnancy and during oral contraceptive and corticosteroid therapy which increases caeruloplasmin levels. Ninety-three per cent of plasma copper is contained in caeruloplasmin, the remainder being loosely bound to albumin. Transport from gut to liver in portal blood is accomplished by binding to albumin. The copper concentration of red blood cells is similar to that in plasma, unlike the situation with zinc. Red cell copper is mostly contained in superoxide dismutase (erythrocuprein).

Copper in soil varies quite widely, producing a considerable geographical variation in dietary copper. Provided soil copper is adequate good dietary sources are animal liver (but not meat) and green vegetables. Oysters and many species of fish are also good sources but most other foodstuffs are low in copper (WHO, 1973). Copper deficiency in infancy is produced by milk formulas providing less than 0.75 μmol/kg body weight; the daily recommended intake in infancy has therefore been raised for safety to 1.25 μmol/kg (WHO, 1973). This 'requirement' falls steadily with age and the average adult male is said to be safe with about 0.5 μmol/kg or about 0.35 mmol (2.2 mg).

Intestinal copper absorption is poorly understood; it is inhibited by sulphide, which forms an insoluble complex, and by zinc, molybdenum and cadmium through an effect at the mucosal level. Copper absorption may be facilitated by amino acids which possibly form absorbable complexes. The metal is bound by two proteins present in intestinal mucosa, superoxide dismutase and a metallothionine; other transition elements compete experimentally for this 'copper-binding protein'.

Copper is excreted almost entirely in bile, as is manganese, and very little appears in urine (0.08–0.04 μmol/day) except in Wilson's disease (see below). Biliary copper is closely associated with the bile salt tauro-cheno-deoxycholate (Lewis, 1973). Enterohepatic recirculation is thought to be negligible.

Infantile syndromes of copper deficiency include anaemia in infants maintained largely on cows' milk who required both copper and iron for an adequate response (Schubert and Lahey, 1959; Sturgeon and Brubaker, 1956); a second syndrome was associated with more variable anaemia, diarrhoea and skeletal rarefaction in which the anaemia responded to copper but not to iron (Graham and Cordano, 1976). Total parenteral feeding has also given rise to copper deficiency disease (Karpel and Peden, 1972). Low plasma copper is also found in malabsorption syndromes and has been reported in nephrotic syndrome.

Menkes' kinky hair syndrome (Menkes *et al.*, 1962) is inherited as a sex-linked recessive disorder characterized by growth retardation, progressive mental deterioration, degeneration of aortic elastin, metaphyseal abnormalities in the skeleton with changes similar to scurvy, hypothermia and a peculiar defect in hair keratin and pigmentation ('kinky hair'). Most of these abnormalities reflect the known activities of copper-containing enzymes already discussed. However, for unknown reasons anaemia is not a feature. The copper-deficient basis of the disease was established by Danks *et al.*, (1972). Excessive copper accumulates in intestinal mucosa; serum copper and caeruloplasmin remain low, oral copper supplements are ineffective but parenteral copper improves the disease.

A second inborn error of copper metabolism, Wilson's disease or hepatolenticular degeneration, is characterized by copper excess. Plasma copper and caeruloplasmin levels are again low but copper steadily accumulates in tissues, particularly the liver, brain, iris and kidneys, and produces progressive toxicity with cirrhosis, mental deterioration, ataxia and choreiform movements. Copper in the iris produces the pathognomonic Kayser-Fleischer ring, and a Fanconi syndrome with vitamin D-resistant osteomalacia develops from proximal renal tubular damage. Urinary copper is increased but biliary and faecal copper excretion is reduced. The cause of this increased tissue uptake is unknown but the copper-binding power of lysosomal metallothionein has been reported as four times greater than normal in Wilson's disease (Evans *et. al.*, 1973). Successful treatment relies on chelating agents, particularly penicillamine, which increase urinary excretion of copper (and zinc).

Raised caeruloplasmin has been found in lymphomas and collagen diseases. Plasma copper may be high in Addison's disease (as is zinc); corticosteroids may increase its biliary excretion. Copper poisoning is rare, but as with zinc it has been reported in patients receiving chronic haemodialysis at home (Lyle *et. al.*, 1976). Cuprous thiocyanate may be used to advantage as an internal faecal marker for metabolic balance studies (Dick, 1969).

## Manganese

Information on manganese derives chiefly from the study of experimental deficiency states and of enzyme systems which appear to be activated by the metal. Considerable problems have surrounded measurement of its minute concentrations free from contamination. Manganese-dependent enzymes may be activated *in vitro* by other metals such as iron, chromium and magnesium, making the true physiological situation difficult to interpret.

Manganese is a cofactor for a number of mammalian enzyme systems including pyruvate carboxylase, mitochondrial superoxide dismutase, a polysaccharide polymerase and N-acetyl-galactosamine transferase. Manganese deficiency impairs gluconeogenesis and experimental deficiency is also associated with diabetic glucose tolerance curves (Leach and Lilburn, 1978). The involvement of manganese in mucopolysaccharide metabolism is related to synthesis of chondroitin sulphate. Manganese deficiency produces growth defects particularly of long bones and tendons, with associated mucopolysaccharide abnormality, and bears some resemblance to human chondrodystrophy (Leach *et. al.*, 1969; Leach, 1971). Manganese may be involved in protein, RNA and DNA synthesis; a DNA-manganese complex has been described (Wiberg and Neuman, 1967) and manganese activates an RNA-polymerase. Manganese is involved in cholesterol synthesis as a necessary cofactor for mevalonate kinase; deficient animals develop hypocholesterolaemia (see below). If manganese is required for steroidogenesis, its general unavailability may conceivably affect the reproductive system; manganese deficiency severely retards sexual development in the young and produces ovarian and testicular degeneration in the adult animal. An inborn error of manganese metabolism may be responsible in mice for a form of hereditary ataxia in which defective mucopolysaccharide synthesis produces abnormal development of the otolith; ataxia in offspring can be prevented by maternal manganese supplementation but offspring will still transmit the ataxia gene (Erway *et. al.*, 1971).

The manganese content of the human body is 0.22–0.36 mmol, about one-fifth that of the copper content. It is widely distributed in soft tissues, particularly brain, kidney, pancreas and liver (Tipton and Cook, 1963). Intracellular distribution is concentrated in the mitochondria. Normal serum manganese levels of 11 pmol/litre have recently been reported by neutron activation analysis (Versieck *et al.*, 1975). Manganese in plasma is transported by a specific globulin transmanganin.

Normal dietary manganese intake in different parts of the world ranges between 36–160 μmol/day, enough to produce positive balances in all subjects, and the lower figure has been given as a recommended intake (WHO, 1973). During the first week of life, faecal manganese loss may be five times the intake from breast milk. In early childhood an intake of 2.7 μmol/kg is considered adequate. Whole cereals, nuts, legumes and green leafy vegetables are rich in manganese and the content in tea is particularly high, one cup providing up to 24 μmol. The mechanism of manganese absorption is unknown. Its excretion is almost entirely in bile.

Accidental production of manganese deficiency by an experimental diet has once been reported in man (Doisy, 1973). The patient suffered weight loss, anorexia and vomiting, transient dermatitis and deterioration of hair; he also developed striking hypocholesterolaemia. Prolonged prothrombin time was not reversed by vitamin K until manganese was provided.

A hypoglycaemic effect of manganese salts in very small dosage has been noted in diabetes (Rubinstein *et. al.*, 1962); the relationship between manganese and glucose tolerance requires further study. Liver manganese is increased in haemochromatosis (Alstatt *et al.*, 1967). Industrial manganese intoxication produces extrapyramidal disease (Parkinsonism).

The human skeleton suffers many poorly classified bone dysplasias which are still 'in search of an inborn error' (Spranger, 1974; Carter, 1976). The involvement of manganese in mucopolysaccharide metabolism is clearly an area of opportunity in clinical research.

## Molybdenum

The unique chemistry of molybdenum makes it the biological catalyst for coupled transfer reactions of proton, electron and possibly oxygen (Coughlan, 1983). Of the dozen or so proteins that contain molybdenum as an essential prosthetic group only three are found in man, xanthine oxidase (which also contains iron), aldehyde oxidase and sulphite oxidase. Molybdenum may play a part in prevention of dental caries but this is far less certain than the situation with fluoride (WHO, 1973).

Dietary molybdenum is derived mainly from vegetables; vegetable content depends on soil content and on other soil characteristics. Root crops are low in molybdenum. A tentative recommended daily intake of 20 pmol/kg body weight has been suggested (WHO, 1973). Dietary intake actually averages 180 μg daily and varies with age, sex and income (Chappell *et al.*, 1979). Molybdenum and copper compete with each other for intestinal absorption but competition may also involve dietary sulphate and its conversion to sulphide with resulting formation of insoluble metal sulphides (Suttle, 1974). The mechanism(s) of molybdenum absorption are unknown although studies of its site, rate and urinary excretion have been made (Chappell *et al.*, 1979). Animal growth may suffer with deficient molybdenum intake.

It has been suggested on epidemiological grounds that hyperuricaemia and gout may result from excessive molybdenum intake via an increase in xanthine oxidase activity: conversely cattle may suffer xanthine stones in molybdenum-poor areas (Rheinhold, 1975). A single case of diet-induced deficiency in man has been reported during prolonged total parenteral nutrition (Abumrad *et al.*, 1981). A molybdenum cofactor is involved in the three molybdenum dependent enzymes. An inborn error characterized by deficiency of these enzymes due to absence of the cofactor has been described (Wadman *et al.*, 1983).

## Cobalt

The only known physiological function of cobalt is as an essential constituent of cyanocobalamin, vitamin $B_{12}$, and man can only utilize the element by ingesting the vitamin in this form. Recommended daily intakes of vitamin $B_{12}$ range from 0.3 μg in infancy to 3 μg in pregnancy (FAO, 1970). Inorganic dietary cobalt is only important from toxicological aspects (WHO, 1973). The vitamin $B_{12}$ enzymes are methyl tetrahydrofolate oxidoreductase, homocysteine transferase, ribonucleotide transferase, and methyl malonyl-GA mutase. They prevent the specific related deficiency diseases pernicious anaemia and subacute combined degeneration of the spinal cord, described in standard textbooks. Pure dietary deficiency of vitamin $B_{12}$ may occur among strict vegans.

Inorganic cobalt salts are of some further clinical interest since they raise haemoglobin levels in the anaemia of chronic renal failure. One recent report has described a possible therapeutic value of cobalt (Duckham and Lee, 1976), which appears to act by stimulating renal erythropoietin through production of histotoxic hypoxia. Undesirable side-effects include gastrointestinal disturbance, tinnitus and reversible deafness, depression of thyroidal iodine uptake, myocardial ischaemia and in high doses, cardiomyopathy. Its value in the anaemia of chronic renal failure is still debated (Lancet, 1976b).

## Chromium

Chromium in biology exists only in its trivalent form and its role has been reviewed (Saner, 1980). It is thought to exist in combination with glutathione and nicotinic acid as a 'glucose tolerance factor' (GTF) which has not to date been characterized. It enhances glucose metabolism by facilitating insulin binding to membrane receptors; chromium is required experimentally for optimal expression of all insulin activity (Hambidge, 1974). In human diabetes, chromium supplementation has improved glucose tolerance and lowered cholesterol and triglyceride levels; pharmacological dosage has no effects and the reported improvement was attributed to pre-existing deficiency.

Food plants are the only satisfactory source of dietary chromium. Recommended safe and adequate intakes range from 10–40 $\mu$g daily in infancy to 50–200 $\mu$g in later life (Committee on Dietary Allowances, 1980). Normal plasma levels are approximately 50–900 ng/litre. The metal is excreted almost entirely in the urine at a rate of approximately 5–10 $\mu$g daily. Two patients have been reported who developed chromium-responsive disease while on prolonged parenteral feeding (Jeejeebhoy *et al.*, 1977; Freund *et. al.*, 1979). Both had grossly impaired glucose tolerance requiring insulin and showed either encephalopathy or peripheral neuropathy. All three features responded markedly to 150 $\mu$g $CrCl_3$ daily.

## Selenium

Selenium is an essential constituent of the enzyme glutathione peroxidase which protects against oxidative damage to membranes and macromolecules including DNA (Young, 1981). It may also have a role in ubiquinone synthesis. Specific deficiency diseases indicate its essential nature in different species of livestock and experimental animals and the presence of selenium-containing glutathione peroxidase in human erythrocytes strongly suggests it to be essential in man. Further evidence derives from the reversible cardiomyopathy seen in selenium-deficient areas of China (Lancet, 1979) and in the fatal cardiomyopathy or severe muscle pains found in three selenium-deficient patients receiving long-term parenteral nutrition (van Rij *et al.*, 1979; Johnson *et al.*, 1981; Fleming *et al.*, 1982).

Most dietary selenium derives from seafoods and fish, poultry, offal and grains but there is wide geographical variation. Dietary recommendations have been suggested (Committee on Dietary Allowances, 1980). Normal levels of selenium in serum, erythrocytes and other tissues have been established by neutron activation analysis.

Experimentally, selenium has anticarginogenic properties. And preliminary studies indicate an inverse correlation between serum selenium and cancer risk in humans (Willett *et al.*, 1983).

## Silicon, vanadium, tin and nickel

Silicon is essential for growth in experimental animals. It is found mainly in connective tissue where it functions as a cross-linking agent. It is also present in certain natural mucopolysaccharide fractions at specific sites in bone metaphyses. There is evidence for a specific silicon requirement, independent of vitamin D, in bone formation (Nutrition Reviews, 1980; Carlisle, 1981). Silicon is a ubiquitous element and its concentration in diets and human tissue is 100–1000 times higher than the other trace elements. Beer is a saturated solution and 250 ml wine contains 143 per cent of the average daily intake. Arguments have been advanced for a protective effect of silicon against atherosclerosis (Schwartz, 1977).

Vanadium is a common, low atomic-weight element which is probably subject to homeostatic control. No vanadium metalloenzymes are known but vanadate inhibits the sodium pump (Na-K ATPase) *in vitro* and is a potent diuretic experimentally; vanadium deficiency has been reported in oedematous patients with kwashiorkor (Golden and Golden, 1981). Experimental vanadium deficiency is also associated with raised cholesterol and triglyceride levels. The richest vanadium-containing foods are fats and vegetable oils, and meat contains ten times more than root crops or pulses.

Nickel metalloenzymes are found in plants and microorganisms but have not to date been found in animals although experimental deficiency produces growth retardation. Nickel is specifically bound to human albumen. Tin deficiency also slows growth experimentally (Mertz, 1974). It rapidly forms coordination complexes with proteins and nucleic acids. Tin accumulates in uraemic patients.

Steady progress in the basic science of metal metabolism continues, aided by further developments in methods of trace element analysis (Fell, 1983). Problems of contamination remain severe. The use of enzyme studies as biochemical markers for trace element nutrition has also gained ground. Further evidence for the essential nature of these elements has come in the past few years from deficiency diseases created in patients receiving long-term parenteral nutrition. Such nutrition is now fully supplemented with trace metals. Certain inborn errors of metabolism, new and old, surely await explanation on the basis of disordered trace element metabolism.

## References

Abumrad, N.N., Schneider, A.J., Steel, D. and Rogers, L.S. (1981). Amino acid intolerance during prolonged total parenteral nutrition reversed by molybdate therapy. *Am. J. Clin. Nutr.*, 34, 2551–9.

Affram, P.A., Hernborg, J. and Nilsson, B.E.R. (1969). The influence of a high fluoride content in the drinking water on the bone mineral mass in man. *Acta Orthop. Scand.*, **40**, 137–42.

Albright, F. and Reifenstein, E.C. (1948). *The Parathyroid Glands and Metabolic Bone Disease.* Williams and Wilkins: Baltimore.

Alcock, N. and MacIntyre, I. (1962). Inter-relationship of calcium and magnesium absorption. *Clin. Sci.*, **22**, 185–93.

Alstatt, L.B., Pollack, S., Feldman, M.H., Reba, R.C. and Crosby, W.H. (1967). Liver manganese in haemochromatosis. *Proc. Soc. Exptl. Biol. and Med.*, **24**, 353–5.

Anast, C., Mohs, J.M., Kaplan, S.L. and Burns, T.W. (1972). Evidence for parathyroid failure in magnesium deficiency. Science, **177**, 606–608.

Avioli, L.V. and Krane, S.M. (1977, 1978). *Metabolic Bone Disease*, Vols I and II. Academic Press: London, New York, San Francisco.

Avioli, L.V. and Raisz, L.G. (1980). Metabolic bone disease. *Clinics in Endocrinol. and Metab.*, 9, no 1

Baker, L.R.I., Ackrill, P., Cattell, W.R., Stamp, T.C.B. and Watson, L. (1974). Iatrogenic osteomalacia and myopathy due to phosphate depletion. *Br. Med. J.*, **3**, 150–52.

Barzel, U.S. (1979). *Osteoporosis II.* Grune and Stratton: New York.

Bernstein, D.S., Sadowsky, N., Hegsted, D.M., Guri, C.D. and Stare, F.J. (1966). Prevalence of osteoporosis in high and low fluoride areas. *J. Am. Med. Assoc.*, **198**, 499–504.

Berry, E.M., Gupta, M.M., Turner, S.J. and Burns, R.R. (1973). Variation in plasma calcium with induced changes in plasma specific gravity, total protein and albumen. *Br. Med. J.*, **4**, 640–43.

Boyle, I.T., Gray, R.W. and De Luca, H.F. (1971). Regulation by calcium of *in vivo* synthesis of 1,25-dihydroxycholecalciferol and 21,25-dihydroxycholecalciferol. *Proc. Nat. Acad. Sci.*, **68**, 2131–4.

Bradfield, R.B. and Hambidge, K.M. (1980). Problems with hair zinc as an indicator of body zinc status. *Lancet*, **i**, 363.

Briançon, D. and Meunier, P.J. (1981). Treatment of osteoporosis with fluoride, calcium and vitamin D. *Orthop. Clin. N. Amer.*, **12**, 629–48.

Brine, C.L. and Johnston, F.A. (1955). Endogenous calcium in the faeces of adult man and the amount of calcium absorbed from food. *Am. J. Clin. Nut.*, **3**, 418–20.

Briscoe, A.M. and Ragan, C. (1967). Relation of magnesium to calcium in human blood serum. *Nature*, **214**, 1126–7.

*British Medical Journal* (1972a). Editorial: Fluorides and the prevention of Dental Decay, **3**, 431.

*British Medical Journal* (1973). Editorial: Disorders of magnesium metabolism in infancy, **4**, 373–4.

Brumbaugh, P.F., Haussler, D.H., Bressler, R. and Haussler, M.R. (1974). Radioreceptor assay for 1 alpha, 25-dihydroxyvitamin $D_3$. *Science*, **183**, 1089–91.

Bruns, E.H. and Avioli, L.V. (1975). The activity and synthesis of calcium binding protein during vitamin D replacement in the ricketic rat. In *Calcium Regulating Hormones*, pp. 336–45. International Congress Series No. 346, Eds. Talmage, R.V., Owen, M. and Parsons, J.A. Excerpta Medica.

Buckle, R.M., Care, A.D., Cooper, C.W. and Gitelman, J.H. (1968). The influence of plasma magnesium concentration on parathyroid hormone secretion. *J. Clin. Endocrinol. and Metab.*, **42**, 529–32.

Bullamore, J.R., Gallagher, J.C., Wilkinson, R., Nordin, B.E.C. and Marshall, D.H. (1970). Effect of age on calcium absorption. *Lancet*, **ii**, 535–7.

Burch, R.E., Hahn, H.K.J. and Sullivan, J.F. (1975). Newer aspects of the roles of zinc, manganese and copper in human nutrition. *Clin. Chem.*, **21**, 501–20.

Burch, R.E. and Sullivan, J.F. (1976). Clinical and nutritional aspects of zinc deficiency and excess. In *Symposium on Trace Elements*, pp. 675–686, **60**, no. 4. Eds. Burch, R.E. and Sullivan, J.F. W.B. Saunders Co.: Philadelphia.

Burkhart, J.M. and Jowsey, J. (1968). Effect of variations in calcium intake on the skeleton of fluoride-fed kittens. *J. Lab. and Clin. Med.*, **72**, 943–50.

Calhoun, N.R., Smith, J.C. and Becker, K.L. (1974). The role of zinc in bone metabolism. *Clin. Orthop. and Rel. Res.*, **103**, 212–34.

Care, A.D., Bell, N.H. and Bates, R.F. (1971). The effects of hypermagnesaemia on calcitonin secretion in vivo. *J. Endocrinol.*, **51**, 381–6.

Carr. T.E., Harrison, G.E. and Nolan, J. (1973). Daily loss of calcium and sodium from the skin of two healthy men. *J. Physiol. (Lond.)*, **235**, 9–15.

Carter, C.O. (1976). Diseases of bone in search of an inborn error. In *Inborn Errors of Calcium and Bone Metabolism*, pp. 214–21. Eds. Bickel, H. and Stern, J. Medical Technical Publishing, Lancaster.

Chappell, W.R., Megler, R.R., Moure-Eraso, R., Solomons, C.C., Tsongas, T.A., Walravens, P.A. and Winston, P.A. (1979). *Human Health Effects of Molybdenum in Drinking Water*. DPA-600/1-79-006. U.S. Environmental Protection Agency.

Clark, I. (1969). Metabolic interrelations of calcium, magnesium and phosphate. *Am. J. Physiol.*, **217**, 871–2.

Clarkson, E.M., McDonald, S.J., De Wardener, H.E. and Anderson, C.K. (1965). Magnesium metabolism in chronic renal failure. *Clin. Sci.*, **28**, 107–115.

Clarkson, E.M., Warren, R.L., McDonald, S.J. and De Wardener, H.E. (1967). The effect of a high intake of calcium on magnesium metabolism in normal subjects and in patients with chronic renal failure. *Clin. Sci.*, **32**, 11–18.

Committee on Dietary Allowances, Food and Nutrition Board (1980). *Recommended Dietary Allowances*, 9th ed. Nat. Acad. Sci., Washington D.C.

Copp, D.H. (1972). *Evolution of calcium regulation in vertebrates. Clinics in Endocrinology and Metabolism*, pp. 21–32. Ed. MacIntyre, I. W.B. Saunders Co.: Philadelphia.

Coughlan, M.P. (1983). The role of molybdenum in human biology. In *Trace Metals and Inherited Metabolic Disease*. Eds. Addison, G.M., Harkness, R.A. and Pollitt, R.J. *J. Inher. Metab. Dis.*, **6** (Suppl. 1), 70–77.

Danks, D.M., Campbell, P.E., Stevens, B.J., Mayne, V. and Cartwright, E. (1972). Menkes' kinky hair syndrome: an inherited defect in copper absorption with widespread effects. *Paediatrics*, **50**, 188–201.

Davies, D.R., Dent, C.E. and Watson, L. (1971). Idiopathic hypercalciuria and hyperparathyroidism. *Br. Med. J.*, **1**, 108.

De Luca, H.F. (1979). The vitamin D system in the regulation of calcium and phosphorus metabolism. *Nutr. Rev.*, **37**, 161–93.

De Luca, H.F., Frost, H.M., Jee, W.S.S., Johnston, C.C.Jr. and Parfitt, A.M. (1981). *Osteoporosis: Recent Advances in Pathogenesis and Treatment*. University Park Press: Baltimore.

Dent, C.E. (1962). Some problems of hyperparathyroidism. *Br. Med. J.*, **2**, 1419–25, 1495–1500.

Dent, C.E. and Stamp, T.C.B. (1970a). Theoretical renal phosphorus threshold in investigation and treatment of osteomalacia. *Lancet*, **i**, 857–860.

Dent, C.E. and Stamp, T.C.B. (1970b). Treatment of primary hyperoxaluria. *Arch. Dis. Child.*, **45**, 735–45.

Dent, C.E. and Smith, R. (1969). Nutritional osteomalacia. *Q. J. Med.*, **38**, 195–209.

Dent, C.E. (1973). Keynote Address: problems in metabolic bone disease. In *Clinical Aspects of Metabolic Bone Disease*, International Congress Series No. 270, pp. 1–6. Eds. Frame, B., Parfitt, A.M. and Duncan, H. Excerpta Medica: Amsterdam.

Dent, C.E. and Winter, C.S. (1974). Osteomalacia due to phosphate depletion from excessive aluminium hydroxide ingestion. *Br. Med. J.*, **1**, 551–2.

Dick, M. (1969). Use of cuprous thiocyanate as a short-term continuous marker for faeces. *Gut*, **10**, 408–12.

Dimich, A., Rizek, J.E., Wallach, S. and Siler, W. (1966). Magnesium transport in patients with thyroid disease. *J. Clin. Endocrinol.*, **26**, 1081–92.

Diplock, A.T. (1974). The nutritional and metabolic roles of selenium and vitamin E. *Proc. Nut. Soc.*, **33**, 315–22.

Dirks, J.H. and Quamme, G.A. (1980). Renal magnesium transport and the effects of hypermagnesaemia, hypercalcaemia, body magnesium stores and parathyroid hormone. In *Phosphate and Minerals in Health and Disease*, pp. 41–9, Eds. Massry, S.G., Ritz, E. and Jahn, H. Adv. Exp. Med. Biol., Plenum Press, New York, 128.

Dixon, A.St.J., Russell, R.G.G. and Stamp, T.C.B. (1983), *Osteoporosis: A Multidisciplinary problem*. R. Soc. Med. Int. Cong. and Symp. Ser. no. 55. Academic Press: London.

Dixon, M. and Webb, E.C. (1964). *Enzymes V*, pp. 421–6. Longmans, Green & Co.: London.

Doisy, E.A.Jr. (1973). Micronutrient control on biosynthesis of clotting proteins and cholesterol. In *Proceedings of the University of Missouri's 6th Annual Conference on Trace Substances in Environmental Health*, p. 193 Ed. Hemphill, D.D. University of Missouri Press: Columbia.

Duckham, J.M. and Lee, H.A. (1976). The treatment of refractory anaemia of chronic renal failure with cobalt chloride. *Q. J. Med.*, **45**, 277–94.

Erway, L.C., Fraser, A.S. and Hurley, L.S. (1971). Prevention of congenital otolith defect in pallid mutant mice by manganese supplementation. *Genetics*, **67**, 97–108.

Evans, G.W., Dubois, R.S. and Hambidge, K.M. (1973). Wilson's disease: identification of an abnormal copper-binding protein. *Science*, **181**, 1175–6.

Evans, G.W. (1973). Copper homeostasis in the mammalian systems. *Physiol. Rev.*, **53**, 535–70.

Evans, G.W., Grace, C.I. and Hahn, C. (1973). Homeostatic regulation of zinc absorption in the rat. *Proc. Soc. Exptl. Biol. and Med.*, **143**, 723–5.

Evans, R.A., Forbes, M.A., Sutton, R.A.L. and Watson, L. (1967). Urinary excretion of calcium and magnesium in patients with calcium-containing renal stones. *Lancet*, **ii**, 958–61.

Faccini, J.M. and Care, A.D. (1965). Effect of sodium fluoride on the ultrastructure of the parathyroid glands of the sheep. *Nature (London)*, **207**, 1399–1401.

Faccini, J.M. (1969). Fluoride-induced hyperplasia of the parathyroid glands. *Proc. R. Soc. Med.*, **62**, 241.

FAO/WHO (1962). Expert group on Calcium requirements. Report . . . . (FAO Nutrition Meetings Report Series, No. 30; Wld. Hlth. Org. techn. Rep. Ser., No. 230).

FAO/WHO (1970). Expert group on requirements of ascorbic acid, vitamin D, vitamin $B_{12}$, folate and iron. Report . . . . (FAO Nutrition Meetings Report Series, No. 41; Wld. Hlth. Org. techn. Rep. Ser., No. 452).

Fell, G.S. (1983). Analytical procedures for diagnosis of trace element disorders. In *Trace Metals and Inherited Metabolic Disease*, pp. 5–8, Eds. Addison, G.M., Harkness, R.A. and Pollitt, R.J. M.T.P Press: Lancaster.

Fleming, C.R., Lie, J.T., McCall, J.T., O'Brien, J.F., Baillie, E.E. and Thistle, J.L. (1982). Selenium deficiency and fatal cardiomyopathy in a patient on home parenteral nutrition. *Gastroenterology*, **83**, 689–93.

Fraser, D.R. (1980). Regulation of the metabolism of vitamin D. *Physiol. Rev.*, **60**, 551–613.

Freund, H., Atamman, S. and Fischer, J.E. (1979). Chromium deficiency during total parenteral nutrition. *J. Am. Med. Assoc.*, **241**, 496–8.

Frieden, E. (1973). The evolution of metals as essential elements. In *Protein–Metal Interactions* pp. 1–32, Ed. Friedman, M. Plenum Press: New York.

Friedman, M., Hatcher, G. and Watson, L. (1967). Primary hypomagnesaemia with secondary hypocalcaemia in an infant. *Lancet*, **i**, 703–705.

Frost, D.V. and Lish, P.M. (1975). Selenium in biology. *Ann. Rev. Pharmacol.*, **15**, 259–84.

Golden, M.H.N. and Golden, B.E. (1981). Trace elements potential importance in human nutrition with particular reference to zinc and vanadium. *Br. Med. Bull.*, **37**, 31–6.

Graham, G.G. and Cordano, A. (1976). Copper Deficiency in Human Subjects. In *Trace Elements in Human Health and Disease*, pp. 363–72. Ed. Prasad, A.S. Academic Press: New York.

Habener, J.F. and Jacobs, J.W. (1982). Biosynthesis and control of secretion of the

calcium-regulating peptides. In *Endocrinology of Calcium Metabolism*, pp. 143–81. Ed. Parsons, J.A. Raven Press: New York.
Haddad, J.G.Jr. and Chuy, K.J. (1971). Competitive protein-binding radio assay for 25-hydroxycholecalciferol. *J. Clin. Endocrinol. and Metab.*, **33**, 992–5.
Haijamae, H. and MacDowell, I.G. (1972). Distribution of divalent cations at the cellular level during primary hypomagnesaemia in infancy. *Acta Paediat. Scand.*, **61**, 591–6.
Halstead, J.A., Smith, J.C.Jr. and Irwin, M.I. (1974). A conspectus of research on zinc requirements of man. *J. Nutrition*, **104**, 345–78.
Hambidge, K.M. (1974). The clinical significance of trace element deficiencies in man. *Proc. Nut. Soc.*, **33**, 249–55.
Hambidge, K.M., Neldner, K.H. and Walravens, P.A. (1975). Zinc, acrodermatitis enterapathica and congenital malformations. *Lancet*, **i**, 577–8.
Hanna, S., MacIntyre, I., Harrison, M. and Fraser, R. (1960). The syndrome of magnesium deficiency in man. *Lancet*, **ii**, 172–6.
Haussler, M.R. and McCain, T.A. (1977). Vitamin D metabolism and action. *N. Eng. J. Med.*, **297**, 974–83; 1041–1050.
Heaton, F.W. and Parsons, F.M. (1961). The metabolic effect of high magnesium intake. *Clin. Sci.*, **21**, 273–84.
Heaton, F.W. and Pyrah, L.N. (1963). Magnesium metabolism in patients with parathyroid disorders. *Clin. Sci.*, **25**, 475–85.
Heaton, F.W., Hogkinson, A. and Rose, G.A. (1964). Observations on the relation between calcium and magnesium metabolism in man. *Clin. Sci.*, **27**, 31–40.
Irving, J.T. (1973). *Calcium and Phosphorus Metabolism*. Academic Press: New York.
Isaksson, B., Lindholm, B. and Sjogren, B. (1967). A critical evaluation of the calcium balance technic. II. Dermal calcium losses. *Metabolism*, **16**, 303–13.
Jackson, M.J. (1977). Zinc and di-iodohydroxyquinoline therapy in Acrodermatitis enteropathica. *J. Clin. Path.*, **30**, 284–7.
Jeejeebhoy, K.N., Chu, R.C., Marliss, E.B., Greenberg, G.R. and Bruce-Robertson, A. (1977). Chromium deficiency, glucose intolerance and neuropathy reversed by chromium supplementation in a patient receiving long-term total parenteral nutrition. *Am. J. Clin. Nutr.*, **30**, 531–8.
Johnson, R.A., Baker, S.S, Fallon, J.T., Maynard, E.P., Ruskin, J.N., Wen, Z., Ge, K. and Cohen, H.J. (1981). An occidental case of cardiomyopathy and selenium deficiency. *N. Engl. J. Med.*, **304**, 1210–12.
Jones, J.E., Desper, P.C., Shane, S.R. and Flink, E.B. (1966). Magnesium metabolism in hyperparathyroidism and hypoparathyroidism. *J. Clin. Invest.*, **45**, 891–900.
Jones, J.E., Manals, R. and Flink, E.B. (1967). Magnesium requirements in adults. *Am. J. Clin. Nut.*, **20**, 632–5.
Jowsey, J., Schenk, R.K. and Reutter, F.W. (1968). Some results of the effect of fluoride on bone tissue in osteoporosis. *J. Clin. Endocrinol. and Metab.*, **28**, 869–74.
Karpel, J.T. and Peden, V.H. (1972). Copper deficiency in long-term parenteral nutrition. *J. Paediat.*, **80**, 32–6.
Kay, R.G., Tasman-Jones, C., Pybus, J., Whiting, R. and Black, H. (1976). A syndrome of acute zinc deficiency during total parenteral alimentation in man. *Ann. Surg.*, **183**, 331–40.
King, R.G. and Stanbury, S.W. (1970). Magnesium metabolism in primary hyperparathyroidism. *Clin. Sci.*, **39**, 281–303.
*Lancet* (1972). Editorial: Treatment of acute hypercalcaemia. **ii**, 314–15.
*Lancet* (1976a). Editorial: Advances in Osteoporosis? **i**, 181–2.
*Lancet* (1976b). Editorial: Cobalt in severe renal failure. **ii**, 26–7.
*Lancet* (1979). Editorial: Selenium in the heart of China. **ii**, 889–90.
Leach, R.M.Jr. (1971). Role of manganese in mucopolysaccharide metabolism. *Fed. Proc.*, **30**, 991–4.
Leach, R.M.Jr. and Lilburn, M.S. (1978). Manganese metabolism and its function. *Wld. Rev. Nutr. Diet.*, **32**, 123–4.
Leach, R.M.Jr., Muenster, A.M. and Wien, E.M. (1969). Studies on the role of

manganese in bone formation. II. Effect upon chondroitin sulfate synthesis in chick epiphyseal cartilage. *Arch. Biochem. Biophys.*, **133**, 22–8.

Lewis, K.O. (1973). The nature of copper complexes in bile and their relationship to the absorption and excretion of copper in normal subjects and in Wilson's disease. *Gut*, **14**, 221–32.

Liberti, P.A., Callahan, H.J. and Maurer, P.H. (1973). Physiochemical studies of $Ca^{++}$ controlled antigen antibody systems. In *Protein–Metal Interactions*, pp. 161–84. Ed. Friedman, M. Plenum Press: New York.

Lingärde, F. (1972). Potentiometric determination of serum ionized calcium in a normal human population. *Clin. Chim. Acta*, **40**, 477–84.

Lingärde, F. (1973). *In vivo* and *in vitro* studies on ionized versus total serum calcium in hyperparathyroidism. *Acta Endocrin.*, **74**, 501–510.

Lotz, M., Ney, R. and Bartter, F.C. (1964). Osteomalacia and debility resulting from phosphorus depletion. *Trans. Ass. Amer. Physns.*, **77**, 281–95.

Lyle, W.H., Paton, J.E. and Hui, M. (1976). Haemodialysis and copper fever. *Lancet*, **i**, 1324–5.

MacIntyre, I. (1963). An outline of magnesium metabolism in health and disease: a review. *J. Chron. Dis.*, **16**, 201–15.

MacIntyre, I., Evans, I.M.A., Hobitz, H.H.G., Joplin, G.F. and Stevenson, J.C. (1980). Chemistry, physiology and therapeutic applications of calcitonin. *Arthritis and Rheumatism*, **23**, 1139–47.

MacIntyre, I., Galante, L.S., Colston, K.W., Evans, I.M.A., Larkins, R.G., MacAuley, S.J., Hillyard, C.J., Greenberg, P.B., Matthews, E.W. and Byfield, P.G.H. (1975). Regulation of vitamin D metabolism. In *Calcium-Regulating Hormones*, pp. 396–404, International Congress Series No. 346; Eds. Talmage, R.V., Owen, M. and Parsons, J.A. Excerpta Medica: Amsterdam.

McCance, R.A. and Widdowson, E.M. (1943). Food tables, their scope and limitations. *Lancet*, **i**, 230–32.

Massry, S.G., Coburn, J.W. and Kleeman, C.R. (1969). Renal handling of magnesium in the dog. *Am. J. Physiol.*, **216**, 1460–67.

Mayer, G.P. (1975) Effect of calcium and magnesium on parathyroid hormone secretion rate in calves. In *Calcium-Regulating Hormones*, pp. 122–4. International Congress Series No. 346; Eds. Talmage, R.V., Owen, M. and Parsons, J.A. Excerpta Medica: Amsterdam.

Menkes, J.H., Alter, M., Steigleder, G.K., Weakley, D.R. and Sung, J.H. (1962). A sex-linked recessive disorder with retardation of growth, peculiar hair and focal cerebral and cerebellar degeneration. *Paediatrics*, **29**, 764–79.

Mertz, W. (1974). The newer essential trace elements, chromium, tin, vanadium, nickel and silicon. *Proc. Nut. Soc.*, **33**, 307–13.

Mertz, W. (1975). Trace-element nutrition in health and disease: contributions and problems of analysis. *Clin. Chem.*, **21**, 468–75.

Morgan, D.B., Paterson, C.R., Woods, C.G., Pulvertaft, C.N. and Fourman, P. (1965). Osteomalacia after gastrectomy: a response to very small doses of vitamin D. *Lancet*, **ii**, 1089–91.

Morgan, D.B., Hunt, G. and Paterson, C.R. (1970). The osteomalacia syndrome after stomach operations. *Q. J. Med.*, **39**, 395–410.

Moynihan, E.J. (1974). Acrodermatitis enteropathica: a lethal inherited human zinc-deficiency disorder. *Lancet*, **ii**, 399–400.

Moynihan, E.J. (1975). Acrodermatitis in two siblings treated with zinc sulphate supplements alone. *Proc. Roy. Soc. Med.*, **68**, 276.

Nagant de Deuxchaisnes, C. (1983). The pathogenesis and treatment of involutional osteoporosis. In *Osteoporosis: a Multi-Disciplinary Problem*, pp. 291–333 R. Soc. Med. Int. Cong. Ser. No. 55, Eds. Dixon, A.St.J., Russell, R.G.G. and Stamp, T.C.B. Academic Press: London.

Nassim, J.R. and Connolly, C.K. (1970). Treatment of calcinosis universalis with aluminium hydroxide. *Arch. Dis. Child.*, **45**, 118–21.

Neuman, W.F. and Ramp, W.K. (1971). The concept of a bone membrane: some implications. In *Cellular Mechanisms for Calcium Transfer and Homeostasis*, pp. 197–209 Eds. Nichols, G. Jr. and Wasserman, R.H. Academic Press: New York.

Nordin, B.E.C., Horsman, A., Marshall, D.H., Simpson, M. and Waterhouse, G.M. (1979). Calcium requirement and calcium therapy. *Clin. Orthop.*, **140**, 216–39.

Nordio, S., Donath, A., Macagno, F. and Gatti, R. (1971). Chronic hypomagnesaemia with magnesium-dependent hypocalcaemia. *Acta Paediat. Scand.*, **60**, 441–8; 449–55.

Norman, A.W. and Ross, F.P. (1979). Vitamin D seco-steroids: unique molecules with both hormone and possible membranophilic properties. *Life Science*, **24**, 759–69.

Nutrition Reviews (1980). Silicon and bone formation. **38**, 194–5.

O'Dell, B.L. (1976). Biochemistry and physiology of copper in vertebrates. In *Trace Elements in Human Health and Disease*, pp. 391–413 Ed. Prasad, A.S. Academic Press: New York.

Omdahl, J.L. and De Luca, H.F. (1973). Regulation of vitamin D metabolism and function. *Phys. Revs.*, **53**, 327–372.

Orimo, H., Chata, M., Fujita, T., Yoshikawa, M., Higashi, T., Abe., J., Watanabe, S. and Otani, K. (1972). Ultimobranchial calcitonin of Anguilla japonica: its chemical properties and physiological significance. In *Endocrinology, 1971*, pp. 48–54. Ed. Taylor, S. William Heinemann: London.

Pak, C.Y.C. (1980). A critical evaluation of treatment of calcium stones. In *Phosphate and Minerals in Health and Disease*, pp. 451–65. Ed. Massry, S.G., Ritz, E. and Jahn, H. *Adv. Exp. Med. Biol.*, **128**, Plenum Press: New York.

Parfitt, A.M. (1983). Dietary risk factors for age-related bone loss and fractures. *Lancet*, **ii**, 1181–4.

Parisi, A.F. and Vallee, B.L. (1970). Isolation of zinc a2-macroglobulin from human serum. *Biochemistry*, **9**, 2421–6.

Parsons, J.A. (1982). *Endocrinology of Calcium Metabolism*. Raven Press: New York.

Peacock, M. and Nordin, B.E.C. (1973). Plasma calcium homeostasis. In *Hard Tissue Growth, Repair and Mineralization*, pp. 409–38. Ciba Foundation Symposium No. 11, Elsevier-Excerpta Medica – North Holland – Associated Science Publishers, Amsterdam.

Pento, J.T., Glick, S.M., Kagan, A. and Gorfein, P.C. (1974). The relative influence of calcium, strontium and magnesium on calcitonin secretion in the pig. *Endocrinology*, **25**, 1176–80.

Prasad, A.S. (1966). Metabolism of zinc and its deficiency in human subjects. In *Zinc Metabolism*, pp. 250–303. Ed. Prasad, A.S. C.C. Thomas: Springfield, Illinois.

Prosser, C.L. and Brown, F.A. (1961). Respiratory functions of body fluids. In *Comparative Animal Physiology*, pp. 195–237. W.B. Saunders Co.: Philadelphia.

Purnell, D.C., Smith, L.H., Schlotz, D.A., Elveback, L.R. and Arnaud, C.D. (1971). Primary hyperparathyroidism: a prospective clinical study. *Am. J. Med.*, **50**, 670–78.

Rasmussen, H. (1972). The cellular basis of mammalian calcium homeostasis. In *Clinics in Endocrinology and Metabolism*, pp. 3–20. Ed. MacIntyre, I. W.B. Saunders Co.: Philadelphia.

Rasmussen, H. and Bordier, P. (1974). *The Physiological and Cellular Basis of Metabolic Bone Disease*. Williams and Wilkins: Baltimore.

Reeve, J., Hesp, R., Williams, D., Hulme, P., Klenerman, L., Zanelli, J.M., Darby, A.J., Tregear, G.W. and Parsons, J.A. (1976). Anabolic effect of low doses of a fragment of human parathyroid hormone on the skeleton in post-menopausal osteoporosis. *Lancet*, **i**, 1035–8.

Rheinhold, J.G. (1975). Trace elements – a selective survey. *Clinical Chemistry*, **21**, 476–500.

Riggs, B.L., Jowsey, J., Kelly, P.J., Hoffman, D.L. and Arnaud, C.D. (1973). Studies on pathogenesis and treatment in post-menopausal and senile osteoporosis. In *Clinics in Endocrinology and Metabolism*, pp. 317–32. W.B. Saunders Co.: Philadelphia.

Riggs, B.L., Seeman, F., Hodgson, S.F., Taves, D. and O'Fallon, W.M. (1982). Effect of the fluoride-calcium regimen on vertebral fracture occurrence in post-menopausal osteoporosis; comparison with conventional therapy. *N. Engl. J. Med.*, **306**, 446–50.

Rubinstein, A.H., Levin, N.W. and Elliot, G.A. (1962). Manganese-induced hypoglycaemia. *Lancet*, **ii**, 1348–51.

Salet, J., Polonovski, C., de Gouyon, F., Pean, G., Melekian, B. and Fournet, J-P. (1966). Tetanie hypocalcemique recidivante par hypomagnesemie congenitale. Une maladie metabolique nouvelle. *Arch.Fr. pediat.*, **23**, 749–68.

Sandstead, H.H., Prasad, A.S., Schulert, A.R., Farid, Z., Miale, A., Bassilly, S. and Darby, A.J. (1967). Human zinc deficiency, endocrine manifestations and responses to therapy. *Am. J. Clin. Nut.*, **20**, 422–42.

Saner, G. (1980). *Chromium in nutrition and disease*. A.R. Liss: New York.

Schubert, W.K. and Lahey, M.E. (1959). Copper and protein deficiency complicating hypoferric anaemia of infancy. *Paediatrics*, **24**, 710–33.

Schwartz, K. (1974). Recent dietary trace element research exemplified by tin, fluoride and silicon. *Fed. Proc.*, **33**, 1748–57.

Shelp, W.D., Steele, T.H., De Luca, H.F. and Reiselbach, R.E. (1966). Influence of exogenous parahormone on urate and magnesium excretion in normal man. *Clin. Res.*, **14**, 448.

Spranger, J.W., Langer, L.O. and Wiedemann, H.R. (1974). *Bone Dysplasias*. W.B. Saunders Co.: Philadelphia.

Silver, J., Rubinger, D., Friedlaender, M.M. and Popovtzer, M.M. (1983). Sodium dependent idiopathic hypercalciuria in renal-stone formers. *Lancet*, **ii**, 484–6.

Stamp, T.C.B. (1972) Phosphorus metabolism in humans. M.D. Thesis, University of Cambridge.

Stamp, T.C.B. (1975). Factors in human vitamin D nutrition and in the production and cure of classical rickets. *Proc. Nut. Soc.*, **34**, 119–30.

Stamp, T.C.B. (1982). The clinical endocrinology of vitamin D. In *Endocrinology of Calcium Metabolism*, pp. 363–422. Ed. Parsons, J.A. Raven Press: New York.

Stamp, T.C.B., Flanagan, R.J., Richens, A., Round, J.M., Thomas, M., Jackson, M., Dupré, P. and Twigg, C.A. (1978). Anticonvulsant Osteomalacia. In *Endocrinology of Calcium Metabolism*, pp. 16–22 Int. Cong. Ser. 421. Eds. Copp, D.H. and Talmage, R.V. Excerpta Medica: Amsterdam.

Stamp, T.C.B., Haddad, J.G.Jr. and Twigg, C.A. (1977). Comparison of oral 25-hydroxycholecalciferol, vitamin D and ultraviolet light as determinants of circulating 25-hydroxyvitamin D. *Lancet*, **i**, 1341–3.

Stamp, T.C.B. and Round, J.M. (1974). Seasonal changes in human plasma levels of 25-hydroxycholecalciferol. *Nature*, **247**, 563–5.

Stanbury, S.W. (1976). Intestinal absorption of calcium and phosphorus in adult man in health and disease. In *Inborn Errors of Calcium and Bone Metabolism*, pp. 21–8. Eds. Bickel, H. and Stern, J. Medical and Technical Publishing: Lancaster.

Sturgeon, P. and Brubaker, C. (1956). Copper deficiency in infants; a syndrome characterized by hypocupremia, iron deficiency anaemia and hypoproteinemia. *Am. Med. Assoc. J. Dis. Child.*, **92**, 254–65.

Suh, S.M., Tashjian, A.H., Matsuo, N., Parkinson, D.K. and Fraser, D. (1973) Pathogenesis of hypocalcaemia in primary hypomagnesaemia: normal end-organ responsiveness to parathyroid hormone, impaired parathyroid gland function. *J. Clin. Invest.*, **52**, 153–60.

Sunderman, F.W. and Sunderman, F.W. Jr. (1967). Chemical measurement of magnesium in biological fluids. In *The Clinical Biology of the Serum Electrolytes*, pp. 56–60. Eds. Sunderman, F.W. and Sunderman, F.W. Jr, C.C. Thomas: Springfield, Ilinois.

Tanaka, Y. and De Luca, H.F. (1973). The control of 25-hydroxyvitamin D metabolism by inorganic phosphorus. *Arch. Biochem. Biophys.*, **154**, 566–74.

Teotia, S.P.S. and Teotia, M. (1973). Secondary hyperparathyroidism in patients with endemic skeletal fluorosis. *Br. Med. J.*, **1**, 637–40.

Tipton, I.H. and Cook, M.J. (1963). Trace elements in human tissue. Part II. Adult subjects from the United States. *Hlth. Phys.*, **9**, 103–45.

Tschöpe, W., Ritz, E. and Schellenberg, B. (1980). Plasma phosphate and urinary calcium in recurrent stone formers. *Min. Elect. Metab.*, **4**, 237–45.

Underwood, E.J. (1977) *Trace Elements in Human and Animal Nutrition*, 4th ed. Academic Press: New York

Vallee, B. and Wacker, W.E.C. (1970). *Metalloproteins. The Proteins*, vol. V. Ed. Neurath, H. Academic Press: New York.

Van Campen, D.R. and Kowalski, T.T. (1971). Studies on zinc absorption: 65Zn binding by homogenates of rat intestinal mucosa. *Proc. Soc. Exptl. Biol. and Med.*, **136**, 294–7.

van Rij, A.M., Thomson, C.D., McKenzie, J.M. and Robinson, M.F. (1979). Selenium deficiency in total parenteral nutrition. *Am. J. Clin. Nut.*, **32**, 2076–85.

Vaughan, J.M. (1975). *The Physiology of Bone*, 2nd ed. Oxford University Press: Oxford. Versieck, J., Barbier, F., Speecke, A. and Hoste, J. (1975). Influence of myocardial infarction on serum manganese, copper and zinc concentrations. *Clin. Chem.*, **21**, 578–81.

Wacker, W.E.B. and Parisi, A.F. (1968). Magnesium metabolism. *New Engl. J. Med.*, **278**, 658–63; 712–17; 772–6.

Wadman, S.K., Duran, M., Beemer, F.A., Cats, B.P., Johnson, J.L., Rajagopalan, K.V., Saudubray, J.M., Ogier, H., Charpentier, C., Berger, R., Smit, G.P.A., Wilson, J. and Krywaych, S. (1983). Absence of hepatic molybdenum cofactor: an inborn error of metabolism leading to a combined deficiency of sulphite oxidase and xanthine dehydrogenase. In *Trace Metals and Inherited Metabolic Disease*, pp. 78–83. Eds. Addison, G.M., Harkness, R.A. and Pollitt, R.J. *J. Inher. Metab. Dis.*, *6*. (suppl. 1). MTP Press: Lancaster.

Walser, M. (1961). Ion association VI. Interaction between calcium, magnesium, inorganic phosphate, citrate and protein in normal human plasma. *J. Clin. Invest.*, **40**, 723–30.

Wasserman, R.H. and Comar, C.L. (1961). The parathyroids and the intestinal absorption of calcium, strontium and phosphate ions in the rat. *Endocrinology*, **69**, 1074–9.

Wasserman, R.H., Taylor, A.N. and Fullmer, C.S. (1974). Vitamin D-induced calcium-binding protein and the intestinal absorption of calcium. In *The Metabolism and Function of Vitamin D*, pp. 55–74. Ed. Fraser, D.R. Biochem. Soc. Special. Publ., No. 3: London,

Watts, R.W.E., Chalmers, R.A., Gibbs, D.A., Lawson, A.M., Purkiss, P. and Spellacy, E. (1979). Studies on some possible biochemical treatments of primary hyperoxaluria. *Q. J. Med.*, **48**, 259–72.

W.H.O. (1970). Fluorides and human health. *World Health Organization (Monograph Series, No. 59)*: Geneva.

W.H.O. (1973) Trace elements in human nutrition. *Wld. Hlth. Org. Techn. Rep. Ser. No. 532.*

Wiberg, J.S. and Neuman, W.F. (1957). The binding of bivalent metals by deoxyribonucleic and ribonucleic acids. *Arch. Biochem. Biophys.*, **72**, 66–83.

Williams, R.J.P. and Wacker, W.E.C. (1967). Cation balance in biological systems. *J. Am. Med. Assoc.*, **201**, 96–100.

Willet, W.C., Polk, B.F., Morris, J.S., Stampfer, M.J., Pressel, S., Rosner, B., Taylor, J.O., Schneider, K. and Hames, C.G. (1983). Prediagnostic serum selenium and risk of cancer. *Lancet*, **ii**, 130–34.

Wills, M.R. and Savory, J. (1983). Aluminium poisoning: dialysis encephalopathy, osteomalacia and anaemia. *Lancet*, **ii**, 29–34.

Yendt, E.R. (1970). Vitamin D: part II. In *International Encyclopedia of Pharmacology and Therapeutics*, pp. 139–95. Section 51. vol. 1. Parathyroid Hormone, Thyrocalcitonin and Related Drugs. Ed. Rasmussen, H. Pergamon Press: Oxford.

Young, V.R. (1981). Selenium; a case for its essentiality in man. *N. Engl. J. Med.*, **304**, 1228–30.

# 15 Nutrition and disorders of the nervous system

John W.T. Dickerson



## Introduction

Normal function in the nervous system is dependent upon an adequate intake and availability of nutrients. The brain, however, differs from other organs like the liver in that it is dependent upon a continuous supply of nutrients, because its capacity for storage is extremely limited. There is, for instance, only a very small, and in energetic terms negligible, amount of glycogen and no detectable neutral fat in the brain. On the other hand, in states of depletion certain of the vitamins, e.g. thiamine, appear to be retained longer in the brain than in almost any other organ.

There are other specific properties of the brain that have relevance to the relationship of nutrition to disturbances in function. Thus, this organ achieves most of its growth early in life, growing most rapidly at a time which differs with respect to birth in different mammalian species (Davison and Dobbing, 1966) but in all species having a growth spurt that is very closely related to chronological age. Moreover, its capacity for growth after this time is extremely limited, and for practical purposes may be negligible. This has profound implications when the effects of nutrition on the brain of the fetus and young child are considered, for damage caused by nutrient deficiencies at this time of life may well be permanent. Furthermore, it is particularly at this period of its growth and development that the brain is affected by its hormonal environment and by the input received from the five senses. The normal growth and development of the brain is, therefore, the result of a complex interplay of all these factors. A discussion of hormonal influences on brain growth and development is outside the scope of this chapter, but it is often difficult to isolate sensory from nutritional deprivation in its effects on the developing brain. Furthermore, the defective structure and function caused by nutritional inadequacy may, in certain conditions, be offset by increased sensory stimulation.

It is well known that the brain of the adult is 'protected' from the effects of noxious and foreign substances that enter the body by virtue of what has long been known as the 'blood-brain barrier'. Dobbing (1968*a*) has emphasized the selective nature of this barrier. Moreover, with respect to its lipid, i.e. its structural components, the adult organ is relatively metabolically inert. It is because of this that the adult brain, in contrast to the developing organ, is resistant to the effects of undernutrition (Dobbing, 1968*b*).

The metabolic compartments of the brain, are, however, highly active, and the entry of substances like amino acids into the free pool is regulated by transport processes similar to those that regulate their transport across the intestinal mucosal cells. These processes are, to some extent, influenced by nutrition and the understanding of this is opening up new possibilities for regulating the availability, or synthesis, of neurotransmitters in the brain, and hence for a possible role for nutrition in the treatment of disorders caused by disturbances in their metabolism.

## Effects of malnutrition on the growth and development of the brain

A number of studies have demonstrated retarded behavioural and mental development in children malnourished in early life (Cravioto and Robles, 1965; Cravioto *et al.*, 1966). Furthermore, the use of appropriate chemical 'markers' has shown that the brains of children who died with protein-energy malnutrition (PEM) contain too few cells, and too little myelin for their chronological age, although probably not for the weight of the brain (Rosso *et al.*, 1970; Winick *et al.*, 1970; Dickerson, 1975). The brains of such children also show evidence of greatly retarded dendritic development (Dickerson *et al.*, 1982). It is tempting to conclude that these structural deficiencies in the brains of malnourished children are a direct consequence of nutritional deprivation, particularly since they are also found in the brains of malnourished experimental animals. Such a direct consequence is, however, by no means certain. Cravioto *et al.*, (1966) drew attention to the complexity of the problem, and to the many factors which operate in an impoverished environment to result in poor growth. The complex interaction of these multiple environmental factors on children in poor countries cannot be ignored (Pollitt and Thomson, 1977; Cravioto and Delicardie, 1979). The condition is also complex in animal experiments for alterations in behaviour and intelligence can follow quite mild undernutrition and may not be closely linked with 'vulnerable periods' (Smart, 1977).

Animal experiments have provided abundant evidence that the effects of undernutrition on the structural components of the brain are likely to be permanent if the nutritional insult occurs at the time of the growth spurt (Davison and Dobbing, 1966). Evidence (Dobbing and Sands, 1973) suggests that the growth spurt of the human brain may extend to two years after birth, and that it remains vulnerable during this time. Support for this conclusion was provided by the study of Hertzig *et al.*, (1972) on the mental development of Jamaican children hospitalized for malnutrition at different ages. There was no correlation of the deficit in mental development with age of hospitalization in the first two years of life.

In rats, the feeding of low protein diets after 21 days of age, i.e. after the brain has completed its growth spurt, results in a changed pattern of free amino acids in the organ (Dickerson and Pao, 1975). The importance of these changes lies in the fact that some of the amino acids are themselves neurotransmitters, or are the precursors of neurotransmitters, and that protein synthesis is impaired. Because of the rapidity with which the composition of the free amino acid pool changes after death, it may not be possible to do similar studies in the brains of malnourished children, but the fact that the changes in the concentrations of amino acids in the brain were paralleled by changes in the concentrations of those in the plasma similar to those found in the plasma of children with PEM makes it reasonable to suppose that these, too, would have a deranged pattern in the brain.

Furthermore, the fact that these changes in amino acids occurred after the completion of the growth spurt is perhaps a warning against complacency about possible effects of poor nutrition on the brain function of the pre-school, or even school-child. This clearly has implications for the socially impoverished in all societies. More attention may also need to be paid to the question of the interaction of nutrition and brain function in those children with the malabsorption syndrome accompanied by some degree of growth retardation.

Even in affluent societies, a number of babies are born who for various reasons have been malnourished *in utero* – the 'light for dates' babies. These babies have brains that are too small for their chronological age, although they are relatively too large for their body weight. Present evidence suggests that the capacity for 'catch-up' is good providing that adequate nutrition in the form of amino acids and glucose is given to the baby within the first few hours of birth. This underlines the importance of the antenatal diagnosis of fetal malnutrition. In rats, deficiencies of specific nutrients such as zinc, manganese, and possibly magnesium during pregnancy have adverse effects on the fetus. There is also evidence of an association of malformations of the central nervous system (CNS), particularly spina bifida, with vitamin deficiencies during early pregnancy (Smithells *et al.*, 1981) and there is evidence to suggest that folic acid deficiency may be responsible (Laurence *et al.*, 1981).

The important question to be answered as far as the brain function of malnourished children is concerned is whether there is capacity for recovery, and to define conditions in which this is likely to be achieved. Of particular interest and importance in this connection are those studies involving an enrichment of the environment. These studies have flowed from the hypothesis that malnutrition and environmental deprivation act synergistically to isolate the infant from the sensory input which is necessary for normal development (Levitsky and Barnes, 1972). Attempts have been made to modify the subsequent environment by keeping the child longer in hospital on a programme of sensory stimulation, or by sending the child home and enrolling it in a special school programme designed to provide enriched experience. Both approaches are successful as long as they are sustained, but reversal occurs when they are stopped (McLaren *et al.*, 1973). A study which provides the most encouraging directive for the future of malnourished children is that carried out by Winick and his colleagues on the effects of early adoption of Korean children into primarily middle-class American homes (Winick *et al.*, 1975). This study showed that severely malnourished children who were adopted before the age of 3 years (mean age 18 months) caught up in height and weight and achieved an IQ and school achievement level that was perfectly normal for children reared in an industrialized society.

For further discussion of the relationship of malnutrition to brain growth and function the reader is referred to the following publications: Birch and Gussow (1970); Manocha (1972); Prescott *et al.*, (1975); Winick (1976); Dickerson, (1981); Dickerson *et al.*, (1982); Brozek and Schürch (1984).

## Relationship of specific nutrients to neurological disorders

### Vitamins

#### The fat-soluble vitamins

Vitamin A deficiency is widespread in many parts of the world and is the largest single cause of blindness in India, South-East Asia, and parts of Central and South America. Blindness results from irreversible keratinizing changes on the conjunctiva and cornea, and finally from keratomalacia. However, before these changes occur, early, but far less dramatic, evidence of vitamin A deficiency is shown by impaired adaptation to vision in the dark (McLaren, 1967). This is said to be evident when the plasma level of vitamin A falls below 150 μg/litre (Hume and Krebs, 1949).

Puppies born to pregnant dogs fed a vitamin A-deficient diet show obstructive hydrocephalus. There is no evidence that this occurs in man. In the classic experiments of Mellanby (1950), puppies fed vitamin A-deficient diets were blind and deaf. These abnormalities were caused by defective bone remodelling of the skull and vertebrae. Raised intracranial pressure has been attributed to hypovitaminosis A (Bass and Caplan, 1955). However,the usual association of raised intracranial pressure and hydrocephalus is with hypervitaminosis A, and may occur in Eskimos who consume polar bear liver with its very high concentration (10 000 μg/g) of vitamin A. Hypervitaminosis A during pregnancy has also been associated with malformations of the CNS in the fetus (Gal *et al.*, 1972).

In severe rickets, the frontal bones may not only fail to unite, but the skull may fail to grow so that the child is microcephalic. In the adult with vitamin D deficiency, muscle weakness may at times antedate changes in the bones (Dent, 1956). Agnes Scott (1916) was probably the first to describe proximal muscle weakness in osteomalacic women in India. In a later detailed study, also in India (Dastur *et al.*, 1972), muscle weakness, initially affecting the pelvic and truncal muscles, was described in 11 women with nutritional osteomalacia, 9 of whom were Muslims. Treatment with vitamin D resulted in early improvement in bone pain and subsequently in muscle power.

A detailed survey at University College Hospital of patients with osteomalacia and with hyperthyroidism (Smith and Stern, 1967) showed that unequivocal muscle weakness was present in 20 out of 45 patients with osteomalacia due to a variety of causes. Present evidence clearly incriminates vitamin D in the aetiology of the myopathy, but the mechanism seems at present to be unclear.

A deficiency of vitamin E has been implicated in the aetiology of the neurological features of abetalipoproteinaemia (Bassen–Kornzweig syndrome). The original link with vitamin E rested on the finding of unrecordable levels of the vitamin in the blood of patients with the syndrome (Kayden *et al.*, 1965), on the occurrence of disorders of the nervous system in rats fed a vitamin E-deficient diet, and on the occurrence of histological changes in the brains of children with defective fat absorption and thus, presumably, reduced absorption of vitamin E. Discussing the evidence for this link between vitamin E and the syndrome, Pallis and Lewis (1974) concluded that it was very tenuous. However, vitamin E is an antioxidant, and deficiency of the vitamin could play a role in the deposition of the intraneuronal pigment, lipofuscin, which has been reported in one autopsied case of the Bassen–Kornzweig syndrome, and which also occurs in the brains of rats fed a vitamin E-deficient diet. There is experimental evidence that feeding rats a diet containing supplemental vitamin E reduces the accumulation of lipofuscin (Rudra *et al.*, 1975). This finding could have some potential significance for man because increased accumulation of this pigment in the brain in old age may be incriminated in senile dementia.

Vitamin E also plays a role in the maintenance of the stability of cell membranes, and Molenaar *et al.*, (1968) have reported an improvement in the appearance of the intracellular membranes of the jejunal epithelium of two patients with the Bassen–Kornzweig syndrome.

### The water-soluble vitamins

Neurological disorders are found in a small proportion of alcoholics and are a direct result of nutritional deficiencies. Peripheral neuropathy is caused principally by a deficiency of thiamine (Fennelly *et al.*, 1964), but deficiencies of other vitamins of the B group (pyridoxine, nicotinic acid, or pantothenic acid) may produce identical signs. It has been estimated that in the United States the condition is found in almost 10 per cent of hospitalized alcoholics (Victor, 1971). Response to treatment with thiamine is variable, and in some patients a neuropathy may persist due to irreversible neurological damage.

Wernicke's encephalopathy develops in alcoholics who have a low intake of thiamine and of normal foodstuffs combined with persistent vomiting. Some of the signs of this condition may disappear with treatment with high doses of vitamins, but there may be persistent evidence of cerebral damage. A large proportion of patients surviving Wernicke's encephalopathy develop Korsakoff's psychosis. The recommended doses of vitamins to be used in treatment are: thiamine, 1000 mg; riboflavin, 10 mg; pyridoxine, 400 mg; nicotinamide, 200 mg; and ascorbic acid, 1500 mg. Since there may be some hindrance to absorption from the alimentary tract, the preferred route of administration is by intravenous injection (Curran *et al.*, 1972). There is, however, some evidence from controlled studies that recovery time is not reduced by vitamin therapy (Victor, 1960). Korsakoff's psychosis may follow Wernicke's encephalopathy due to degeneration of the mamillary bodies. However, the memory disturbance of this condition is often strikingly improved by massive doses of thiamine usually with other vitamins of the B complex. It has been suggested that the difference between Wernicke's encephalopathy and Korsakoff's psychosis is only in the age of the glial and vascular lesions, and that the disease should be referred to as the Wernicke–Korsakoff syndrome (Victor, 1971).

A disorder of the optic nerves may develop either alone or in conjunction with the Wernicke–Korsakoff syndrome. This disorder generally responds to a good diet supplemented with B group vitamins.

Although usually considered a complication of alcoholism, the Wernicke–Korsakoff syndrome may occur as a complication of any gastrointestinal disease in which there is severe vomiting, independent of alcoholism (Pallis and Lewis, 1974). The syndrome has been reported in patients with carcinoma of the stomach, carcinoma of the head of the pancreas and rectum, metastatic melanoma of the stomach and with post-operative peritonitis, intestinal obstruction, 'chronic gastritis', and ascending cholangitis and gastric ulceration.

Many of the effects of vitamin deficiencies are somewhat non-specific for particular vitamins. This is true of the corneal vascularization which has been attributed to riboflavin deficiency. This disorder, often associated with lacyrymation and photophobia, angular stomatitis, vasolabial seborrhoea, and scrotal and vulval dermatitis, may respond to riboflavin supplements. Favourable response to supplements has also been reported for other corneal diseases including superficial punctate keratitis, corneal ulcer, and catarrhal infiltration (Stern, 1974).

Niacin deficiency causes pellagra, a disease which is characterized classically by the three 'D's – dermatitis, diarrhoea, and dementia. Irritability, headaches, sleeplessness, loss of memory, or other signs of emotional instability are often early clinical signs of niacin deficiency. In some cases psychoneurosis, dementia, and acute encephalopathy (Jolliffe's syndrome) may develop. Various other neurological disturbances such as peripheral neuropathy, myelopathy, and amblyopia have been described. It is difficult to isolate the signs due to pure niacin deficiency from those due to the multiple deficiencies that may develop in an anorectic patient. There is some indication of this in the response to therapy, for whereas the administration of niacin produces a striking and prompt improvement in the mental symptoms, it has no effect on symptoms of the peripheral nervous system, and may, in fact, exacerbate them (Pallis and Lewis, 1974). These symptoms have, in fact, been thought to be due to an associated thiamine deficiency. Jolliffe's syndrome is due to acute nicotinic acid deficiency and is characterized by clouding of consciousness, marked sucking, and grasping reflexes, and rigidity of the extrapyramidal type. Clinical signs of pellagra are often absent because there has not been time for them to develop. Jolliffe *et al.*, (1940) stressed that the syndrome more often occurred in chronic alcoholics and other malnourished individuals than in endemic pellagrins. It may occur in such patients when they develop acute intercurrent illnesses like pneumonia, lung abscess, perforated ulcer, or subarachnoid haemorrhage. From what has been said above about the association of both thiamine and niacin deficiencies with acute illness, it would seem that supplements of B-group vitamins might well constitute part of the therapy for these disorders, particularly in malnourished or elderly patients.

Epileptic seizures occur in animals maintained on a pyridoxine-free diet, and there is evidence that in man pyridoxine deficiency, particularly in infancy (Coursin, 1954), also causes seizures. The seizures are thought to result from a depression of the conversion of glutamic acid to $\gamma$-aminobutyric acid (GABA) by the pyridoxine-dependent enzyme, glutamic acid decarboxylase. Seizures may also be a symptom of isonicotinic acid hydrazide (INAH)-induced pyridoxine deficiency. A peripheral neuropathy, with symptoms of the 'burning feet' syndrome has been described in patients treated with INAH (Biehl and Vilter, 1954).

There is evidence from supplementation studies (Gopalan, 1946; Bibile *et al.*, 1957) that the 'burning feet' syndrome encountered in malnourished populations may be due to a deficiency of pantothenic acid. In normal circumstances a deficiency of this vitamin is most unlikely to occur because of its ubiquitous distribution in food. It has, however, been produced in human volunteers by the combined administration of a semi-synthetic diet and a pantothenic acid antagonist ($\omega$-methylpantothenic acid).

Vitamin $B_{12}$, or cyanocobalamin, is an essential nutrient for man. The clinical manifestations of deficiency, whether they be due to the diet itself, or to the inability to absorb the vitamin due to a deficiency of intrinsic factor, are seen in haemopoietic tissue, epithelial surfaces, and the nervous system. In the latter the deficiency produces profound changes in the peripheral nerves and spinal cord, but the biochemistry of the changes remains to be elucidated (Silber and Moldow, 1970). Pallis and Lewis (1974) have given an extensive review of the older cases reported in the literature and of the various clinical manifestations.

Peripheral neuropathy seems to be the least well known of the neurological signs of vitamin $B_{12}$ deficiency, but is perhaps the commonest. It may occur with, or without, evidence of myelopathy or subacute combined degeneration of the cord (SCD). Psychosis has been reported in patients with pernicious anaemia, but it seems that the two conditions may coexist rather than the psychosis be due to vitamin $B_{12}$ deficiency. On the other hand, optic neuritis is well known as a complication of the disease, although it is today a rarity. The treatment of the neurological complication of vitamin $B_{12}$ deficiency is the same as for pernicious anaemia except that the dose of cyanocobalamin should be two or three times as large as for uncomplicated cases.

Vitamin $B_{12}$ is only synthesized by microorganisms and is present in only minute amounts in *clean* vegetables. It follows that a dietary deficiency may occur in strict vegetarians (vegans) who do not consume any food of animal origin. However, myelopathy due to dietary vitamin $B_{12}$ deficiency is extremely rare, and in their review of the literature, Pallis and Lewis (1974) were able to find reports of only two cases. High folic acid status may reduce the requirement for vitamin $B_{12}$ (Sanders *et al.*, 1978). Vegetarians have lower serum $B_{12}$ values than non-vegetarians, but the difference seems to be of no clinical importance. Vitamin $B_{12}$ deficiency is almost always due to malabsorption of the vitamin. The situation is complicated by the fact that dietary folate and iron deficiency interfere with the ileal absorption of vitamin $B_{12}$.

The milk of vegan mothers contains a lower concentration of vitamin $B_{12}$ than that of omnivores, and there has been one report from India of encephalopathy in infants breast-fed by vegan mothers (Jadhav *et al.*, 1962).

Vitamin $B_{12}$ is, in some way, involved in the metabolism of cyanide, and it is possible, therefore, that in $B_{12}$ deficient subjects the plasma concentration may tend to rise excessively, particularly if they are heavy smokers. There is some evidence that Leber's optic atrophy is due to an inborn error of cyanide metabolism, and it has been suggested (Adams *et al.*, 1966) that massive doses of hydroxocobalamin may be of therapeutic value. Cyanide is detoxicated in the body by conversion to thiocyanate with sulphur derived from the sulphur-containing amino acids, methionine, cysteine, and cystine. Low levels of these amino acids have been found in patients with tropical or nutritional ataxic neuropathy whose staple diet was cassava which contains a cyanogenetic glycoside (Osuntokun *et al.*, 1968). There was no evidence of $B_{12}$ deficiency in these patients.

The relationship of folic acid to the nervous system, and to neurological disorders in particular, is still a matter of uncertainty, and the literature is somewhat misleading. The association of low folate status with a disorder in the same individual clearly does not mean that the relationship is causal. However, it seems possible that in patients with senile dementia a deficiency of folate and of the water soluble vitamins may contribute to the condition (Thomas *et al.*, 1986). Improvement of general nutritional status following folate supplementation may be a contributing factor to the clinical improvement of an elderly patient with dementia. The synthesis of the neurotransmitters, dopamine and noradrenaline, in the brain is dependent on the activity of tyrosine hydroxylase, and this is in turn regulated by the concentration of the hydroxylase cofactor tetrahydrobiopterin ($BH_4$). There is a defect in $BH_4$ metabolism in the brains of patients with senile dementia of the Alzheimer type (Barford *et al.*, 1984).

A report by Manzoor and Runcie (1976) suggested that the relationship of folic acid deficiency to neuropathy should be taken seriously. Ten patients aged 52 to 93 years with a severe neurological disease clinically indistinguishable from subacute combined degeneration had normal serum vitamin $B_{12}$ levels but low serum folate concentrations ($< 1\ \mu g$/litre). Two weeks of treatment with oral folic acid (10 mg three times a day) caused an improvement in psyche and knee jerks returned in eight of the ten patients and six of the patients that had been bedfast. The authors were of the opinion that in patients with undiagnosed myelopathy with normal vitamin $B_{12}$ levels, folic acid supplementation is mandatory.

In patients presenting to general physicians with megaloblastic anaemia two-thirds of those with either vitamin $B_{12}$ or folic acid deficiency had neuropsychiatric disorders (Shorvon *et al.*, 1980). However, the fact that one-third of patients with deficiency of either vitamin severe enough to cause megaloblastic anaemia had no nervous system complications suggests that other factors may play a role in the evolution of such disorders (Reynolds, 1984).

The relationship of anticonvulsant therapy to folate metabolism is discussed elsewhere (p 409).

Ascorbic acid deficiency has been reported (Kinsman and Hood, 1971) to cause personality changes corresponding to the 'neurotic triad' of hysteria, depression and hypochondriasis. These changes preceded decreased psychomotor performance associated with decreased arousal and motivation.

### Minerals

Brain function and behaviour is affected by deficiencies of a number of minerals (Oberleas *et al.*, 1972). Severe iron deficiency anaemia could considerably interfere with the oxygen supply to the brain, and thus produce symptoms similar to those of anaemia, but there seems to be no quantitative information about these effects. Copper deficiency has not been described in man except in cases where its absorption from the gut is impaired as a result of sprue, lymphosarcoma, scleroderma, or kwashiorkor. Excess deposition of copper, along with iron, occurs in the brain of patients with Wilson's disease and is associated with impaired brain function. Brain function improves when the brain copper levels are reduced by treatment with a chelating agent such as penicillamine. Hypomagnesaemia is characterized by nervousness, anorexia, muscular twitchings, unsteady gait, increased salivation, frothing and muscular tetany. Convulsions may also occur. Neuromuscular signs of magnesium deficiency have been reported in a number of conditions including cancer, diabetic acidosis, chronic renal disease, congestive heart failure, epilepsy, and pancreatitis. It also occurs in chronic alcoholics and in post-operative patients fed parenterally with solutions not containing magnesium. A deficiency of zinc causes apathy, anorexia, lethargy, and hypomagnesaemia in children (Hambidge *et al.*, 1972). Patients respond to oral zinc sulphate (1–2 mg $ZnSO_4$/kg). Pica, manifested by geophagia, has been associated with zinc deficiency and there is evidence that this may respond dramatically to dietary zinc supplementation (Hambidge and Silverman, 1973).

Lead is an enzyme poison which occurs as a pollutant in the environment. In high doses it has serious effects on the central nervous system, but chronic entry of the element into the body, either as the result of oral ingestion, or by inhalation through the lungs, causes elevated levels of lead in the blood which are associated with hyperactivity or hyperkinesis, particularly in children (David *et al.*, 1972), and the percentage of children having this disorder is higher in cities than in rural areas (Rutter, 1973). According to a review by Bryce-Smith and Waldron (1974), children having blood lead levels greater than 250 μg/litre who are hyperactive for no known cause can be completely cured of their hyperactivity, and improved in their general conduct, by treatment with penicillamine or calcium EDTA.

## Nutrition, mental retardation and psychiatric disorders

### Down's syndrome

The life expectancy of patients with trisomy 21 remains less than that of the general population (Oster *et al.*, 1975) but is steadily increasing, probably due to better standards of care. Deficiencies of both water and fat-soluble vitamins (Matin *et al.*, 1981) and minerals (Barlow *et al.*, 1981) have been reported in adults with Down's syndrome. There is also evidence of abnormal vitamin $B_6$ metabolism in this condition (Coburn *et al.*, 1983). It seems possible that such deficiencies may result from malabsorption rather than dietary lack since xylose absorption was found to be low (Williams *et al.*, 1985). These findings apparently lend support to the possibility that nutritional supplements might benefit Down's syndrome subjects. Harrell *et al.*, (1981) reported improvements in I.Q. in eight mentally subnormal children, five of whom had Down's syndrome, after receiving large doses of multivitamins for eight months. An attempt (Smith *et al.*, 1983) to repeat this study failed to reproduce the findings. A similar study (Ellman *et al.*, 1984) of vitamin-mineral supplements failed to improve the I.Q. of mentally retarded young adults. Most of the studies of the effects of supplements in Down's syndrome have used amounts of vitamins and minerals greatly in excess of those contained in a normal diet, that is, they were so-called 'mega' amounts. It is therefore of particular interest that an oral non-pharmacological supplement of zinc (1 mg zinc /kg body weight/day) has been reported (C. Franceschi, personal communication) to improve immunocompetence and reduce infection rate in children with Down's syndrome.

## Alzheimer's disease and senile dementia

The disease known as Alzheimer's disease is so named after the German neurologist who first described the condition in 1907. For a long time the disease was considered to be a presenile dementia but in recent years it has become clear that the brains of most old people who die with dementia show the characteristic signs of Alzheimer's disease. It is of considerable interest that individuals with Down's syndrome show evidence of Alzheimer's disease earlier in life (Sylvester, 1984). Interest in a link with nutrition in this disease stems from the finding that the hippocampus and cerebral cortex of patients with Alzheimer's disease contain low levels (as little as 10 per cent of control values) of the enzyme choline acetyltransferase which catalyses the synthesis of acetylcholine from its precursors choline and acetyl coenzyme A.

More recently there has been interest in the possibility that serotoninergic transmission may also be depressed in at least some patients with senile dementia. Low plasma levels of tryptophan, the precursor of serotonin, have been reported (Shaw *et al.*, 1981) in patients with senile dementia. These observations have been confirmed (Thomas *et al.*, 1986) and evidence of nutritional deficiencies, particularly of thiamine, ascorbic acid and folic acid have been found. Whilst these cannot be the cause of senile dementia, they may nevertheless contribute to the clinical picture by modifying the manifestations of other metabolic abnormalities. It remains to be shown whether patients with senile dementia will respond to vitamin supplements. A preliminary study (Shaw *et al.*, unpublished observation) has yielded encouraging results.

## Depression

Tryptophan plays a key role in brain function by virtue of the fact that it is a precursor of 5-HT (Fig. 15.1). There is some evidence that brain amine metabolism may be disturbed in some kinds of depression, and that defective synthesis of 5-HT may be involved (Lapin and Oxenkrug, 1969). Indeed, low levels of 5-HT (Shaw *et al.*, 1967) and its metabolite, 5-hydroxyindoleacetic acid (5-HIAA) (Bourne *et al.*, 1968), have been reported in the hind-brain of depressive suicides. Women with depressive illness have been reported to have very significantly reduced plasma concentrations of free, but not total, tryptophan (Coppen *et al.*, 1973).

Oral doses of L-tryptophan have been used in the treatment of depression (Coppen *et al.*, 1967). The claim that L-tryptophan on its own may be effective has been critically examined (Carroll, 1972) and it seems that it does not possess significant antidepressant properties in severely ill patients. In a further study (Herrington *et al.*, 1974) administration of doses of L-tryptophan of up to 8 g per day was found not to be as effective as other treatments, including electroconvulsive therapy. Interest in this treatment now centres on the possible role of three factors; tryptophan, nicotinamide, and pyridoxine. In some patients the administration of 5 g L-tryptophan per day may cause a remission of depression in about two weeks (Winston, 1975), and a dose of 3 g of L-tryptophan per day may be effective if combined with nicotinamide (MacSweeney, 1975), since this vitamin inhibits the activity of tryptophan pyrrolase (Young and Sourkes, 1974; Badawy and Evans, 1975) and blocks the metabolism of tryptophan along the kynurenine pathway. We have seen elsewhere that pyridoxine supplements may cause remission of depression in some women taking oral contraceptives of the combined oestrogen-progestogen type. When pyridoxine is combined with 5 g L-tryptophan, however, in the treatment of depression, the disorder is exacerbated (Winston, 1975).

The rate at which amines are synthesized in the brain depends on the

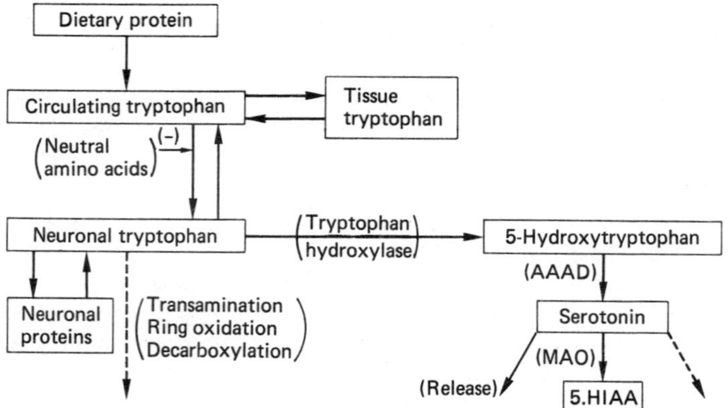


Fig. 15.1 Control of serotonin synthesis in brain neurons (Wurtman and Fernstrom, 1975). AAAD, aromatic L-amino acid decarboxylase; MAO, monoamine oxidase; ---- indicates unproved pathway.

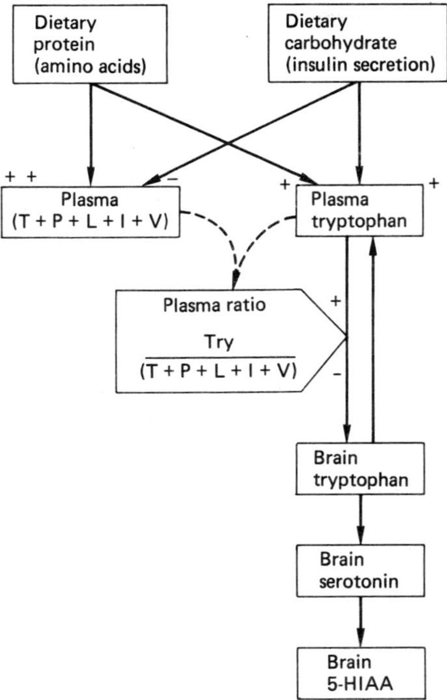


Fig. 15.2 Proposed interaction of dietary protein and dietary carbohydrate in regulating brain serotonin concentrations in the rat (Wurtman and Fernstrom, 1975). The entry of tryptophan into the brain is thought to be regulated by the ratio of the concentration of tryptophan (Try) in the plasma to the combined concentrations of tyrosine (T), phenylalanine (P), leucine (L), isoleucine (I) and valine (V).

amount of the precursor amino acid entering the blood-stream and also on the regulation of the passage of the amino acid into the brain (see Wurtman and Fernstrom, 1975). Thus, entry of tryptophan into the brain is suppressed by feeding protein which contributes to plasma considerably larger amounts of neutral amino acids (e.g. leucine, phenylalanine) which compete with tryptophan (see Fig. 15.1) whereas entry is facilitated by feeding carbohydrate, or giving insulin (Fig. 15.2) (Dickerson and Pao, 1975). It is of interest that a survey of 215 healthy dentists and their wives suggested that the higher the tryptophan intake, the better the psychic rating (Cheraskin and Ringsdorf, 1971).

Patients suffering from endogenous depression have been found to have significantly greater proportions of long chain polyunsaturated fatty acids, docosahexaenoic acid and eicosapentaenoic acid and a reduced proportion of linoleic acid in their plasma choline phosphoglycerides compared with those in age-sex-matched healthy controls (Fehily *et al.*, 1981). Similar, but smaller, changes were found in red cell membranes. There was no evidence that these changes were due to diet.

Changes in mood may be associated with anticonvulsant-induced folate depletion (Reynolds, 1967; Trimble *et al.*, 1980). Up to one-third of psychiatric in-patients (Thornton and Thornton, 1977) and a higher proportion of psychogeriatric patients (Runcie, 1979) had folate deficiency associated with depression and dementia. Whilst in some patients the folate deficiency was probably secondary to a poor diet, in others a primary role for folate deficiencies was possible. Clearly, the role of folate deficiency in depression merits further investigation, particularly in the light of the fact that methyl folate may exert a modulatory role on neurotransmission (Hommes *et al.*, 1979).

Physiological variations of the choline content of the diet, within the range that omnivorous humans may consume from day to day, are associated with parallel changes in brain acetylcholine concentrations in the rat (Cohen and Wurtman, 1976). This clearly raises the possibility of the dietary treatment of disorders in which there is defective acetylcholine synthesis such as tardive dyskinesia (Davis *et al.*, 1975) and also the use of diet to raise the potency of drugs acting at cholinergic synapses.

In a study of elderly people receiving 'meals on wheels' (Davies, *et al.*, 1973), 69% of the subjects had daily potassium intakes below the recommended minimum of 60 mmol (2.3g) per day (Judge, 1968). A blind assessment for depression by a psychiatrist showed that 35 of the subjects considered to be depressed had a lower mean energy intake (1600 kcal) than the remainder (1920 kcal). There was a highly significant correlation between depression and low potassium intake. The authors pointed out that this did not establish a cause and effect relationship, for it could be that depression caused the individual to take a monotonous low energy diet which resulted in potassium depletion, rather than that the depression was the direct result of the diet.

Studies in a Psychiatric Hospital (Horwitt *et al.*, 1946) showed that patients receiving a diet yielding 2200 kcal, but containing only 400 μg of thiamine, gradually restricted their activity with increased dulling of interest and ambition. There was also a diminished desire to please and a lessened tendency to bantering and playfulness. The psychiatric complaints of patients transferred to a low (200 μg) thiamine diet also became exaggerated and changes in behaviour obvious.

## Schizophrenia

It seems clear that there is a genetic predisposition towards the development of schizophrenia because relatives of schizophrenics are afflicted with the disease more frequently than members of the general population. This suggests a metabolic basis for the disease and quite a bit of literature exists describing biochemical changes in this condition. Difficulty in the interpretation of some of the studies arises from the problem of diagnosis, and in some of the older studies from the fact that the patients were malnourished and had abnormal liver function. Modern drugs, such as the phenothiazines used in the treatment of schizophrenia, appear to have resulted in patients having a predisposition towards obesity rather than the reverse.

Tryptophan metabolism, or the uptake of the amino acid into the brain, may be deranged in some forms of schizophrenia (Frohman *et al.*, 1969; Gottlieb and Frohman, 1974). These observations may not be unconnected with the claim that high doses of niacin have proved beneficial in some cases of schizophrenia (*see* Hoffer, 1973). This form of treatment, which still awaits adequate evaluation, is a development of Pauling's 'orthomolecular' concept (Pauling, 1968), and involves the administration of large amounts of a number of vitamins. Some psychiatrists practising orthomolecular therapy adjust the doses of the vitamins to suit the individual patient, and use the vitamins as an adjuvant to normal drug therapy, making it possible to reduce the level of intake of the drugs.

Autism has been considered by some to be a childhood form of schizophrenia, and again as with schizophrenia, criteria for its diagnosis are by no means uniform with different clinicians, and it is doubtful if all children treated as 'autistic' fulfil the criteria laid down by Rutter (1974). However, Rimland (1973) reported the results of a trial in which about 300 autistic children were treated with daily doses of vitamin C (1.0 g), nicotinamide (1.0 g), pyridoxine (150 mg), and pantothenic acid (200 mg) together with small amounts of iron, inositol, thiamine, folic acid, and vitamin $B_{12}$. Reports are available on 190 of these children and showed that 45 per cent showed 'definite improvement' and a further 41 per cent a 'possible improvement'. A 'double-blind' trial of this form of therapy has been carried out by Dr Rimland and Professor Dreyfus of the Department of Neurology, University of California, and has fully confirmed the previous findings (Rimland, personal communication).

The incidence of new cases of schizophrenia differed in countries where food rationing was imposed during the Second World War, and those in which such rationing was not necessary (Dohan, 1966a), and this has led to the suggestion of a link between wheat consumption and schizophrenia. Coeliac disease, which is caused by a fraction of wheat gliadin (Townley *et al.*, 1973) has a higher incidence in patients with schizophrenia than in the general population (Dohan, 1966b). In a clinical trial of their hypothesis (Dohan *et al.*, 1969), schizophrenics were reported to improve more rapidly on a milk and cereal-free diet. These observations have been confirmed (Singh and Kay, 1976) in a study in which 14 schizophrenics were kept in a locked research ward with strict dietary control. A reversal of therapeutic progress which was not due to variations in doses of neuroleptic drugs, was noted when the patients were challenged with wheat gluten.

## Hyperactivity or hyperkinesis

Behaviour disorders are not uncommon in children and as long ago as 1945, Schneider suggested that they might be caused by food. Kittler (1970) described some children with 'minimal brain dysfunction' whose difficult behaviour had improved when certain foods, such as chocolate and milk, were excluded. In the US such children would be described as 'hyperactive'. Indeed, the hyperactive child syndrome has included other conditions such as 'minimal brain damage', 'hyperactivity' or 'hyperkinesis' and 'overactivity'. In the UK child psychiatrists recognize the hyperkinetic syndrome as a condition characterized by hyperactivity, impulsivity, intractability and excitability (Sandberg *et al.*, 1978).

It is perhaps necessary for a nutritionist who may be approached by a parent for help with a hyperactive child to appreciate something of the difficulties in arriving at a diagnosis of the hyperactivity syndrome. The term 'hyperactive' is also used to describe children who are badly behaved, unruly and find it very difficult to be attentive and keep still. Thus, it becomes necessary to distinguish between the true hyperactivity syndrome and hyperactivity as a symptom.

The condition has attracted considerable attention since Feingold (1975) claimed that 30–50 per cent of hyperactive children show significant improvement in behaviour when placed on a special diet eliminating foods containing salicylates and additives, particularly dyes and flavours. A number of attempts have been made to investigate Feingold's hypothesis (*see* Dickerson and Pepler, 1980) with at best equivocal results. However, these investigations have been criticized on a number of counts (Rippere, 1983). It is difficult on the basis of this published work to see how the US Nutrition Foundation could confidently state that studies 'provide sufficient evidence to refute the claim that artificial flavourings and natural salicylates produce hyperactivity'.

It would rather seem prudent at present to state that Feingold's hypothesis remains unconfirmed.

It is a matter of empirical observation, however, that a number of children with a short attention span, tantrums and outbursts of aggressive behaviour improve when highly coloured fruit drinks and iced lollies, etc., are excluded from their diet. It seems clear that such children have an ideosyncratic response to certain additives. However, a wide variety of foods may cause hyperactivity in susceptible children. Thus, in a controlled trial (Egger *et al.*, 1985), involving 76 children, 62 were found to improve and 21 to achieve a normal range of behaviour on an oligoantigenic diet. Other symptoms, such as headaches, abdominal pain and fits also improved. A total of 48 foods were incriminated. Artificial colourants and preservatives were the commonest provoking substances but no child was sensitive to these alone. It was of interest that of the nine children who reacted to sugar, three reacted to cane sugar only and one to beet sugar only. Clearly, on the basis of this study the possibility that diet may be responsible for overactivity in children should be carefully investigated.

## Alcoholism

This subject is discussed in Chapter 20.

## Sleep

Two classes of sleep can be distinguished with reference to the EEG patterns. Non-REM sleep (NREM; REM stands for Rapid Eye Movements) is further divided into stages according to its EEG characteristics, varying from light to deep sleep, the depth being assessed by the threshold to an auditory stimulus. REM sleep is characterized by a low voltage EEG activity, similar to that found in light NREM sleep, presence of rapid eye movements (REM) and a marked fall in muscle activity. Crisp and Stonehill (1976) have reviewed their own contributions and those of others to the inter-relationship of sleep, nutrition, and mood.

It seems clear that the amount and kind of sleep can be affected by changes in body weight and by diet, and particularly by the amount of carbohydrate consumed. Subjects with anorexia nervosa experience changes in sleep pattern in the second half of the night which may be related to carbohydrate starvation (Crisp, 1967). Other patients with anorexia nervosa have achieved starvation by vomiting and lose protein as well as carbohydrates and other nutrients. These patients then suffer general starvation and are, in fact, the most restless.

There is a direct association between the concentration of free tryptophan in the blood and the amount of REM sleep (Chen *et al.*, 1974). As pointed out earlier, dietary carbohydrate affects blood tryptophan levels but also, and perhaps more importantly for the present discussion, by regulating the concentration of other amino acids, controls the entry of tryptophan into the brain (*see* Wurtman and Fernstrom, 1975; Fig. 15.2). It may be that the beneficial effect on the amount of sleep, and its depth, of a bedtime hot milk cereal drink reported by Southwell and Evans (1972), and Brezinova and Oswald (1972) is related to this mechanism. It is of interest, too, in this connection that Fara *et al.*, (1969) found that fat introduced into the duodenum of cats enhanced their sleep. Using isocaloric diets containing different ratios of carbohydrate and fat, Phillips and her colleagues (Phillips *et al.*, 1975) found that REM sleep was especially significantly increased by a high carbohydrate/low fat diet.

## Relationship of nutrition to other disorders of the nervous system

### Multiple sclerosis

The true aetiology of multiple sclerosis (MS) remains obscure. The geographical distribution of the disease strongly suggests that a dietary factor may be involved (Agranoff and Goldberg, 1974). Since the disease involves degeneration and destruction of myelin it seemed logical to suppose that lipids and, in particular, fatty acids might be involved. Thompson and his colleagues (Baker *et al.*, 1966) reported that the serum of patients with MS contained lower concentrations of linoleic acid than that of controls. These findings led to a double-blind trial of linoleic acid supplementation in London and Belfast (Millar *et al.*, 1973) and later in Newcastle (Bates *et al.*, 1978) which showed a decrease in frequency and duration of relapses in the treated groups. However, of the two essential fatty acids (EFA) linoleic (18:2W6) and $\alpha$-linolenic acid (18:3W3) the evidence has been suggested (Bernsohn and Stephanides, 1967) to point more to dietary deficiency of $\alpha$-linolenic acid. The background to a rational approach to dietary management in multiple sclerosis has been reviewed by Crawford *et al.*, (1979). They concluded that both EFA families may be involved and that long chain derivatives of these EFA when supplied in the diet can be used by the brain. Moreover, there is evidence that the rate of conversion of the parent EFA to their long chain derivatives is slow and that the preformed derivatives arachidonic acid (20:4W6) and docosahexaenoic acid (22:6W3) can be supplied in the diet. Dietary sources of EFA and their derivatives are shown in Table 15.1. Conversion of the EFA to their long-chain derivatives involves chain elongation and desaturation. These reactions involve B vitamins and the minerals zinc, copper and iron. Polyunsaturated fatty acids are prone to peroxidation and Crawford and his colleagues suggested that important sources, if not supplements, of the biological

Table 15.1 Dietary sources of essential fatty acids and their long chain derivatives (From Crawford *et al.*, 1979)

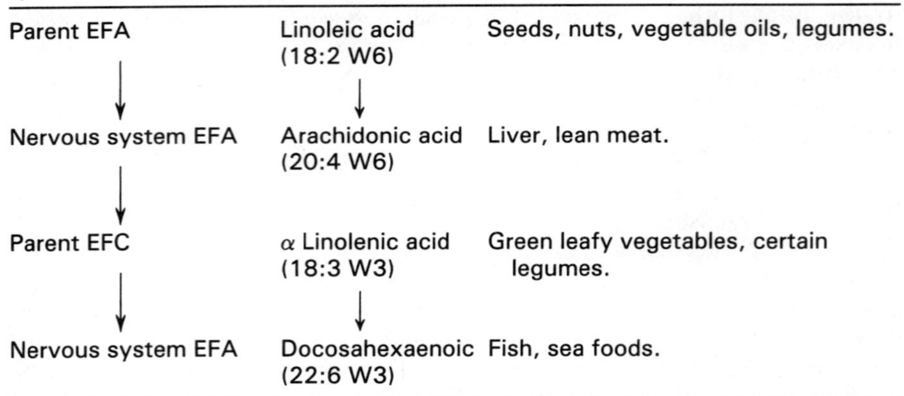

| | | |
|---|---|---|
| Parent EFA | Linoleic acid (18:2 W6) | Seeds, nuts, vegetable oils, legumes. |
| ↓ | ↓ | |
| Nervous system EFA | Arachidonic acid (20:4 W6) | Liver, lean meat. |
| ↓ | | |
| Parent EFC | α Linolenic acid (18:3 W3) | Green leafy vegetables, certain legumes. |
| ↓ | ↓ | |
| Nervous system EFA | Docosahexaenoic (22:6 W3) | Fish, sea foods. |

anti-oxidants vitamins E and C should be included. Wheat germ is a rich source of vitamin E.

Crawford and his colleagues have recently published (Hewson *et al.*, 1984) the results of a study of the food intake of people with multiple sclerosis. Future work may, indeed, show that people with this disease have specific nutritional requirements and need nutritional guidance.

Wheat gluten has been implicated as an aetiological factor and it has been suggested that patients might benefit from a gluten-free milk-free diet with suitable mineral supplements particularly of magnesium (Matheson, 1974) and there are isolated reports of almost complete 'cures' in persons who have received this kind of regime. A diet of this sort is not easy to follow but there has been a tendency for many sufferers to put themselves on to a gluten-free regime. However, an attempt to find gluten antibodies in the serum of patients with multiple sclerosis (Hunter, *et al.*, 1984) failed to find any support for the use of a gluten-free diet. These findings are supported by a study of patients following gluten-free regimes (Hewson, 1984).

## Migraine

Migraine is a multifactorial condition which in some individuals is associated with hypertension and hypertensive headaches. In some patients migraine may be associated with dietary factors. Certain foods contain varying quantities of tyramine, a powerful pressor amine, and can be lethal to patients receiving monoamine oxidase inhibitors. In other susceptible individuals they produce migraine. However, in a double-blind, placebo-controlled trial of nearly 100 patients Moffett *et al.*, (1974) were unable to find an association between oral tyramine, whole chocolate, and phenylethylamine and headaches, in spite of the fact that the patients were convinced that the materials caused headaches. They did find, however, that oral tyramine caused unexplained changes in the EEG pattern in migrainous subjects. It may be that combinations of foods act synergistically to produce the effect, and in some people severe headaches result from the consumption of wine and cheese.

Migraine may also be due to an allergic response to more than one food in adults (Grant, 1979; Monro *et al.*, 1980) and in children (Egger *et al.*, 1983). In the latter study, 93 per cent of 88 children with severe frequent migraine recovered when the causative foods were omitted. More detailed study of 40 of the children confirmed the findings in a double-blind trial.

## Conclusion

The normal growth and function of the brain is dependent upon a continuous supply of adequate amounts of the various nutrients. If these are witheld during the growing period, the effects on the structural components of the brain may well be permanent. The effects of malnutrition on the metabolically active components of the brain are, however, likely to be transient, but if a child is malnourished at a time when certain skills are normally being acquired there may be some disadvantage to learning.

Neurological and psychiatric disorders account for a considerable proportion of human ill health. We are now beginning to understand links between such diseases and nutrition which could have considerable potential for the treatment of these diseases.

## References

Adams, J. H., Blackwood, W. and Wilson, J. (1966). Further clinical and pathological observations on Leber's optic atrophy. *Brain*, **89**, 15–26.

Agranoff, B.W. and Goldberg, D. (1974). Diet and the geographical distribution of multiple sclerosis. *Lancet*, **ii**, 1061–6.

Badawy, A. A.-B. and Evans, M. (1975). Tryptophan plus a pyrrolase inhibitor for depression. *Lancet*, **ii**, 869.

Baker, R. W. R., Thompson, R. H. S. and Zilkha, K. J. (1966). Changes in the amounts of linoleic acid in the serum of patients with multiple sclerosis. *J. Neurol. Neurosurg. Psychiat.*, **29**, 95–8.

Barford, P.A., Blair, J.A., Eggar, C., Hamon, C., Morar, C. and Whitburn, S.B. (1984). Tetrahydrobiopterin metabolism in the temporal lobe of patients dying with senile dementia of Alzheimer type. *J. Neurol. Neurosurg. Psychiat*, **47**, 736–8.

Barlow, P.J., Sylvester, P.E. and Dickerson, J.W.T. (1981). Hair trace metal levels in Down's syndrome patients. *J. Ment. Def. Res.*, **25**, 161–8.

Bass, M.H. and Caplan, J. (1955). Vitamin A deficiency in infancy. *J. Pediat.*, **47**, 690–95.

Bates, D., Fawcett, P.R., Shaw, D.A. and Weightman, D. (1977). Trial of polyunsaturated fatty acids in non-relapsing multiple sclerosis. *Br. Med. J.*, **2**, 932–3.

Bernsohn, J. and Stephanides, L.M. (1976). Aetiology of multiple sclerosis. *Nature*, **215**, 821–3.

Bibile, S.W., Lionel, N.D.W., Dunuwille, R. and Perera, G. (1957). Pantothenol and the burning feet syndrome. *Br. J. Nutr.*, **11**, 434–9.

Biehl, J.P. and Vilter, R.W. (1954). Effect of isoniazid on vitamin $B_6$ metabolism–its possible significance in producing isoniazid neuritis. *Proc. Soc. Exp. Biol. Med.*, **85**, 389–92.

Birch, H.G. and Gussow, J.D. (1970). *Disadvantaged Children*. Grune and Stratton: New York.

Bourne, H.R., Bunney, W.E.Jr., Colbourn, R.W., Davis, J.M., Davis, J.N., Shaw, D.M. and Coppen, A.J. (1968). Noradrenaline, 5-hydroxytryptamine, and 5-hydroxyindoleactic acid in hindbrains of suicidal patients. *Lancet*, **ii**, 805–8.

Brezinova, V. and Oswald, I. (1972). Sleep after a bedtime beverage. *Br. Med. J.*, **ii**, 431–3.
Brozek, J. and Schürch, B. (1984). *Malnutrition and Behaviour: Critical Assessment of Key Issues*. Nestlé Foundation: Lausanne, Switzerland.
Bryce-Smith, D. and Waldron, H.A. (1974). Lead, behaviour and criminality. *Ecologist*, **4**, No. 10.
Cabak, V. and Najdanvic, R. (1965). Effect of undernutrition in early life on physical and mental development. *Archs Dis. Child.*, **40**, 532–4.
Carroll, B.J. (1972). In *Depressive Illness*. Eds. Davies, B., Carroll, B.J. and Mowbray, R.M. Thomas: Springfield.
Chen, C.N., Kalucy, R.S., Hartmann, M.K., Lacey, J.H., Crisp, A.H., Bailey, J.E., Eccleston, E.G. and Coppen, A. (1974). Plasma tryptophan and sleep. *Br. Med. J.*, **iv**, 564–6.
Cheraskin, E. and Ringsdorf, W.M. (1971). Daily tryptophan consumption and psychologic state. *Nutr. Rep. Int.*, **3**, 135–41.
Coburn, S.P., Schaltenbrand, W.E., Mahuren, J.D., Clausman, R.J. and Townsend, D. (1983). Effect of megavitamin treatment on mental performance and plasma vitamin $B_6$ concentration in mentally retarded young adults. *Am. J. Clin. Nutr.*, **38**, 352–5.
Cohen, E.L. and Wurtman, R.J. (1976). Brain acetylcholine: control by dietary choline. *Science*, **191**, 561–2.
Coppen, A., Eccleston, E.G. and Peet, M. (1973). Total and free tryptophan concentration in the plasma of depressive patients. *Lancet*, **ii**, 60–63.
Coppen, A., Shaw, D.M., Herzeberg, B. and Maggs, R. (1967). Tryptophan in the treatment of depression. *Lancet*, **ii**, 1178–80.
Coursin, D.B. (1954). Convulsive seizures in infants with pyridoxine-deficient diet. *J. Am. Med. Ass.*, **154**, 406–8.
Cravioto, J. and Delicardie, E.R. (1979). Nutrition, mental development. In *Human Growth*, p.481. Eds. Falkner, F. and Tanner, J.M. Plenum: New York.
Cravioto, J., Delicardie, E.R.. and Birch, H.G. (1966). Nutrition, growth and neurointegrative development: An experimental ecological study. *Pediatrics*, **38**, 319–72.
Cravioto, J. and Robles, B. (1965). Evolution of adaptive and motor behaviour during rehabilitation from kwashiorkor. *Am. J. Orthopsychiat.*, **35**, 449–64.
Crawford, M.A., Budowski, P. and Hassam, A.G. (1979). Dietary management of multiple sclerosis. *Proc. Nutr. Soc.*, **38**, 373–89.
Crisp, A.H. (1967). The possible significance of some behavioural correlates of weight and carbohydrate intake. *J. Psychosom. Res.*, **11**, 117–31.
Crisp, A.H. and Stonehill, E. (1976). *Sleep, Nutrition and Mood*. Wiley: London.
Curran, D., Partridge, M. and Storey, P. (1972). *Psychological Medicine*. Churchill Livingstone: London.
Dastur, D.K., Wadia, N.H. and Bharucha, E.P. (1972). *Studies of Nutritional Disorders of the Nervous System*. (NIH Project 01–011–1; Interim Report) Neuropathology Unit, Grant Medical College and J.J. Group of Hospitals, Bombay 8. Quoted by Pallis and Lewis (1974).
David, O., Clark, J. and Voeller, K. (1972). Lead and hyperactivity. *Lancet*, **ii**, 900.
Davies, L., Hastrop, K. and Bender, A.E. (1973). Potassium intake of the elderly. *Mod. Geriat.*, **3**, 482–8.
Davis, K.L., Berger, P.A. and Hollister, L.E. (1975). Choline for tardive dyskinesia. *N. Engl. J. Med.*, **293**, 152.
Davison, A.N. and Dobbing, J. (1966). Myelination as a vulnerable period in brain development. *Br. Med. Bull.*, **22**, 40–44.
Dent, C.E. (1956). Discussion on surgical aspects of disordered calcium metabolism. *Proc. R. Soc. Med.*, **49**, 715–27.

Dickerson, J.W.T. (1981). Nutrition, brain growth and development. In *Maturation and Development: Biological and Psychological Perspectives*. p. 110. Eds. Connolly, K.J. and Prechtl, H.F.R. Heinemann Medical: London.

Dickerson, J.W.T., Merat, A. and Yusuf, H.K.M. (1982). Effects of malnutrition on brain growth and development. In *Brain and Behavioural Development*, p. 73. Eds. Dickerson, J.W.T. and McGurk, H. Blackie (Surrey University Press): Glasgow.

Dickerson, J.W.T. and Pepler, F. (1980). Diet and hyperactivity. *J. Hum. Nutr.*, **34**, 167–74.

Dickerson, J.W.T. (1975). Effect of growth and undernutrition on the chemical composition of the brain. *Proc. 9th Int. Congr. Nutrition*, **2**, 132–8.

Dickerson, J.W.T. and Pao, S.-K. (1975). The effect of a low protein diet and exogenous insulin on brain tryptophan and its metabolites in the weanling rat. *J. Neurochem.*, **25**, 559–64.

Dobbing, J. (1968*a*). The blood-brain barrier. In *Applied Neurochemistry*, pp. 317–31. Eds. Davison, A.N. and Dobbing, J. Blackwell: Oxford.

Dobbing, J. (1968*b*). Vulnerable periods in developing brain. In *Applied Neurochemistry*, pp. 287–316. Eds. Davison, A.N. and Dobbing, J. Blackwell: Oxford.

Dobbing, J. and Sands, J. (1973). Quantitative growth and development of the human brain. *Archs Dis. Child.*, **48**, 757–67.

Dohan, F.C. (1966*a*). Wartime changes in hospital admissions for schizophrenia: a comparison of admissions for schizophrenia and other psychoses in six countries during World War II. *Acta Psychiat. Scand.*, **42**, 1–23.

Dohan, F.C. (1966*b*). Cereals and schizophrenia data and hypothesis. *Acta Psychiat. Scand.*, **42**, 125–52.

Dohan, F.C., Grasberger, J.C., Lowell, F.M., Johnston, H.T. and Arbegast, A.W. (1969). Relapsed schizophrenics: more rapid improvement on a milk and cereal-free diet. *Br. J. Psychiat.*, **115**, 595–6.

Egger, J., Carter, C.M., Graham, P.J., Gumley, D. and Soothill, J.F. (1985). Controlled trial of oligoantigenic treatment in the hyperkinetic syndrome. *Lancet*, **i**, 540–45.

Egger, J., Carter, C.M., Wilson, J., Turner, M.W. and Soothill, J.F. (1983). Is migraine food allergy? A double-blind controlled trial of oligoantigenic diet treatment. *Lancet*, **ii**, 865–9.

Ellman, G., Silverstein, C.I., Zingarell, G., Schafer, E.W. and Silverstein, L. (1984). Vitamin–mineral supplement fails to improve IQ of mentally retarded young adults. *Am. J. Ment. Defic.*, **88**, 688–91.

Fara, J.W., Rubinstein, E.H. and Sonnenschein, R.R. (1969). Visceral and behavioural responses to intraduodenal fat. *Science*, **166**, 110–11.

Feingold, B. (1975). *Why Your Child is Hyperactive*. Random House: New York.

Fehily, A.M.A., Bowey, O.A.M., Ellis, F.R., Dickerson, J.W.T. and Meade, B.W. (1981). Plasma and erythrocyte membrane long chain polyunsaturated fatty acids in endogenous depression. *Neurochem. International*, **3**, 37–42.

Fennelly, J., Frank, O., Baker, H. and Leevy, C.M. (1964). Peripheral neuropathy of the alcoholic. 1. Aetiological role of aneurin and other B-complex vitamins. *Br. Med. J.*, **ii**, 1290–92.

Frohman, C.E., Warner, K.A., Yoon, H.S., Arthur, R.E. and Gottlieb, J.S. (1969). The plasma factor and transport of indoleamino acids. *Biol. Psychiat.*, **i**, 377–85.

Gal, I., Sharman, I.M. and Pryse-Davies, J. (1972). Vitamin A in relation to human congenital malformations. *Adv. Teratology*, **5**, 143–55.

Gopalan, C. (1946). Burning feet syndrome. *Indian Med. Gaz.*, **81**, 22–6.

Gottlieb, J.S. and Frohman, C.E. (1974). Towards a biologic mechanism in schizophrenia. In *Biological Mechanisms of Schizophrenia and Schizophrenia-like psychoses*, pp. 156–66. Eds. Mitsuda, H. and Fakuda, T. Igakushoin: Tokyo.

Grant, E.C.G. (1979). Food allergies and migraine. *Lancet*, **i**, 966–8.
Hambidge, K.M., Hambidge, C., Jacobs, M. and Baum, J.D. (1972). Low levels of zinc in hair, anorexia, poor growth, and hypogeusia in children. *Pediat. Res.*, **6**, 858–74.
Hambidge, K.M. and Silverman, A. (1973). Pica with rapid improvement after dietary zinc supplementation. *Archs Dis. Child.*, **48**, 567–8.
Harrell, R.F., Capp, R.H., Davis, D.R., Peerless, J. and Ravitz, L.R. (1981). Can nutritional supplements help mentally retarded children? An exploratory study. *Proc. Nat. Acad. Sci.* (Wash.) **78**, 574–8.
Herrington, R.N., Bruce, A., Johnstone, E.C. and Lader, M.H. (1974). Comparative trials of L-tryptophan and ECT in severe depressive illness. *Lancet*, **ii**, 731–4.
Hertzig, M.E., Birch, H.G., Richardson, S.A. and Tizard, J. (1972). Intellectual levels of school children severely malnourished during the first two years of life. *Pediatrics*, **49**, 814–24.
Hewson, D.C. (1984). Is there a role for gluten-free diets in multiple sclerosis? *Hum. Nutr.: Appl. Nutr.*, **38A**, 417–20.
Hewson, D., Phillips, M.A., Simpson, K.E., Drury, P. and Crawford, M.A. (1984). Food intake in multiple sclerosis. *Hum. Nutr.: Clin. Nutr.*, **3**, 142–3.
Hoffer, A. (1973). Mechanism of action of nicotinic acid and nicotinamide in the treatment of schizophrenia. In *Orthomolecular Psychiatry*, pp. 202–62. Eds. Hawkins, D. and Pauling, L. Freeman: San Francisco,
Hommes, O.R., Hollinger, J.L., Jansen, M.J.T., Schoofs, M., van der Weil, T. and Kok, J.C.N. (1979). Convulsant properties of folate compounds: Some considerations and speculations. In *Folic Acid in Neurology, Psychiatry and Internal Medicine*, pp. 285–316. Eds. Botez, M.I. and Reynolds, E.H. Raven Press: New York.
Horwitt, M.K., Liebert, E., Kreisler, O. and Wittman, P. (1946). Studies of vitamin deficiency. *Science*, **104**, 407–8.
Hume, E.M. and Krebs, H.A. (1949). Vitamin A requirements of human adults. *Medical Research Council, Special Report Series*, No. 264. HMSO: London.
Hunter, A.L., Rees, B.W.G. and Jones, L.T. (1984). Gluten antibodies in patients with multiple sclerosis. *Hum. Nutr.: Appl. Nutr.*, **38A**, 142–3.
Jadhav, M., Webb, J.K.G., Vaishnava, S. and Baker, S.J. (1962). Vitamin $B_{12}$ deficiency in Indian infants. A clinical syndrome. *Lancet*, **ii**, 903–7.
Jolliffe, N., Bowman, K.M., Rosenblum, L.A. and Fein, H.D. (1940). Nicotinic acid deficiency encephalopathy. *J. Am. Med. Ass.*, **114**, 307–12.
Judge, T.G. (1968). Hypokalaemia in the elderly. *Geront. Clin.*, **10**, 102–7.
Kayden, H.J., Silber, R. and Kossmann, C.E. (1965). The role of vitamin E deficiency in the abnormal autohemolysis of acanthocytosis. *Trans. Ass. Am. Physns*, **78**, 334–42.
Kinsman, R.A. and Hood, J. (1971). Some behavioural effects of ascorbic acid deficiency. *Am. J. Clin. Nutr.*, **24**, 455–64.
Kittler, F.J. (1970). The effect of allergy on children with minimal brain damage. In *Allergy of the Nervous System*. Ed. Speer, F. Thomas: Springfield.
Lapin, I.R. and Oxenkrug, G.F. (1969). Intensification of the central serotoninergic processes as a possible determinant of the thymoleptic effect. *Lancet*, **i**, 132–6.
Laurence, K.M., James, N., Miller, M.H., Tennent, E.G. and Campbell, H. (1981). Double blind randomised controlled trial of folate before conception to prevent recurrence of neural tube defects. *Br. Med. J.*, **282**, 1509–11.
Levitsky, D.A. and Barnes, R.H. (1972). Nutritional and environmental interactions in the behavioral development of the rat: long-term effects. *Science*, **176**, 68–73.
Matin, M.A., Sylvester, P.E., Edwards, D. and Dickerson, J.W.T. (1981). Vitamin and zinc status in Down's syndrome. *J. Ment. Def. Res.*, **25**, 121–6.
McLaren, D. (1967). Vitamin A and carotene: effects of vitamin A deficiency in man.

In *The Vitamins: Chemistry, Physiology, Pathology, Methods*, Vol. 1, Ch. 1. Ed. Sebrell, W.H. and Harris, R.S. Academic Press: London.

McLaren, D.S., Yaktin, U.S., Kanawati, A.A., Sabbagh, S. and Kadi, Z. (1973). The subsequent mental and physical development of rehabilitated marasmic infants. *J. Ment. Defic. Res.*, **17**, 273–81.

MacSweeney, D.A. (1975). Treatment of unipolar depression. *Lancet*, **ii**, 510.

Manocha, S.L. (1972). *Malnutrition and Retarded Human Development*. Thomas: Springfield.

Manzoor, M. and Runcie, J. (1976). Folate responsive neuropathy: report of 10 cases. *Br. Med. J.*, **i**, 1176–8.

Matheson, N.A, (1974). Multiple sclerosis and diet. *Lancet*, **ii**, 831.

Mellanby, E. (1950). *A Story of Nutritional Research*. Williams & Wilkins: Baltimore.

Millar, J.H.D., Zilkha, K.J., Langman, M.J.S., Wright, H.P., Smith, A.D., Belin, J. and Thompson, R.H.S. (1973). Double-blind trial of linoleate supplementation of the diet in multiple sclerosis. *Br. Med. J.*, **i**, 765–8.

Moffett, A.M., Swash, M. and Scott, D.F. (1974). Migraine and diet. *Lancet*, **ii**, 897.

Molenaar, I., Hommes, F.A., Braams, W.G. and Polman, H.A. (1968). Effect of vitamin E on membranes of the intestinal cell. *Proc. Natn. Acad. Sci.*, U.S.A., **61**, 982–8.

Monro, J.A., Brostoft, J., Cai, C. and Zilka, K. (1980). Food allergy in migraine. Study of dietary exclusion and RAST. *Lancet*, **ii**, 1–4.

Monro, J.A. (1983). Food allergy in migraine. *Proc. Nutr. Soc.*, **42**, 241–6.

Oberleas, D., Caldwell, D.F. and Prasad, A.S. (1972). Trace elements and behaviour. *Int. Rev. Neurobiol.*, Suppl. 1, 83–103.

Oster, J., Mikkelsen, M. and Nielsen, A. (1975). Mortality and life table in Down's syndrome. *Acta Paediatr. Scand.*, **64**, 322–6.

Osuntokun, B.O., Durowoju, J.E., McFarlane, H. and Wilson, J. (1968). Plasma amino acids in the Nigerian nutritional ataxia neuropathy. *Br. Med. J.*, **iii**, 647–9.

Pallis, C.A. and Lewis, P.D. (1974). *The Neurology of Gastrointestinal Disease*. Saunders: London.

Pauling, L. (1968). Orthomolecular psychiatry. *Science*, **160**, 265–71.

Phillips, F., Chen, C.N., Crisp, A.H., Koval, J., McGuinness, B., Kalucy, R.S., Kalucy, E.C. and Lacey, J.H. (1975). Isocaloric diet changes and electroencephalographic sleep. *Lancet*, **ii**, 723–5.

Pollitt, E. and Thomson, C. (1977). Protein-calorie malnutrition and behaviour : a review from psychology. In *Nutrition and the Brain, Vol. 2*, p.261. Eds. Wurtman, R.J. and Wurtman, J.J. Raven Press: New York.

Prescott, J.W., Read, M.S. and Coursin, D.B. (Eds.) (1975). *Brain Function and Malnutrition*. Wiley: New York.

Reynolds, E.H. (1967). Effects of folic acid on the mental state and fit frequency of drug-treated epileptic patients. *Lancet*, **i**, 1086–88.

Reynolds, E.H. (1984). Folic acid, vitamin $B_{12}$ and neuropsychiatry. *Clin. Neuropharmacol.*, **7**, 98–107.

Prescott, J.W., Read, M.S. and Coursin, D.B. (Eds.) (1975). *Brain Function and Malnutrition*. Wiley: New York.

Rimland, B. (1973). High-dosage levels of certain vitamins in the treatment of children with severe mental disorders. In *Orthomolecular Psychiatry*, pp. 513–39. Eds. Hawkins, D. and Pauling, L. Freeman: San Francisco.

Rippere, V. (1983). Food additives and hyperactive children: A critique of Connors. *Br. J. Clin. Psychol.*, **22**, 19–32.

Rosso, P., Hormazabal, J. and Winick, M. (1970). Changes in brain weight, cholesterol, phospholipid, and DNA content in marasmic children. *Am. J. Clin. Nutr.*, **23**, 1275–9.

Rudra, D.N., Dickerson, J.W.T., Walker, R. and Chayen, J. (1975). The effect of some antioxidants on lipofuscin accumulation in rat brain. *Proc. Nutr. Soc.*, **34**, 122A.

Runcie, J. (1979). Folate deficiency in the elderly. In *Folic Acid in Neurology, Psychiatry and Internal Medicine*. Eds. Botez, M.I. and Reynolds, E.H. pp. 493–9. Raven Press: New York.

Rutter, M. (1973). Why are London children so disturbed? *Proc. Roy. Soc. Med.*, **66**, 1221–5.

Rutter, M. (1974). The development of infantile autism. *Psychol. Med.*, **4**, 147–63.

Sanberg, S.T., Rutter, M. and Taylor, E. (1978). Hyperkinetic disorder in psychiatric clinic attenders. *Develop. Med. Child Neurol.*, **20**, 279–99.

Sanders, T.A.B., Ellis, F.R. and Dickerson, J.W.T. (1978). Haematological studies in vegans. *Br. J. Nutr.*, **40**, 9–15.

Scott, A.C. (1916). A contribution to the study of osteomalacia in India. *Ind. J. Med. Res.*, **4**, 140–68.

Shaw, D.M., Tidmarsh, S.F., Sweeney, A.E., Williams, S., Karajgi, B.M., Elameer, M. and Twining, C. (1981). Pilot study of amino acids in senile dementia. *Br. J. Psychiat.*, **139**, 580–82.

Shaw, D.M., Camps, F.E. and Eccleston, E.G. (1967). 5-Hydroxytryptamine in hindbrain of depressive suicides. *Br. J. Psychiat.*, **113**, 1407–11.

Shorvon, S.D., Carney, M.W.P., Chanarin, I. and Reynolds, E.H. (1980). The neuropsychiatry of megaloblastic anaemia. *Br. Med. J.*, **281**, 1036–8.

Silber, R. and Moldow, C.F. (1970). The biochemistry of $B_{12}$ mediated reactions in man. *Am. J. Med.*, **48**, 549–54.

Singh, M.M. and Kay, S.R. (1976). Wheat gluten as a pathogenic factor in schizophrenia. *Science*, **191**, 401–2.

Smart, J.L. (1977). Early life malnutrition and later learning ability. A critical analysis. In *Genetics, Environment and Intelligence* p. 215. Ed. Oliverio, A. Elsevier: Holland.

Smith, R. and Stern, G. (1967). Myopathy, ostemalacia and hyperparathyroidism. *Brain*, **90**, 593–602.

Smith, G.F., Spiker, D., Peterson, C. and Cicchetti, D. (1983). Failure of vitamin/mineral supplementation in Down's syndrome. *Lancet*, **ii**, 8340–41.

Smithells, R.W., Sheppard, C., Schorah, C.J., Seller, M.J., Nevin, M., Harris, R., Read, A.P. and Fielding, D.W. (1981). Apparent prevention of neural tube defect by periconceptional vitamin supplementation. *Arch. Dis. Child.*, **56**, 811–918.

Southwell, P.R., Evans, C.R. (1972). Effect of hot milk drink on movements during sleep. *Br. Med. J.*, **2**, 429.

Stern, J.J. (1974). Nutrition in Opthalmology. In *Modern Nutrition in Health and Disease*, pp. 997–1011. Eds. Goodhart, R.S. and Shils, M.E. Lea & Febiger: Philadelphia.

Sylvester, P.E. (1984). Nutritional aspects of Down's Syndrome with special reference to the Nervous System. *Br. J. Psychiat.*, **145**, 115–20.

Thomas, D.E., Chung-a-On, K.O., Dickerson, J.W.T., Tidmarsh, S.F. and Shaw, D.M. (1986). Tryptophan and nutritional status of patients with senile dementia. *Psychol. Med.*, **16**, 297–305.

Thornton, W.E. and Thornton, B.P. (1977). Geriatric mental function and serum folate: a review and survey. *South Afr. Med. J.*, **70**, 919–22.

Townley, R.R.W., Bhathal, P.S., Cornell, H.J. and Mitchell, J.D. (1973). Toxicity of wheat gliadin fractions in coeliac disease. *Lancet*, **i**, 1363–4.

Trimble, M.R., Corbett, J. and Donaldson, D. (1980). Folic acid and mental symptoms in children with epilepsy. *J. Neurol. Neurosurg. Psychiatry.*, **43**, 1030–34.

Victor, M. (1960). The role of nutrition in alcoholic neurological diseases. *J. Clin. Invest.*, **39**, 1037–8.

Victor, M. (1971). Deficiency diseases of the nervous system secondary to alcoholism. *Postgrad. Med. J.*, **50**, 75–9.

Williams, C.A., Quinn, H., Wright, E.C., Sylvester, P.E., Gosling, P.J.H. and Dickerson, J.W.T. (1985). Xylose absorption in Down's syndrome. *J. Ment. Def. Res.*, **29**, 173–7.

Winick, M. (1976). *Malnutrition and Brain Development*. Oxford University Press: New York.

Winick, M., Meyer, K.K. and Harris, R.C. (1975). Malnutrition and environmental enrichment by early adoption. *Science*, **190**, 1173–5.

Winick, M., Rosso, P. and Waterlow, J. (1970). Cellular growth of cerebrum, cerebellum, and brain stem in normal and marasmic children. *Exp. Neurol.*, **26**, 393–400.

Winston, F. (1975). Treatment of unipolar depression. *Lancet*, **ii**, 868.

Wurtman, R.J. and Fernstrom, J.D. (1975). Control of brain monoamine synthesis by diet and plasma amino acids. *Am. J. Clin. Nutr.*, **28**, 638–47.

Young, S.N. and Sourkes, T.L. (1974). Antidepressant action of tryptophan. *Lancet*, **ii**, 897–8.

# 16 Nutrition and cancer

John W.T. Dickerson and
Christine M. Williams



## Introduction

It is now considered that possibly 80% or more of human cancers are attributable to environmental factors (Doll, 1977). The lowest overall incidence of cancer in the world-wide figures available occurs in Honduras with a death rate of 24.5 per 100 000 population. By contrast the figure for Scotland is 269.8, for England and Wales 251.5 and for the United States 213.6. If we assume that the lowest value is the natural basic incidence of the disease, then the residue in each country represents the proportion of the total due to environmental factors. Thus, in Scotland environmental factors account for 245.3/269.8 × 100 = 90.9 %, in England and Wales 227.0/251.5 × 100 = 90.2 and in the USA 189.1/213.6 × 100 = 88.5 %. Superficially, these calculations and deductions appear convincing. However, environmental factors will vary considerably from one country to another and even within a single country from one part to another. Interpretation of such crude values must also be affected by the life-expectancy of the population for it is well-known that the incidence of cancer increases with increasing age. In Honduras in 1974, life expectancy was 52 years for men and 56 years for women compared with 68 and 76 years respectively, in the United States. It is difficult to know how the crude proportion of cancer deaths in the United States attributed by the above calculation (88.5 %) can be adjusted for the fact that in the US 83 % of deaths from cancer occur after 55 years of age.

To some extent the problem of differences in life expectancy can be controlled by considering death rates from cancer in different parts of a large country like the US. In 1982, values ranged from 63 per 100 000 inhabitants in underpopulated Alaska to 293 per 100 000 in the urban district of Columbia. In the predominantly Mormon community in Utah, with their abstemious life-style, the cancer death rate was 85 per 100 000 whilst Florida with its large proportion of retirees had a cancer mortality of 210 per 100 000.

Smoking is the best identified factor involved in the aetiology of lung cancer. Smoking may also be involved in conjunction with atmospheric pollution in the aetiology of cancers of the larynx, pharynx, pancreas and bladder. When all these factors are excluded it has been claimed (Wynder, 1976) that one half of all cancers in women and one-third of all cancers in men are associated with dietary factors. These factors fall into several categories. There are a few foods which contain naturally occurring carcinogens (Miller and Miller, 1976). Then there are substances that are deliberately added to foods, such as nitrite (Issenberg, 1976) or are present as contaminants. Moreover, variations in fat, protein, fibre, vitamins and minerals may predispose to or prevent some forms of cancer (Werther, 1980). Furthermore, there are items which are either ingested or chewed which are not strictly dietary components. These items include alcoholic beverages, betel nuts, tobacco and tea.

Defining the role of dietary components in the carcinogenic process is not easy. The process occurs in a number of stages and takes a long time to progress from initiation to the manifestation of the disease. Moreover, dietary factors may not act independently but are carcinogenic only in combination with other factors. Examples are oral and oesophageal cancers which show a strong correlation with the combination of alcoholic beverages and smoking (Veena, 1982; Hunter *et al.*, 1980). It also seems unlikely that dietary factors, except perhaps contaminants and natural carcinogens, act at the initiation phase of cancer development but rather that they act by promoting or moderating processes initiated in some other way.

The more clearly we can identify the causes of cancer the better position we are in to actively prevent it. If, as was suggested earlier, environmental factors do play a major role in the aetiology of cancers at certain sites then it should be possible by modifying the appropriate factors to reduce the incidence of the disease. However, nutrition is involved in the management of the patient with cancer, for both the disease process and its treatment may compromise nutritional status in various ways – increasing requirements, physically interfering with the ingestion of food, causing psychological disturbance including aversions to foods and causing profound metabolic disturbances including the genesis of cachexia. Moreover, nutritional support is often a necessary adjunct to active treatment, rehabilitation and continuing care, making a major contribution to the quality of the life (Holmes and Dickerson, 1986) that may remain. These aspects of nutrition in relation to cancer have now assumed an even greater emphasis with dietary modification being considered as part of an 'alternative' or 'holistic' treatment programme for the disease.

The role of nutrition in the aetiology of cancer is probably coupled with no single factor having a direct affect but rather the disease resulting from a complex interplay of factors. Some of these are examined in relation to cancers at specific sites. The nutritional management of the cancer patient is also discussed.

## Epidemiology of cancer

Studies of the international variations in the incidence of cancers have given valuable clues to the possible involvement of diet in the aetiology of cancer in different parts of the body. The evidence is stronger for some cancers than others and not unexpectedly evidence of association, at least, is strongest for cancers of the alimentary tract than those at other sites.

### Oesophagus

A belt of high incidence of cancer of the oesophagus runs from the Middle East through central Asia to China. East and South Africa are other regions of high risk and high rates also occur in Normandy and Brittany. In the West there is a consistent high association with alcohol consumption (Chilvers *et al.*, 1979) and a high correlation between deaths from oesophageal cancer and hepatic cirrhosis due to alcoholism (Lipworth and Rice, 1979). The association with alcohol has been confirmed in case-control studies after controlling for cigarette smoking, but there is evidence also of a synergistic action between smoking and ingestion of alcohol (Tuyns *et al.*, 1977).

The pattern of oesophageal cancer in Africa and Asia, in contrast to that in the West, is not explained by alcohol consumption. High risk regions in the Caspian Littoral region in Iran are associated with lower intakes of pulses, green vegetables, fresh fruit and animal and fish protein. Low intakes of vitamins A and C and riboflavin are particularly evident. In China low intakes of trace elements, animal products, fat, fruits, vegetables, calcium and riboflavin and high intakes of pickles, mouldy foods and consumption of foods at very high temperatures have been implicated. In Japan Segi (1975) reported a positive correlation between oesophageal cancer mortality and the consumption of tea-cooked rice gruel. The possibility of the involvement of specific nutrient deficiency being associated with high risk of oesophageal cancer has been examined (Van Rensberg, 1981) and it seems that relative deficiencies of zinc, magnesium, nicotonic acid and probably riboflavin may be involved. Thus, whatever the dietary association it seems possible that throughout the world the common factor may be deficiencies of specific nutrients.

### Stomach

Stomach cancer occurs with high frequency in Japan and other parts of Asia and South America but with a low and diminishing frequency in North America and Europe (Werther, 1980). Epidemiological studies suggest a link with diet. Japanese immigrants to the US seem to keep a high risk of cancer of the stomach compared to the local population (Haenszel and Kurihara, 1968). However, the first generation of Japanese living in the US has a diminished risk and with successive generations the risk falls to a level found in the US population. Studies of the diets of the Japanese immigrants and their offspring have shown that the changes in incidence are associated with a change to a more American-type diet (Hankin *et al.*, 1975).

Animal studies have shown that alkyl nitrosamines are potent gastric carcinogens. These can be ingested with food or formed in the stomach from nitrate and a suitable amine. This reaction can be inhibited by vitamin C (Hill *et al.*, 1973). Nitrate is widely present in vegetables and fruits, in particular beetroot, celery, lettuce, spinach, radishes and rhubarb. Nitrate is also present in water and is used in the curing and preserving of meat. The hypothesis that nitrate is involved in the aetiology of human gastric cancer is strongly supported by epidemiological studies. However, direct evidence of *in vivo* formation of N-nitroso compounds in high risk populations is still insufficient for nitrosamines to be unequivocally involved in human gastric cancer.

The high incidence of stomach cancer in Iceland is associated with a high consumption of smoked food (Dungal, 1966). In Japan, stomach cancer has been associated with chronic gastritis (Imai *et al.*, 1971) and with the consumption of spiced and pickled foods. In Hawaii, Japanese migrants continue to show an increased risk of stomach cancer but the offspring who consume Western-type diets do not (Haenszel *et al.*, 1972). Consumption of pickled vegetables and dried or salted fish appears to increase risk whereas consumption of Western vegetables, many eaten raw, decrease it.

## Colon and rectum

Cancer of the colon, in contrast to that of the stomach, is tending to rise in England and Wales. At the present time cancers of the colon and rectum are amongst the commonest neoplasms in industrialized societies whereas they are uncommon in the poorer developing countries. As with stomach cancer, the incidence in migrants changes within one generation. Investigations have focused on four dietary constituents as possible contributors to the disease. These are high meat, fat and alcohol, and low fibre consumption. However, evidence from case-control studies tends not to support epidemiological evidence for the involvement of high animal fat and protein consumption. Evidence for an involvement of fibre intake would seem to be stronger (Burkitt, 1971; Graham *et al.*, 1978). A major problem in studies of this kind is the estimation of dietary fibre consumption. In a more recent study, using new estimates of dietary fibre as non-starch polysaccharides (NSP), Bingham *et al.*, (1985) examined the relationship between regional intakes of NSP and age truncated (35–64 years) average annual death rate during 1969–1973. The NSP consumption varied over a rather narrow range of 11.8 to 13.2 g per day but nevertheless intakes were lowest in Scotland where the death rate from colon cancer was highest. The values overall showed a negative correlation between NSP and deaths from colon cancer. Thus, the results were in keeping with the hypothesis that low NSP consumption, possibly via altered microbiological metabolism, longer transit time and concentrated colonic contents resulted in high risk. It is likely that the greatest protection will always occur when such protective factors operate throughout life. Moreover, the contribution of dietary fibre is likely to be complicated by the usually complex nature of the fibre in the diet. There is some evidence that in Britain the major factor affecting death rates is the pentose fraction of dietary fibre. It is also likely that fibre acts synergistically with other dietary factors, such as low fat. The incidence of chemically induced tumours may also be affected by the dietary intake of substances which promote the metabolic inactivation of the carcinogen. Green vegetables, for instance, contain indoles which induce the activity of drug-metabolizing enzymes (Pantuck *et al.*, 1976).

Possible induction of colon cancer is a hazard of drug and dietary treatment of hypercholesterolaemia (Lancet, 1980a; Marenah *et al.*, 1983). Persons, particularly women, who have cholecystectomies have a higher risk of right-sided colon cancer and this is probably associated with the increased concentration of secondary bile salts (Lancet, 1981).

## Liver

Primary liver cancer is comparatively rare in Britain but is amongst the commonest tumours in south-east Asia and Africa. Whilst chronic infection with hepatitis B virus is a major cause, aflatoxin, a carcinogen produced by the fungus Aspergillus flavus, has also been implicated (Werther, 1980). It seems that poorly stored grain and ground nuts are mainly responsible.

## Pancreas

The main risk factors identified in epidemiological studies appear to be dietary fat and protein, cigarette smoking and possibly coffee and alcohol consumption (Cummings, 1978).

## Breast

Per capita fat intake correlates strongly with age-adjusted rates of breast cancer and this association is confirmed by studies of migrant populations. However, case-control studies are less convincing. One complicating factor is the different ages at which breast cancer occurs, that is before and after the menopause. It is unlikely that the risk factors are the same in these two groups and it seems likely that a high fat intake operates via its effects on female sex hormones, and particularly oestrogen and prolactin levels. The interaction between dietary fat, hormones and breast cancer has been reviewed elsewhere (Williams and Dickerson, 1987). Case-control studies of breast cancer patients consistently report elevated levels of total lipids, phospholipids and cholesterol, particularly in post-menopausal patients (Dickerson, 1979a). In one such study (Bani *et al.*, 1986) in which comparisons were made between patients with cancerous and non-cancerous breast disease, pre-menopausal but not post-menopausal cancer patients were found to have significantly higher levels of plasma prolactin. It has been suggested that the higher lipid levels in breast cancer patients reflect a disturbance of lipid metabolism associated with the disease rather than reflecting risk-related dietary influences. However, women taking part in a prospective cardiovascular risk screening programme in Iowa who subsequently developed breast cancer were also found to have higher mean cholesterol levels (Wallace *et al.*, 1982). Evidence from animal studies (Chan and Cohen, 1974) suggests that the tumorigenic effects of dietary fat are mediated via prolactin. There are a number of ways in which dietary fat may influence the carcinogenic potential of hormones, including direct stimulation of hormone synthesis and secretion, influence at the target organ via membrane effects and also by acting as a carrier for lipid carcinogens. The high incidence of breast cancer in overweight menopausal women has been attributed to hyperoestrogenic stimulation of breast tissue with the increased synthesis and availability of oestrogen reported in these women (Grodin *et al.*, 1973; Edman and MacDonald, 1978; Hill *et al.*, 1980). Prolactin has been reported to be higher in overweight subjects but no significant difference has been demonstrated between obese and non-obese subjects (Kwa *et al.*, 1981). Prolactin levels have been reported to be raised by feeding a high fat diet. This has been observed in women switched from a vegetarian to an animal based diet (Hill *et al.*, 1980) and in animals fed a diet containing 20% corn oil (Chan and Cohen, 1975; Chan *et al.*, 1977).

It is tempting to suggest that the relationships between diet and hormones briefly discussed above and more fully discussed elsewhere (Williams and Dickerson, 1986) offers scope for the primary prevention of breast cancer in at risk women such as those with a familial history of the disease or for secondary prevention in women successfully treated. However, there are a number of points that need clarification before such manipulation is attempted. These include better understanding of the susceptibility of hormone levels to dietary fat intake and the level of dietary fat at which significant reduction of hormone levels occurs. We also need information about the nature of dietary fat-saturated or unsaturated that will be most beneficial. Very low fat diets are not very acceptable to most people and therefore a level must be chosen which will result in the greatest compliance.

### Endometrium and prostate

Attempts to link diet with cancer of the endometrium and prostate are somewhat tenuous and certainly indirect.

## Effects of cancer on nutrition

### Malnutrition and the anorexia–cachexia syndrome

Many patients with cancer lose weight and have a reduced body fat and muscle mass (Soukop and Calman, 1979; Brennan, 1981). However, deterioration in nutritional status occurs late in the progress of cancers at some sites, e.g. the breast (Whittaker and Clark, 1971; Stein *et al.*, 1976) but at all stages in patients with gastro-intestinal cancer (Bolton *et al.*, 1975; Jubert *et al.*, 1977). Weight loss may be the first indication to the patient of the presence of a tumour. The causes of weight loss are many. Decreased food intake is probably the most important factor and may be insidious in its onset and often denied by the patient. Anorexia, a failure of appetite, is the most important cause of a low food intake. The aetiology of anorexia is, however, often complex with a number of interacting factors, rather than one single factor, being responsible in different patients.

The factors responsible for anorexia may be loosely identified as psychological, physical and metabolic and we can distinguish three main kinds

Table 16.1 Anorexia in the cancer patient (Dickerson, 1983)

1. *Transient, caused by emotional distress*
   (a) During diagnostic workup
   (b) At the time of diagnosis of recurrence or metastases
   (c) During times of pain or discouragement
2. *Introgenic, related to treatment*
   (a) Following surgical procedures
   (b) Side effect of chemotherapy
   (c) Consequence of radiation sickness
3. *Pathological, related to disease*
   (a) Occurs early with tumours of the gastrointestinal tract
   (b) As part of the anorexia – cachexia syndrome of advanced disease

of anorexia (Table 16.1). It seems important to assess the contribution of psychological factors such as feelings of worthlessness, loss of self-esteem, pessimism, guilt and suicidal ideas (Holland *et al.*, 1977). The importance of these factors may decrease with the progress of the disease as physical factors become more prominent, but they may nonetheless make a substantial contribution to the appetite failure. Schmale (1979) has suggested that anorexia with the consequent cachexia is sometimes the physical result of the cancer patient's own beliefs and attitudes about his disease and its treatment. Left to themselves, patients are unable to overcome a sense of fear and hopelessness which leads to an adaptive biological reaction called conservation-withdrawal.

In health, a number of mechanisms interact to control food intake. Internal as well as external factors affect the amount of food consumed. Despite this, however, body weight stays reasonably constant over long periods of time. In experimental animals, such as the rat, the feeding and satiety centres in the hypothalamus play an important role in controlling food intake. Wurtman and his colleagues have explored an important relationship between specific nutrients and the synthesis of certain neurotransmitters particularly serotonin (5-hydroxytryptamin) in the brain. It is of interest that a number of investigations have suggested that serotonin is, itself, involved in the regulation of food intake. Thus, increased serotonin turn-over has been associated with decreased food intake (Samanin *et al.*, 1980) while decreased serotonin concentration induces hyperphagia (Saller and Stricker, 1976; Breisch *et al.*, 1976). Studies in rats bearing the Walker 256 carcinoma (Krause *et al.*, 1979) showed that anorexia was associated with a significant rise in brain tryptophan and serotonin concentrations. The changes in brain tryptophan and serotonin metabolism were thought to reflect disturbed peripheral tryptophan metabolism with raised free tryptophan concentrations and an elevated ratio of free tryptophan: the sum of neutral amino acids. These changes have been suggested by Wurtman to facilitate the entry of tryptophan into the brain. Preliminary studies in Holland with a serotonin antagonist, BC 105 (Krause and Meyenfeldt, 1982) suggest that at a dose level of 12 mg/day of this compound increases food intake and body weight with a concomitant improvement of depressive symptoms.

Morrison (1979) has pointed out that the primary nutritional problem of cancer is that the patient doesn't eat. Evidence derived from animal experiments indicates that the growth of tumours deletes various feeding controls, and that this deletion process starts early in the growth of the tumour. Normally, rats respond to a dilution of their food by consuming a greater bulk so that the total amount of energy consumed remains practically constant. This response was found to be impaired in Sprague-Dawley rats bearing Walker-256 carcinomas. On the other hand, the hyperphagic response of normal rats to insulin which is mediated by the hypothalamus was not impaired in the tumour-bearing animals. Morrison suggested that the failure of extrahypothalamically mediated control of energy intake contributes to the anorexia-cachexia syndrome in cancer patients.

In some cancer patients the resting metabolic energy expenditure (RME) has been reported to be raised (Warnold *et al.*, 1978; Bozetti *et al.*, 1980) and since the rise in RME is unlikely to be accompanied by a corresponding rise in energy intake it will contribute to the patient's weight loss. However, a rise in RME is not an invariable finding (Dempsey and Mullen, 1985) and this may indicate that the effect is tumour and site specific.

In accordance with this suggestion, it is a matter of empirical observation that patients with some, but not all, kinds of cancer develop the syndrome known as 'cancer cachexia'. This syndrome, while possessing some features that are similar to those resulting from starvation, has other features peculiar to it (Table 16.2) The distinguishing features are the result of a failure of adaptation to a reduced food intake. Clinically the patient is emaciated, weak, anaemic and psychologically depressed. The prevention of this condition presents a challenge and its development may be interpreted as a failure on the part of the Care Team to meet the challenge.

The cause of cancer cachexia is unknown. According to ideas summarized by Theologides (1979) these changes result from disturbances in cellular

Table 16.2 Metabolic effects of starvation and 'Cancer cachexia' (Dickerson, 1983)

| | Starvation | Cancer cachexia |
|---|---|---|
| Appetite | Good | Poor |
| Energy expenditure | ↓ | ↑ |
| Protein metabolism | ↓ | ↑ |
| Body fat | ↓ | ↑ |
| Carbohydrate metabolism | | |
| Glycogen stores | ↓ | ↓ |
| Glucose tolerance | Normal | Diabetic type |
| Weight | ↓ | ↓ |
| Body water | | |
| Total | ↑ | ↑ |
| Extracellular | ↑ | ↑ |
| Intracellular | No change | ↑ |
| Electrolytes: Sodium | No change | ↓ |
| Anaemia | None unless condition is severe and chronic | Present and multifactorial |

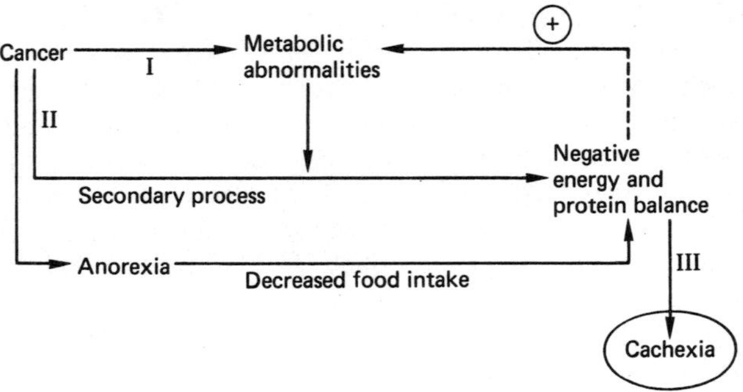


Fig. 16.1 Proposed evolution of cancer cachexia (Heber *et al.*, 1985).

enzyme systems (aptly described as 'metabolic chaos') consequent upon the entry into cells of hormone-like substances produced by cancers. Since not all tumours cause cachexia, it is suggested that some but not all tumours produce these toxic substances.

Heber *et al.*, (1985) suggested that the development of cancer cachexia can be viewed as occurring in three phases (Fig. 16.1). In the first phase, as in the hypothesis outlined above, the tumour causes metabolic or nutritional changes by some remote effect of the tumour on the host. In the second phase, these early proposed effects of the tumour are increased by secondary effects such as oropharyngeal lesions or intestinal obstruction which can lead to malnutrition. The effects of radiation or chemotherapy on gastrointestinal functions are also part of this phase. These changes and also any accompanying mineral or vitamin deficiencies, are potentially reversible. The third phase is characterized by signs of marked negative energy and protein balance, including hypoalbuminaemia, weight loss and leucopenia.

More recently, attention has focused on a substance known as 'cachectin' or 'tumour necrosis factor', a polypeptide hormone secreted by macrophages. A considerable body of evidence (reviewed by Beutler and Cerami, 1986) has implicated cachectin as a central mediator of the wasting that occurs in chronic invasive states. Whether this substance is identical with the 'toxohormones' is not known. Interest in cachectin is now centred in its possible use as an antineoplastic agent.

More work is necessary to develop techniques that can be used to identify the patient at risk of malnutrition so that cachexia can be prevented, remembering that it is often easier to prevent malnutrition than it is to try to rehabilitate the severely malnourished patient. The most hopeful indication may well come from the elucidation of the complex metabolic changes in carbohydrate protein and fat metabolism outlined below.

A further hypothesis to account for weight loss in the cancer patient depends on the possible key role played by the enzyme pyruvate dehydrogenase (PDH) (Fields *et al.*, 1982). During fasting, the oxidation of tissue fat leads to inactivation of PDH, preventing irreversible loss of pyruvate precursors which would have to be replaced by protein breakdown. A tumour in which PDH remains high in the fasting state would cause loss of lean body mass thus leading to decrease in body weight with loss of muscle mass. It still remains for this hypothesis to be tested.

An additional factor contributing to low food intake in cancer patients is the disturbances in the sense of taste which often accompany the disease. Taste thresholds can be quantitatively assessed using a technique originally described by Henkin *et al.*, (1963). This threshold for sweetness is determined with solutions of sucrose, that for bitterness with urea, that for sourness with hydrochloric acid and that for saltiness with solutions of sodium chloride. Abnormalities summarized by De Wys (1978) are shown in Table 16.3. The incidence of abnormalities is directly proportional to the tumour burden, being most common in those whose tumours are most extensive. De Wys (1977) reported that changes in taste sensation were inversely correlated with energy intake and that if the intake was raised the abnormalities became less obvious. These taste aberrations have important consequences for the feeding of cancer patients. Those with a reduced bitter threshold find beef and pork less desirable, poultry and fish intermediate, but cheese and eggs pleasurable.

A study of taste thresholds in patients with cancer of the oesophagus showed no significant differences from controls for the four major tastes (bitter, sweet, sour and salty). The authors (Kamath *et al.*, 1983) warned that no general statement can be made about taste in cancer patients.

Deficiencies of zinc, vitamins of the B group and vitamin A have been associated with aberrations of taste (Schiffman, 1983). The relationship of taste with zinc deficiency has been confirmed in some clinical conditions but no in depth study appears to have been done in cancer patients in spite of the fact that mineral and vitamin deficiencies are common in these patients.

Cancer anorexia may be caused by learned food aversions in rats (Bernstein and Sigmundi, 1980). The same workers have reported that children receiving cancer chemotherapy developed aversions to familiar foods in their usual diet when these foods were consumed prior to drug treatments (Bernstein *et al.*, 1982). These aversions were evidently learned by association of the particular foods with the symptoms of the drug treatment. Many of these aversions

Table 16.3 Abnormalities of taste recognition thresholds in cancer patients

| Reference | Cancer | Increased for sweet | Increased for bitter | Increased for sour | Increased for salt |
|---|---|---|---|---|---|
| De Wys and Walters (1975) | Not specified | 17/50 | 8/50 | 1/50 | 5/50 |
| Gershein (1977) | Disseminated malignancy | 5/5 | 1/5 | 0/5 | 0/5 |
| Williams and Cohen (1978) | Lung | 9/30 | 3/30 | 1/30 | 6/30 |
| Carson and Gormican (1977) | Breast and colon | 3/48† | NR* | NR** | 8/48 |

* Data shown as number abnormal in the number studied. From De Wys (1978).
† Three abnormal values among 11 patients with recurrent or metastatic colon cancer.
** Not reported.

proved to be persistent lasting for several months. It was suggested that a novel taste, presented in association with the antitumour drugs, might act as an interference stimulus and prevent or attenuate aversions to normal dietary components. Bernstein (1982) has discussed the physiological and psychological mechanisms involved in cancer anorexia.

## Protein metabolism

Muscle wasting is clear evidence of altered protein metabolism. The changes in protein metabolism induced by cancer were reviewed by Scherstén *et al.*, (1982). Most of the studies have been done on experimental animals, but the few studies done in patients appear to confirm the experimental observations. The conclusions, as summarized by Scherstén and his colleagues, are that cancer causes increased whole body protein turnover, with an increased rate of protein synthesis in the liver, but a decreased rate of synthesis in skeletal muscle with a simultaneous increase in net degradation of skeletal muscle protein.

The energy costs of protein synthesis in the body account for possibly about 20 per cent of the negative energy balance (Warnold *et al.*, 1978) of the tumour host. Increased activity of the Cori cycle (see below) also makes a contribution. In the study of protein metabolism, as with every aspect of the nutrition of the cancer patient, much more attention needs to be directed to understanding the importance of tumour specificity, the staging of the tumour and possibly the age, sex and previous nutritional condition of the patient.

The biggest challenge in the nutritional management of the cancer patient is to reverse the changes in protein metabolism which result in the severe muscle wasting seen in the cachectic patient.

Hypoalbuminaemia is common in patients with cancer and is often interpreted as evidence of malnutrition. However, there are other reasons for a low albumin concentration in cancer patients. These are decreased synthesis, increased plasma volume and the passage of protein-rich fluid into the gut, that is, protein-losing enteropathy (Waldmann *et al.*, 1974). Clearly, interpretation of a low albumin concentration requires knowledge of these possibilities (Moore *et al.*, 1982). Raines *et al.*, (1982) have suggested that knowledge of albumin metabolism could be of help in the management of the cancer patient. This suggestion is based on the fact that albumin is involved in the transport of drugs and specifically of chemotherapeutic agents and knowledge of albumin metabolism could be of importance in relation to drug transport and actions.

## Fat metabolism

One of the most noticeable features of cancer cachexia is a depletion of body fat and a development of lipaemia (Fenninger and Mider, 1954). Patients with progressive disease metabolize more fat than those with non-progressive disease. Studies by Mueller and Watkin (1961) in which plasma free fatty acids (FFA) were used as an indirect index of the mobilization of fat stores seemed to suggest that a significant increase correlated with the clinical activity of the tumour, those patients with the more aggressive tumours having the higher

FFA concentrations. However, this study can be criticized because of lack of homogeneity in the patient population. Some patients were febrile whilst others were receiving corticosteroids or other forms of chemotherapy. In addition, there was no control of the dietary intake of the patients or the degree of weight loss at the time of the determination of the plasma FFA. The results have not been confirmed (Holroyde *et al.*, 1975; Schein *et al.*, 1979).

FFA have been reported to be reduced less by glucose in cancer patients than in controls (Waterhouse and Kemperman, 1971), and this has been interpreted as evidence of continuous intracellular oxidation of FFA after glucose loading. This suggests that patients with metastatic cancer retain a fasting state of oxidative metabolism in the fed condition. Thus there is failure of normal homeostatic mechanisms, possibly due to insulin insensitivity (Lundholm *et al.*, 1978).

## Glucose metabolism

The altered glucose metabolism of the cancer patient who is losing weight is the result of glucose intolerance, changed $\beta$ cell function and decreased sensitivity and responsiveness to insulin (Lundholm *et al.*, 1977; Lundholm *et al.*, 1978). The mechanisms by which these changes are brought about are not known but it seems likely that decreased food intake, protein loss and hormone changes contribute as also do specific characteristics of the tumour. These first reactions can lead sometimes to increased gluconeogenesis and increased glucose turnover. Studies by Lundholm *et al.*, (1982) led to the conclusion that lactate is quantitatively more important than alanine and glycerol as a precursor for gluconeogenesis in patients with progressive cancer. The increased glucose turnover has been found to be a composite of increased Cori cycle activity (80 per cent), glucose oxidation (15 per cent) and lipid synthesis, ketone formation, etc. (5 per cent). It was suggested that the increased Cori cycle activity could explain the greater part of the increased oxygen uptake in weight-losing, as compared with depleted weight stable patients.

## Effects of cancer on specific nutrients

Numerous studies have been made of the blood and tissue levels of a variety of minerals and vitamins in the hope that the results might provide a clue about a possible link between deficiency and aetiology of specific tumours, the metabolic requirements of tumours and the nutrient requirements of patients (Dickerson, 1983). The results are, however, difficult to interpret in these terms without other supporting evidence. Studies of this sort are of little value unless designed to answer a specific question, the samples taken under tightly controlled conditions and the patients carefully chosen and described.

Possible difficulties are also caused by interaction between nutrients. This is well illustrated from studies on vitamin A status in cancer patients. There is epidemiological evidence suggesting that vitamin A deficiency or more strictly carotene deficiency, may be involved in the aetiology of cancers at a number of sites e.g. lung, bladder and cervix (Peto *et al.*, 1981). In the case of lung cancer, measurements of plasma retinol levels in newly diagnosed patients showed lower values in patients than in matched non-cancer bearing controls (Basu *et al.*, 1976; Atukorala *et al.*, 1979). However, in the latter study the values for plasma retinol of both patients and controls were significantly correlated with those for retinol binding protein (RBP). It seemed that the low RBP values could in turn have been due to a reduced zinc–copper ratio since zinc is necessary for the hepatic synthesis of RBP. However, RBP is a protein with a short half-life and therefore its synthesis is susceptible to protein energy malnutrition and lung cancer has been described as 'a starving disease' (Griffin *et al.*, 1985). Patients with bladder cancer were generally found to have similar plasma retinol values to age sex matched controls (Tyler *et al.*, 1986). The only patients with low values were those with invasive tumours. Similar results were obtained in patients with cervical cancer (Tyler *et al.*, 1988) with those with more advanced, but not those with early, disease having low retinol and RBP levels. A case-control study in Finland has suggested that low serum selenium levels predispose individuals to developing cancer and that this risk is enhanced if vitamin E levels are also low (Salonen *et al.*, 1985). These findings are in agreement with a role for free radicals in the aetiology of cancer.

## Vitamins and the cancer patient

The determination of vitamin requirements is difficult (Dickerson, 1979b) and routine assessment of vitamin status seldom undertaken. Most studies on the nutrition of the cancer patient and indeed on other critically ill patients have tended to concentrate on the need for the provision of energy and protein. Vitamin deficiencies are, however, common in cancer patients (Soukop and Calman, 1979).

Vitamin C has attracted considerable attention. Early studies suggested that the low vitamin C status of cancer patients was similar to that found in patients with other chronic diseases. However, more recent work on patients with advanced disease (Basu *et al.*, 1974) pointed to an increased requirement for the vitamin because low plasma and leucocyte levels were found in patients who had been receiving an oral supplement of 50 mg/day. The findings by Soukop and Calman of low leucocyte vitamin C values in over 50 per cent of their cancer patients and the vulnerability of the vitamin in institutional catering suggests that all patients with cancer should receive a vitamin C supplement or receive it in orange juice. Apart from its well-known role in wound healing, vitamin C also plays an important role in the brain (see Chapter 15 page 409) and in skeletal muscle. Its role in skeletal muscle relates to its effect on carnitine synthesis (Hughes, 1981) with deficiency causing muscle weakness, a not uncommon occurrence in cancer patients.

Is there a role for vitamin C in 'mega' doses, that is, as a drug in the management of the cancer patient? Cameron and Pauling (1976) reported that 'mean survival times of 100 terminal cancer patients' who received 10 g of ascorbic acid per day was 210 days, compared with an average survival time of 50 days for 1000 matched controls. Following criticisms of the controls in this study a further set was identified, and essentially similar findings reported in a further paper (Cameron and Pauling, 1978). Subsequently, a randomized double-blind trial (Creagan *et al.*, 1979) failed to demonstrate any therapeutic value of high doses of vitamin C. However, these patients had all received anti-cancer therapy which could have interfered with the suggested mode of action of vitamin C in promoting immunocompetence. A further study (Moertel *et al.*, 1985) has failed to demonstrate any therapeutic value of high doses of vitamin C in patients with advanced cancer who had received no prior chemotherapy. The study by Basu *et al.*, (1976) suggested that high doses of vitamin C might be beneficial in patients with metastatic bone disease due to breast cancer. One gram of vitamin C was found to decrease the urinary excretion of hydroxyproline in these patients. However, a case-control trial (Poulter *et al.*, 1984) did not show any increase in the 5-year survival rate of patients with breast cancer who received 3 g vitamin C/day.

The possibility that vitamin C supplements might stimulate tumour growth is raised by the observation that lung tumours contain higher concentrations of vitamin C than normal tissue and may have a high requirement for this vitamin (Anthony and Schorah, 1982). The inter-relationships of vitamin C and cancer are discussed in more detail elsewhere (Dickerson, 1981).

Cytotoxic drugs may increase the requirements for some vitamins. Thus the drug 5-fluorouracil when given alone or in combination with other cytotoxics decreases the thiamin status in 4 weeks (Aksoy *et al.*, 1980). Further work is necessary to establish whether patients taking this drug would derive any benefit from thiamin supplementation. Cancer chemotherapy often involves courses of drugs separated by treatment-free days. With one such regimen involving intermittent vinblastine and bleomycin ('Samuel's regimen') for metastatic testicular teratome we found fluctuations in vitamin status with the treatment cycle (Atukorala *et al.*, 1982).

Reference has already been made above to a possible role for vitamin A and/or carotene in the prevention of cancer at certain sites. High doses of retinol are extremely toxic but there is a possibility that synthetic retinoids might be of use in the treatment of cancer (Sporn and Newton, 1979; Lancet, 1980b; Bollag, 1983; Hicks, 1983). These retinoids have the advantage that they are not taken up avidly by the liver and therefore are not hepatotoxic. There are some indications of promising results and the results of more trials are awaited with interest.

The possible roles of vitamins in preventing cancer are discussed by Willet and MacMahon (1984).

## Feeding the cancer patient

The patient with cancer should be fed. Although starvation has been shown to reduce tumour growth in experimental animals, it cannot form part of an ethical programme of treatment. Concern is often expressed that feeding the patient increases the nutrient supply to the tumour and accelerates its growth. There is little firm evidence for this presently available in man. In fact, early claims for support by total parenteral nutrition (TPN) were rather the reverse with impressive claims for usefulness and therapeutic advantage (Copeland *et al.*, 1975, 1977; Lanzotti *et al.*, 1975).

However, nutrition is supportive and not therapeutic. It may well have an adjunctive role, increasing the effectiveness, or decreasing the side-effects, of specific antitumour regimes. However, in spite of some rather enthusiastic claims that well-fed patients do not suffer so many set-backs, it is probably prudent to be somewhat cautious at present (Brennan, 1981). Be this as it may, nutritional support of the right kind, be it enteral (Dickerson, 1981) or parenteral, can play a very important role in restoring or maintaining some sense of well-being, be it physical or psychological. The role of nutritional support in maintaining or improving the quality of life of cancer patients merits further study. The first step towards investigating this important matter must be the development of a suitable method of assessment of quality of life. Such an assessment must, by the nature of the enquiry, be subjective and depend largely on questionnaires (Selby *et al.*, 1984; Holmes and Dickerson, 1987).

The need for this kind of support often continues long after the possibilities for active anti-cancer treatment have been exhausted. The aim of rehabilitation and continuing care must be to maintain the greatest quality of life of which the patient is capable for as long as possible (Fig. 16.2). To achieve this objective it is necessary to combine nutritional support with appropriate occupational and psychotherapy. It is, however, important to realize that nutrition is a potent life-support system and there may come a time with some patients when further aggressive nutritional support is no longer desirable and the patient is allowed to die with dignity.

From a practical point of view the feeding of cancer patients presents a challenge. We have seen that appetite is often poor and the sense of taste deranged with the patient easily satisfied with small amounts of food. The patient's problems are, in fact, partly the result of his disease and partly the result of treatment (Fig. 16.3; from Dickerson, 1985). Anorexia is often exacerbated by radiotherapy and chemotherapy. Surgery which completely

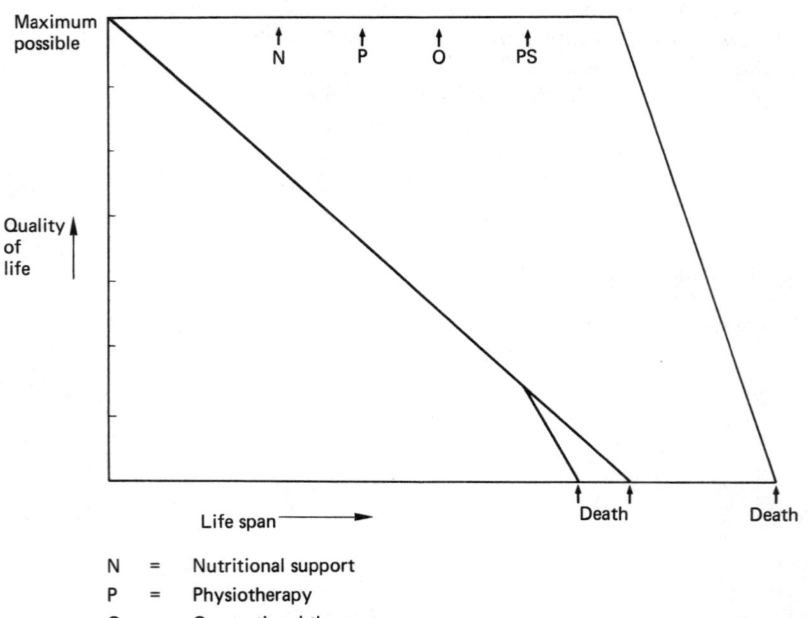


Fig. 16.2 Survival profile.

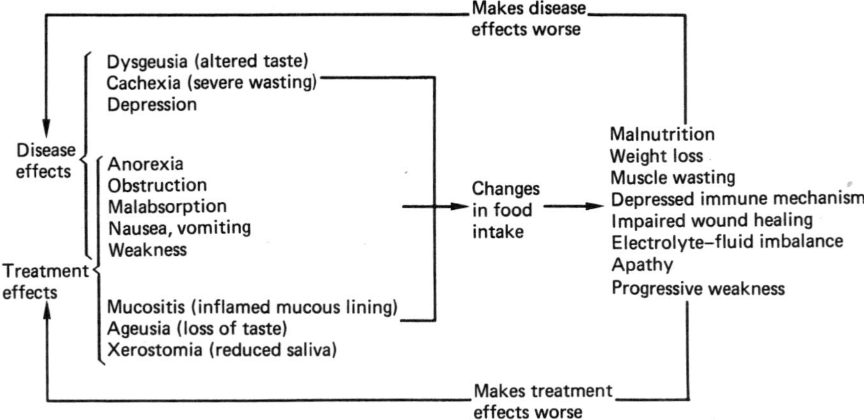


Fig. 16.3 Nutritional implications of cancer and cancer therapy (Dickerson, 1985).

removes a tumour may well reduce the patient to a life-long nutritional cripple requiring careful advice, selective supplements and frequent psychological support. In spite of indications that changes in metabolism induced by cancer are specific, it seems that the consequent changes in indices of nutritional status are not different from those in undernourished patients with non-malignant disease (Lennard *et al.*, 1983).

Although there have been discussions as to whether the nutritional management of these patients should differ from that of other malnourished patients (Buzby *et al.*, 1980), Lennard *et al.*, (1983) concluded that the nutritional support for cancer patients should follow the principles established (MacBurney and Wilmore, 1981) for the management of any malnourished patient. It may be that in the future we will know the optimum concentrations of amino acids and other constituents for TPN solutions for the cancer patient (Landel *et al.*, 1985).

The nutritional support of the cancer patient should be seen as part of his therapeutic programme and suitably planned. Oral or enteral feeding is always desirable. Suggestions for the dietary management of undesirable effects of the treatment of cancer are shown in Table 16.4, and for increasing energy and protein intake in Table 16.5. Preparation of nutritious and attractive dishes such as mousses, blancmanges and trifles based on a ready prepared enteral feed such as Clinifeed, Ensure or Osmolite can sometimes tempt a poor appetite whilst at the same time conveying a message of interest and care. Long term dependence on tube feeding may be necessary in, for instance, patients having surgery for head and neck cancer. Enteral feeding through a jejunostomy is useful following oesophagectomy and reconstruction (Schattenkerk *et al.*, 1984) and patients may be sent home with a jejunostomy pending reconstruction.

The surgeon is often faced with a malnourished cancer patient and has to decide whether to provide nutritional support before as well as after surgery. Nitrogen balance studies in patients with obstructive carcinoma of the oesophagus (Moghissi *et al.*, 1977) showed that patients given a high energy and nitrogen regimen before and after surgery were in positive nitrogen

Table 16.4 Undesirable effects of the treatment of cancer and their dietary treatment

| Therapy | Possible undesirable effects | Possible palliative dietary treatment |
|---|---|---|
| Radiation of mouth and throat | Nausea | Small frequent meals, reduced fat content |
| | Vomiting | TPN |
| | Severe anorexia | Tube feeding |
| | Anorexia | Small meals, served attractively to fit patients' desires where feasible |
| | Loss of taste sensation | Emphasis on aroma of food |
| | Dental deterioration | Reduced concentrated sweet intake |
| | Sore mouth | Bland, soft, or full liquid or tube feeding |
| | Lack of saliva | Avoidance of dry foods |
| | General swallowing and chewing difficulties | Soft, semi-solid small frequent meals served at correct temperatures – between meal supplements |
| Radiation of upper abdominal area | Nausea and vomiting | As above |
| | Sense of fullness | Small frequent meals reduced in fat |
| | Diminution in secretion of digestive enzymes | Soft moist easily digested foods |
| Radiation of lower abdominal area | Intestinal cramping | Soft, low residue, bland |
| | Diarrhoea – dehydration | Low residue with a high fluid intake to replace intestinal losses |
| | Malabsorption | Low fat? Lactose free? elemental diet. TPN |
| Surgery in oropharyngeal area | Mechanical difficulties with food ingestion | Long-term dependence on tube feeding |
| Oesophageal surgery | Gastric stasis | As above |
| | Malabsorption | As above |
| | Fistulae | Tube feeding |
| Gastrectomy | Dumping syndrome | Reduced carbohydrate, increased protein and fat – avoidance of fluids at mealtimes |
| | Steatorrhoea | Reduced fat intake |
| | Loss of intrinsic factor | Parenteral $B_{12}$ |
| Gastrostomy, jejunostomy | No food by oral route | Lifelong dependence on tube feeding |
| Resected ileum, colostomy | Malabsorption | Progression from TPN to a normal diet as tolerated |
| Chemotherapy (effects in general) of special note: | Nausea, vomiting, anorexia, diarrhoea | As above |

Table 16.4 *Continued*

| Therapy | Possible undesirable effects | Possible palliative dietary treatment |
|---|---|---|
| Nitrogen mustard | Metallic taste in mouth | Elimination of any foods accentuating this taste – individual tolerance |
| Cyterabine | Abdominal pain | Bland, low residue |
| Hydroxyurea | Intermittent constipation | Prune juice, large fluid intake (at least 3 litres/day) |
| Vinca alkaloids | Intermittent constipation | As above |
| | Abdominal pain | As above |

Table 16.5 Suggestions for increasing energy and protein intake

1. Plan a definite eating schedule and then adhere to it. Do not omit meals or between meal snacks.
2. Add cereal with banana or other fruit, sugar, and cream to your breakfast menu.
3. Butter toast or bread when it is hot because more butter can be used.
4. Use jam, marmalade or cheese with toast or bread.
5. Add cream to milk beverages.
6. Add skim milk powder to milk, soups, pudding, mashed potatoes etc.
7. Add ice cream or whipped cream to desserts (cake and ice cream, apple pie with whipped cream etc.).
8. Use mayonnaise, salad dressing, butter or margarine with sandwiches, salads and vegetables.
9. Serve thickened gravy with meat and potatoes.
10. Have bacon, ham or sausages with eggs at breakfast.
11. Add eggs to beverages or recipes to increase the protein.
12. Use milk instead of water to prepare canned condensed cream soups.

balance and had satisfactory postoperative progress. This was in contrast to the findings of negative nitrogen balance and unsatisfactory progress in a control group given glucose and saline until resumption of normal feeding. In a larger study, Muller *et al.*, (1982) reported on the effects of 10 days preoperative TPN in patients with gastrointestinal carcinoma. The authors reported that patients treated in this way had a significantly low incidence of major complications and mortality. Taken at face value the results of this study which involved 66 patients having TPN compared with a control group of 59 receiving the hospital diet, are impressive. However, the way in which the study was done has been severely criticized (Koretz, 1983) and it seems that the value of preoperative TPN in patients with gastrointestinal cancer is still an open question.

After major surgery nutritional advice and support for the patients and relatives must continue after the patient leaves hospital and the dietitian has a key role to play. The nutritional care team might be extended to include general practitioners and health visitors as well as relatives (Tredger, 1982) and communication between hospital and community services is essential. Patients often express the need for simple dietary advice and specially prepared attractive bookets have been very acceptable (M. Slevin, personal communication).

## Does diet cure cancer?

There are at least three ways in which diet might form the basis of a treatment for cancer. Theoretically, it should be possible to devise a diet on which healthy tissues could survive and cancer cells cease to grow. This would be feasible only if the nutritional requirements of cancer cells differ greatly from those of normal cells. Considerable research has failed to identify differences that are large enough to be manipulated in this way. Diet affects immunocompetence and it might therefore be considered that dietary manipulation would help the body to 'fight' the disease. Then, it is possible that major dietary changes, such as the adoption of a wholly vegetarian diet with its high 'roughage' content might remove 'toxic' substances from the body.

A number of dietary programmes based on a combination of these suggestions have gained considerable popularity. In spite of anecdotal reports of their success, none of the programmes have been submitted to proper trial and therefore they must be treated with some scepticism. Wholly vegetarian diets may, in fact, be dangerous in malnourished patients and simply exacerbate the malnutrition.

## Conclusion

Cancer patients are at considerable risk of malnutrition. Their adequate nutrition presents a challenge to the Care Team but is essential to the promotion and maintenance of the best possible quality of life.

## References

Aksoy, M., Basu, T.K., Brient, J. and Dickerson, J.W.T. (1980). Thiamin status of patients treated with drug combinations containing 5-fluorouracil. *Eur. J. Cancer*, **16**, 1041–5.

Anthony, H.M. and Schorah, C.J. (1982). Severe hypovitaminosis C in lung cancer patients: the utilisation of vitamin C in surgical repair and lymphocyte – related host resistance. *Br. J. Cancer*, **46**, 354–67.

Atukorala, S., Basu, T.K., Dickerson, J.W.T., Donaldson, D. and Sakula, A. (1979). Vitamin A, zinc and lung cancer. *Br. J. Cancer*, **40**, 927–31.

Atukorala, S., Dickerson, J.W.T., Basu, T.K. and McElwain, T.J. (1983). Longitudinal studies of nutritional status in patients having chemotherapy for testicular teratomas. *Clin. Oncol.*, **9**, 3–10.

Bani, I.A., Williams, C.M., Boulter, P.S. and Dickerson, J.W.T. (1986). Plasma lipids and prolactin in breast cancer patients. *Br. J. Cancer.*, **54**, 439–46.

Basu, T.K., Raven, R.W., Dickerson, J.W.T. and Williams, D.C. (1974). Leucocyte ascorbic acid and urinary hydroxyproline levels in patients bearing breast tumour with skeletal metastases. *Eur. J. Cancer*, **10**, 507–11.

Basu, T.K., Donaldson, D., Jenner, M., Williams, D.C. and Sakula, A. (1976). Plasma vitamin A in patients with bronchial carcinoma. *Br. J. Cancer.*, **33**, 11.

Bernstein, I.L. (1982). Physiological and psychological mechanisms of cancer anorexia. *Cancer Res.*, **42**, 715.

Bernstein, I.L. and Sigmundi, R.A. (1980). Tumour anorexia: A learned food aversion? *Science*, **209**, 416–18.

Bernstein, I.L., Webster, M.M. and Bernstein, I.D. (1982). Food aversions in children receiving chemotherapy for cancer. *Cancer*, **50**, 2961–3.

Beutler, B. and Cerami, A. (1986). Cachectin and tumour necrosis factor as two sides of the same biological coin. *Nature* (London), **320**, 584–8.

Bingham, S.A., Williams, D.R.R. and Cummings, J.H. (1985). Dietary fibre consumption in Britain: new estimates and their relation to large bowel cancer mortality. *Br. J. Cancer*, **52**, 399–402.

Bollag, W. (1983). Vitamin A and retinoids: From nutrition to pharmecotherapy in dermatology and oncology. *Lancet*, **i**, 860–63.

Bolton, P.M., Mander, A.M., Davidson, J.M., James, S.L., Newcombe, R.G. and Hughes, L.E. (1975). Cellular immunity in cancer: comparison of delayed hypersensitivity skin tests in three common cancers. *Br. Med. J.*, **iii**, 18–20.

Bozzetti, F., Pagnoni, A.M. and Del Vecchio, M. (1980). Excessive calorie expenditure as a cause of malnutrition in patients with cancer. *Surg. Gynacol. Obstet.*, **150**, 229–34.

Breisch, S.T., Zemlan. F.P. and Hoebel, B.G. (1976). Hyperphagia and obesity following serotonin depletion by intraventricular p – chlorophenylalanine. *Science*, **192**, 382–5.

Brennan, M.F. (1981). Total parenteral nutrition in the management of the cancer patient. *Acta. Chir. Scand. Suppl.*, **507**, 428–34.

British Medical Journal Editorial (1983). Fat and cancer. *Br. Med. J.*, **286**, 1081–2.

Burkitt, D.P. (1971). Epidemiology of cancer of the colon and rectum. *Cancer*, **28**, 3–13.

Buzby, G.P., Mullen, J.L., Stein, T.P., Miller, E.E., Hobbs, C.L. and Rosato, E.F. (1980). Host tumour interaction and nutrient supply. *Cancer*, **45**, 2940–48.

Cameron, E. and Pauling, L. (1976). Supplemental ascorbate in the supportive treatment of cancer: prolongation of survival times in terminal human cancer. *Proc. Natl. Acad. Sci.* (Wash.), **73**, 3685–9.

Cameron, E. and Pauling, L. (1978). Supplemental ascorbate in the supportive treatment of cancer: reevaluation of prolongation of survival times in terminal human cancer. *Proc. Natl. Acad. Sci.* (Wash.), **75**, 4538–42.

Carson, J.A.S. and Gormican, A. (1977). Taste acuity and food attitudes of selected patients with cancer. *J. Am. Diet Ass.*, **70**, 361–4.

Chan, P.C. and Cohen, L.A. (1974). Effect of dietary fat antioestrogen and antiprolactin on the development of mammary tumours in rats. *J. Natl. Cancer Inst.*, **52**, 25–30.

Chan, P.C. and Cohen, L.A. (1975). Dietary fat and growth promotion of rat mammary tumours. *Cancer Res.*, **35**, 3384–6.

Chan, P.C., Head, J.F., Cohen, L.A. and Wynder. E.L. (1977). Influence of dietary fat on the induction of rat mammary tumours by N-nitrosomethylurea: Associated hormone changes and differences between Sprague Dawley and F344 rats. *J. Natl. Cancer Inst.*, **59**, 1279–83.

Chilvers, C., Fraser, P. and Beral, V. (1979). Alcohol and oesophageal cancer: an assessment of the evidence from routinely collected data. *J. Epidemiology Community Health*, **33**, 127–33.

Copeland, E.M., Daly, J.M. and Dudrick, S.J. (1977). Nutrition as an adjunct to cancer treatment in the adult. *Cancer Res.*, **37**, 2451–6.

Copeland, E.M., MacFadyen, B.V. Jr., Lanzotti V. and Dudrick, S.J. (1975). Intravenous hyperalimentation as an adjunct to cancer chemotherapy. *Am. J. Surg.*, **129**, 167–73.

Creagan, E.T., Moertel, C.G., O'Fallon, J.R., Schutt, A.J., O'Connell, M.J. and Rubin, J. (1979). Failure of high dose vitamin C (ascorbic acid) therapy to benefit patients with advanced cancer. A controlled trial. *N. Engl. J. Med.*, **301**, 687–90.

Cummings, J.H. (1978). Dietary factors in the aetiology of gastro-intestinal cancer. *J. Hum. Nutr.*, **32**, 455–65.

Dempsey, D.T. and Mullen, J.L. (1985). Macronutrient requirements in the malnourished cancer patient: How much of what and why? *Cancer*, **55**, 290–94.

De Wys, W.D. (1977). Changes in taste sensation in cancer patients: correlation with caloric intake. In *The Chemical Senses and Nutrition*, pp. 381–9. Eds. Kane, M.R. and Maller, O. Academic Press: London.

De Wys, W.D. (1978). Changes in taste sensation and feeding behaviour in cancer patients. *J. Human Nutr.*, **32**, 447–53.

De Wys, W.D. and Walters, K. (1975). Abnormalities of taste sensation in cancer patients. *Cancer*, **36**, 1888–96.

Dickerson, J.W.T. (1979a). Nutrition and breast cancer. *J. Human Nutr.*, **33**, 17–23.

Dickerson, J.W.T. (1979b). Man's needs for vitamins – a need for review? In *The Importance of Vitamins to Human Health*, pp. 1–7. Ed. Taylor, T.G. MTP Press: Lancaster.

Dickerson, J.W.T. (1981). The role of enteral nutrition in malignant disease. *Acta Chir. Scand.* (Suppl. 1507). Eds. Wright, P.D. and Elliott, M. Almqvist & Wiksell Periodical Co: Stockholm.

Dickerson, J.W.T. (1982). Vitamin C and cancer. In *Vitamin C.*, pp. 349–59. Eds. Counsell, J.N. and Hornig, D.H. Applied Science Publishers: London.

Dickerson, J.W.T. (1983). Nutrition of the cancer patient. In *Advances in Nutritional Research*, Vol. 5, pp. 105–31. Ed. Draper, H.H. Plenum Press: New York.

Dickerson, J.W.T. (1985). Nutrition of elderly patients with cancer. In *Vitamin Deficiency in the Elderly*, pp. 138–44. Eds. Kemm, J.R. and Ancill, R.J. John Wiley: Chichester.

Dickerson, J.W.T. and Tredger, J. (1978). Nutrition and the cancer patient. In *Oncology for Nurses and Health Care Professionals*, pp. 63–81. Ed. Tiffany, R. Allen & Unwin : London.

Doll, R. (1977). Strategy for detection of cancer hazards to man. *Nature*, **256**, 589–96.

Dungal, N. (1966). Stomach cancer in Iceland. *Canad. Cancer Conf.*, **6**, 441–50.

Edman, C.D. and MacDonald, P.C. (1978). Effects of obesity on conversion of plasma and osteredrone to oestrone in ovulatory and anovulatory young women. *Am. J. Obstet. Gynaecol.*, **130**, 456–61.

Fenninger, L.D. and Mider, G.B. (1954). Energy and nitrogen metabolism in cancer. *Adv. Cancer Res.* **2**, 229–34.

Fields, A.L.A., Cheema-Dhadli, S., Wolman, S.L. and Halperin, M.L. (1982). Theoretical aspects of weight loss in patients with cancer. *Cancer*, **50**, 2183–8.

Gershein, D. (1977). Posthypophysectomy taste abnormalities: their relationship to remote effects of cancer. *Cancer*, **39**, 1700–703.

Graham, S., Dayal, H., Swanson, M. *et al.*, (1978). Diet in the epidemiology of cancer of the colon and rectum. *J. Nat. Cancer Inst.*, **61**, 701–14.

Griffin, C., Royce, C., De La Hunt, M. and Karran, S.J. (1985). Lung cancer: a starving disease? *Proc. Nutr. Soc.*, **45**, 3A.

Grodin, J.M., Silteri, P.K. and MacDonald, P.C. (1973). Sources of oestrogen production in postmenopausal women. *J. Clin. Endocrinol. Metab.*, **36**, 207–14.

Haenszel, W. and Kurihara, M. (1968). Studies of Japanese migrants: Mortality from cancer and other diseases among Japanese in the United States. *J. Nat. Cancer Inst.*, **40**, 53–68.

Haenszel, W., Kurihara, M., Segi, M. and Lee, R.K.C., (1972). Stomach cancer among Japanese in Hawaii. *J. Nat. Cancer Inst.*, **49**, 969–88.

Hankin. J.H., Nomura, A. and Rhoads, G.G. (1975). Dietary patterns among men of

Japanese ancestry in Hawaii. *Cancer Res.*, **35**, 3259–64.
Heber, D., Byerly, L.O. and Chlebowski, R.T. (1985). Metabolic abnormalities in the cancer patient. *Cancer*, **55**, 225–9.
Henkin, R.I., Gill, J.R. and Bartter, F.C. (1963). Studies on taste thresholds in normal man and in patients with adrenal cortical insufficiencies. The role of adrenal cortical steroids and the serum sodium concentration. *J. Clin. Invest.*, **42**, 727.
Hicks, R.M. (1983). The scientific basis for regarding vitamin A and its analogues as anti-carcinogenic agents. *Proc. Nutr. Soc.*, **42**, 83–93.
Hill, M.J., Hawksworth, G. and Tattersall, G. (1973). Bacteria, nitrosamines and cancer of the stomach. *Br. J. Cancer*, **28**, 562–7.
Hill, P., Garbaczewski, L., Helman, P., Huskisson, J., Sporangisa, E. and Wynder, E.L. (1980). Diet, lifestyle and menstrual activity. *Amer. J. Clin. Nutr.*, **33**, 1192–8.
Holland, J.C., Rowland, D.J. and Plumb, M. (1977). Psychological aspects of anorexia in cancer patients. *Cancer Res.*, **37**, 2425–8.
Holmes, S. and Dickerson, J.W.T. (1987). The quality of life: design and evaluation of a self assessment instrument for use with cancer patients. *Internat. J. Nursing Studies*. **24**, 15–24.
Holroyde, C.P., Gabuzda, T.G., Putman, R.C., Paul, P. and Reichard, G.A. (1975). Altered glucose metabolism in metastatic carcinoma. *Cancer Res.*, **35**, 3710–14.
Hughes, R.E. (1981). Recommended daily amounts and biochemical roles – the vitamin C, carnitine, fatigue relationship. In *Vitamin C*, pp. 75–86. Eds. Counsell, J.N. and Hornig, D.H. Applied Science Publishers: London.
Hunter, K., Linn, M.W. and Harris, R. (1980). Dietary patterns and cancer of the digestive tract in older patients. *J. Am. Geriatr. Soc.*, **28**, 405–409.
Imai, T., Kubo, T. and Watanabe, H. (1971). Chronic gastritis in Japanese with reference to high incidence of gastric carcinoma. *J. Natl. Cancer Inst.*, **47**, 179–95.
Issenberg, P. (1976). Nitrite, nitrosamines and cancer. *Fed. Proc.*, **35**, 1322–6.
Jubert, A.V., Talbott, T.M., Mazier, P. *et al.*, (1977). Correlation of immune responses with Dukes classifications in colorectal carcinoma. *Surgery*, **82**, 452–9.
Kamath, S., Mams, P.B., Lad, T.E., Kohrs, M.B. and McGuire, W.P. (1983). Taste thresholds of patients with cancer of the oesophagus. *Cancer*, **52**, 386–9.
Koretz, R.L. (1983). Parenteral nutrition before surgery for gastro-intestinal cancer. *Lancet*, **i**, 180.
Krause, R., James, J.H., Ziparo, V. and Fischer, J.E. (1979). Brain tryptophan and the neoplastic anorexia–cachexia syndrome. *Cancer*, **44**, 1003–1008.
Krause, R. and Von Meyenfeldt, M.F. (1982). Tumour metabolism and anorexia. In *Clinical Nutrition 1981*, pp. 166–71. Eds. Wesdorp, R.I.C. and Soeters, P.B. Churchill–Livingstone: Edinburgh.
Kwa, H.G., Cleton, F., Bulbrook, R.D., Wang, D.Y. and Hayward, J.L. (1981). Plasma prolactin levels and breast cancer: relation to parity, weight and height, and age at first birth. *Int. J. Cancer*, **28**, 31–4.
Lancet Editorial (1980a). The link between cholesterol and cancer. *Lancet*, **ii**, 243–4.
Lancet Editorial (1980b). Vitamin A and cancer. *Lancet*, **i**, 575–6.
Lancet Editorial (1981). Large bowel cancer after cholecystectomy. *Lancet*, **ii**, 562–3.
Landel, A.M., Hammond, W.G., Meguid, M.M. (1985). Aspects of amino acid and protein metabolism in cancer-bearing states. *Cancer*, **55**, 230–37.
Lanzotti, V.J., Copeland, E.M., George, S.L., Dudrick, S.J. and Samuels, M.L. (1975). Cancer chemotherapeutic response and intravenous hyper-alimentation. *Cancer Chemother. Rep.*, **59**, 437–9.
Lennard, T.W.J., Rich, A.J., Wright, P.D. and Johnston, I.D.A. (1983). Cancer cachexia – a clinical entity? *Clin. Nutr.*, **2**, 27–9.
Lipworth, L.L. and Rice, C.A. (1979). Correlating in mortality data involving cancers of the colorectum and oesophagus. *Cancer*, **43**, 1927–33.
Lundholm, K., Bylund, A. -C. and Schersten, T. (1977). Glucose tolerance in relation

to skeletal muscle enzyme activities in cancer patients. *Scand. J. Clin. Lab. Invest.*, **37**, 267–72.

Lundholm, K., Holm, G. and Schersten, T. (1978). Insulin resistance in patients with cancer. *Cancer Res.*, **38**, 4665–70.

Lundholm, M., Bennegard, K., Eden, E., Edström, S. and Schersten, T. (1982). Glucose metabolism in cancer disease. In *Clinical Nutrition 1981*. pp. 153–9. Eds. Wesdorp, R.I.C. and Soeters, P.B. Churchill–Livingstone: Edinburgh.

MacBurney, M. and Wilmore, D.W. (1981). Rational decision-making in nutritional care. *Surg. Clin. N. America*, **61**, 571–82.

Marenah, C.B., Lewis, B., Hassall, D. *et al.*, (1983). Hypocholesterolaemia and non-cardiovascular disease: metabolic studies on subjects with low plasma cholesterol concentrations. *Br. Med. J.*, **286**, 1603–6.

Miller, J.A. and Miller E.C. (1976). Carcinogens occurring naturally in foods. *Fed. Proc.*, **35**, 1316–21.

Moertel, C.G., Fleming, T.R., Creagen, E.T., Rubin, J., O'Connell, M.J. and Ames, M.M. (1985). High dose vitamin C versus placebo in the treatment of patients with advanced cancer who have had no prior chemotherapy: a randomised double-blind trial. *N. Engl. J. Med.*, **312**, 137–41.

Moghissi, K., Hernshaw, J., Teasdale, P.R. and Dawes, E.A. (1977). Parenteral nutrition in carcinoma of the oesophagus treated by surgery: nitrogen balance and clinical studies. *Br. J. Surg.*, **64**, 125–8.

Moore, P.J., Margrall, D. and Clark, R.G. (1982). The significance of hypoalbuminaemia. In *Clinical Nutrition 1981*, pp. 227–32. Eds. Wesdorp, R.I.C. and Soeters, P.B. Churchill–Livingstone: Edinburgh.

Morrison, S.D. (1979). Anorexia and the cancer patient. In *Nutrition and Cancer*, pp. 31–47. Eds. Van Eys, J., Seelig, M.S. and Nichols, B.L. S.P. Medical and Scientific Books: New York.

Mueller, P.S. and Watkin, D.M. (1961). Plasma unesterified fatty acid concentrations in neoplastic disease. *J. Lab. Clin. Med.*, **57**, 95–108.

Müller, J.M., Brenner, U., Dienst, C. and Pichlmaier, H. (1982). Preoperative parenteral feeding in patients with gastrointestinal carcinoma. *Lancet*, **1**, 68–71.

Pantuck, E.J., Hsiao, K.C., Loub, W.D. *et al.*, (1976). Stimulatory effect of vegetables on intestinal drug metabolism in the rat. *J. Pharmacol. Exp. Ther.*, **198**, 278–83.

Peto, R., Doll, R., Buckley, J.D. and Sporn, M.B. (1981). Can dietary beta-carotene materially reduce human cancer rates? *Nature* (London), **290**, 201–208.

Poulter, J.M., White, W.F. and Dickerson, J.W.T. (1984). Ascorbic acid supplementation and five year survival rates in women with early breast cancer. *Acta Vitaminol. Enzymol.*, **6**, 175–82.

Raines, G.E., Calman, K.C., Fleck, A., Trotter, J.M. *et al.*, (1982). Albumin metabolism in cancer. In *Clinical Nutrition 1981*. pp. 160–65. Eds. Wesdorp, R.I.C. and Soeters, P.B. Churchill–Livingstone: Edinburgh.

Saller, C.F. and Stricker, E.M. (1976). Hyperphagia and increased growth in rats after intraventricular injection of 5, 7-dihydroxytryptamine. *Science*, **192**, 385–7.

Salonen, J.T., Salonen, R., Lappeteläinen, R., *et al.*, (1985). Risk of cancer in relation to serum concentrations of selenium and vitamins A and E: matched case control analysis of prospective data. *Br. Med. J.*, **290**, 417–20.

Samanin, R., Mennini, T. and Garattini, S. (1980). Evidence that it is possible to cause anorexia by increasing release and/or directly stimulating postsynaptic receptors in the brain. *Prog. Neuropsychopharma acol.*, **4**, 363–9.

Schattenkerk, M.E., Obertop, H., Bruining, H.A., Van-Rooyen, W. and Van-Houten, H. (1984). Early postoperative enteral feeding by a needle catheter jejunostomy after 100 oesophageal resections and reconstructions for cancer. *Clin. Nutr.*, **3**, 47–9.

Schein, P.S., Kisner, D., Haller, D., Blecher, M. and Hannoch, M. (1979). Cachexia of malignancy. *Cancer*, **43**, 2070–76.

Schersten, T., Bennegard, K., Ekman, I., Karlberg, I., *et al.*, (1982). Protein metabolism in cancer. In *Clinical Nutrition 1981*, pp. 143–52. Eds. Wesdorp, R.I.C. and Soeters, P.B. Churchill–Livingstone: Edinburgh.

Schiffman, S.S. (1983). Taste and smell in disease. *N. Engl. J. Med.*, **308**, 1337–43.

Schmale, A.H. (1979). Psychological aspects of anorexia. *Cancer*, **43**, 2067–92.

Segi, M. (1975). Tea gruel as a possible factor for cancer of the oesophagus. *Gann*, **66**, 199–202.

Selby, P.J., Chapman, J.A.W., Etazadi-Amoli, J., Dalley, D. and Boyd, N.F. (1984). Development of a method for assessing the quality of life of cancer patients. *Br. J. Cancer*, **50**, 13–22.

Soukop, M. and Calman, K.C. (1979). Nutritional support in patients with malignant disease. *J. Human Nutr.*, **33**, 179–88.

Sporn, M.B. and Newton, D.L. (1979). Chemoprevention of cancer with retinoids. *Proc. Fedn. Am. Socs. exp. Biol.*, **38**, 2528–34.

Stein, J.A., Adler, A., Efrao,. S.B. and Maor, M. (1976). Immunocompetence, immunosuppression and human breast cancer. *Cancer*, **38**, 1171–87.

Theologides, A., (1979). Cancer cachexia. *Cancer*, **43**, 2004–12.

Tredger, J. (1982). Feeding the patient – a team effort. Nursing, (Second Series). **4**, 92–3.

Tuyns, A.J., Pequignot, G. and Jensen, O.M. (1977). Le cancer de l' l'oesophage en Ille-et-Vilsine en fonction des niveaux de consommation d'alcool et de tabac. Des risques qui se multiplient. *Bull. Cancer (Paris)*, **64**, 45–60.

Tyler, H.A., Dalley, V.M. and Dickerson, J.W.T. (1988.) Serum retinol and related factors in relation to stage of cervical cancer. (In Preparation).

Tyler, H.A., Notley, R.G., Schweitzer, F.A.W. and Dickerson, J.W.T. (1986). Vitamin A status and bladder cancer. *Europ. J. Surg. Oncol.*, **12**, 35–41.

Van Rensberg, S.J. (1981). Epidemiologic and dietary evidence for a specific predisposition to esophageal cancer. *J. Natl. Cancer Inst.*, **67**, 243–51.

Veena, J.E. (1982). Air pollution as a risk factor in lung cancer. *Am. J. Epidemiology*, **116**, 42–56.

Waldmann, T.A., Broder, S. and Strober, W. (1974). Protein-losing enteropathias in malignancy. *Am. N.Y. Acad. Sci.*, **230**, 306–17.

Williams, C.M. and Dickerson, J.W.T. (1987). Dietary fat, hormones and breast cancer: the cell membrane as a possible site of interaction of these two risk factors. *Eur. J. Surg. Oncol.*, **13**, 89–104.

Williams, L.R. and Cohen, M.H. (1978). Altered taste thresholds in lung cancer. *Am. J. Clin. Nutr.*, **31**, 122–5.

# 17 Food intolerance

E. Bruce Mitchell



## Introduction

In recent years, few areas of medicine have been the subject of as much debate and controversy as that of adverse reactions to ingested substances. It is quite clear that such reactions can exist with records of this type of problem dating back to the time of Hippocrates (460–370 BC). More recently, the whole basis of understanding of allergy has changed following the discovery of IgE immunoglobulin, the search for which emanated from the demonstration of a serum reaginic activity (Ishizaka and Ishizaka, 1967). This activity was demonstrated by Prauznitz and Kustner (1921). Immediate skin reactivity to cooked fish was elicited by intradermal injection of serum from a fish sensitive individual into the skin of a nonsensitive individual followed by subsequent antigen challenge 24 hours later. This observation led to the science of *allergy*, where much effort has been put into the investigation of allergic diseases. In spite of this, the prevalence of adverse reactions to foods remains unknown, as is their contribution to a wide variety of clinical disease states. Confusion abounds, even in the area of terminology. The recent report from the Royal College of Physicians and the British Nutrition Foundation (1984), signifiying a reawakening of interest in this area, has directly addressed the problem of terminology, The report recommends that the general term of food intolerance be used, and that other terms such as food allergy and hypersensitivity be reserved for those situations where a pathogenetic mechanism is known or presumed.

In the decades immediately prior to the 1980s, interest in food as a factor in symptom induction had waned among medical practitioners perhaps because of the great advances in pharmacologic management of most diseases. The result, an important clinical area becoming identified with 'alternative medicine' practitioners, has been accompanied by the development of a myriad of unproven techniques both in the diagnosis and treatment of 'supposedly affected' patients. It is essential, therefore, that medical science has adequate resources to define the issues which must be addressed. Technology allowing confirmation of a supposed food reaction must be developed. It is only through fundamental and clinical research that the extent of this problem can be determined and meaningful treatment modalities developed.

## Definitions

The term food intolerance, as defined in the recent Royal College of Physicians/British Nutrition Foundation Report (1984), means 'a reproducible, unpleasant (i.e. adverse) reaction to a specific food or food ingredient which is not psychologically based'. Some food intolerance has an allergic basis and deserves to be termed food allergy or food hypersensitivity, there being 'evidence of an abnormal immunological reaction to the food'. However, as it is not known what constitutes a normal immunological reaction to food, it is not always possible to make a distinction between intolerance and allergy. In other circumstances, the adverse reaction is due to enzyme defects, pharmacological effects, irritant reactions, fermentation, and mechanisms as yet unidentified (Table 17.1). Furthermore, the possibility that more than one reaction may be underway at the same time also exists, further compounding difficulties in understanding. The definition of food intolerance excludes reactions which are psychologically based, where either 'avoidance for psychological reasons' or 'unpleasant bodily reactions caused by emotions associated with the food rather than the food itself and which do not occur when the food is given in an unrecognisable form', are present. A psychological component to an adverse food reaction is not excluded by this definition, however.

Table 17.1 Food intolerance

| |
|---|
| Allergic |
| Pharmacological |
| Enzyme deficiency |
| Storage |
| Irritant |
| Psychological |

## The immune response to foods

### Absorption

Digestion and subsequent absorption of ingested food represents the primary function of the digestive tract. While food stuffs are usually reduced, enzymatically, to disaccharides, short chain peptides and fatty acids, antigenically intact material can be transported across the mucosal barrier. Both food antigens and immune complexes (i.e. food antigen complexed to specific antibody) have been demonstrated in the circulation (Paganelli *et al.*, 1979; Inganas *et al.*, 1980). It is unclear how antigenic material crosses the mucosal wall; animal studies have demonstrated that antigenic macromolecules can cross the mature gut wall by a process of pinocytosis and other non-specific mechanisms, the rate of antigen entry being related to the load of antigenic material in the gut lumen (Walker, 1981). The presence of specialized membraneous epithelial cells overlying the Peyers Patches in the gastrointestinal wall appears to allow active transport of antigen across the mucosa even when concentrations of antigen are low (Owen and Jones, 1974). In the neonatal period, it is suggested that immaturity in structure and function of the mucosa and the secretory immune system enables a greater absorption of food antigens. With maturation, permeability to antigenic material is markedly reduced, but does not cease entirely.

The constant uptake of antigen is balanced by a number of immune and non-immune processes that reduce antigen entry. Physicochemical barriers to the uptake of antigen include enzyme and acid degradation, mucus secretion, and *gut* movement, which together act to reduce adherence and absorption.

Immunological responses reducing antigen entry are also present. Local *gut* immunity is provided by a blanket of gut associated lymphoid tissue (GALT) comprising nodular formations of lymphocytes in the Peyers Patches and mesenteric lymph nodes and a diffuse population of lymphocytes and plasma cells underlying the mucosal epithelium (Biemenstock and Befus, 1980). There is evidence that mucosal T and B cells represent a separate population, derived from lymphocytes activated in the Peyers Patches that have migrated via the systemic circulation into the mucosal tissues, selective switching of IgM surface positive B cells occurs in the mucosal tissue (Strober, 1982). The processes allowing antigen independent homing and differentiation of these cells remains unknown.

### Secretory immune system

A high proportion of plasma cells (80 per cent) found in mucosal tissue secrete IgA. This is reflected in the high levels of IgA relative to other immunoglobulins found in the gastrointestinal tract, and other mucosal secretions and can be contrasted with the situation in serum where IgA forms a much smaller percentage of the total immunoglobulin present. There are two IgA subclasses (IgA 1 and IgA 2) with differences being found in the ratios present in serum and secretions. Serum IgA contains 70 per cent subclass 1 whereas secretions contain equal concentrations of the two subclasses. Functional differences have yet to be described for the two subpopulations.

The majority of serum IgA is found as the 7S monomer whereas IgA in secretions is found predominantly as the 11S dimer molecule.

These dimers comprise monomeric subunits covalently linked to J chain, a 22000 molecular weight polypeptide (Brandtzaeg and Prydz, 1984). Active secretion of polymeric IgA is achieved by covalent linkage via J chain to secretory component (SC), a specific receptor expressed on the serosal surface of mucosal epithelial cells. Bound IgA crosses the cell and is extruded into the gut lumen retaining secretory component, which appears to increase the resistance of the IgA polymer to enzyme degradation.

Pentameric IgM, possessing J chain, is also secreted by this process which allows free secretory piece to enter the secretions. Some antibody irrespective of isotype or the presence of J chain enters the secretions via the tight junctions of the epithelial cells. In the rat it has also been demonstrated that polymeric IgA enters the bowel lumen via the biliary tract having been cleared from the systemic circulation by liver parenchymal cells, (Jackson *et al.*,1978). Other immunoglobulins present in secretions appear identical to their serum counterparts with neither secretory component nor J chain being associated. Secreted dimeric IgA in conjunction with the non-immune processes already outlined is thought to play a major role in reducing the entry of antigen to the circulation. As sIgA is known to cross-link antigen (Newcomb and Sutoris, 1974), does not activate complement by the classical pathway, and is a poor opsonin, its major action appears to be the inhibition of interaction between antigen and mucosa. Furthermore, absence of sIgA leads to an increase in antigen entry and the presence of circulating immune complexes (Cunningham–Rundles *et al.*, 1979).

## Tolerance

Animal studies suggest that ingested antigen usually gives rise to an antigen specific tolerance, i.e. hyporesponsiveness in which the animal fails to mount an appropriate immune response (Chase, 1946; Thomas and Parrot, 1974; Tomasi, 1980). In the gut associated lymphoid tissue (GALT) this tolerance appears selective and involves the activation of cells which are presumed to be suppressor cells (Mowat *et al.*, 1982). In such circumstances, cells with this phenotype appear in the Peyers Patches (Strober, 1982). However, lymphocytes with suppressor function may also be induced by non-specific mechanisms e.g. bacterial lipopolysaccharide (McGhee *et al.*, 1980). The induction of tolerance is dependent upon a variety of features including the age of first exposure, antigenic load, and the form in which the antigen is presented. The ability to induce specific tolerance by directed entry of antigen into the portal system and the finding that suppression of a response to ingested antigen can be avoided by performing a portacaval shunt suggests that the liver also plays a role in this regulation.

## Antibody production

The presence of serum antibody responses to food antigens has been known for some time and can be detected in the majority of individuals (Peterson and Good, 1963; Rothberg and Farr, 1965). These responses have been shown to include all classes of immunoglobulin. Elevated titres have been shown in a variety of disease states including coeliac disease, inflammatory bowel disease, Wiscott–Aldrich syndrome, systemic lupus erythematosis, iron deficiency anaemia (in children), Down's syndrome and conditions in which frequent aspiration of food may occur e.g. familial dysautonomia. The significance of these raised serum levels in the pathogenesis of specific disease remains unresolved and at the present time they are of little diagnostic importance.

Antibodies are assumed to aid elimination of food antigens from the circulation by the formation of immune complexes which subsequently are phagocytosed by the cells of the reticuloendothelial system (Mannik and Arend, 1971). Immune complexes containing specific food antigens have been demonstrated in the sera of both normal and disease subjects and it has been suggested that failure to remove these complexes could result in their tissue deposition with subsequent inflammation involving complement activation (Brostoff *et al.*, 1979). Indeed, complement activation presumably giving rise to inflammation has been reported in food sensitive children (Matthews and Soothill, 1970; Berrens *et al.*, 1977).

## IgE antibody

A number of animal studies have shown that oral administration of food antigen in the presence of adjuvant can stimulate an IgE antibody response. IgE antibody is the allergic type antibody present in some serum and was shown to be the antibody giving rise to the reaginic activity initially demonstrated by Prauznitz and Kustner (1921). Unlike IgG antibody, IgE does not activate complement by the classical pathway. It does, however, bind to cells such as Mast cells via a receptor specific for the Fc portion of the molecule. In the animal model where IgE antibody to food has been induced, re-exposure to very small quantities will induce a secondary IgE antibody response whereas large quantities suppress this response (Jarrett *et al.*, 1976). This work implies that early feeding regimes may be of importance in determining the subsequent antibody response. Clinical studies have demonstrated the presence of IgE antibody to food antigens in various individuals (Foucard, 1973; Kaplan and Soli, 1979; Hill *et al.*, 1981; Barnetson *et al.*, 1981). The variety of foods involved is great but antibodies to egg, milk, nuts, and fish occur most commonly. The frequency of adverse reactions to food appears greatest in the first year of life apparently waning thereafter. However, in some individuals the problems persist and often so does the IgE antibody. Its demonstration in serum may be difficult, in part because of the high levels of other antibody classes directed against food proteins (Rowntree *et al.*, 1986). While skin testing as a means of demonstrating the presence of IgE antibody is effective in the case of inhalant allergens, this is not the case where foods are concerned (Rowntree *et al.*, 1985). Indeed, early in life the skin test response to foods may be lost even though IgE antibody remains present.

## Cellular mechanisms

Cellular immune mechanisms appear to be involved in the histological changes seen in the gut mucosa of patients with food hypersensitivity diseases such as coeliac disease (Jewell and Thomas, 1983). Similarly cellular infiltrates are seen in the skin of patients with atopic dermatitis, an allergic disease often associated with food hypersensitivity (Leung *et al.*, 1981). It has been suggested that the cellular infiltrate in the animal model of coeliac disease is responsible for the tissue necrosis and crypt changes seen (MacDonald and Ferguson, 1976; Ferguson, 1980). Other evidence for food induced hypersensitivity responses involving cellular mechanisms include the suggestion that human peripheral blood lymphocytes from patients with certain diseases, when exposed *in vitro* to food antigens will proliferate (May and Alberto, 1972; Valverde *et al.*, 1980). This has not been an agreed finding, however (Scheinmann *et al.*, 1976). Food antigens have also been reported to stimulate release of the lymphocyte product, migration inhibition factor (Ashkenazi *et al.*, 1980). The presence of such a response is considered to be indicative of cell mediated immunity.

## The Mast cell

The Mast cell, first identified by Von Recklinhausen in the 19th century, is the cell upon which the allergic process appears to depend (Holgate, 1983). This cell is ubiquitously distributed throughout the body, being particularly predominant around blood vessels and in the gastrointestinal tract (Ishizaka *et al.*, 1972). Recent developments in fixation and staining techniques have revealed that Mast cell heterogeneity exists (Pearce, In Press). A mucosal and a connective tissue Mast cell have now been recognized in experimental animals and there is evidence that similar differences may exist in man (Jarrett and Haig, 1984; Wardlaw *et al.*, 1986). Crucially these differences may include responsiveness to various pharmacological compounds as well as mucopolysaccharide content.

As outlined above, the cell possesses surface receptors for the Fc fragment of IgE antibody (Ishizaka *et al.*, 1972). Binding occurs with a high affinity. Cross linking of IgE bound to the cell results in a membrane perturbation, calcium ion influx, and cell activation. Specific antigen represents the main trigger. However, the cell can also be activated by a variety of non-immunological stimuli (i.e. not involving IgE antibody), including enzymes, ionophores, opiates, physical factors and radio contrast dyes. The potency of the cell is vested in its wide range of mediators, which are liberated into the microenvironment following activation. It is now realized that the preformed mediators, such as histamine, do not adequately explain all the effects induced and a wide range of newly generated mediators are now recognized (Matthews, 1974).

These are the products of membrane phospholipid metabolism, with arachidonic acid metabolism occurring through two main enzyme dependent pathways, the cyclo-oxygenase and lipoxygenase pathways. The wide variety of effects attributed to the particular prostaglandins and Leukatrienes produced includes humoral effects, with smooth muscle contraction and vessel permeability occurring early following activation, to cellular recruitment developing some hours later. These accessory cells such as eosinophils and neutrophils are required to augment the early inflammatory response and are deemed to give rise to the late phase response (LPR). The cell also appears to generate platelet activating factor (PAF), identified as AGEPC**, another lipid mediator which has the property of activating platelets to release their contained mediators. Finally the cells contain a variety of enzymes, including proteases and exoglycosidases among others (Ishizaka *et al.*, 1972) which further enlarge the range of activities regulated by Mast cells.

It has been reported that Mast cell hyperplasia occurs in many chronic inflammatory states including coeliac disease (Pearce, In Press), renal allograft rejection (Dvorak *et al.*, 1974) and atopic dermatitis (Mihm, 1976). These diseases, primarily involving cell mediated immune mechanisms must also depend upon the presence of the Mast cell. Recent work indicates that, in experimental animals, Mast cell function is crucial to the elicitation of cellular infiltration, based upon its ability to enhance vessel permeability (Askenase, *et. al.*, 1983). It is now clear that an antigen specific T cell product can induce Mast cell activation, in a manner analogous to IgE antibody AGEPC (Van Asperen *et al.*, 1983). This observation has opened a whole new area of study seeking cellular products which can regulate the function of this most important cell type (Fig. 17.1).

## Clinical features of food intolerance

When considering the clinical features associated with food intolerance, the

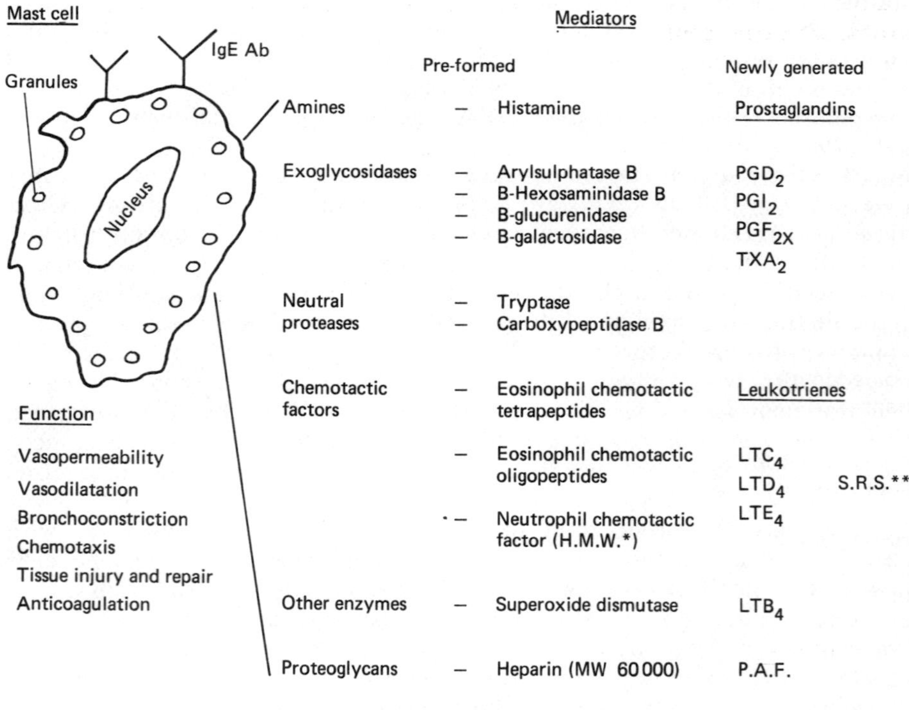


Fig. 17.1 Possible regulations of Mast cell function.

confusion concerning definition and mechanism must be remembered. Similarly, as many organ systems can be involved, albeit with one predominating, a simple list of syndromes and diseases is wholly inadequate. However, within these constraints it is possible to identify certain clinical presentations and diseases which can be due to a food reactivity. The most readily identified are 'immediate' reactions where symptoms develop within a fixed time period, often minutes following food ingestion. In this circumstance it is often possible to identify the offending food and eliminate it. Symptoms and signs such as anaphylaxis, with cardiovascular collapse, bronchospasm, laryngeal oedema, urticaria, and gastrointestinal symptoms of nausea, vomiting, abdominal pain and diarrhoea can develop and represent the most florid example (Table 17.2). However, one of these problems may occur to the exclusion of the remainder.

In contrast it is recognized that delayed reactions can develop, taking from hours to days to become manifest. Unfortunately consensus has not been achieved on methods to be utilized in establishing 'cause and effect' where a prolonged delay is suspected. In the absence of appropriate diagnostic tests, subjectivity rather than objectivity in diagnosis can become the norm.

## Skin

Urticaria is, perhaps, the most frequently associated clinical disorder (Matthews, 1974). However, unlike the acute situation outlined above, chronic urticaria occurring regularly over months and years does not lend itself to the identification of a single provoking food. The disorder appears to be one of dysregulation or a lowering of the threshold of Mast cell releasability. In these patients, an intercurrent event such as a viral infection, or the taking of medication, e.g. aspirin or other non-steroidal anti-inflammatory drug, can unmask an urticaria. It is known that certain drugs, as well as biological factors produced by the host's cells in response to viral infection, can induce alterations in mast cell function. In a percentage of such patients, exclusion

Table 17.2 Clinical features

| |
|---|
| Angioedema |
| Anaphylaxis |
| Urticaria |
| Atopic dermatitis |
| Allergic rhinitis |
| Bronchial asthma |
| Arthralgia/arthritis |
| Diarrhoea |
| Vomiting |
| Abdominal pain |
| Malabsorption |
| Migraine |
| Hyperactivity |
| ? Epilepsy |
| ? Depression |

diets give rise to a clinical remission. It is rare to find an underlying IgE dependent mechanism of disease in these individuals. The suggestions that colourant and preservatives represent the most frequently implicated foods (Juhlin, 1981; Michaelsson and Juhlin, 1973) may suggest that a pharmacological, rather than an immunological effect is underway. Against this is the finding of multiple foods being implicated in the same individual.

Atopic dermatitis represents a fascinating disorder in which the majority of patients have the capacity to mount IgE mediated immunological responses to a wide variety of inhaled, and sometimes ingested, antigens (Atherton, 1982). The inflammatory response in the skin, however, is one of a delayed cellular infiltrate. Foods are often implicated in the pathogenesis of this disorder, especially in the earliest years of life (Atherton, 1982; Van Asperen *et al.*, 1983).

It is now becoming apparent that the presence of IgE antibody to antigen does not dictate that the ensuing response is immediate in nature. Rather the capacity to mount one type of immune response is often paralleled by the capacity to mount other types of reactivity. Proof that foods can exacerbate atopic dermatitis is possible only in a small number of patients, and, in these, it is not always possible to delineate mechanism.

## Respiratory tract

Both allergic rhinitis and bronchial asthma can be manifestations of an acute reaction to food. Recently, it has been shown that bronchial reactivity, a measure of airway responsiveness to non-specific stimuli, is increased following the ingestion of particular foods (Wilson *et al.*, 1982). The observation shows that, in the absence of an immediate episode of bronchospasm, foods can alter events in the bronchial wall, but does not indicate how this effect is mediated. Other work shows that T-lymphocytes comprise a part of the airway inflammatory response indicating, at the very least, that the capacity to mount a delayed immune response to allergen can exist in the airway.

## Joints

It is quite clear that joint inflammation can develop as part of the acute inflammatory response to a food antigen (Denman *et al.*, 1983). However, reports conflict as to whether a chronic destructive process, as is involved in the disorder rheumatoid arthritis, can be induced in this manner (Walport *et al.*, 1983; Little *et al.*, 1983). Exclusion diets, necessary to prove an association, are very difficult to evaluate in the presence of a chronic disease, characterized by remission and exacerbation. It would be necessary to follow a dietary protocol for six months or more before assessment could be made. Not surprisingly, patient compliance becomes a major problem. Furthermore, it is possible that a secondary acute event, as might be induced by food intolerance, could exacerbate a primary inflammatory process, even though the aetiology of both is unrelated.

## Bowel disease

The classical model of food 'allergy' is coeliac disease (Jewell and Thomas, 1983), a disorder in which a gluten sensitivity in genetically susceptible individuals can give rise to mucosal damage, presumed to be dependent upon the cellular infiltrate which is present. Symptoms associated with malabsorption predominate. Removal of the offending antigen (by avoidance of wheat products) results in a clinical remission. It is fascinating that reintroduction can take from days to months to induce exacerbation. Cell mediated immune mechanisms appear to predominate, and no evidence of IgE production to this food antigen in coeliac subjects exists.

A very similar clinical disorder appears to exist in young children, associated with a cows' milk protein intolerance (Harrison *et al.*, 1976). Again the cellular infiltrate in the small bowel mucosa predominates, with diarrhoea and a 'failure to thrive' as the major findings. Colic also can develop. Again IgE antibody does not appear to play the major role.

Chronic bowel disease, as evidenced by the irritable bowel syndrome (IBS) has been reported to respond well to food elimination diets (Jones *et al.*, 1982). The mechanism underlying the clinical response awaits elucidation, and other workers have suggested that only a minority of subjects respond (Bentley *et al.*, 1983). Similarly inflammatory bowel disease (IBD) may benefit from a dietary alteration with the response to an elemental diet of particular interest (O'Morain and Levi, 1981). Whether the response represents withdrawal of an immunological stimulus, alteration in bowel flora, or a change in residue is unclear.

## Central nervous system (CNS)

Migraine represents a CNS disorder in which certain foods can have a role in exacerbation (Hanington, 1983). Those foods, containing tyramine (e.g. wine, cheese) have been identified for some time. More controversial is the suggestion that a food intolerance, rather than an undue sensitivity to a substance with a pharmacological effect, can induce this disorder. In children almost any food has been implicated (Egger *et al.*, 1983), withdrawal giving rise to clinical benefit. Similar claims have been made for the clinical problems of hyperactivity in children as well as epilepsy (Leading Article, 1979; Soothill, personal communication). Both with migraine, and hyperactivity, a more generalized clinical experience suggests that a food association is present in only a minority of subjects. The situation with regard to epilepsy is entirely unclear at this time, but, given its emotional potential, must be clarified without delay.

## **Psychological factors in food intolerance**

It is clear that psychological factors influence our attitude to foods. In particular societies, certain foods might be frequently eaten which in others may cause revulsion. In addition, food fads are common especially in children. It is only when food fadism becomes severe that the spectre of psychiatric illness looms in the minds of those managing such cases. Often the patients or a member of the family will consider that the syndrome is a manifestation of food 'allergy', a situation which raises problems for the physicians involved. It has been suggested that the most common reason for failing to tolerate specific foods is psychological. The proponents of this thesis would suggest that 'psychological processes can bring about pathophysiological changes identical to those of genuine immunological reactions'. It is essential to consider this area in detail.

At the present time, we do not know the range of symptoms that can be attributed to adverse food reactivity. As outlined above, disorders from hyperactivity and irritable bowel syndrome to migraine and epilepsy may involve a food intolerance mechanism. All of these clinical areas are under investigation from a 'food point of view', and hopefully in the not too distant future the prevalence of food reactions in these disorders will be clear. Whether disorders such as depression and lethargy can be attributed to foods on a primary basis or be reactive in association with food induced inflammation elsewhere is unclear. Certainly some of the popular paperback self-help books which attribute almost all possible symptoms and syndromes to food allergy have done a lot of harm. Many patients have quite inappropriately withdrawn food from their diets and in extreme cases malnourishment has resulted. However, these works have found ready acceptance from a population which has an ever expanding appetite for knowledge on preventive health care. Unfortunately, this need has not been fully met by the medical establishment, leaving a void which has been filled mainly by alternative medicine practitioners. Most of us will on occasion have noted unusual symptoms associated with ingestion of particular foods. These can include agitation and irritability following coffee (or other caffeine containing foods) to alteration in bowel habit following spiced food, changes in residue ingestion, and alcohol. It is easy to suggest that in particularly sensitive subjects, a small quantity of such foods on a continuing basis may give rise to similar symptoms on a chronic basis. In the absence of a mechanism to prove or disprove such an association one is dependent on the patient's subjective impression of the response to food avoidance. All too often this is favourable. It is clear that the attitude of the practitioner managing such patients is of relevance, objective assessment representing a crucial requirement. If diagnostic techniques or measurements were available which could reliably identify adverse reactions, involving immunological mechanisms or otherwise, it would then be possible to categorize symptoms following ingestion on an objective basis.

That psychological factors may contribute to the perception of symptoms by an individual cannot be disputed. In most circumstances this may be a minor factor but in a proportion it will assume major significance. Similarly if foods can induce vague or minor symptoms, in some affected individuals the discomfort will assume a major importance. In these cases the problem is not purely one of food intolerance or of psychological disease; however, the treatment involves the removal of the offending food or foods from the diet. Providing that any dietary inadequacy is corrected, a clinical improvement obtained in this fashion may represent a valid treatment end-point.

Certain syndromes are clearly psychological in nature, and though involving foods, are clearly the province of psychologists and psychiatrists. Anorexia nervosa (Crisp and Kalucy, 1974), in young girls particularly and bulimia (Kalucy, 1976), eating with a 'bingeing' quality, fall into this category. Often these patients come to attention through requests for food allergy assessment, and in particularly complex cases present all the difficulties in sorting out purely psychological disease from possible food related symptoms. In such cases food avoidance can create major problems, with an ever increasing number of foods added to the list of those inducing symptoms. Given the inability to modulate clinical responses to foods, it is not surprising that a focus on the psychological disease is the only beneficial approach. 'Total Allergy Syndrome' is considered by some clinicians to represent the extreme end of this disease spectrum.

In most cases, vague 'psychiatric type' or purely subjective symptoms attributed to foods occur in women. This fact has been used to support the claim that psychiatric factors are mainly involved. However, such interpretation ignores the fact that many immune disorders such as systemic lupus erythematosis and rheumatoid arthritis are more common in women. Further, such diseases are affected by changing hormonal factors such as pregnancy, and menopause. It is therefore feasible that similar hormonal factors may induce some of the symptoms attributed to adverse food reactions. Indeed there is a surprising overlap between symptoms of premenstrual tension and the common features of supposed psychological food intolerance.

In summary, the issue of psychological factors and supposed food intolerance in patients with symptoms not usually accepted as allergic in nature is highly contentious. It is becoming accepted that in at least some patients symptoms previously unrecognized as food related may indeed represent an adverse food reactivity. The absence of objective tests to confirm an adverse reaction would indicate that until further research corrects this deficiency, it will not be possible to determine the role that food might play in the pathogenesis of a variety of clinical problems.

## Diagnosis

*Laboratory.* Immediate symptoms following food ingestion or contact usually involve IgE antibody. There are now a number of techniques available for measurement of this antibody, the most popular being the solid phase radioallergosorbent test (RAST), or enzyme linked immunoassay (ELIZA) (Kemeny and Lessof, 1982). This test is useful in certain circumstances, in particular where antigens known to be effective in the test have been coupled to the discs used, e.g. milk, egg, fish, and nuts. Other antigens are less effective. Very high levels of total IgE in the serum will influence the test result with false positive results occurring in some tests (Kemeny and Lessof, 1982). Tests for other antibody classes or sub-classes have not been shown to be of diagnostic use. Neither have tests for cellular immunity. Most interesting has been the recent use of sensitive tests for inflammatory mediators, such as histamine, different tests being shown to be of advantage in different clinical situations. Cytotoxic food testing, a much advertised and used test has been shown to have no useful place in the diagnosis of food intolerance (Royal College of Physicians, 1984).

*Clinical.* Skin testing is a valid method for determining the presence of IgE antibody but is dependent upon the skill of the tester and the particular reagents used. Futhermore, in the case of food antigens, it has been shown that skin test reactivity can be lost while IgE antibody remains in the circulation (Rowntree *et al.*, 1986). The clinical relevance of this finding is unknown. A variety of unproven tests are in use, which upon investigation have been shown to be of no diagnostic use. These include the Pulse test, Sublingual testing and Rinkel type intradermal testing (Royal College of Physicians, 1984).

## Elimination diets

The most important approach to the diagnosis of food intolerance involves carefully controlled challenge and avoidance studies. Such studies must involve a team approach in which the physician is assisted by a dietician and in certain circumstances a psychiatrist. The role of the dietician is crucially important, with the diet history and involvement in planning and control of elimination diets and challenge studies representing the major contributions. Often from the clinical history or the diet history (including a diary card) the single or limited number of foods can be identified and a simple nutritionally adequate exclusion diet structured. More frequently, such an approach is not possible and a more restrictive diet has to be structured. Here an oligo-allergenic diet is structured in which a limited number of foods are allowed for a set period of time and if no improvement occurs the diet is either terminated or a second group of foods, unrelated to the first group, is given again for a set period. The choice of food is arbitrary but can include lamb and rice +/− pears or a vegetable. Other approaches are less restrictive, but it must be remembered that the more liberal one is, the less the chance of success becomes. At all times nutritional requirements must be maintained with adequate supplementation of vitamins, minerals and essential elements.

The most extreme end of the spectrum of elimination diets involves the use of elemental diets in which nutritional support is maintained by a liquid preparation including protein derived from free amino acids or oligopeptides and a source of calories.

## Challenge studies

If a patient improves after a set period on an elimination diet it is essential that an attempt be made to identify the food or foods involved in the adverse reactivity. Similarly it is important to show if possible that symptoms can be reproducibly induced by exposure to implicated foods. These objectives are met by the gradual re-introduction of particular foods or groups of foods at stated intervals, according to a pre-arranged protocol. Following the identification of a particular food and after an appropriate symptom-free interval double blind challenge studies are organized in which the results of food ingestion or placebo in a disguised form over a period of time are assessed by a 'blinded' clinician!

Following successful challenge studies a maintenance diet is structured in which the implicated foods or groups of foods are eliminated from the diet. Again the structuring of this maintenance diet must involve an experienced dietician who is aware of the nutritional requirements of a particular situation especially those involving children (Fig. 17.2).

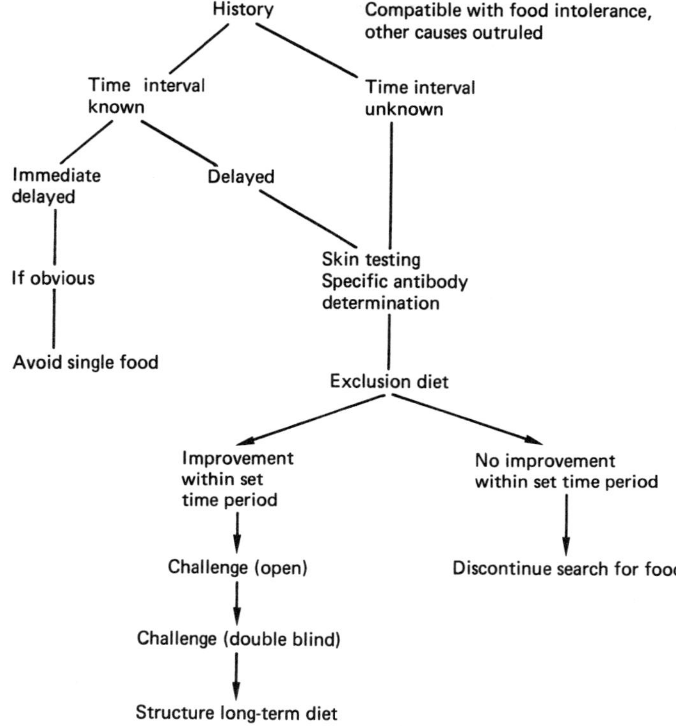


Fig. 17.2 Approach to food intolerant patient.

## Management

Once a diagnosis of food intolerance has been confirmed, the issue of an appropriate management strategy must be addressed. The simplest, and most effective approach, involves avoidance of the offending foods. Coeliac disease, and gluten avoidance, represents an example. The need to avoid a certain foodstuff may not be permanent, with individuals subsequently tolerating foods to which they were previously intolerant. This is particularly evident in, though not restricted to young children, and can occur where both immunological and non-immunological mechanisms are involved. Problems can develop where many foods are suspected, either because an individual is truly intolerant of all, or as is more usual, a particular constituent common to all. In this case, and as outlined above, the role of the dietician assumes an additional importance.

While nature has effectively induced tolerance to food in most individuals, we do not understand the mechanisms sufficiently well to emulate them. Consequently no method of iatrogenic manipulation of food exposure can be shown to beneficially affect the food intolerant individual. Many such methods are utilized, but where carefully studied, have not been of proven benefit in man. In certain individuals, who have a salicylate sensitivity, aspirin desensitization can be effective.

In a small subgroup of these subjects reactivity to certain Azo dyes also develops and this procedure may alter the response to these food constituents also.

Drugs which affect the allergic response can have a varied outcome in food intolerance. The anti-mediator agents, mainly comprising anti-histamines, can be useful where pruritus and other symptoms develop as a part of the clinical presentation. Antagonists of the other more potent Mast cell mediators are awaited. Unlike sodium cromoglycate and perhaps Ketotifen, the anti-histamines appear to be ineffective in preventing the induction of the immune response. Cromolyn acts as a membrane stabilizing agent, preventing the activation of the cell. Varied reports of clinical efficacy abound.

Corticosteroids are only rarely used in the management of food reactivity. Certainly no place for long-term usage exists. However, complex situations, where cellular infiltration of an organ system indicates chronic inflammation of the skin, gastrointestinal mucosa or respiratory tract, occur, in which the potent anti-inflammatory agents may be necessary. In conclusion, pharmacological management of food intolerance problems is somewhat empirical, and has not replaced the need to carefully identify and avoid offending foods.

## References


Askenase, P.W., Van Loveren, H., Rosenstein, R.W., and Ptak, W. (1983). Immunologic specificity of antigen binding T cells – derived factors that transfer mast cell dependent immediate-like reactions. *Monogr. Allergy*, **18**, 249–55.

Ashkenazi, A., Levin, S., Idar, D., Or. A., Rosenberg, I, and Handz, El, Zt. (1980). In vitro cell-mediated immunologic assay for cow's milk allergy. *Pediatrics*, **66**, 399–402.

Atherton, D.J. (1982). Atopic eczema. *Clinics in Immunology and Allergy*, **2**, 77–100.

Barnetson, R. Stc., Merrett, T.G. and Ferguson, A. (1981). Studies on hyperimmunoglobulinaemia E in atopic diseases with particular reference to food allergens. *Clin. Exp. Immunol.*, **46**, 54–60.

Bentley, S.J., Pearson, D.J., Rix, K.J.B., and Roberts, C. (1983). Food hypersensitivity and irritable bowel syndrome. *Lancet*, **2**, 746–7.

Berrens, L., Koers, W.J. and Bruynzeel, P.L.B. (1977). IgE and IgG4 antibodies in specific allergies. *Lancet*, **2**, 92.

Biemenstock, J. and Befus, A.D. (1980). Mucosal immunology. *Immunology*, **41**, 249–70.

Brandtzaeg, P. and Prydz, H. (1984). Direct evidence for an integrated function of J chain and secretary component in epithelial transport of immunoglobins. *Nature*, **311**, 71–3.

Brostoff, J., Carini, C., Wraith, D.G., Paganelli, R. and Levinsky, R.J. (1979). Immune-complexes in atopy. In *The Mast Cell: Its Role in Health and Disease*, pp. 380–93 Eds. Pepys, J. and Edwards, A.M. Pitman Medical: Tunbridge Wells.

Cantor, H.M. and Dumont, A.E. (1967). Hepatic suppression of sensitization to antigen absorbed into the portal system. *Nature*, **215**, 744–5.

Crisp, A.H., and Kalucy, R.S. (1974). Aspects of the perceptional disorder in anorexia nervosa. *Br. J. Med. Psychol.*, **47**, 349–61.

Cunningham-Rundles, C., Brandeis, W.E., Good, R.A. and N.K. Day, (1979). Bovine antigens and the formation of circulating immune complexes in selective immunoglobulin A deficiency. *J. Clin. Invest.*, **64**, 272–9.

Denman, A.M., Mitchell, E.B. and Ansell, B.M. (1983). Joint complaints and food allergic disorders. *Annals of Allergy*, **41**, 260–63.

Dvorak, H.F., Mihm, M.C., Jr., Dvorak, A.M., Johnson, R.A., Manseau, E.J., Morgan, E., and Coluin, R.B. Morphology of delayed type hypersensitivity reactions in man. I. Quantitative description of the inflammatory response. *Lab. Invest.*, **31**, 111–30.

Egger, J., Wilson, J., Carter, C.M., Turner, M.W. and Soothill, J.F. (1983). Is migraine food allergy? A double-blind controlled trial of oligoantigenic diet treatment. *Lancet*, **2**, 865–9.

Ferguson, A. (1980). Pathogenesis and mechanisms in the gastro-intestinal tract. In *Proceedings of the First Food Allergy Workshop*, p.28. Med. Ed. Services Ltd: Oxford.

Foucard, T. (1973). Follow-up study of children with asthmatic bronchitis. I. Skin test reactions and IgE antibodies to common allergens. *Acta Paediatr. Scand.*, **62**, 633–44.

Hanington, E. (1983). Migraine. In *Clinical Reactions to Food.*, pp. 155–80. Ed. Lessof, M.H. Wiley: Chichester.

Harrison, M., Kilby, A., Walker-Smith, J.A., France, N.E. and Wood, C.B.S. (1976). Cow's milk protein intolerance: a possible association with gastroenteritis, lactose intolerance and IgA deficiency. *Br. Med. J.*, **1**, 1501–4.

Hill, D.J., Balloch, A. and Hosking, C.S. (1981). IgE responses to environmental antigens in atopic children. *Clin. Allergy*, **11**, 541–7.

Holgate, S.T. (1983). Mast cells and their mediators. In *Immunology in Medicine*, 2nd ed. Eds. Holborrow, E.J. and Reeves, W.G. pp. 79–84. Academic Press: London.

Inganas, M.S., Johansson, S.G.O. and Dannaeus, A. (1980). A method for estimation of circulating immune complexes after oral challenge with ovalbumin. *Clinical Allergy*, **10**, 293–302.

Ishizaka, K. and Ishizaka, T. (1967). Identification of $^{2}$/E-antibodies as a carrier of reaginic activity. *J. Immunol.*, **99**, 1187–98.

Ishizaka, T., Ishizaka, K. and Tomioka, H. (1972). Release of histamine and slow reacting substance of anaphylasius (SRS-A) by IgE-Anti-IgE reactions on monkey mast cells. *J. Immunol.*, **108**, 513–20.

Jackson, C.D.F., Lemaitre-Coelho, I., Vaerman, J.P., Bazine, H., Beckers, A. (1978). Rapid disappearance from serum of intravenously injected rat myeloma IgA and its secretion into the bile. *Europ. J. Immunol.*, **8**, 122–6.

Jarrett, E.E.E. and Hall, E. (1984). The development of IgE suppressive immunocompetence in young animals: influence of exposure to young antigen in the presence and absence of maternal antibody. *Immunol.*, **53**, 365–73.

Jarrett, E.E.E., Haig, D.M., McDougall, W. and McNulty, E. (1976). Rat IgE production. II. Primary and booster reaginic antibody responses following intradermal or oral immunization. *Immunology*, **30**, 671–7.

Jewell, D.P. and Thomas, H.C. (1983). Coeliac disease. In *Immunology in Medicine*, 2nd edn, p. 324, 616.097. Eds. Holborrow, E.J. and Reeves, W.G. Grune & Stratton: London.

Jones, V.A., McLaughlan, P., Shorthouse, M., Workman, E. and Hunter, J.O. (1982). Food intolerance: a major factor in the pathogenesis of irritable bowel syndrome. *Lancet*, **2**, 1115–17.

Juhlin, L. (1981). Recurrent urticaria: clinical investigation of 330 patients. *Br. J. Dermatol.*, **104**, 369–81.

Kalucy, R.S. (1976). Obesity: an attempt to find a common ground among some of the biological, psychological and sociological phenomenon of obesity/overeating syndromes. In *Psychosomatic Approach to the Prevention of Disease*, pp. 616–896. Eds. Carruthers, M. and Priest, R. Pergamon Press: Oxford.

Kaplan, M.D. and Soli, N.J. (1979). IgE to cows milk protein in breast fed atopic children. *J. All. Clin. Immun.*, **64**, 122–6.

Kemeny, D.M. and Lessof, M.H. (Eds.) (1982). I.C.A.C.I. Satellite meeting on: Recent developments in RAST and other solid phase immunoassay systems. *Excerpta Medica*: Oxford.

Leading Article (1979). Feingold's regimen for hyperkinesis. *Lancet*, **2**, 617–18.

Leung, D.Y.M., Rhodes, A.R. and Geha, R.S. (1981). Enumeration of T cell subsets in atopic dermatitis using monoclonal antibodies. *J. All. Clin. Immunol.*, **67**, 450–55.

Little, C.H., Stewart, A.G. and Fennessy, M.R. (1983). Platelet serotonin release in rheumatoid arthritis: a study in food-intolerant patients. *Lancet*, **2**, 297–9.

MacDonald, T.T. and Ferguson, A. (1976). Hypersensitivity reactions in the small intestine. 2. Effects of allograft rejection on mucosal architecture and lymhpoid cell infiltrate. *Gut*, **17**, 81–91.

McGhee, J.R., Kiyono, H., Michalek, S.M. *et al.*, (1980). Lipopolysaccharide (RPS) regulation of the immune response: T lymphocytes from normal mice suppress mitogenic and immunogenic responses to LPS. *J. Immunol.*, **124**, 1603–1611.

Mannik, M. and Arend, W.P. (1971). Fate of preformed immune complexes in rabbits and rhesus monkeys. *J. Exp. Med.*, **134**, (Suppl). 195–315.

Matthews, K.P. (1974). Urticaria. *Med. Clin. North America*. 185–205.

Matthews, T.S. and Soothill, J.F. (1970). Complement activation after milk feeding in children with cow's milk allergy. *Lancet*, **2**, 893–5.

May, C.D. and Alberto, R. (1972). In vitro responses of leucocytes to food proteins in allergic and normal children: lymphocyte stimulation and histamine release. *Clin. Allergy*, **2**, 335–44.

Michaelsson, G. and Juhlin, L. (1973). Urticaria induced by preservatives and dye additives in food and drugs. *Br. J. Dermatol.*, **88**, 525–32.

Mihm, M.C. Jr., Soter, N.A., Dvorak, H.F. *et al.*, (1976). The structure of normal skin and the morphology of atopic eczema. *J. Invest. Derm.*, **67**, 305–12.

Mowat, A. McI., Strobel, S., Drummond, H.E. and Ferguson, A. (1982). Immunological responses to fed protein antigens in mice. I. Reversal of oral tolerance to ovalbumin by cyclophosphamide. *Immunology*, **45**, 105–113.

Newcomb, R.W. and Sutoris, C.A. (1974). Comparative studies on human and rabbit exocrine IgA antibodies to an albumin. *Immunochemistry*, **11**, 623–32.

O'Morain, C. and Levi, A.J. (1981). Elemental diets in the treatment of acute Crohn's disease. In *Recent Advances in Crohn's Disease*, p. 507. Eds. Peno, A.S., Waterman, I.T., Booth, C.C. and Strober, W. Martinus Nijhoff: London.

Owen, R.L. and Jones, A.L. (1974). Epithelial cell specialization within human Peyer's patches: an ultrastructural study of intestinal lymphoid follicles. *Gastroenterology*, **66**, 189–203.

Paganelli, R., Levinsky, R.J., Brostoff, J. and Wraith, D.G. (1979). Immune complexes containing food proteins in normal and atopic subjects after oral challenge and effect of sodium cromoglycate on antigen absorption. *Lancet*, **1**, 1270–72.

Peterson, R.D.A. and Good, R.A. (1963). Antibodies to cow's milk proteins. Their presence and significance. *Pediatrics*, **31**, 209–21.

Prauznitz, C. and Kustner, H. (1921). Studien uber die Uberemfindlichkeit Zentralbl Bakteriol. (B) **86**, 160–69.

Rothberg, R.M. and Farr, R.S. (1965). Anti-bovine serum albumin and anti-alpha lactalbumin in the serum of children and adults. *Pediatrics*, **35**, 571–88.

Rowntree, S., Cogswell, J.J., Platts-Mills, T.A. and Mitchell, E.B. (1985). Development of IgE and IgG antibodies to food and inhalant allergens in children at risk of allergic disease. *Arch. Dis. Child.*, **60**, 727–35.

Rowntree, S., Mitchell, E.B., Platts and Mills, T.A.E. (1986). Assessment of skin reactivity and specific antibody to egg and milk proteins in patients with atopic dermatitis: comparison with responses to the house dust mite antigen. *Int. Arch. All. appl. Immunol.*, **79**, 132–9.

Royal College of Physicians (1984). Food intolerance and food aversion. A Joint Report of the Royal College of Physicians and the British Nutrition Foundation. *J. Roy. Coll. Physicians Lond.*, **18**, No. 2.

Scheinmann, P., Gendrel, D., Charles, J. *et al.*, (1976). Value of lymphoblast transformation test in cow's milk protein intestinal intolerance. *Clin. Allergy*, **6**, 515–21.

Strober, W. (1982). The regulation of mucosal immune system. *J. All. Clin. Immunol.*, **70**, 225–30.

Valverde, E., Vich, J.M., Garcia-Caleron, J.V. and Garcia-Calderon, P.A. (1980). In vitro stimulation of lymphocytes in patients with chronic urticaria induced by additives and food. *Clin. Allergy*, **10**, 691–8.

Van Asperen, P.P., Kemp, A.S. and Mellis, C.M. (1983). Immediate food hypersensitivity reactions on the first known exposure to the food. *Arch. Dis. Child.*, **58**, 253–6.

Walker, W.A. (1981). Antigen uptake in the gut: immunologic implications. *Immunol. Today*, **2**, 30–34.

Walport, M.H., Parke, A.L. and Hughes, G.R.V. (1983). Food and the connective tissue diseases. In *Food Allergy*, pp. 113–20. Eds. Brostoff, J. and Challacombe S.J. Saunders: London.

Wardlaw, A.J. (1986). Morphological and secretory properties of bronchoalveolar lauage mast cells in respiratory diseases. *Clin. Allergy*, **16**, 163–73.

Wilson, N., Vickers, H., Taylor, G. and Silverman, M. (1982). Objective test for food sensitivity in asthmatic children: increased bronchial reactivity after cola drinks. *Br. Med. J.*, **284**, 1226–8.

# 18 The interrelationships of nutrition and drugs

John W.T. Dickerson



## Introduction

Most of the drugs in use today for the treatment of human disease owe their activity to a selectively toxic effect on an infective or invasive agent, or to the selective inhibition of an enzyme system. Their effect may be modified by various factors in the host such as age, sex, nutritional status, pregnancy, disease, and the pre-administration of other drugs or 'foreign compounds' (Parke, 1968). They are metabolized in the body by a non-specific mixed function oxidase system involving reduced nicotinamide adenine dinucleotide (NADPH) and cytochrome P-450 located primarily, but not exclusively, in hepatic microsomes. Deficiencies of energy, protein, vitamins, or minerals may modify the activity of these enzymes so that the toxicity of the drug is increased or decreased. An increase in toxicity occurs when the drug exerts a direct action, and a decrease when the drug must first be converted into its active derivative.

The enzymatic metabolism of drugs takes place in two stages (Williams,

1967). The first stage is asynthetic and results in the formation of a polar compound by N-dealkylation, deamination, hydroxylation, oxidation, or reduction. The second, synthetic phase consists of the conjugation of the polar compound formed in the first phase with glucuronic acid, sulphate, or glycine. The final process is the elimination of the conjugate in the urine or bile. The enzyme system that carries out the Stage 1 reaction also catalyses the hydrolysis of a number of endogenous compounds such as steroid hormones and fatty acids. Regardless of the species, the activity of these enzymes is low in the liver of the new-born animal and develops in a characteristic manner to reach mature values by 4 to 6 weeks after birth.

The nutrition of the sick is often impaired as the result of a disease process or by the treatment of disease, and this may have a profound effect upon the body's response to drugs. On the other hand, the drugs themselves may interfere with nutrition in various ways (*vide infra*) some of which are desirable and others undesirable. An understanding of these interrelationships may lead to a more rational approach to drug dosage and the reduction in adverse drug reaction and interaction.

This chapter will be concerned with the effect of food on the absorption and metabolism of drugs, the interaction of drugs and foods, the effects of drugs on the metabolism of nutrients, the use of nutrients as drugs and groups vulnerable to drug-nutrient interaction.

## The effects of food on the absorption of drugs

Patients may be told to take their drugs 'before', 'with' or 'after' meals. The consumption of food before taking a drug may increase or decrease its pharmacological action depending on the nature of the drug and particularly on its chemical properties (Toothaker and Welling, 1980). Food may also influence drug absorption as a result of physiological changes induced in the GI tract. These changes include effects on splanchnic blood flow, gastric motility and gastric secretion.

### Splanchnic blood flow (SBF)

High protein liquid meals increase, while high glucose liquid meals cause a transient small decrease, in SBF. The effect of these changes on drug absorption depends on whether the absorption is passive, in which case it may be affected by a change in transluminal concentration gradient, or active, in which case it should not be affected. Changes in SBF may also affect the absorption of drugs that are extensively metabolized in the liver (McLean *et al.*, 1978).

### Gastric motility

The principal effect of food ingestion is to delay stomach emptying due to feed-back mechanisms from the osmoreceptors, acid receptors and fat and fatty acid receptors in the proximal small intestine. Stomach emptying is delayed by hot meals, by solutions of high viscosity and by high fat and to a lesser extent high protein and carbohydrate meals. In rats, solid meals almost double gastric emptying time. The effect of such changes on the absorption of drugs will clearly depend on their chemical nature. Prolonged residence in the acid medium of the stomach is likely to delay dissolution of acidic, and accelerate that of basic compounds. Since the optimal site of drug absorption is in the intestine delayed gastric emptying will delay absorption. However, if the drug is absorbed actively by a saturable process, delayed gastric emptying will tend to enhance absorption.

### Gastric secretion

The increased secretion of hydrochloric acid, and of many enzymes, which follows food ingestion may affect drug dissolution and degradation. Increased bile secretion after food may accelerate the dissolution of poorly soluble compounds. However, the combination of drugs with bile salts may hinder their absorption.

### Drug-fluid and drug-food interactions

Since drugs are often absorbed by a passive process it might be supposed that they would be absorbed more readily from concentrated solutions. However, studies in both experimental animals and man have indicated that the reverse is the case. Thus, sodium pentobarbital and salicylate are both absorbed more readily from dilute solutions (Borowitz *et al.*, 1971). Similar effects have been demonstrated in the human (Welling, 1977).

The chelation of drugs to polyvalent metal ions inhibits drug bioavailability. Some drugs chelate to proteins (Kohn, 1961). There is also the possibility that food may inhibit drug absorption simply by forming a physical barrier at the absorptive surface.

## The effects of food on drug metabolism

### Induction of intestinal drug metabolism

The mixed function oxidase (MFO) system responsible for drug metabolism is at its highest activity in the liver but it is also present in other tissues including the small intestine. In this organ it is possible for food constituents to induce the enzyme activity and for drugs and other 'foreign' substances to undergo biotransformation before entering the blood stream as well as subsequently as the result of metabolism in the liver. Smoked food, in particular, may contain substances which induce drug metabolizing enzymes. Studies in experimental animals have shown that ingestion of the polycylic hydrocarbons of broiled beef resulted in an increase in *in vitro* metabolism by the intestine (Pantuck *et al.*, 1975). Similar observations have been made in man (Conney *et al.*, 1976).

Many foods normally contain substances which act as inducers of the MFO system in the intestine. Thus, indoles present in cabbage and Brussel sprouts (Fig. 18.1) have this action and their consumption by rats has been shown to stimulate the *in vitro* metabolism of phenacetin, 1-ethoxycoumarin, hexobarbital and benzo-(α)pyrene by the intestine (Pantuck *et al.*, 1976).

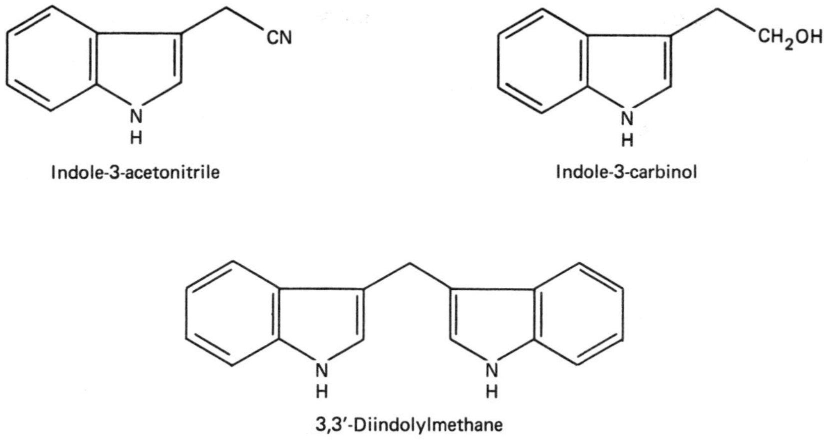

Indole-3-acetonitrile

Indole-3-carbinol

3,3′-Diindolylmethane

Fig. 18.1 Indoles present in cabbage and Brussels sprouts (Dickerson, 1980).

## The effects of protein-energy malnutrition (PEM)

Primary PEM resulting from the ingestion of insufficient food of the right kind, is presently the most widespread nutritional disease in children, but secondary malnutrition, arising from certain disease states, may affect individuals of all ages even in affluent societies. The effect of PEM on the toxicity of drugs depends on the severity of the nutritional deprivation, the age of the individual, the presence of infection, diarrhoea, or deranged renal and circulatory function. Nutrition can affect the metabolism of drugs in at least two ways. If the dietary intake of energy is low, tissue protein will be catabolized and used as a source of energy, thus reducing the availability of amino acids for protein synthesis. This may reduce the amounts of the different enzymes in the tissues, including those involved in the metabolism of drugs. Secondly, the substrates used for the conjugation of drugs are derived from nutrients, and there could be competition between the metabolism of drugs and the needs of the tissues for particular nutrients.

Much of our knowledge of the effects of energy and protein deficiency on the metabolism of drugs has been derived from animal experiments and must be extrapolated to man with caution. However, analysis of post-mortem samples of human liver has shown that similar enzymes are present to those found in the livers of experimental animals (Nelson *et al.*, 1971).

In adult rats, the rate of drug metabolism and the activity of drug metabolizing enzymes in the liver is closely related to the amount of protein in the diet (Kato *et al.*, 1968). Administration of phenobarbital to rats fed a low protein diet also induces a smaller increase in hepatic cytochrome P-450 than in well-fed controls (Marshall and McLean, 1969). It seems that in the malnourished animal, cytochrome P-450 and the drug metabolizing enzymes increase more slowly than other liver proteins when the animals are being nutritionally rehabilitated (Marshall and McLean, 1969). Anutrients other than drugs are metabolized by the drug-metabolizing enzymes, and two of these, dimethylnitrosamine and aflatoxin, that are likely to occur in areas of the world where protein deficiency is common, have their carcinogenic action enhanced by the suppressed enzyme activity resulting from a low protein diet (McLean and McLean, 1969).

In contrast, low protein diets reduce the toxicity of compounds which must first be converted into a toxic derivative. Thus young male rats are protected by a low protein diet from the toxic effect of carbon tetrachloride ($CCl_4$), judged by the mortality and by indices of liver damage (McLean and McLean, 1966), but the protective effect is reversed by the administration of an enzyme-inducer such as phenobarbitone. It seems possible that antioxidants such as butylated hydroxytoluene (BHT) that are commonly added to food, may protect against the adverse effects of $CCl_4$ by preventing the formation of the toxic metabolite.

In children with kwashiorkor there is evidence of an adaptive response of amino acid activating enzymes in the liver which is mediated by the gluco-corticoids (Waterlow, 1968). In young rats a low protein diet produces a similar adaptive response of the hepatic microsomal drug metabolizing enzymes involved in stage I (Dickerson *et al.*, 1976) and stage II reactions (Woodcock and Wood, 1971), and there is evidence that this adaptive response, at least as far as the stage I enzymes are concerned, is mediated by corticosteroids (Basu *et al.*, 1971).

The clinical problems related to the use of drugs in malnourished subjects have been reviewed by Poskitt (1974). The pharmacological response to a drug depends in the first instance on the rate at which it is absorbed and distributed, and nutrition is one of the factors that may affect the rate of absorption of drugs from the gastrointestinal tract (see above).

A reduced activity of hepatic drug-metabolizing enzymes in children with kwashiorkor may be inferred from the finding that they excrete a higher ratio of the antimalarial drug, chloroquine, to its liver-formed metabolites. Chloramphenicol is a useful drug for the study of stage II (conjugation) reactions because in normal adult humans 90 per cent of the drug excreted in the urine is in the form of its glucuronide (Glazko, 1949). After a test dose (25 mg/kg body weight), this drug has been found to take longer (30 hours) to clear from the plasma of children with PEM than it did from controls (12 hours) (Mehta *et al.*, 1975). Further evidence of slower hepatic metabolism of the drug was obtained from the urinary excretion of the glucuronide, for whereas the control subjects excreted 75–85 per cent of the drug as the conjugate, the patients excreted only 35–55 per cent of the drug in this form. Liver biopsies in two patients showed low activities of bilirubin-UDP transferase. A slower rate of disappearance of penicillin from the plasma of children with kwashiorkor, which increases on recovery, has been attributed (Buchanan and Hansen, 1976) to the inadequate renal function which is characteristic of this condition (Alleyne, 1967).

Tetrachloroethylene is used to treat hookworm infestations in children with kwashiorkor. It seems possible that depressed activity of drug metabolizing enzymes in the livers of children with kwashiorkor may protect them from the toxic effects of this drug by reducing the rate of transformation to toxic metabolites.

Trimethoprim is an antibacterial drug that owes its action to its inhibition of dihydrofolate reductase. This inhibition is greater in bacteria than in man; nevertheless, trimethoprim can produce biochemical and clinical folate deficiency in the human. Dihydrofolate reductase is also inhibited with consequent clinical folate deficiency, by the antimalarial drug pyrimethamine. This drug also inhibits the conversion of phenylalanine to tyrosine. This inhibition may be of particular importance in patients with kwashiorkor, for in this condition the metabolism of phenylalanine is impaired and if they are treated with a high protein diet and the drug, there could be a risk that elevated plasma levels of the amino acid might cause brain damage.

There is some evidence that protein intake may modify the action of levodopa in patients with Parkinson's disease (Gillespie *et al.*, 1973; Mena and Cotzias, 1975). A diet containing 0.5 g of protein per kg body weight per day tended to potentiate and stabilize the therapeutic effects of the drugs, and also reduce the amount of the drug excreted as the methylated derivative, homovanillic acid.

## Effects of minerals and vitamins

As with the major food components, energy and protein, so too with minor components, minerals and vitamins; we know more about the effects of deficiency states in experimental animals than in man (for review see Basu and Dickerson, 1974). In the weanling rat, dietary deficiencies of calcium, zinc, and magnesium depress the metabolism of a number of drugs; deficiencies of zinc and magnesium both result in lower levels of hepatic cytochrome P-450 and hence could lead to lower activity of the electron transport system required for drug metabolism.

Because of the extreme dietary deficiencies used, these experimental studies may have little significance for man beyond showing that the particular minerals are involved in the metabolism of drugs. However, the body content of potassium significantly affects the toxicity of digitalis in patients with cardiac failure. Thus, any treatment which reduces serum potassium level in a digitalized patient will increase the risk of digitalis-induced cardiac arrhythmias (D'Arcy and Griffin, 1972). Diuretics, particularly those of the thiazide group, and adrenal steroids may precipitate digitalis toxicity by depleting the body of potassium. This interaction is of particular importance in old people. A reduction in the plasma potassium ions may also result from the infusion of glucose solutions since potassium ions move into skeletal muscle with glucose. According to D'Arcy and Griffin, the treatment of digitalis-induced arrhythmia may require the oral administration of 5–7 g of potassium chloride which acts in 30 minutes. It may be necessary to follow this with 1 g of potassium chloride orally three times a day for two to three days. In unskilled hands, however, the $\beta$-adrenergic blocker, propanolol, is probably safer than potassium. Kwashiorkor is often complicated by anaemia and cardiac failure (Wharton *et al.*, 1967) and the low body content of potassium in these children may also modify the response to digoxin. In animals, calcium increases the response to digitalis, and thus caution must be exercised when intravenous calcium is given to digitalized patients (D'Arcy and Griffin, 1972).

Ascorbic acid (AA) interacts with drugs in various ways and plays an important role in drug metabolism (Wilson, 1974). Thus in the rat, enzyme-inducing drugs such as phenobarbitone increase the urinary excretion of the vitamin, and in the guinea-pig, deficiency increases the toxicity of the muscle relaxant drug, zoxazolamine, due to a decreased activity of drug-metabolizing enzymes. Scorbutic animals can be anaesthetized more rapidly and recover more slowly than those receiving ascorbic acid supplements, and the sleeping time of rats given vitamin C supplements is reduced due to the stimulating effect of the vitamin on hydroxylating enzymes in hepatic microsomes.

Many arguments have been advanced in favour of the use of large doses of ascorbic acid both prophylactically and therapeutically. These arguments have been countered by claims that ascorbic acid is toxic in large quantities. Most of these claims are now considered doubtful (Hornig and Moser, 1981). However, it has been found that in the guinea-pig high doses of AA reduced the concentration of the cytochromes P-450 and B5 (Sutton *et al.*, 1983). It seems that when given in high doses AA ceases to act as a vitamin and should be considered a drug.

### Effects of other substances

Some drugs, such as phenobarbitone, are potent inducers of drug-metabolizing enzymes. Other substances, though they are weak inducers themselves, nevertheless enhance induction by phenobarbitone, and have been said to have a 'permissive' role (Marshall and McLean, 1971). Linoleic acid appears to act in this way.

As we shall see later, oral contraceptive agents (OCA) affect nutrition in a number of different ways which may contribute to the fact that they also reduce the rate at which the body metabolizes various drugs such as meperidine (Pethidine) and promazine (Sparine) (Crawford and Rudofsky, 1966) and antipyrine (O'Malley *et al.*, 1972).

## Interaction of drugs and foods

Foods contain a number of non-nutrient substances. Some of these are additives, others occur naturally. Additives are generally metabolized by the hepatic mixed function oxidase system whereas others are metabolized by enzymes concerned with other metabolic pathways. In this latter group of substances, sympathomimetic tyramines are of particular interest and importance. These substances are normally metabolized by the enzyme, monoamine oxidase (MAO). It follows therefore that drugs which inhibit this enzyme will inhibit the metabolism of these amines and allow them to enter the circulation with very unpleasant consequences. It is essential that patients receiving MAO inhibitors (Table 18.1) are told not to consume the following foods: cheese (especially strong cheddar, camembert and stilton), game, yoghurt, stored liver, 'Marmite', 'Bovril', pickled herrings, broad beans, certain wines and chocolate. Amphetamine, sometimes used in the treatment of obesity, is a mild MAO inhibitor, and thus may also cause headache, nausea, and hypertension, if taken with any of the foods mentioned above.

## Alcohol

Alcohol is a drug in its own right. If taken with carbohydrate it may cause delayed hypoglycaemia due to potentiation of the action of insulin (O'Keefe and Marks, 1977). This is a problem that may be experienced for instance by a

Table 18.1 Monoamine oxidase inhibitors reported to interact with tyramine-containing foods (From Dickerson, 1980a)

| |
|---|
| Phenelzine (Nardil) |
| Tranylcypromine (Parnate, Parstelin) |
| Iproniazid (Marsilid) |
| Nialamide (Niamid) |
| Mebanazine (Actomol) |
| Pargyline (Eutonyl) |

commercial traveller who stops for a gin and tonic and sandwich for lunch and may feel sleepy 3 to 4 hours later due to hypoglycaemia.

Heavy drinking may potentiate the action of the hypoglycaemic drug, tolbutamide, due to inhibition of its metabolism. On the other hand, alcohol may hasten the removal of propanolol from the blood so that its effect on blood pressure may be reduced. Even small amounts of alcohol can increase the effects of central nervous system depressants such as barbiturates and benzodiazepines. Persistent heavy drinking induces the hepatic mixed function oxidase system and consequently leads to accelerated metabolism of a number of drugs such as tolbutamide, anticonvulsants and the anti-coagulant, warfarin. Doctors should be aware that a wide spectrum of drugs – diuretics, antirheumatics, hypoglycaemics, hypotensives, antidepressants, tranquilizers and antibiotics may interact with alcohol.

## Effects of drugs on the metabolism of nutrients

### Effects on appetite

#### Drugs which decrease appetite

Obese patients often have considerable difficulty in adhering to a reducing diet and certain drugs such as diethylproprion (Tenuate), fenfluramine (Ponderal), amphetamine (Benzedrine), dexamphetamine (Dexedrine), and mazindol (Terenoc) are used as anorectic agents (Pawan, 1974). There are dangers of addiction, abuse, and the development of side-effects with most of these drugs. Amphetamine is also used to stimulate appetite in patients with anorexia nervosa. Since it is a sympathomimetic amine, severe side-effects and even death may result from its use in depressed patients who are being treated with monoamine oxidase inhibitors (see above).

Biguanides, eg., phenethyl biguanide (Phenformin) and dimethyl biguanide (Metformin) are used as oral hypoglycaemic agents. The depression of appetite is a useful side-effect in adult-onset diabetes as many of the patients are overweight.

There are a number of other drugs that may cause anorexia. These include digitalis, glucagon, indomethacin, morphine and cyclophosphamide. The latter cytotoxic drug is used in the treatment of cancer patients who may already be malnourished. In many patients threatened with it, the effects disappear when administration of the drug is stopped. In a few patients, however, the effect may be of much longer duration and these patients should be identified and attempts made to help them.

**Drugs which increase appetite**

The sulphonylureas (eg., tolbutamide, chlorpropamide, and glibenclamide) increase appetite, possibly by a stimulating effect on the release of pancreatic insulin. Increased appetite and consequent weight gain is often seen in depressed patients following the administration of antidepressants. Similarly, anxious or agitated patients often put on weight when treated with tranquilizers, such as the phenothiazines (eg., Largactil), and benzodiazepines (eg., Valium, Librium and Nobrium).

Some antihistamine drugs affect appetite. One of these, cyproheptadine (Periactin), a serotonin-antagonist used in the treatment of pruritus, may act by virtue of its hypoglycaemic effect or by directly affecting the hypothalamus (Pawan, 1974). This drug now tends to be used more for it side-effect than for its original purpose (Noble, 1969). Hormones, such as oral contraceptives, the androgens, corticosteroids, insulin and anabolic agents like Durabolin also act as appetite stimulants.

A small amount of alcohol taken before a meal may act as a useful appetite stimulant in sick patients by stimulating the sense of taste, increasing the flow of saliva, gastric, and pancreatic secretions, and producing relaxation and a feeling of well-being.

## Effects on carbohydrate metabolism

Drugs that affect the metabolism of carbohydrate can be divided into those that tend to raise the fasting blood sugar level and reduce glucose tolerance (predominantly hyperglycaemia), and those that tend to lower the fasting blood sugar generally with little or no improvement of glucose tolerance (Marks, 1974).

**Drugs causing hyperglycaemia**

Thiazide diuretics induce hyperglycaemia in normal animals, but the results of clinical investigation are not so definite. It seems that generally these have shown that the thiazides are potentially diabetogenic in high doses to patients who have recently developed diabetes, to those with a family history of diabetes, to those with hypertension and during pregnancy (D'Arcy and Griffin, 1972). Early studies (Dinon *et al.*, 1958) yielded no evidence of altered carbohydrate metabolism in 121 oedematous and hypertensive patients treated with chlorothiazide at dose levels of 0.5–2 g/day. Goldner *et al.*, (1960) found no increase in fasting blood sugar levels in non-diabetics treated with chlorothiazide, hydrochlorothiazide, and dihydroflumethiazide and raised blood sugar levels were only found in diabetics on high doses of the drugs.

Diabetes, or an inherited tendency to it, may not necessarily be a prerequisite for diabetic response to chlorothiazide, however, for Brown and Brown (1967) found that three of five normal men with negative family histories of diabetes who received 50 mg of hydrochlorothiazide daily for 14 months showed an abnormal oral glucose tolerance.

These findings are sufficiently suggestive for D'Arcy and Griffin (1972) to recommend that knowledge of carbohydrate tolerance before starting thiazide therapy would be a wise precaution.

Another diuretic, frusemide, has also been reported to cause impaired glucose tolerance which is not necessarily related to existing diabetes, and which may disappear on stopping the drug.

Diazoxide structurally resembles chlorothiazide, but has only the antihypertensive properties of the latter, and not its diuretic properties. Diazoxide is a potent diabetogenic agent in man inhibiting the release of insulin, and its effect is increased by combining it with a thiazide diuretic (Dollery *et al.*, 1962; Okun *et al.*, 1963). Occasionally, the unwanted and even potentially dangerous side-effects of drugs can be used therapeutically. Diazoxide is a good example, for children with leucine-sensitive hypoglycaemia have been satisfactorily treated with the drug (Samols and Marks, 1966).

Corticosteroids induce hyperglycaemia in a proportion of patients. Thus, Matsunaga *et al.*, (1963) found that 5.5 per cent of a group of 235 patients receiving steroids developed diabetes. This included 7 per cent of patients treated with prednisolone, 23 per cent of those treated with paramethasone, and 20 per cent of those treated with betamethasone, but none of the patients treated with corticotrophin or cortisone. In another series, Schubert and Schulte (1963) reported that 14 per cent of 214 patients treated with corticosteroids for longer than 3 days developed diabetes. These authors noted that disturbances of carbohydrate metabolism occurred earlier in patients on higher doses of steroids, and in those who had liver disease in whom excretion of the glucuronide conjugate was reduced. It appears that patients with diabetes may absorb enough of at least some topically applied steroids to upset their management. Thus, Kershbaum (1963) reported on four patients with diabetes whose insulin or tolbutamide requirements were increased following treatment with fluocinolone acetonide for skin conditions.

Impaired glucose tolerance was one of the earliest metabolic consequences of taking oral contraceptives to be described. Many of the early reports suggested that these drugs upset the control of diabetics necessitating an increase in the amount of insulin to be used. It is also unwise to be complacent about the use of oral contraceptives in women with potential diabetes (Szabo *et al.*, 1970). In the study reported by these authors the glucose tolerance of fifteen women that had been abnormal during the last trimester of pregnancy returned to normal on delivery. Five of the women subsequently received a combination of norethindrone (1 mg) and mestranol (0.05 mg) as an oral contraceptive cyclically. In all five women, abnormal glucose tolerance recurred and three of them remained diabetic after ceasing to use the contraceptive agent. The authors concluded that screening tests for diabetes should be performed early during contraceptive treatment so that women with latent diabetes can be excluded from the use of hormones.

Wynn and Doar (1969) carried out a longitudinal study on a group of normal women treated with combined oral contraceptive agents. Of 91 women tested before and during medication 13 per cent developed chemical diabetes mellitus as a result of the medication. These authors concluded that the impaired glucose tolerance was steroid diabetes caused by elevated plasma cortisol levels secondary to the oestrogen component of the oral contraceptive.

It would be reasonable to conclude from these studies that the risk of precipitating permanent diabetes by the use of combined oral contraceptives cannot be ignored. D'Arcy and Griffin (1972) recommend a routine investigation of the status of carbohydrate metabolism as a wise and sensible precaution, particularly in those with a family history of diabetes mellitus.

Diphenylhydantoin (Phenytoin) and other anticonvulsants can cause hyperglycaemia. The mechanism by which they may do so has not been established. It has variously been suggested that diphenylhydantoin acts directly on the hypothalamus, stimulates the pituitary and adrenal cortex, and that it causes an impaired insulin response to carbohydrate.

Pharmacological doses (up to 3 g per day) of nicotinic acid have been used, particularly in the United States, as a hypolipidaemic agent in the treatment of hypercholesterolaemia. There are a number of unpleasant side-effects to taking these large amounts of the vitamin including unpleasant flushing, itching, liver damage, and impaired glucose tolerance (Gey and Carlson, 1971).

An analogue of nicotinic acid, $\beta$-pyridylcarbinol (Ronicol) when given in large (Marks *et al.*, 1971) but not in small doses, also causes a rise in fasting blood glucose and a moderate to severe impairment of glucose tolerance. The impairment of glucose tolerance appears not to be due to suppression of pancreatic $\beta$-cell activity. Current evidence suggests that nicotinic acid causes impaired tissue utilization of glucose, possibly due to an increase in intracellular free fatty acids (Marks, 1974).

Experiments aimed at demonstrating a hyperglycaemic effect of caffeine have yielded conflicting results. Experiments by Marks and his colleagues (Marks, 1974) in which moderate amounts of caffeine were given as tea revealed no consistent effect upon oral glucose tolerance in normal individuals or those suffering from chemical diabetes.

**Drugs causing hypoglycaemia**

Overdosage of sulphonylureas can cause serious or fatal hypoglycaemia, particularly in elderly malnourished patients in whom the ability to metabolize and excrete the drug may be impaired. It is important to consider the question of drug interaction when sulphonylureas are being used. The amount of the drug reaching the tissues may be greatly increased by other drugs such as phenylbutazone and warfarin which displace the sulphonylureas from their binding sites on plasma proteins. Alternatively, other drugs such as sulphaphenozol, dicoumarol, and phenyramidole may compete with the sulphonylureas for metabolism by hepatic drug-metabolizing enzymes, thus decreasing their rate of degradation and potentiating their hypoglycaemic effects (Marks, 1974).

In normal doses (i.e., sufficient to produce a blood alcohol level of less than 1 g/litre) alcohol does not affect blood glucose levels. In the alcohol-naive subject, whether recently fed or fasted overnight, large intoxicating amounts produce a rise in blood sugar concentrations (Marks, 1975). This change, which does not occur in the alcohol-habituated subject, is due to activation of hepatic glycogenolysis.

The much more important effect of alcohol is that when taken in non-intoxicating amounts it can produce severe, and occasionally fatal, hypoglycaemia in both alcohol-naive and habituated subjects (Marks and Medd, 1964). The hypoglycaemia results from the inhibition of hepatic gluconeogenesis and therefore most often occurs in situations in which this process is the main source of glucose entering the blood. Thus it occurs in overnight-fasted children, or 36–72 hour acutely starved or chronically malnourished adults.

Administration of acetylsalicylic acid to diabetic and normal humans causes a profound hypoglycaemia, which is probably due to an inhibition of gluconeogenesis (Madapally *et al.*, 1972).

## Effects on lipid metabolism

### Drugs that lower plasma lipids

A number of drugs affect the absorption of fat and other nutrients from the gastrointestinal tract to varying degrees (Truswell, 1973). The antibiotics neomycin and kanamycin cause mild morphological changes in the jejunal villi and fat malabsorption, and lower the serum cholesterol level by binding bile acids in the gut. Colchicine, phenindione, p-aminosalicylic acid (PAS) and indomethacin can have similar effect. Tygstrup and his colleagues (1959) reported that PAS in tuberculous patients lowered plasma cholesterol levels and caused malabsorption of triolein from the gut. The intestinal symptoms caused by PAS are reduced if the drug is crystallized in the presence of ascorbic acid. Levine (1968) studied the effects of PAS-C in young adult male volunteers and found that 6 g per day failed to produce malabsorption of fats, whereas 12 g per day for 4 weeks induced moderate steatorrhoea without diarrhoea. Malabsorption of vitamin $B_{12}$ may also occur in patients treated with PAS.

Cholestyramine resin is used to bind bile acids and is the drug of choice in the treatment of Type IIA hyperlipoproteinaemia. In large doses it can induce steatorrhoea in man and loss of fat-soluble vitamins. The absorption of fat-soluble vitamins is also reduced by liquid paraffin.

The incorporation of triglyceride from circulating chylomicrons into adipose tissue involves the action of lipoprotein lipase. This enzyme is released by heparin, inhibited by protamine sulphate, and its action is potentiated by insulin in physiological amounts. Sugar taken with fat facilitates the clearing of the postabsorptive lipaemia, and the clearing is more rapid when the sugar is taken as glucose rather than sucrose, because glucose is the more effective stimulant of insulin secretion (Mann *et al.*, 1971). The female sex hormones reduce lipoprotein lipase activity and this partly explains the action of oestrogens and oestrogen-progestagen oral contraceptives in increasing plasma triglyceride concentrations.

Ethanol is the commonest cause of drug-induced fatty liver. The condition has also been reported in patients given large doses of adrenal corticosteroids, and acute fatty liver can occur when tetracycline is given intravenously in late pregnancy.

A large number of drugs increase lipolysis. These include the catecholamines, methyl xanthines, and appetite suppressants such as the amphetamines which are in use as anorexigenic drugs in doses of 5 to 20 mg per day depending on the patient. Of the drugs that decrease lipolysis, nicotinic acid is the best known. Nicotinamide is ineffective. There are several chemical analogues of nicotinic acid that have a similar action. One of these, 5-fluoro-3-hydroxymethylpyridine hydrochloride which is metabolized to 5-fluoronicotinic acid, does not cause the troublesome flushing which follows ingestion of nicotinic acid, and has been found to lower the plasma free fatty acid concentrations in patients who have had a myocardial infarction (Rowe *et al.*, 1973).

Some drugs that lower plasma lipid concentrations are used clinically in the treatment of hyperlipidaemias. No drugs are available for use in the rare Type I hyperlipidaemia. Cholestyramine is useful for Type II and lowers only the plasma cholesterol concentration. This drug has no effect on very low density lipoproteins (VLDL). D- but not L-thyroxine also reduces the plasma cholesterol concentration, but by a different mechanism, for it acts by increasing hepatic catabolism of cholesterol. Clofibrate (Atromid) is effective in the treatment of Types IIb, III, IV and V hyperlipidaemia and reduces plasma concentration of cholesterol, VLDL and triglyceride. In spite of the large amount of work done on this drug its mode of action does not seem to be known. It was originally introduced by Thorp who suggested (Thorp *et al.*, 1963) that it acted by displacing thyroxine from its binding sites on plasma albumin, thus increasing the circulating levels of free thyroxine. Nicotinic acid can be used as an alternative to clofibrate in the treatment of Types IV and V and is effective because of its inhibitory effect on adipose tissue lipolysis. The progestogen norethisterone acetate is also effective in the familial variety of Type V.

A variety of other drugs incidentally lower plasma lipid concentration. These include aspirin, PAS, chlortetracycline, colchicine, fenfluramine, phenformin, glucagon, phenindione, trifluperidol and sulphinpyrazone. Tryptophan lowers the hyperlipidaemia that occurs in the nephrotic syndrome (Schapel *et al.*, 1974).

**Drugs that raise plasma lipids**

An increase in the plasma concentration of certain lipids may occur as an incidental result of the administration of some drugs. Thus, oral contraceptives, large doses of adrenal corticosteroids, ethanol, and growth hormones raise plasma triglyceride concentrations, and oral contraceptives, chlorpromazine, thiouracil and vitamin D raise plasma cholesterol concentrations. In human volunteers (Miller and Nestel, 1973) phenobarbitone causes a rise in plasma triglyceride and cholesterol concentrations, the latter being due to increased cholesterol synthesis.

The effects of oral contraceptives on plasma lipids are perhaps the most disturbing feature of their use. In fact, any metabolic disturbance caused by these agents must be evaluated in the light of the fact that they are now being freely made available to teenage girls both for use as contraceptive agents and also as a treatment of dysmenorrhoea. Elevated plasma concentrations of cholesterol and triglycerides are significantly correlated in men with the development of atherosclerosis and coronary heart disease. The concentrations found in pre-menopausal women are lower and this correlates with a smaller risk of sudden death. The increase in plasma triglycerides and cholesterol in women receiving oral contraceptive agents (Wynn *et al.*, 1969) reduces the sex differential between men and women of similar ages. The prospect of metabolic consequences of long-term use of such agents is one which responsible doctors cannot ignore. It may be possible, however, to manipulate the diet to reduce, or entirely obliterate, the changes in plasma lipids caused by the oral contraceptive agents. A diet containing a relatively high ratio of polyunsaturated to saturated fatty acids is used for this purpose in individuals at risk of coronary thrombosis (see p. 20) and experiments in rats have shown that the incorporation of sunflower oil in the diet mitigated the changes in blood lipids caused by the oral contraceptives, particularly when the diet was also low in cholesterol (Tabacchi and Kirksey, 1973).

## Effects on protein and amino acid metabolism

A number of drugs such as corticosteroids, thyroid hormones, and tetracyclines increase the urinary excretion of nitrogen and thus cause a negative nitrogen balance. In an analysis of 1957 patients of mean age 61 years included in the Boston Collaborative Drug Surveillance Programme (1972), it was found that when tetracyclines were used in conjunction with diuretics a significant rise in blood urea levels occurred. Anabolic steroids, and possibly insulin have an opposite effect and stimulate protein synthesis.

The response of the fasting amino acid pattern to the administration of only a few drugs has been investigated. The changes produced are often complex with the concentrations of some amino acids being affected more than others. Oral contraceptives cause a significant reduction in the concentration of total free amino acids in the second half of the menstrual cycle, with reductions in the concentration of proline, glycine, alanine, valine, leucine, and tyrosine (Craft and Peters, 1971). After completing one course of oral contraceptives and before starting another the plasma total amino acid concentration rises to normal values but a significant reduction in the concentration of glycine persists.

Insulin causes a reduction in the plasma concentration of amino acids, and particularly affects glycine and alanine, while tranylcypromine has the reverse effect, causing a rise in total amino acids. The cytotoxic drug methotrexate is a folic acid antagonist, and interferes with phenylalanine metabolism probably by preventing the formation of tetrahydrobiopterin, which is a cofactor for phenylalanine hydroxylase.

## Effects on mineral metabolism

The decrease in body potassium that may occur when thiazide diuretics are used has already been mentioned. Many of the patients receiving these drugs are likely to be elderly and therefore the condition may be aggravated by a low intake of potassium which has been reported in the elderly (Judge, 1968; Davies *et al.*, 1973b). Depletion of body potassium also occurs due to the regular use of purgatives, and again the elderly, with their often almost pathological obsession with bowel evacuation, are probably most at risk. Judge (1968) has recommended that the potassium intake of an adult should be 60 mmol/day. Cases of hypokalaemia can be treated with 'Slow K' separately or in combination.

Salt and water retention are common in patients treated with corticosteroids and are partly responsible for the weight gain, oedema, and hypertension that frequently develop. The sodium retaining properties of cortisone, deoxycorticosterone, and aldosterone are far greater than those of prednisone, prednisolone, and the newer steroid analogues.

The retention of salt and water accompanies medication with the combined oestrogen-progestogen oral contraceptive and leads to weight gain with oedema and the possible development of hypertension. Similar side-effects commonly occur in patients treated with phenylbutazone and oxyphenbutazone. Hypertension, oedema, or potassium loss has also been reported in up to 50 per cent of patients receiving 300 mg/day of carbenoxolone sodium for the treatment of peptic ulcer.

The absorption of iron from the gut is influenced by a number of factors such as the form in which it is present, the presence of other food constituents with which it may form insoluble chelates, and other factors which may affect the mucosal cells themselves. Thus, ascorbic acid facilitates the absorption of iron, and this effect is partly, but not entirely (Hughes, 1974) accounted for by the ascorbic acid keeping the iron in the ferrous state. Fructose also facilitates iron absorption, whilst absorption is decreased by phosphates, antacids, and tetracyline. Combined oral contraceptives do not affect the absorption of iron from the intestine, but they do cause a rise in the concentration of iron in the plasma, and in the total iron binding capacity (Norrby *et al.*, 1972). These changes are probably due to increased mobilization of iron from stores mediated by the elevated transferrin concentrations.

Sulphonylureas, phenylbutazone, cobalt, and lithium interfere with $^{131}I$ uptake or release and can cause goitre. Oral contraceptive use causes a reduction in plasma zinc concentrations and an associated increase in plasma copper, changes which are similar to those that occur in pregnancy. Osteoporosis is a common adverse effect of long-term treatment with adrenal steroids. Pathological fractures and collapses of vertebrae may occur in elderly patients in whom the effect of the steroids is superimposed on senile osteoporosis. Aseptic necrosis of bone in the head of the femur has also been reported (D'Arcy and Griffin, 1972). The exact mechanism by which steroids bring about these changes does not seem to have been elucidated yet.

Thiazide diuretics increase the tubular reabsorption of calcium and thus lead to a fall in the urinary excretion of this mineral.

## Effects on vitamins

The allowance of various nutrients recommended by government agencies such as the UK Department of Health and Social Security and the US Food and Nutrition Board are, for practical purposes, the amounts that will maintain a normal population free from the corresponding deficiency diseases. They do not take account of the effects of the disease, or the iatrogenic effects of the treatment of disease. It is particularly important to have this in mind when considering the possible effects of drugs on the requirements for specific vitamins. There is now an extensive literature showing that drugs reduce the absorption, increase the excretion, or interfere with the utilization of these micronutrients in such a way as to increase the amounts required to levels that cannot be supplied from the diet.

Alcohol, whether in the blood or in the intestinal lumen, interferes with the absorption of thiamine (Thomson *et al.*, 1970) and this is one factor contributing to the clinical evidence of thiamine deficiency, such as peripheral neuropathy, seen in alcoholics. These patients are often malnourished and this further exacerbates the condition because malnutrition may also interfere with the absorption of the vitamin.

Drug-induced riboflavin deficiency has so far been demonstrated only in laboratory animals. However, the biochemical evidence of deficiency without clinical manifestations has been reported in Thai women on oral contraceptives, and this interaction could be important in areas where riboflavin deficiency is common (Sanpitok and Chayutimonkul, 1974).

Pellagra-like symptoms have been described in patients undergoing treatment for tuberculosis with isoniazid. The symptoms disappear following combined treatment with niacin and pyridoxine (DiLorenzo, 1967). In these patients a deficiency of niacin may be secondary to that of pyridoxine since isoniazid is a pyridoxine antagonist and interferes with the availability of this vitamin for the synthesis of niacin from tryptophan. This complication is most likely to occur in communities where maize is the staple diet.

The vitamin, pyridoxine, exists in three forms in food – pyridoxal, pyridoxine, and pyridoxamine. These are converted in the cells to the active phosphate form of the vitamin, pyridoxine-5-phosphate or pyridoxamine 5-phosphate. The antagonistic effect of isoniazid on pyridoxine has been mentioned. The result of this effect is that isoniazid pyridoxine hydrazone is excreted in the urine in amounts sufficient to deplete body stores of pyridoxal phosphate (Vilter, 1964). The peripheral neuropathy that may develop in tuberculosis patients treated with this drug responds to oral pyridoxine, and administration of the vitamin does not reduce the antituberculosis action of the drug (Ungar *et al.*, 1954).

More recent studies (Standal *et al.*, 1974) have shown that measurements of erythrocyte glutamic oxaloacetic transminase (EGOT) gave evidence of pyridoxine deficiency in tuberculous patients treated with isoniazid who selected their own diets in hospital. These diets contained less than 2 mg of pyridoxine per day. The patients were given supplements of 50 mg/day, and at this level of supplementation remained in optimum pyridoxine status despite high doses of isoniazid. It could be questioned, however, whether this level of supplementation daily may, in fact, be necessary as the patients did not show evidence of pyridoxine deficiency for 17 days after the supplement was withdrawn. Penicillamine may also cause symptoms of pyridoxine deficiency by forming a complex with pyridoxal phosphate (Aposhian, 1971).

Ingestion of pyridoxine nullifies the beneficial effect of L-dopa in the control of Parkinson's disease, but this is probably unlikely to occur on a normal dietary intake of about 2 mg/day of the vitamin. The most probable explanation of this effect seems to be that an accelerated decarboxylation of L-dopa to dopamine in extracerebral tissues reduces the amount of L-dopa entering the brain to replenish striatal dopamine which is deficient in Parkinson's disease.

Depression occurs in 5–30 per cent of women taking oral contraceptives of the combination type. On the other hand, 10–20 per cent of women receiving this medication experience relief from pre-menstrual tension. Complaints of depression are most often associated with contraceptives with a high progestogen content and diminish with a change to a more oestrogenic composition (Editorial, 1969). A proportion of women complaining of depression as a result of taking oral contraceptives show biochemical evidence of a disturbance of tryptophan metabolism in response to an orally administered tryptophan load. In such patients, the excretion of tryptophan metabolites returns to normal on administration of 20 mg pyridoxine t.d.s. (Adams *et al.*, 1973). The mechanism of the effect of oral contraceptives on tryptophan metabolism has been thought to be by way of an induction of tryptophan pyrrolase (Fig. 18.2). Since this enzyme is the rate-limiting enzyme in the nicotinic acid pathway, pyridoxine would be utilized for the synthesis of nicotinic acid at the expense of the serotonin pathways, thus interfering with the synthesis of this neurotransmitter. Widespread supplementation with pyridoxine of women taking oral contraceptives would not seem to be justified, however, since only those showing evidence of a disturbance in tryptophan metabolism respond to the supplement. Indeed, a study of 215 women receiving this medication (Brown *et al.*, 1975) using three biochemical indices of pyridoxine status failed to find evidence of deficiency on intakes of 0.8–2.0 mg/day (see also Bender, 1983). Depression may also occur with evidence of a disturbance of tryptophan metabolism in patients treated with corticosteroids, and this, too, may be prevented by pre-medication with pyridoxine.

Venous thrombosis may occur as a serious side-effect of the use of oral contraceptives, and McCully (1975) has made the interesting suggestion that pyridoxine supplements may prevent this complication. The argument for its use hinges on the suggested involvement of homocysteine derivatives in the aetiology of arteriosclerosis (McCully and Wilson, 1975).

There is now a considerable literature describing the effects of drugs on folic acid metabolism. This vitamin plays a role in one-carbon transfer mechanisms, an important example of which occurs in the synthesis of DNA. There are a number of different ways in which drugs may induce folic acid deficiency. Thus, they may interfere with the absorption of the vitamin by

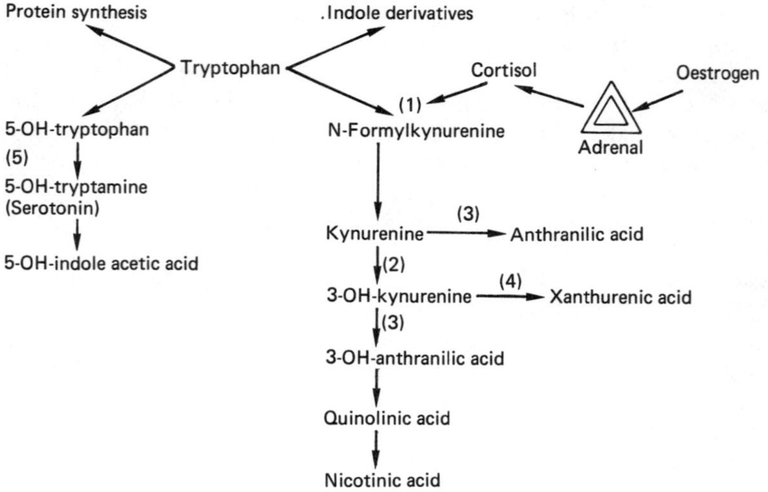


Fig. 18.2 Tryptophan metabolism. Enzymes (and vitamins involved) shown: 1. Typtophan pyrrolase (thiamin); 2. Kynurenine hydroxylase (riboflavin); 3. Kynureninase (pyridoxine); 4. Aminotransferase (pyridoxine); 5. Tryptophan decarboxylase (pyridoxine).

inhibiting the intestinal conjugase enzyme in the intestinal mucosa which reduces the dietary polyglutamate form to monoglutamate before absorption. This was originally reported to occur with diphenylhydantoin and will be discussed below. The cytotoxic drug methotrexate binds irreversibly to the enzyme dihydrofolate reductase which catalyses the conversion of dihydrofolate to tetrahydrofolate, the cofactor necessary for DNA synthesis. Drugs which induce vitamin $B_{12}$ deficiency interfere with the conversion of homocysteine to methionine which involves the removal of a methyl group from methyl folate. Methyl folate is the dominant form of folate in serum and liver, but is metabolically useless until made available by demethylation. Pyridoxine is required for the production of methionine from homocysteine and also acts with folic acid in the interconversion of glycine and serine. This is then the site of action on folate metabolism of drugs that induce pyridoxine deficiency.

Ethanol inhibits the absorption of folic acid, and so too does the biguanide, metformin, and oral contraceptives.

Low serum and red cell folate levels, and occasionally overt megaloblastic anaemia, occur in a majority of patients receiving long-term anticonvulsant therapy (Reynolds, 1974). Diphenylhydantoin has been most studied, but folate deficiencies have also been reported with phenobarbital and primidone. Studies in psychiatric patients (Labadarios *et al.*, 1977) indicated that other drugs such as the phenothiazines and tricyclics also induce biochemical evidence of folic acid deficiency. As mentioned above, the early work on this problem suggested that diphenylhydantoin reduced the absorption of the vitamin from the intestine. There is now some doubt about this mechanism (Fehling *et al.*, 1973) and the present balance of evidence involves an effect on hepatic microsomal drug metabolizing enzymes which are known to require folate as cofactor (Maxwell *et al.*, 1972). The determination of folic acid intakes presents a number of problems, principally because of the difficulty of assessing the concentration of folic acid in foods (Poh Tan *et al.*, 1984). Estimates from standard tables of food composition, however, suggest (Dickerson *et al.*, 1974) that the folate intake of patients in British psychiatric hospitals may be low, and thus a dietary deficiency would further exacerbate the drug-induced deficiency. Furthermore, if as has been suggested (Labadarios *et al.*, 1977) folic acid plays a role not only as a coenzyme for drug-metabolizing enzymes, but also in the synthesis of the enzymes themselves, a vicious circle could be visualized (Fig. 18.3) in which chronic administration of any enzyme-inducing drug would be increasingly likely to cause folate deficiency and consequently increased toxicity. It remains controversial as to whether folic acid supplements should be given therapeutically or prophylactically to epileptic patients receiving anticonvulsant drugs. The administration of folic acid to epileptics has been reported to aggravate their condition, disturb the drug control of seizures, and even to precipitate a deficiency of vitamin $B_{12}$. However, red cell folate levels below 260 ng/ml in epileptics respond to regular yeast tablet supplements without causing adverse side-effects and with the benefit of eliminating the need to monitor red cell folate levels (Eastham *et al.*, 1975).

Isolated malabsorption of vitamin $B_{12}$ may be induced by a number of drugs including PAS, metformin, slow release potassium iodide, colchicine,

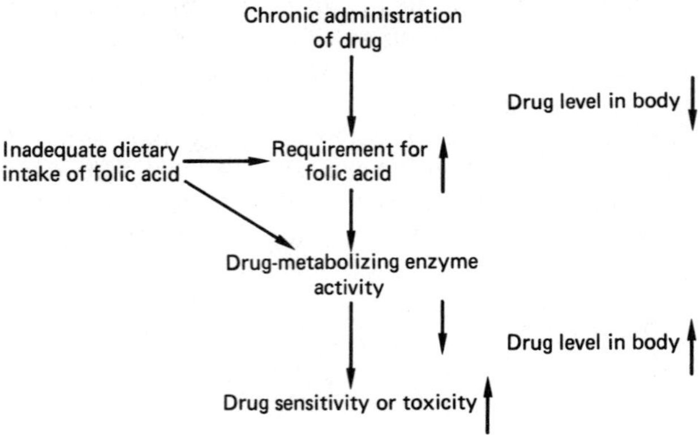


Fig. 18.3 Possible interrelationship of chronic administration of enzyme-inducing drug, nutritional status, and drug toxicity (Labadarios *et al.*, 1977).

trifluoperazine (Stelazine), and ethanol (Truswell, 1973). In the case of PAS, studies on patients with tuberculosis have confirmed that the drug does not interfere with intrinsic factors, but causes malabsorption in some other way. Low serum levels of vitamin $B_{12}$ can be induced quickly by certain oral contraceptives (Wertalik *et al.*, 1972) and this may have particular significance for women in developing countries where the diet consists predominantly of vegetables. Serum levels of vitamin $B_{12}$ are also reduced by smoking due to the utilization of the vitamin in the detoxication of cyanide.

Tetracycline reduces the ascorbic acid content of leucocytes and increases the urinary excretion of the vitamin. This effect could be important in old people, many of whom are at risk of deficiency. Oral contraceptives, by virtue of their oestrogen components, reduce the levels of ascorbic acid in plasma, leucocytes and platelets. Accelerated breakdown of the vitamin and a change in tissue distribution (Rivers, 1975) have been suggested as possible mechanisms. Blood levels of ascorbic acid are also reduced by smoking and high doses of aspirin. The latter has been shown to depress the entry of ascorbic acid into platelets (Sahud and Aggeler, 1970), and leucocytes (Loh *et al.*, 1973). In spite of these effects, however, it would seem to be desirable for patients with rheumatoid arthritis receiving 12 tablets or more per day of aspirin to be given ascorbic acid supplements (Sahud and Cohen, 1971). This is also true for patients being treated with corticosteroids, because these increase the excretion of ascorbic acid, and there is one report (Bartholomew, 1972) of frank scurvy in a 43-year-old patient with rheumatoid arthritis given 10 mg prednisone t.b.d. Confirmation of this effect of prednisone has been obtained in guinea-pigs on a borderline intake of the vitamin (Labadarios, 1975). The excretion of ascorbic acid is also increased in patients receiving phenylbutazone, sulphinpyrazone, and chlorcyclizine.

Studies on mentally handicapped children in long-stay hospitals (Dawson and Duncan, 1975; Heald *et al.*, 1976) have not identified any effect of anticonvulsant drugs on ascorbic acid requirements.

The effects of anticonvulsant drugs on vitamin D metabolism resulting in rickets and osteomalacia are described elsewhere (Stamp, p. 300).

Haemolytic anaemia due to vitamin E deficiency occurs in premature babies, and administration of iron may aggravate the condition. Warfarin, an antimetabolite of vitamin K, is used in patients with atherosclerosis to reduce the risk of thrombosis. Vitamin K deficiency can sometimes occur following treatment with purgatives or intestinal antibiotics. The latter removes the colonic bacteria which synthesize the vitamin.

## Nutrients as drugs

Some nutrients, when taken in amounts larger than the recommended dietary intakes, have an established, or claimed, pharmacological action. Thus, nicotinic acid is effective in some types of hyperlipidaemia at a dose of 100 or more times the normal intake and may also be used as a treatment for chilblains because of its vasodilator effect. Tryptophan has been used as an antidepressant (Jensen *et al.*, 1975). One gram doses of ascorbic acid lower blood cholesterol levels (Horsey *et al.*, 1981). Larger doses (3 to 8 g) may reduce bone pain in patients with Paget's disease (Basu *et al.*, 1978) and have been claimed to have a role in the treatment of cancer (Cameron *et al.*, 1979) (see p. 362).

Claims have also been made that high doses of vitamins are effective in the treatment of psychiatric diseases (see p. 339). Vitamins can be purchased from health food shops in preparations which contain many times the recommended daily allowance. Media claims for beneficial effects of large, 'mega', or 'pharmacological', doses have resulted in a number of people taking them. There are, in fact, few conditions for which megavitamin treatment is definitely justified (Table 18.2; Evans and Lacey, 1986). Physicians should be aware that patients may not admit to consuming large doses of vitamins as a form of self-medication whilst at the same time complaining of some of their toxic effects (Table 18.3; Evans and Lacey, 1986).

Toxic effects of high doses of the fat-soluble vitamins A and D are well-known, but satisfactory evidence for some of the described toxic effects of

Table 18.2 Conditions for which treatment with megadoses of vitamins appears well supported (Adapted from Evans and Lacey, 1986)

| | |
|---|---|
| Vitamin $B_3$ | Peripheral vasodilation (chilblains). |
| Vitamin $B_6$ | Pyridoxine dependency; infantile convulsive disorders; sideroblastic anaemia; urinary oxidate stones; homocystinuria; cystathioninuria. |
| Folic acid | Congenital megaloblastic anaemia, homocystinuria and homothioninuria; formiminotransferase deficiency; malabsorption with megaloblastic anaemia. |
| Vitamin $B_{12}$ | Juvenile pernicious anaemia; transcobalamin II deficiency; methylmalonic acidiaria; homocystinuria; hypomethioninaemia. |
| Vitamins A, D, E, K | Definite fat malabsorption syndromes. |
| Vitamin E | Peripheral vasodilation (Intermittent claudication); prevention of haemolytic anaemia, intraventricular haemorrhage and retrolental fibroplasia in pre-terms. |
| Vitamin K | Coagulopothies of liver disease after parturition. |

Table 18.3 Toxic effects of vitamin overdoses (From Evans and Lacey, 1986)

| | |
|---|---|
| Vitamin A | Raised intracranial pressure; chronic liver disease; skin changes; hair loss; tenderness of bones. |
| Vitamin $B_3$ (niacin, nicotinamide) | Peptic ulcer; alopecia; pruritus; hepato-toxicity; arrhythmias; hypotension. |
| Vitamin $B_6$ (pyridoxine) | Dependency; peripheral sensory neuropathy and ataxia; decrease in therapeutic effect of levodopa. |
| Vitamin C (ascorbic acid) | Dependency; oxalate stones in predisposed individuals; possible teratogenesis and carcinogenesis with very high doses; multiplicity of minor idiosyncratic symptoms. |
| Vitamin D (cholecalciferol) | Hypercalcaemia; hypertension; renal calcinosis; metastatic calcification. |
| Vitamin E (tocopherols) | Increased anticoagulant action of warfarin. |
| Vitamin K | Haemolytic anaemia; neonatal jaundice. |

water-soluble vitamins, particularly vitamin C (Hornig and Moser, 1981; Sutton *et al.*, 1983) may not be available. Pyridoxine in doses of 5–20 mg or even up to 150 mg may be necessary in some women before the symptoms, including nausea and depression, disappear. Pyridoxine supplements were recommended as a treatment for the premenstrual syndrome (Barr, 1984). The first report of sensory neuropathy from pyridoxine abuse (Schaumberg *et al.*, 1983) was in adults who were taking mean daily doses of 2–6 g. More recently, however, adverse effects, sensory neuropathy as evidenced by burning, shooting, tingling pains, paraesthesiae of the limbs, clumsiness, ataxia or peri-oral numbness has been reported in 23/58 women with elevated serum $B_6$ levels (Dalton, 1985). Some of the affected women were taking only 50 mg per day.

## Population groups vulnerable to drug-nutrient interactions

### Pregnant women

During pregnancy a mother's diet must provide the nutrients necessary for her own body and that of the fetus. There is abundant experimental evidence that the fetus is particularly susceptible to nutrient deficiencies. If these occur during the period of organogenesis they result in congenital abnormalities. Thus deficiencies of vitamin A, vitamin E, riboflavin, pantothenic acid and folic acid may all be teratogenic. There is no reason to believe that these deficiencies would not cause malformations in the human.

Thalidomide was withdrawn from the market for reasons which are only too well known. What may not be so widely appreciated is the possibility that the devastating effects of this drug may well have resulted from interaction with one or more vitamins of the B-group, with riboflavin and nicotinic acid being the most likely (Robertson, 1962). It is possible that other drugs, such as tetracycline, which are associated with fetal malformations may cause them by virtue of interactions with nutrients.

There have been a number of reports suggesting that there is an excess of congenital malformations amongst infants born to epileptic mothers. Since the administration of anticonvulsants is associated with low folic acid status it seemed possible that the congenital abnormalities were due to interference with folate availability by the drugs. We were able to demonstrate that giving phenytoin and phenobarbitone to pregnant rats fed a diet deficient in folate produced a variety of fetal abnormalities including spina bifida (Labadarios, 1975).

The possibility that such tragedies can occur is obviously a reason for thinking carefully about the administration of drugs to pregnant women. Furthermore, since it is possible that interference with nutrients only becomes important if the nutrient intake is of border-line adequacy, it is necessary to give careful consideration to diet during pregnancy. It cannot be assumed that because a patient does not show evidence of deficiency diseases, vitamin status is adequate. Careful enquiry about the kinds of foods eaten and frequency of consumption may help to identify likely deficiencies.

For the purposes of the present discussion, alcohol must be considered a drug. There is historical evidence that alcoholic mothers often gave birth to infants with malformations and in more recent times the characteristics of such infants have been carefully described (Hanson *et al.*, 1976; Clarren and Smith, 1978). The 'fetal alcohol syndrome' includes growth retardation, small head size, mental and psychomotor retardation, craniofacial peculiarities and cardiovascular defects. A range of other defects has been less consistently described. It seems that if a woman consumes more than 2 g of alcohol per kg body weight per day during gestation her offspring will show the whole range of defective growth and malformation. The vital question to be answered is whether there is a safe limit and whether infrequent binge drinking is likely to have the same effect as more consistent drinking of smaller amounts. Undoubtedly, the wisest recommendation would be not to drink alcohol but there is a need for a more sympathetic approach to those women who feel it impossible to abstain for various reasons. The effects of alcohol may be mediated by the effects of alcohol on nutritional status (Morgan, 1982).

## The elderly

The degenerative diseases that become increasingly evident with increasing age are responsible for twice as many prescriptions as the national average (Royal College of Physicians, 1984) and they consume far more drugs than the young. It is not surprising, therefore, that adverse reactions are common in the elderly (Hurwitz, 1969) and contribute to some 10 per cent of admissions to geriatric units in hospitals (Williamson and Chaplin, 1980). The possibility of drug-drug interactions and failure to understand or follow instructions on how the drugs should be taken increases the risk of adverse reactions. Prescribing errors are also a cause of drug-induced morbidity (Gosney and Tallis, 1984).

These factors operate at a time when age-related changes in the hepatic mixed function oxidase system and its inducibility may well be reduced (Kato and Takanaka, 1968). Furthermore, in man deficiencies of a number of nutrients–protein, ascorbic acid, folic acid and potassium that occur in old people may further reduce the activity of this system. The products of the metabolism of drugs and in some cases unchanged drugs are excreted in the bile and in the urine. Thus, the fall in renal function which occurs with increasing

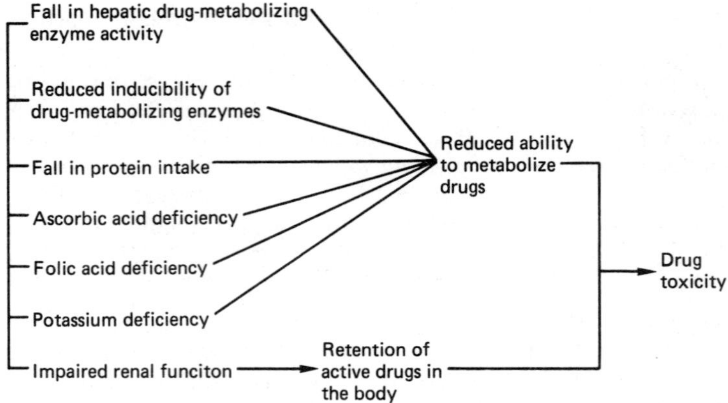


Fig. 18.4 Nutritional and other factors which may lead to increased drug toxicity in the elderly.

age may lead to the longer retention in the body of drugs and their degradation products (Fig. 18.4).

Drugs commonly given to elderly patients with their possible nutritional interactions are shown in Table 18.4.

Table 18.4 Nutritional interaction with drugs commonly given to elderly patients

| | | |
|---|---|---|
| Appetite | Depressed | Biguanides (e.g. phenformin and metformin); digitalis |
| | Increased | Sulphonylureas (e.g. tolbutamide, chlorpropamide, glibenclamide); phenothiazine (e.g. Largactil); benzodiazepines (e.g. Valium, Librium, Nobrium); anabolic agents (e.g. Durabolin) |
| Carbohydrate metabolism | Hyperglycaemia | Thiazide diuretics (?); Diazonide; corticosteroids; Phenytoin |
| | Hypoglycaemia | Sulphonylureas when given with phenylbutazone, warfarin or dicoumarol; alcohol; aspirin |
| Lipid metabolism | Hyperlipidaemia | Chlorpromazine (cholesterol ↑); Phenobarbitone (cholesterol ↑); triglycerides ↑ |
| Protein metabolism | Negative nitrogen balance | Corticosteroids; tetracyclines |
| Mineral metabolism | Potassium depletion | Thiazide diuretics; purgatives |
| | Sodium depletion | Diuretics |
| | Iron depletion | Aspirin |
| Vitamins | Thiamin | Alcohol; antacids |
| | Folic Acid | Alcohol, anticonvulsants |
| | Ascorbic Acid | Aspirin; tetracyclines |
| | Vitamin D | Anticonvulsants |
| | Vitamin K | Purgatives; intestinal antibiotics |

Table 18.5 Adverse effects of 'Over the Counter' drugs used by the elderly, (Dickerson 1985)

| Drugs | Indication for prescription | Reasons for self medication | Adverse effects |
|---|---|---|---|
| Antacids | Hyperphosphataemia | Indigestion<br>Flatulence<br>'Heart problems' | Milk alkali syndrome<br>Hypophosphataemia<br>Sodium overload |
| | Reduce gastric pH | Gas and bloating<br>Gastric discomfort | Magnesium overload<br>Folate malabsorption<br>Low thiamin status |
| Laxatives | Constipation | Constipation<br>Bowel obsession | Hypokalaemia<br>Potassium deficiency |
| | Diseases of colon and rectum | Intake of drugs that are constipating | Malabsorption of fat soluble vitamins (A, D and K) particularly due to mineral oil |
| Analgesics | Pain relief particularly for prevention of myocardial infarcts | Headache<br>Insomnia<br>Nervousness<br>Hangover | Iron deficiency anaemia due to gastric bleeding |
| | | Cold and cough<br>Sore throat<br>Pain | Folid acid deficiency<br>Vitamin C deficiency |

Roe (1984) has discussed in some detail the problem of drug-nutrition interaction in the elderly and has commented that up to 60 per cent of the drugs consumed by elderly people may be purchased by them over the counter in Chemist shops. Few of these are taken for specific diseases and most are consumed for relief of rather vague symptoms such as indigestion, flatulence, gastric discomfort, constipation, headache or hangover. The importance of this self medication in causing nutritional disturbances should not be overlooked (Table 18.5).

## Conclusion

Drugs interact with food in a variety of ways. Disregard of these interactions can result in drugs being ineffective, producing adverse effects, malformations and even death. There is a real need for all members of the health care team to be aware of the importance to their patients of these reactions.

## References

Adams, P.W., Wynn, V., Rose, D.P., Seed, M., Folkard, J. and Strong, R. (1973). Effect of pyridoxine hydrochloride (vitamin $B_6$) upon depression associated with oral contraception. *Lancet*, **i**, 897–904.

Agate, J. (1970) *The Practice of Geriatrics*, 2nd ed. Heinemann: London.

Alleyne, G.A.O. (1967). The effect of severe protein–calorie malnutrition on the renal function of Jamaican children. *Pediatrics*, **39**, 400–11.

Aposhian, H.V. (1971). Penicillamine and analogous chelating agents. *Ann. N.Y. Acad. Sci.*, **179**, 481–6.

Barr, W. (1984). Pyridoxine supplements in the premenstrual syndrome. *Practitioner*, **228**, 425–7.

Basu, T.K. and Dickerson, J.W.T. (1974). Interrelationships of nutrition and the metabolism of drugs. *Chem.-Biol. Interactions*, **8**, 193–206.

Basu, T.K., Dickerson, J.W.T. and Parke, D.V. (1971). Effect of diet on rat plasma corticosteroids and liver aromatic hydroxylase activity. *Biochem J.*, **125**, 16p.

Basu, T.K., Smethurst, T.M., Gillett, M.B., Donaldson, D., Jordan, S.J., Williams, D.C. and Hucklin, J.A. (1978). Ascorbic acid therapy for the relief of bone pain in Paget's disease. *Acta Vitaminol. Enzymol.* (Milano) **32**, 45–9.

Bartholomew, C. (1972) Rheumatoid arthritis and prednisone-treated scurvy. *Post-Grad. Med. I.*, **48**, 243–5.

Bender, D.A. (1983). Effect of oestradiol and vitamin $B_6$ on tryptophan metabolism in the rat: implications for the interpretation of the tryptophan load test for vitamin $B_6$ nutritional status. *Br. J. Nutr.*, **50**, 33–42.

Borowitz, J.L., Moore, P.F., Yim, G.K.W., Miya, T.S. (1971). Mechanism of enhanced drug effects produced by dilution of the oral dose. *Toxicol. Appl. Pharmacol.*, **19**, 164–8.

Boston Collaborative Drug Surveillance Programme (1972). Tetracycline and drug-attributed rises in blood urea nitrogen. *J. Am. Med. Ass.*, **220**, 377–9.

Brown, R.R., Rose, D.P., Leklem, J.E., Linkswiler, H. and Anand, R. (1975). Urinary 4-pyridoxic acid, plasma pyridoxal phosphate, and erythrocyte aminotransferase levels in oral contraceptive users receiving controlled intakes of vitamin $B_6$. *Am. J. Clin. Nutr.*, **28**, 10–19.

Brown, W.J. Jr. and Brown, F.K. (1967). Thiazide-induced alteration of carbohydrate tolerance in normal men. *Curr. Ther. Res.*, **9**, 200–7.

Buchanan, N. and Hansen, J.D.L. (1976). Chloramphenicol metabolism in children with PCM. *Am. J. Clin. Nutr.*, **29**, 327–30.

Budd, G. (1840) Scurvy. In *The Library of Medicine*, p. 94. Ed. Tweedie, A. Whittaker: London.

Cameron, E., Pauling, L. and Liebovitz, B. (1979). Ascorbic acid and cancer. A review. *Cancer Res.*, **39**, 663–81.

Conney, A.H., Pantuck, E.J., Hsiao, K-C., Garland, W.A., Anderson, K.E., Aluares, A.P. and Kappas, A. (1976). Enhanced phenacetin metabolism in human subjects fed charcoal-broiled beef. *Clin. Pharmacol. Ther.*, **20**, 633–42.

Craft, I.L. and Peters, T.J. (1971). Quantitative changes in plasma amino acids induced by oral contraceptives. *Clin. Sci.*, **41**, 301–7.

Crawford, J.J. and Rudofsky, S. (1966). Some alteration in the pattern of drug metabolism associated with pregnancy, oral contraceptives and the newly born. *Br. J. Anaesth.*, **38**, 446–54.

Dalton, K. (1985). Pyridoxine overdose in premenstrual syndrome. *Lancet*, **1**, 1168–9.

D'Arcy, P.F. and Griffin, J.P. (1972). *Iatrogenic Diseases*. Oxford University Press: London.

Davies, L., Hastrop, K. and Bender, A.E. (1973*a*). Ascorbic acid in meals on wheels. *Mod. Geriat.*, **3**, 390–94.

Davies, L., Hastrop, K. and Bender, A.E. (1973*b*). Potassium intake of the elderly. *Mod. Geriat.*, **3**, 482–8.

Dawson, K.P. and Duncan, A. (1975). Ascorbic acid and long-term anticonvulsant therapy in children. *Br. J. Nutr.*, **33**, 315–18.

Dickerson, J.W.T. (1985). Interaction of drugs and nutrition in elderly. In *Vitamin Deficiency in the Elderly*, pp. 145–53. Eds. Kemm, J. and Ancill, R.J. Blackwell Scientific Publ.: Oxford.

Dickerson, J.W.T. (1980a). Nutrition and drugs. In *Symposium on Nutrition*, pp. 42–62. Ed. Davies, S.H. The Royal College of Physicians of Edinburgh.

Dickerson, J.W.T. (1980b). Interrelationships between diet and drugs. In *Topics in*

*Therapeutics*. *6*. 27–136. Ed. Wood, H.F. Pitman Medical: Tunbridge Wells.
Dickerson, J.W.T., Basu, T.K. and Parke, D.V. (1976). Effect of protein-energy nutrition on the activity of hepatic microsomal drug metabolizing enzymes in growing rats. *J. Nutr.*, **106**, 258–64.
Dickerson, J.W.T., Heald, M. and Torrens, P.E. (1974). Dietary intakes of elderly patients at Graylingwell Hospital, Chichester. *Report to South West Thames Regional Health Authority*.
DiLorenzo, P.A. (1967). Pellagra-like syndrome associated with isoniazid therapy. *Acta Derm.-vener., Stockh.*, **47**, 318–22.
Dinon, L.R., Kim, Y.S. and Vander Veer, J.B. (1958). Clinical experience with chlorothiazide (diuril) with particular emphasis on untoward responses. A report of 121 cases studied over a 15 month period. *Am. J. Med. Sci.*, **236**, 533–45.
Dollery, C.T., Pentecost, B.L. and Samaan, N.A. (1962). Drug-induced diabetes. *Lancet*, **ii**, 7356.
Doluisio, J.T., Tan, G.H., Billups, N.F. and Diamond, L. (1969). Drug absorption II; Effects of fasting on intestinal drug absorption. *J. Pharm. Sci.*, **58**, 1200–2.
Eastham, R.D., Jancar, J. and Cameron, J.D. (1975). Red cell folate and macrocytosis during long-term anticonvulsant therapy in non-anaemic mentally retarded epileptics. *Br. J. Psychiat.*, **126**, 263–5.
Editorial (1969). Oral contraception and depression, leading article. *Br. Med. J.*, iv, 380–81.
Evans, C.D.H. and Lacey, J.H. (1986). Toxicity of vitamins: complications of a health movement. *Br. Med. J.*, **292**, 509–10.
Exton-Smith, A.N. (1974). Vitamins and the elderly. In *Geriatric Medicine*, pp. 247–67. Eds. Anderson, W.F. and Judge, T.G. Academic Press: London.
Fehling, C., Jagerstad, M., Lindstrand, K. and Westesson, A.-K. (1973). The effect of anticonvulsant therapy upon the absorption of folates. *Clin. Sci.*, **44**, 595–600.
Gey, K.F. and Carlson, L.A. (1971). *Metabolic Effects of Nicotinic acid and its Derivatives*, Hans Huber: Bern.
Gillespie, N.G., Mena, I., Cotzias, G.C. and Bell, M.A. (1973). Diets affecting treatment of parkinsonism with laevodopa. *J. Am. Diet. Ass.*, **62**, 525–8.
Glazko, A.J. (1949). Biochemical studies on chloramphenicol II. Tissue distribution and excretion studies. *J. Pharmacol. Exp. Ther.*, **96**, 445–59.
Goldner, M.G., Zarowitz, H. and Akgun, S. (1960). Hyperglycaemia and glycosuria due to thiazide derivatives administered in diabetes mellitus. *N. Engl. J. Med.*, **262**, 403–5.
Gosney, M. and Tallis, R. (1984). Prescription of contraindicated and interacting drugs in elderly patients admitted to hospital. *Lancet*, **2**, 564–7.
Hanson, J.W., Jones, K.L. and Smith, D.W. (1976). Fetal alcohol syndrome. Experience with 41 patients. *JAMA*, **235**, 1458–60.
Heald, L.M., Barnett, P.M., Sethi, P.C. and Dickerson, J.W.T. (1976). A survey of the diets, nutrient intake and nutritional status of patients at Botley's Park Hospital, Chertsey, Surrey, *Report to South West Thames Regional Health Authority*.
Hornig, D.H. and Moser, U. (1981). The safety of high vitamin C intakes in man. In *Vitamin C (Ascorbic acid)*, pp. 225–48. Eds. Counsell, J.S. and Hornig, D.H. Applied Science Publishers: London.
Horsey, J., Livesley, B. and Dickerson, J.W.T. (1981). Ischaemic heart disease and aged patients: effects of ascorbic acid on lipoproteins. *J. Hum. Nutr.*, **35**, 53–8.
Hughes, R.E. (1974). Nutritional interactions between vitamin C and heavy metals. In *Vitamin C*, pp. 68–76. Eds. Birch, G.G. and Parker, K. Applied Science Publishers: London.
Hurwitz, N. (1969). Predisposing factors in adverse reactions to drugs. *Br. Med. J.*, **i**, 536–9.

Jensen, K., Fruensgaard, K., Ahlfors, U.G., *et al.*, (1975). Tryptophan imipramine in depression. *Lancet*, **2**, 920.
Judge, T.G. (1968). Hypokalaemia in the elderly. *Geront. clin.*, **10**, 102–7.
Kato, R., Oshima, T. and Tomizawa, S. (1968). Toxicity and metabolism of drugs in relation to dietary protein. *Jap. J. Pharmac.*, **18**, 356–66.
Kato, R. and Takanaka, A. (1968). Effect of phenobarbital on electron transport system, oxidation and reduction of drugs in liver microsomes of rats of different ages. *J. Biochem.* (Tokyo) **63**, 406–408.
Kershbaum, A. (1963). Diabetogenic effect of fluorine-containing steroids. *Br. Med. J.*, **ii**, 253.
Kohn, K.W. (1961). Mediation of divalent metal ions in the binding of tetracycline to macromolecules. *Nature*, **191**, 1156–8.
Labadarios, D. (1975). Studies on the effects of drugs on nutritional status. *Ph.D. Thesis*, University of Surrey.
Labadarios, D., Obuwa, G., Lucas, E.G., Dickerson, J.W.T. and Parke, D.V. (1978). The effects of chronic drug administration on hepatic enzyme induction and folate metabolism. *Br. J. Clin. Pharmac.*, **5**, 167–73.
Levine, R.A. (1968). Steatorrhea induced by *para*-aminosalicylic acid. *Ann. Intern. Med.*, **68**, 1265–70.
Loh, H.S., Watters, K. and Wilson, C.W.M. (1973). The effects of aspirin on the metabolic availability of ascorbic acid in human beings. *J. Clin. Pharmac.*, **13**, 480–86.
McCully, K.S. (1975). Homocystine, atherosclerosis and thrombosis: implications for oral contraceptive users. *Am. J. Clin. Nutr.*, **28**, 542–9.
McCully, K.S. and Wilson, R.B. (1975). Homocysteine theory of arteriosclerosis. *Atherosclerosis*, **22**, 215–27.
McLean, A.E.M. and McLean, E.K. (1966). The effect of diet and 1,1,1,-trichloro-2,2-bis-(*p*-chlorophenyl)ethane (DDT) on microsomal hydroxylating enzymes and on sensitivity of rats to carbon tetrachloride poisoning. *Biochem. J.*, **100**, 564–71.
McLean, A.E.M. and McLean, E.K. (1969). Diet and toxicity. *Br. Med. Bull.*, **25**, 278–81.
McLean, A.J., McNamara, P.J., du Souich P. *et al.*, (1978). Food, splanchnic blood flow, and bioavailability of drugs subject to first-pass metabolism. *Clin. Pharmacol. Ther.*, **24**, 5–10.
Madapally, M.M., Mackerer, C.R. and Mehlman, M.A. (1972). The inhibitory effects of acetylsalicylic acid feeding on gluconeogenic enzymes in rat liver and kidney. *Life Sci.*, **11**, 77–85.
Mann, J.I., Truswell, A.S. and Pimstone, B.L. (1971). The different effects of oral sucrose and glucose on alimentary lipaemia. *Clin. Sci.*, **41**, 123–9.
Marks, V. (1974) Effect of drugs on carbohydrate metabolism. *Proc. Nutr. Soc.*, **33**, 209–14.
Marks, V. (1975). Alcohol and changes in body constituents; glucose and hormones. *Proc. R. Soc. Med.*, **68**, 377–80.
Marks, V., Frizel, D., Twycross, R.G. and Buchanon, K.D. (1971). Effect of β-pyridylcarbinol on glucose tolerance, plasma glucagon, insulin and growth hormone in man. In *Metabolic Effects of Nicotinic Acid and its Derivatives*, pp. 961–76. Eds. Gey, K.F. and Carlson, L.A. Hans Huber: Bern.
Marks, V. and Medd, W.E. (1964). Alcohol-induced hypoglycaemia. *Br. J. Psychiat.*, **110**, 228–32.
Marshall, W.J. and McLean, A.E.M. (1969). The effect of nutrition and hormonal status on cytochrome P-450 and its induction. *Biochem J.*, **115**, 27.
Marshall, W.J. and McLean, A.E.M. (1971). A requirement for dietary lipids for

induction of cytochrome P-450 by phenobarbitone in rat liver microsomal fraction. *Biochem. J.*, **122**, 569–73.

Matsunaga, F., Kubo, A., Katakura, G. *et al.*, (1963). Steroid diabetes, diabetes mellitus appearing during treatment with pituitary-adrenal hormones. *J. Ther., Tokyo*, **45**, 1988–95.

Maxwell, J.D., Hunter, J., Stewart, D.A. and Williams, R. (1972). Folate deficiency after anticonvulsant drugs: An effect of hepatic enzyme induction? *Br. Med. J.*, **i**, 297–9.

Mehta, S., Kalsi, H.K., Jayaraman, S. and Mathur, V.S. (1975). Chloroamphenicol metabolism in children with protein-calorie malnutrition. *Am. J. Clin. Nutr.*, **28**, 977–81.

Mena, I. and Cotzias, G.C. (1975). Protein intake and treatment of Parkinson's disease with levodopa. *N. Engl. J. Med.*, **292**, 181–4.

Miller, N.E. and Nestel, P.J. (1973). Altered bile acid metabolism during treatment with phenobarbitone. *Clin. Sci. Molec. Med.*, **45**, 257–62.

Morgan, B.L.G. (1982). Effects of hormonal and other factors on growth and development. In *Brain and Behavioural Development*, pp. 109–30. Eds. Dickerson, J.W.T. and McGurk, H. Surrey University Press: Glasgow.

Murty, H.S., Caasi, P.I., Brooks, S.K. and Nair, P.D. (1970). Biosynthesis of haem in the vitamin E deficient rat. *J. Biol. Chem.*, **245**, 5498–504.

Nelson, E.B., Prithvi Raj, P., Belfi, K.J. and Masters, B.S.S. (1971). Oxidative drug metabolism in human liver microsomes. *J. Pharmac. Exp. Ther.*, **178**, 580–88.

Noble, R.E. (1969). Effect of cycloheptadine on appetite and weight gain in adults. *J. Am. Med. Ass.*, **209**, 2054–5.

Norrby, A., Rybo, G. and Sölvell, L. (1972). The influence of a combined oral contraceptive on the absorption of iron. *Scand. J. Haemat.*, **9**, 43–51.

O'Keefe, J.D. and Marks, V. (1977). Lunchtime gin and tonic a cause of reactive hypoglycaemia. *Lancet*, **i**, 1286.

Okun, R., Russell, R.P. and Wilson, W.R. (1963). Use of diazoxide with trichlormethiazide for hypertension. *Archs intern. Med.*, **112**, 882–8.

O'Malley, K., Stevenson, I.J. and Crooks, J. (1972). Impairment of human drug metabolism by oral contraceptive steroids. *Clin. Pharmac. Ther.*, **13**, 552–7.

Pantuck, E.J., Hsiao, K.C., Kuntsman, R. and Conney, A.H. (1975). Intestinal metabolism of charcoal-broiled beef and rat chow. *Science*, **187**, 744–6.

Pantuck, E.J., Hsiao, K.C., Loub, W.D. Wattenberg, L.W., Kuntzman, R. and Conney, A.H. (1976). Stimulatory effect of vegetables on intestinal drug metabolism in the rat. *J. Pharmacol. Exp. Ther.*, **198**, 278–83.

Parke, D.V. (1968). The biochemistry of foreign compounds. *International Series of Monographs in Pure and Applied Biology*. Vol. 5. Pergamon: Oxford.

Pawan, G.L.S. (1974). Drugs and appetite. *Proc. Nutr. Soc.*, **33**, 239–44.

Platt, B.S., Eddy, T.P. and Pellett, P.L. (1963). *Food in Hospitals*. Oxford University Press: London.

Poh Tan, S., Wenlock, R.W. and Buss, D.H. (1984). Folic acid content of the diet in various types of British household. *Human Nutrition: Applied Nutrition*, **38A**, 17–22.

Poskitt, E.M.E. (1974). Clinical problems related to the use of drugs in malnutrition. *Proc. Nutr. Soc.*, **33**, 203–7.

Reynold, E.H. (1974). Iatrogenic nutritional effects of anticonvulsants. *Proc. Nutr. Soc.*, **33**, 225–9.

Rivers, J.M. (1975). Oral contraceptives and ascorbic acid. *Am. J. Clin. Nutr.*, **28**, 550–54.

Robertson, W.F. (1962). Thalidomide (Distaral) and vitamin B deficiency. *Br. Med. J.*, **1**, 792–3.

Roe, D.A. (1984). Adverse nutritional effects of OTC drug use in the elderly. In *Drugs and nutrition in the geriatric patient*, pp. 121–33. Ed. Roe, D.A. Churchill-Livingstone: Edinburgh.

Rowe, M.J., Dolder, M.A., Kirby, B.J. and Oliver, M.F. (1973). Effect of a nicotinic acid analogue on raised plasma-free-fatty-acids after acute myocardial infarction. *Lancet*, **ii**, 814–17.

Royal College of Physicians (1984). Medication for the elderly. *J.R. Coll. Phys. Lond.*, **18**, 7–17.

Sahud, M.A. and Aggeler, P.M. (1970). Utilization of ascorbic acid during platelet aggregation. *Proc. Soc. Exp. Biol. Med.*, **134**, 13–16.

Sahud, M.A. and Cohen, R.J. (1971). Effect of aspirin ingestion on ascorbic acid levels in rheumatoid arthritis. *Lancet*, **i**, 937–8.

Samols, E. and Marks, V. (1966). The treatment of hypoglycaemia with diazoxide. *Proc. R. Soc. Med.*, **59**, 811–14.

Sanpitok, N. and Chayutimonkul, L. (1974). Oral contraceptives and riboflavine nutrition. *Lancet*, **i**, 836–7.

Schapel, G.J., Edwards, K.D.G. and Neale, F.C. (1974). Factorial study of the efficiency of cholestyramine, L-tryptophan and clofibrate in human nephrotic hyperlipidaemia. *Prog. Biochem. Pharmac.*, **9**, 82–98.

Schaumberg, H., Kaplan, J., Winderbank, A. *et al.*, (1983). Sensory neuropathy from pyridoxine abuse – a new megavitamin syndrome. *N. Engl. J. Med.*, **309**, 445–8.

Schubert, G.E. and Schulte, H.D. (1963). Contributions to the clinical picture of steroid diabetes. *Dtsch. Med. Wschr.*, **88**, 1175–88.

Standal, B.R., Kao-Chen, S.M., Yang, G.Y. and Char, D.F.B. (1974). Early changes in pyridoxine status of patients receiving isoniazid therapy. *Am. J. Clin. Nutr.*, **27**, 479–84.

Sutton, J.L., Basu, T.K. and Dickerson, J.W.T. (1983). Effect of large doses of ascorbic acid in man on some nitrogenous components of urine. *Hum. Nutr.: Appl. Nutr.*, **37A**, 136–40.

Sutton, J.L., Basu, T.K. and Dickerson, J.W.T. (1983). Effect of pharmacological doses of ascorbic acid on the hepatic microsomal haemoproteins in the guinea-pig. *Br. J. Nutr.*, **49**, 27–33.

Szabo, A.J., Cole, H.S. and Grimaldi, R.D. (1970). Glucose tolerance in gestational diabetic women during and after treatment with a combination-type oral contraceptive. *N. Engl. J. Med.*, **282**, 646–50.

Tabacchi, M.H. and Kirksey, A. (1973). Influence of dietary lipids on plasma and hepatic lipids and on blood clotting properties in rats fed oral contraceptives. *J. Nutr.*, **103**, 1270–78.

Thomson, A.D., Baker, H. and Leevy, C.M. (1970). Pattern of $^{35}$S-thiamine hydrochloride absorption in malnourished alcoholic patients. *J. Lab. Clin. Med.*, **76**, 34–45.

Thorp, J.M. (1963). An experimental approach to the problem of disordered lipid metabolism. *J. Atheroscl. Res.*, **3**, 351–60.

Toothaker, R.D. and Welling, P.G. (1980). The effect of food on drug bioavailability. *Ann. Revs. Pharmacol. Toxicol.*, **20**, 173–99.

Truswell, A.S. (1973). Effects of drugs on nutrition. *Update*, July, 179–86.

Tygstrup, N., Winkler, K. and Warburg, E. (1959). Effect of *p*-aminosalicylic acid on serum-cholesterol. *Lancet*, **i**, 503.

Ungar, J., Parkin, K.R., Tomich, E.G. and Muggleton, P.W. (1954). Effect of pyridoxine on the action of isoniazid. *Lancet*, **ii**, 220–21.

Vakil, B.J., Kulkarni, R.D., Chabria, N.L., Chadha, D.R. and Deshpande, V.A. (1975). Intense surveillance of adverse drug reactions. *J. Clin. Pharmac.*, **15**, 435–41.

Vestal, R.E., Norris, A.H., Tobin, J.D., Cohen, B.H., Shock, N.W. and Andres, R.

(1975). Antipyrine metabolism in man: influence of age, alcohol, caffeine, and smoking. *J. Clin. Pharmac. Ther.*, **18**, 425–32.

Vilter, R.W. (1964). The vitamin $B_6$ hydrazide relationship. *Vitams Horm.*, **22**, 797–805.

Viswanathan, C.T. and Welling, P.G. (1983). Food effects on drug absorption in the elderly. In *Drugs and Nutrition in the Geriatric Patient*, pp. 47–70. Ed. Roe, D.A. Churchill Livingstone: Edinburgh.

Waterlow, J.C. (1968). Observations on the mechanism of adaptation to low protein intakes. *Lancet*, **ii**, 1091–7.

Wertalik, L.F., Metz, E.N., Lobuglio, A.F. and Balcerzak, S.P. (1972). Decreased $B_{12}$ levels with oral contraceptive use. *J. Am. Med. Ass.*, **221**, 1371–4.

Wharton, B.A., Howells, G.R. and McCance, R.A. (1967). Cardiac failure in kwashiorkor, *Lancet*, **ii**, 384–7.

Williams, R.T. (1967). Comparative patterns of drug metabolism. *Fedn Proc.*, **26**, 1029–39.

Williamson, J. and Chaplin, J.M. (1980). Adverse reactions to drugs in the elderly: a multicentre investigation. *Age and Ageing*, **9**, 73–80.

Wilson, C.W.M. (1974). Vitamins and drug metabolism with particular reference to vitamin C. *Proc. Nutr. Soc.*, **33**, 231–8.

Wood, G.C. and Woodcock, B.G. (1970). Effects of dietary protein-deficiency on the conjugation of foreign compounds in rat liver. *J. Pharm. Pharmac.*, **22**, (Suppl), 605.

Woodcock, B.G. and Wood, G.C. (1971). Effect of protein-free diet on UDP-glucuronyl transferase and sulphotransferase activities in rat liver. *Biochem. Pharmac.*, **20**, 2703–13.

Wynn, V. and Doar, J.W.H. (1969). Some effects of oral contraceptives on carbohydrate metabolism. *Lancet*, **ii**, 761–6.

Wynn, V., Doar, J.W.H., Mills, G.L. and Stokes, T. (1969). Fasting serum triglyceride, cholesterol, and lipoprotein levels during oral contraceptive therapy. *Lancet*, **ii**, 756–60.

# 19 Nutritional aspects of different dietary practices

Celia A. Williams and Bashir Qureshi



## Introduction

It is very important that health professionals acknowledge the wide range of dietary practices which occur in the United Kingdom. Certain dietary practices have associated health problems. To give effective nutritional advice to an individual, for whatever reason, requires an understanding of the diet and of the foods used by the patient.

For the purposes of this chapter the omnivorous diet will be taken as the usual diet but it should never be seen as the 'ideal' dietary pattern; this still remains elusive! The omnivorous meat containing diet is the most common and widely catered for in the UK but is by no means acceptable to all the population. It is the aim of this chapter to consider alternative diets, the majority of which embrace some form of vegetarianism, and to consider ethnic diets and food choices.

Of increasing concern is the use of highly restrictive dietary practices e.g. macrobiotic diets, fruitarianism, and this is especially so in the susceptible, or vulnerable, groups of the population such as young babies, children, pregnant and lactating women. The implications of such diets will be considered.

The use of nutritional supplements and administration of large quantities of vitamins would appear to be of increasing popularity in the UK; it is likely that not all the effects of this trend will be beneficial. In so far as the problems can be considered to be nutritional in origin, they will be considered briefly.

## Vegetarianism

To know an individual is vegetarian gives no more nutritional information than that the individual exerts some discretion over the inclusion of animal products in the diet. Strict vegetarians or vegans exclude all animal products from their diets; lactovegetarians include dairy products whereas ovo-vegetarians include eggs, and pescovegetarians include fish. Combinations of these inclusions and therefore prefixes are used.

The nutritional quality of vegetarian diets is highly variable, probably more so than that of omnivorous diets. If dairy produce is included the nutrient composition of the diet can be similar to that of the average non vegetarian diet. Care must be taken to ensure an adequate intake of vitamin $B_{12}$ if dairy produce and eggs are restricted or excluded from the diet. In children, the intake of vitamin D may give cause for concern. The more restricted the food choice the more likely there are to be problems with the diet.

The vegetarian population of the UK is large and includes a number of ethnic groups; problems encountered by these groups will be discussed after a general consideration of vegetarian diets as eaten in the UK for reasons not related to culture or religion. An increasing proportion of individuals and families are choosing to eliminate animal and/or animal produce from their diet. This trend is found most frequently among professional people and those with tertiary education. Practitioners of homeopathy, osteopathy and naturopathy often recommend vegetarian diets. It is not just the eating practices of this group which sets them apart from the rest of the population. They tend to be more health conscious, take frequent exercise and abstain from alcohol and tobacco. A vegetarian regime is often followed for philosophical, ethical or health reasons. The vegan diet invariably contains less energy, protein, fat, saturated fat, calcium, vitamin $B_{12}$ and riboflavin but more polyunsaturated fatty acids, vitamins C and A, folate, iron, fibre and unrefined carbohydrate than a non vegetarian diet (Sanders, 1983; Sanders and Purves, 1981). Although the protein content is less, the percentage of energy derived from protein is similar to that of a non vegetarian diet (Miller and Mumford, 1972). Generalizations about other vegetarian diets are impossible. The vegan diet is notably different from other vegetarian diets in that it contains less fat and very little cholesterol (Carlson *et al.*, 1985). The fat content of vegetarian diets is very variable and ethnic influences are notable; it is wrong to assume all plant oils are rich in polyunsaturated fats and low in saturated fats. Coconut oil, palm oil, cheaper blends of vegetable oils and processed vegetable oils are the commonly used exceptions.

Vegetarian diets contain more fibre than omnivorous diets (Burr and Sweetnam, 1982; Carlson *et al.*, 1985) and although this might be beneficial in adults, it can pose problems for children and infants as the fibre effectively dilutes the nutrient content of the diet. The higher fibre content of the vegetarian diet and the predominance of foods with a low energy density could explain the lower energy intake commonly found with most vegetarian diets.

The major sources of protein in the vegetarian diets are cereals, nuts and pulses; with the notable exception of soya protein, plant proteins are of a lesser quality than animal proteins. However, the proteins of these three food groups are complementary – if foods from all three groups are used then the protein quality of the diet is assured. From the information given in Table 19.1 it can be seen that foods that have certain limiting amino acids can be taken with those that are good sources of these particular amino acids in order to yield, in the mixed diet, adequate amounts of all the essential amino acids. Most

Table 19.1 Protein sources in the vegetarian diet – meat given for comparison

| | Protein | | |
|---|---|---|---|
| | g/100 g | % energy | Essential amino acids |
| *Cereals* | | | |
| Wheat (wholemeal) | 13.2 | 16.6 | Limiting amino acid is lysine. |
| Oats – rolled | 13.0 | 13.5 | Good sources of methionine |
| Rye | 11.0 | 13.8 | and cystine.* Tryptophan |
| Maize – wholemeal | 9.5 | 10.6* | also limiting.†† Threonine |
| Rice – husked | 6.5 | 7.2†† | also limiting |
| *Pulses* | | | |
| Soya bean – raw | 38 | 45.2 | |
| Lentils – raw | 23.8 | 31.3 | Limiting amino acids – |
| Haricot beans – raw | 21.4 | 31.5 | methionine and cystine. |
| Red kidney beans – raw | 22.1 | 32.5 | Good sources of lysine. |
| Butter beans – raw | 19.1 | 27.9 | |
| *Nuts* | | | |
| Almonds | 16.9 | 11.9 | Limiting amino acids – |
| Peanuts | 24.3 | 17.0 | methionine and cystine. |
| Hazelnuts | 7.6 | 8.0 | Good sources of lysine. |
| Brazil | 12.0 | 7.8 | Limiting amino acid is lysine. Good source of methionine and cystine. |
| *Meat* | | | |
| Beef rumpsteak grilled | 27.3 | 51.0 | |
| Chicken – roast | 22.6 | 41.7 | |

Based on data taken from Paul and Southgate (1978) and Davidson *et al.* (1979)

vegetarian meals combine foods from more than one of these groups.

The vitamin A content of the vegan diet will be entirely in the form of carotenoids with provitamin A activity i.e. $\alpha$-carotene, $\beta$-carotene and cryptoxanthin. Pre-formed vitamin A or retinol is only found in animal products. Vitamin D is found only in animal products – but it is added to margarines and some breakfast cereals and this is acceptable to most vegetarians. Vitamin D is added to soya milks e.g. Plamil. Vitamin D can also be synthesized in the body by the action of sunlight on the skin; it is not normally a problem with vegetarians with the exception of those in some Asian communities.

Vitamin $B_{12}$ is found exclusively in animal products and is a cause of concern for all vegetarian diets. Dairy produce and eggs contain vitamin $B_{12}$ and a range of foods supplemented with $B_{12}$ is available specifically for vegetarians, (see Table 19.2). The adult daily minimum requirement for vitamin $B_{12}$ is 1 $\mu$g.

Evidence of vitamin $B_{12}$ deficiency is rare in most vegetarians, although recently a number of cases have been reported amongst ethnic minorities (see p. 284). It is possible that $B_{12}$ requirements are met by alternative sources. Thus, it may be present on poorly washed fruit and vegetables as a microbial contaminant, some drinking water contains vitamin $B_{12}$, the microflora of the large intestine can synthesize vitamin $B_{12}$ and possibly some of this is absorbed (Immerman, 1981). Often the low intakes of vitamin $B_{12}$ are accompanied by

Table 19.2 Valuable sources of riboflavin, vitamin $B_{12}$ and Vitamin D in vegetarian diets

| Food | Portion g | Riboflavin mg | Vitamin $B_{12}$ μg | Vitamin D μg |
|---|---|---|---|---|
| Milk: cows' | 142 (¼ pt) | 0.27 | 0.43 | 0.02–0.04 |
| soya Plamil-concentrate | 71 | 0.45 | 2.27 | 1.07 |
| Butter | 10 | tr | tr | 0.06–0.10 |
| Margarine | 10 | tr | tr | 0.07–0.09 |
| Cheese: cheddar | 56 | 0.17–0.45 | 0.84 | 0.15 |
| cottage | 113 | 0.21 | 0.57 | 0.03 |
| Yogurt | 150 | 0.35–0.41 | tr | 0* |
| Egg | 50 | 0.24 | 0.85–1.30 | 0.88 |
| Breakfast cereal: All Bran | 40 | 1.12 | 0 | 0 |
| Grapenuts | 42 | 0.67 | 2.10 | 1.47 |
| Weetabix | 38 | 0.57 | 0 | 0 |
| Special K | 30 | 0.57 | 0 | 0 |
| Rice K | 30 | 0.51 | 0 | 0 |
| Cornflakes | 30 | 0.48 | 0 | 0 |
| Green leafy veg: boiled | 113 | 0.17–0.34 | 0 | 0 |
| Mushrooms: cooked | 56 | 0.20 | 0 | 0 |
| Almonds | 28 | 0.26 | 0 | 0 |
| Savoury spreads: Marmite | 5 | 0.55 | 0.05 | 0 |

* fortified yogurts can be found

high intakes of folate and this might explain why when clinical vitamin $B_{12}$ deficiency is described in vegetarian populations it is often the neurological and not the haematological form. The high folate intakes can possibly mask or antagonize the effect of vitamin $B_{12}$ deficiency and this emphasizes the need for vitamin $B_{12}$ supplements. Prolonged cooking can destroy both vitamin $B_{12}$ and folic acid.

Caucasian vegans have been reported to have lower serum $B_{12}$ and higher erythrocyte folate levels than non vegetarians; male vegans, users and non users of vitamin $B_{12}$ supplements were found to have lower erthrocyte counts, and higher MCV and MCHb levels than non vegetarians (Sanders *et al.*, 1977). However, the authors concluded that a mixed vegan diet using foods supplemented with vitamin $B_{12}$ could promote normal blood formation. Vitamin $B_{12}$ supplementation is essential during pregnancy, lactation and childhood. The riboflavin intake of vegetarians can be lower than that of non vegetarians especially if dairy foods are not used, alternative sources are leafy vegetables, nuts and pulses (see Table 19.2). The maternal intake of both riboflavin and vitamin $B_{12}$ is reflected in the milk produced; supplements should be recommended during lactation. Riboflavin and vitamin $B_{12}$ supplements should also be given to vegetarian children.

The calcium intake of vegetarians who do not use dairy produce is often less than that of omnivores. However, metabolic studies have shown that adaptation to low calcium intakes occurs in vegetarians and faecal calcium losses are reduced (Nnakwe and Kies, 1985). During pregnancy and lactation when the requirements for calcium increase, additional sources of calcium will be needed e.g. soya milk. Although the iron intake of vegans and vegetarians can exceed that of omnivores, the iron will be in a non-haem form and therefore less well absorbed; iron absorption can also be impaired by phytate and vegetable fibre and facilitated by vitamin C. There is no medical evidence to suggest an increased incidence of iron deficiency anaemia exists amongst caucasian adult vegetarians (Sanders, 1983).

Legumes, a valuable protein source in the vegetarian diet, can contain a number of toxic compounds including lectins (haemagglutinins), aflatoxin, cyanogens and favism and lathyrus factors. Mostly these occur due to changes during poor storage and are not encountered in the UK. However, the incidence of food poisoning due to lectins might be under-estimated in the UK (Bender and Readi, 1982). Kidney beans, *Phaseolus vulgaris*, are popular legumes with a high lectin content. These beans must be boiled for at least 10 minutes prior to simmer cooking. If the water temperature does not reach 100°C the lectin content can in fact increase (Bender and Readi, 1982). Symptoms of lectin food poisoning usually occur 2 hours after ingestion of the contaminated food and include nausea, vomiting and diarrhoea.

Adults who follow a strict vegetarian regime are lighter and have a lower proportion of body fat than non vegetarians (Sanders *et al.*, 1978). It is common to lose weight on initiation of a vegan diet. Vegetarians are often used to illustrate the benefits of long term consumption of dietary fibre; vegetarians who eat 30 g or more fibre per day suffer from less constipation (Davies *et al.*, 1986). A lower prevalence of diverticular disease has been reported in vegetarians compared to non vegetarians (Gear *et al.*, 1979). A prospective study in the UK found vegetarians to be less likely to die from IHD than non vegetarians – the effect was most notable in men; fibre intake and cigarette smoking were not found to be related factors (Burr and Sweetnam, 1982).

Reports have shown vegetarians have different serum lipid profiles to non vegetarians. Fasting serum cholesterol levels can be lower or similar between the two groups but the HDL/LDL ratio is higher in the vegetarian group. Vegans have significantly lower fasting plasma cholesterol and triglyceride levels than non vegetarians (Sanders *et al.*, 1978; Dickerson and Fehily, 1979; Sanders, 1983).

Female vegans can follow their diets and produce normal healthy offspring. Vitamin $B_{12}$ and riboflavin supplementation should be strongly recommended during lactation. The majority of vegetarians breast feed their children – however, if this is not possible a range of soya-based modified milk formulas are available. These milks should be included in a young child's diet if cows' milk is not acceptable. Modified formula milk substitutes suitable for infants and children include Velactin (Wander), Prosobee (Mead Johnson), Wysoy (Wyeth) and Formula S (Cow & Gate).

There is no evidence that vegan diets can significantly impair growth in children. A recent American study on the growth of pre-school children found the growth curves of vegetarians to be 0.5–1.0 kg and 1.0–2.0 cm lower than omnivores and girls to be more affected than boys (Dwyer *et al.*, 1983). A study on the same age group in Holland also found vegetarian children to be significantly lighter and shorter than omnivores but within normal limits (van

Straveren *et al.*, 1985). Both studies describe serious effects on growth of highly restrictive macrobiotic vegetarian diets.

## Dietary practices of ethnic minorities in the United Kingdom

The aim of this section is to describe the diet and associated problems of a limited number of the ethnic groups found in the UK. All ethnic groups usually eat a balanced diet, and do not depend solely on the foods associated with their country of origin, and allowance should be made for this. Ethnic diets contribute towards the quality of life of the individuals and communities (Mann, 1980). But there are problems which, if one is aware of them, can be dealt with. A good hospital menu should cover all ethnic diets with allowances for local and personal preferences, and for various religious taboos.

Variations in food choice within particular ethnic minority groups occur and can be partially explained by the four generation concept.

1. *The first generation, A* – The migrants who came as dependent relatives of the migrant workers. They are mostly retired people, who prefer to eat their native foods rather than adapt to English-style foods.
2. *The first generation, B* – The migrant workers who sought employment in the UK. They are aged 21–65 and will accept English food and their native food equally.
3. *The second generation* – The young generation who went to school in Britain. Aged 7–21 most were born in the UK and prefer to adhere to an English diet. They will strongly resist attempts to force them to consume their native food, which to them is alien. It is folly to bracket them with their grandparents in matters of nutrition; they have different needs as well as different demands, therefore provisions should differ accordingly.
4. *The third generation* – The children who feel British but become interested in tracing their roots. They are dependent upon their parents for food – English as well as native diet.

It is interesting to note that the first generation adhere to their native culture, whereas the second generation adhere to English culture. Moreover, the second generation, under the impact of a 'two-culture conflict' may even reject their native food and this point should be borne in mind. The third generation of all migrants enjoy retracing their roots.

Not only do food choices and preferences differ between ethnic minorities, but dietary habits also vary. For example, for eating rice, the English will use a fork, Afro-Caribbeans and Asians will use a spoon, and the Chinese prefer chopsticks. First and third generations of ethnic minority groups may follow their native custom of eating whereas the second generation will follow their English peers. If an Asian or Chinese patient is given a knife and fork, he may refuse to eat and may be too embarrassed to attempt to explain the reason why. Ethnic Asians and Afro-Caribbeans prefer a spoon for rice, but most of the food is eaten with clean hands, spiced meats being wrapped in chapatis, hence protecting the buccal mucosa. According to religious and cultural customs they wash their hands before eating, and after eating they not only wash their hands again but also rinse their mouths, thereby cleaning their teeth. It is said that this habit is the reason for their strong, healthy teeth. Some children who do not wash their hands or have long nails which they have not cleaned can get intestinal problems. Moreover their hands, even after being washed, may remain stained with turmeric and other spices. The ethnic Chinese, Malaysians and Indonesians all use chopsticks (Goodwin, 1980). In this way they can take only small amounts of food at one time, allowing more time for the food to mix with the saliva. They appear to reach satiety with smaller amounts of food with this method, and over-eating is not normally a problem.

A health professional should not take it for granted that all his ethnic patients will be eating by one method. It is important for a patient to use his ethnic method of eating when he is ill, rather than be forced to eat with a knife and fork.

The attitude of an individual to the role of foods in maintaining health and preventing or curing an illness should be recognized or the patient might be disillusioned by the attitude of the health professional. Asian healers such as Hakims and Vaids were aware of food allergies. In fact in treating any disease, the avoidance of certain foods was usually advised. In Asian countries a patient is used to receiving such advice and medication from his conventional doctor. Sometimes the doctor asks him to avoid spices or curries for a few days and take 'khichri', a rice dish. Such a doctor may also advise a patient to avoid red and green chillies and to use black pepper instead. As a result, an ethnic Asian may well ask his doctor what foods he should avoid; this is called 'perhaiz'. If a health professional simply dismisses this customary question from an ethnic Asian or Chinese patient, the patient may lose faith in him and turn to alternative medicine.

In Afro-Asian cultures, milk, orange juice, lemonade and Ribena are considered drinks which aggravate colds and coughs. Therefore patients may ask the health professional if these should be avoided. Similarly, hot curries and meat dishes, especially 'paya', a local Punjabi dish, are considered 'hot' and therefore beneficial in the treatment of colds and coughs, but harmful in cases of epistaxis. Although this area needs further research, lack of explanation by a health professional may lead to lack of faith in the treatment prescribed and again, patients may turn to alternative medicine.

In an investigation of the nutritional status of a patient from an ethnic minority it is important not to overlook racial differences of genetic origin, for example in measurements of heights and weights. The standard height and weight charts for British children who are mostly omnivores do not apply to Gujrati Hindu children who are vegetarians. They also do not apply to the Chinese and Malaysians as well as Bangladeshis and South Indians or Sri Lankans, who are smaller and lighter than Europeans, Africans, Pakistanis and North Indians. Their normal babies are of light birth weight and small (Table 19.3).

The majority of non-caucasian adults are lactose intolerant; this can result in chronic diarrhoea and occasionally acute diarrhoea and vomiting if milk is taken. Lactose intolerance should always be considered as a possibility when an infant presents with these symptoms.

There are chronic and acute disease patterns in the various ethnic minority groups found in the United Kingdom which are possibly related to the staple foods of the diet.

Cassava (mohogo) is mainly consumed by Africans. It contains very small amounts of thiocyanates, and when eaten in excess over a long period can cause pancreatic diabetes.

Chapati is eaten exclusively by ethnic Asians as their main bread, in unlimited amounts. Chapati flour, often imported from India, contains phytic acid which combines with dietary calcium to form calcium phytate which is inedible and cannot be absorbed (O'Riordan, 1974). This factor, in addition to lack of vitamin D and calcium supplements in the diet, is possibly involved in the aetiology of: fetal rickets, childhood rickets (1–4 years of age – this is the time when an Asian infant is introduced to chapatis) and osteomalacia in adults. Moreover, rickets is more common in ethnic Asian toddlers than in ethnic Africans or Europeans, although all have the same exposure to British sunshine (Dunnigan *et al.*, 1981). It is not enough to give vitamin D; it is essential also to supplement the calcium in the diet.

Rice is the main carbohyrate of Chinese food, and for reasons yet to be discovered, it may cause post-bulbar duodenal ulcers. However, rice is also consumed by Bangladeshis, South Indians, Sri Lankans and Afro-Caribbeans, who are also liable to develop this condition.

There are three ethnic foods which can cause medical emergencies. Karela (*Mormodica charantia*) is a popular choice of vegetarian Hindus (Indians) and is cooked in a curry. This vegetable has a marked hypoglycaemic effect; it has been used in place of insulin by Hakims in old Indian therapies. It can potentiate the action of oral hypoglycaemics and cause prolonged hypoglycaemia (Aslam, 1979), resulting in faintness or coma. In the differential diagnosis of fainting or coma, this possibility should be included.

In mild cases, a patient may come to the doctor complaining of feeling weak. This should be differentiated from the symptoms of anaemia or depression before embarking on investigation or treatment. A diabetic patient would do well either to avoid karela curry altogether, or to make an allowance for the amount of karela he eats, and adjust his medication accordingly, and this should be taken into account when taking the history of a patient in an ethnic minority.

Ackee is a fruit eaten as a native delicacy in Jamaica. If picked unripe from plants and cooked, it is so poisonous that it can kill. The pod and the film dividing the fruit contain two poisonous chemicals, hypoglycin A and hypoglycin B which cause severe hypoglycaemia. However, when it is ripe and cooked well the pulp is delicious. 'Bushtea' contains this fruit and can cause 'Jamaican vomiting sickness'. Approximately 75 per cent of the ethnic West Indians in the UK are from Jamaica. It is customary for them, after visiting their native country, to bring back ackee as a present for relatives and this possibility should be borne in mind in any cases of apparent food poisoning.

Vetsin, a food additive, can be present in sauces provided in Chinese restaurants. It contains monosodium glutamate (Kenny, 1979) and some people are allergic to it. This allergy can cause severe headache lasting for up to an hour, a condition known as the 'Chinese Restaurant Syndrome' (Kenny, 1980).

Although these are rare emergencies, in multi-ethnic areas such information can be life-saving.

Table 19.3 Regional differences among ethnic Asians

| Origin | Physical features: Colour | Height | Weight | Cultural features: Religion | Language |
|---|---|---|---|---|---|
| *Pakistan* | | | | | |
| 1. Punjabis | Fair | Tall | Medium | Muslim | Urdu or Punjabi |
| 2. Pathans | White | Tall and well built | Large | Muslim | Pushtu or Persian |
| *India* | | | | | |
| 1. Punjabis | Fair | Tall | Medium | Sikh or Hindu | Punjabi or Hindi |
| 2. Gujratis | Fair | Short | Light | Hindu | Gujrati |
| 3. Bengalis | Dark | Short | Light | Hindu | Bengali |
| 4. South Indians | Dark | Short | Light | Hindu or Christian | Tamil or Malyalam |
| *Bangladesh* | | | | | |
| Bangladeshis | Dark | Short | Light | Muslim | Bengali |
| *Sri Lanka* | | | | | |
| Sri Lankans | Dark | Short | Light | Buddhist or Hindu | Sinhalese or Tamil |
| *Kenyan or Ugandan Asians* | | | | | |
| 1. Punjabis | Fair | Tall | Medium | Hindu or Muslim | Punjabi, Hindi or Urdu |
| 2. Gujratis | Fair | Short | Light | Hindu | Gujrati |

(Qureshi 1986)

## Ethnic Asian Groups

Regional differences found amongst ethnic Asians are summarized in Table 19.3. Their food choices can be strongly influenced by religion. However, they are also susceptible to certain dietary practices that they encounter in the UK. This can lead to problems, especially in the young, i.e. second and third generations (see p. 427), when the ethnic foods are shunned in favour of such foods as jam sandwiches, crisps and chocolate bars (Jivani, 1984).

### Muslim

The Muslims' faith is Islam in which eating is seen as a worship of Allah. According to the Qur'an there are two types of food. Haram – prohibited and Hallal – lawful. Muslims are not allowed to eat pork or take alcohol. Meat and animal fats have to be prepared ritually according to Islamic faith in order to be hallal. Many convenience foods are not permitted as the contents are not hallal; this includes proprietary baby foods. Ismailis of East African origin can also follow these rules.

### Hindu

Hindus follow ahisma – not killing animals for food. They are strictly forbidden to eat beef, pork, lamb, chicken, fish, shellfish, animal fats and alcohol. Dairy produce and eggs are acceptable to most, but not all, Hindus. Those of the higher castes are often strict vegetarians.

**Sikhism**

This faith combines certain concepts of Hinduism and Islam. Sikhs do not eat beef and rarely eat pork; many Sikhs are lactovegetarians.

**Buddhism**

The followers of Buddha eat a rice based diet, meat and fish are eaten exceptionally and only when it has not been killed specifically for eating.

Asian children are a group at nutritional risk today in the UK. Parents can be confused over the feeding of babies and infants, familiar foods might be unavailable or too expensive; those to whom they would normally turn to for advice are no longer with them. Asian parents can misunderstand or misinterpret the advice of health professionals which takes no account of their dietary practices; unless understanding advice is given they can lose confidence in their own foods and cooking practices.

Although breast feeding is becoming increasingly popular in the UK, the incidence of bottle feeding remains high amongst the Asian community. This must be a cause for concern. In their indigenous country the majority of Asian women would have almost certainly breast fed their infants.

Immigrant Asians introduce cows' milk into the diet of infants earlier than is advisable – this is probably done as a matter of convenience because fresh cows' milk is readily available locally (Jivani, 1984). One consequence of this practice is an increased risk of iron deficiency because the iron content of cow's milk is considerably less than that of modified formulas and of breast milk. Iron deficiency anaemia is, in fact, common amongst Asian children. Health professionals will often recommend tinned or packet foods as part of the weaning regime because these foods are sterile. However, Hindus and Muslims will not use those which contain meat or meat products and as a consequence the babies are often weaned on to poor protein starchy foods which are alien to their mothers. This can undermine the confidence of the mother in the suitability of her own foods for the infant and the infant will not be introduced to the family's natural diet.

Biochemical vitamin D deficiency and clinical rickets occur in Asian children, and the incidence of rickets is biphasic, occurring in toddlers and in pre-adolescents. It is advisable that all Asian children should receive daily vitamin D supplements of 400 IU especially during periods of growth. Routine supplements of 1000 IU have been recommended for pregnant Asian women in whom clinical and biochemical osteomalacia is common (Brooke *et al.*, 1980). No one factor appears to be responsible for the susceptibility of Asian women and children to vitamin D deficiency – however, the following might be involved:

1. increased requirement;
2. a dietary deficiency of vitamin D;
3. the high phytate content of chapatis might impair calcium absorption;
4. lack of exposure to UV light of required intensity to allow endogenous production of vitamin D;

5. cultural differences;
6. a genetic predisposition.

Asian families should be encouraged to use familiar foods when possible. Spiced meat dishes which do not contain chilli can be given to infants. Legumes and seeds can be purέed and mixed with milk to provide a valuable protein source. Although most cereals have a poor mineral content, ragi or finger millet is a good source of calcium and bajra or spruce millet is a good source of iron; both foods are familiar to Asian families (Jivani, 1984). Asians who follow a strict vegetarian diet or restrict the use of dairy produce and eggs can encounter some nutritional problems as previously described in the section on vegetarianism (p. 422). Megaloblastic anaemia due to nutritional vitamin $B_{12}$ deficiency has been reported in male and female vegetarian Hindus in the UK. A high frequency of iron deficiency anaemia was also described in this group and it was suggested that this might be associated with the vitamin $B_{12}$ deficiency (Chanarin *et al.*, 1985).

The diet of Asian vegetarians can contain more fat than that of other vegetarians possibly due to the emphasis on the use of oils in cooking. Intakes of sugar especially in beverages have been reported to exceed normal levels in some Asian communities. Asian immigrants from the Indian subcontinent have a higher morbidity and mortality from coronary heart disease than average (Tunstall-Pedoe *et al.*, 1975; Editorial, 1980; Marmot *et al.*, 1984). However, a recent study of Asians living in London who had a higher incidence of coronary heart disease and a lower incidence of cancer of the colon than average failed to associate the incidence of these diseases with high fat and saturated fat intakes. The four main groups involved were Gujratis, Punjabis, Southern Indians and Muslims. A dietary survey of a mixed group comprising vegetarians and non-vegetarians found lower intakes of saturated fats and cholesterol and higher intakes of polyunsaturated fats and vegetables compared to normal UK levels. The total fat intake of the vegetarians was similar to that of non vegetarian households (McKeigue *et al.*, 1985).

Vegetarianism, as practised in Asian groups, in contrast to that practised by Caucasians, does not appear to be protective against obesity.

## Afro-Caribbeans

Their diet contains predominantly pork, chicken, rice and peas, and bananas. The diet is economical, easy to prepare and has a high fibre content. However, along with herbs and spices, large amounts of salt are used. Afro-Caribbeans have an ethnic predisposition to hypertension, said to be due to their genetic hypersensitivity to sodium chloride (Swales, 1980). However, the incidence of CHD in immigrants from the Caribbean living in London was found to be lower than average (Tunstall–Pedoe *et al.*, 1975).

## Rastafarian diet

Rastafarianism is a religious sect started in Jamaica in the 1930s. It has now spread from the West Indies to North America and Europe, and its popularity amongst young black people in the UK appears to be increasing. Rastafarians are a diverse group and dietary practices vary considerably. The male is dominant in the family and is likely to adhere most strictly to the dietary laws and insist that such practices are followed by his children. Foods acceptable to a Rasta must be 'total' or 'natural'. As 'I' is the most powerful letter in the alphabet to Rastafarians such foods are referred to as 'I-tal'. Foods of animal origin are regarded as 'dead' and therefore are undesirable; foods of vegetable origin are 'I-tal'. The Old Testament is also used as a source of food laws. Meat is considered of no benefit, expensive, unhygienic and capable of making a man violent and aggressive. Some Rastafarians will eat fish. Strict Rastafarian women will do so on a doctor's advice during pregnancy. Preserved foods are regarded as 'chemical' and are avoided. Salt and alcohol are limited or prohibited according to interpretation of the Bible (Springer and Thomas, 1983).

The orthodox Rastafarian diet represents a strict vegan regime but unlike many strict vegans living in the UK the Rastafarians can be considered to be at greater nutritional risk for a number of reasons. Their nutritional knowledge is more likely to be poorer than that of other vegans. The choice of food items might be restricted as the preference is for vegetables and fruit of an Afro/Caribbean nature. These are considerably more expensive than more readily available produce. Their cooking practices are more likely to reduce the nutritional value of foods and they tend to under use pulses and legumes – valuable protein sources in a vegan regime. If followed closely, as it is by orthodox Rastafarians, then the diet represents a strict vegan regime and as such can be deficient in vitamin $B_{12}$ due to the absence of foods of animal origin. Unlike other strict vegans – orthodox Rastafarians have a strong aversion to the use of foods supplemented with vitamin $B_{12}$. To date, there have been no reports concerning $B_{12}$ deficiencies in Rastafarians living in the UK, but megaloblastic anaemia and neurological changes have been reported to be associated with low serum $B_{12}$ levels in the male Rastafarians living in Jamaica (Campbell *et al.*, 1982). Also unlike other strict vegans in the UK the folate intake of Rastafarian vegans might be low due to poor cooking practices involving the lengthy boiling of vegetables and discarding of cooking water. Folate deficiency might also contribute to the development of megaloblastic anaemia in Rastafarians.

Rickets has been reported in children born in the UK to Rastafarian parents of Jamaican origin. Of 42 Rastafarian children under the age of five, twenty were identified as being at risk of developing rickets. On investigation, seven were found to have clinical signs associated with rickets. This represents an incidence of 17 per cent. All these children had been breast-fed for more than 6 months and were then weaned on to a strict I-tal diet containing no animal products and limited fats and oils. None had received vitamin supplements because it was believed that such supplements were of animal origin and therefore non I-tal. Analysis of the diets of four children who developed rickets showed an intake of vitamin D of less than 3 $\mu$g/day. Calcium intakes were considered adequate (James *et al.*, 1985).

Biochemical evidence of iron deficiency was also present in 14/18 children investigated. Concern has also been expressed for the health of Rastafarian mothers who might consume a poor diet during pregnancy followed by a prolonged period of breast feeding.

## Restrictive dietary practices

Restriction of foods available to an individual can produce a diet that might be considered hazardous to health. Food choices are restricted for a number of reasons but two major factors are a restriction due to cultural influences or for philosophical reasons, e.g. Zen macrobiotic diet or a restriction in the belief that health will improve, or benefit. This latter category is almost without end. The excessive number of bizarre and unusual diets which are suggested to be either a panacea for all ailments or as cures for specific disorders must be a cause of concern for all health care professionals.

The manifestation of an actual hazard to health is dependent on the length of time for which the diet is followed. It is highly likely that it is only due to the lack of success of the majority of these diets that they are not followed for sufficient time to allow their hazardous nature to become fully obvious.

There are times in life during which the individual can be considered to be more susceptible to the hazardous effects of a restrictive diet. Young infants, for example, are vulnerable to the hazardous effects of diet especially if they are weaned on to an inappropriate diet by parents who follow a restrictive dietary practice. In times of illness an individual can be considered to be metabolically more vulnerable to the hazardous effects of a restrictive diet and also more susceptible to follow diets of questionable nutritional quality. There are occasional reports of children on vegetarian diets suffering severe malnutrition; this results from a poor understanding of the need for a mixed diet and the adoption of highly restrictive practices (Dickerson and Fehily 1979; Roberts *et al.*, 1979).

### The Zen macrobiotic diet

These diets were popularized by George Ohsawa (1893–1966) and can represent an extremely restrictive diet. Generally, the Zen macrobiotic diet is based on wholegrain cereals supplemented with beans and vegetables. Processed foods and stimulant drinks, for example, alcohol or caffeine-containing beverages, are all avoided. Drinking liquids of any description is restricted. The diet ranges in extremity and the individual is responsible for discerning what may or may not be eaten (MacLean and Graham, 1980).

Followers of the macrobiotic way of life believe that life can become more ordered through the strict regulation of food habits. There are ten diets that are rated from −3 to 7 and become increasingly restricted, level 7 being the purest and composed only of whole grain cereals. Followers of these regimes use tables listing the percentage contribution of various food groups to the different diets. Cereals are strongly emphasized in the diet with a preference for wholegrain rice. Normally two-thirds of the daily vegetables are cooked and one third eaten raw. Animal foods can only be used in diets −3 to 2. Shell fish, fresh fish and wild game are preferred. The potential nutritional problems of adults and children increase as the higher levels of diet are used. Strict adherence to diet 7 can result in scurvy, anaemia, hypoproteinaemia, hypocalcaemia, and loss of kidney function. Severe malnutrition has been reported in the UK in infants fed on macrobiotic diets and can result in marasmus and even in cases of frank kwashiorkor (Roberts *et al.*, 1979); scurvy and anaemia have also been reported. Parents following strict macrobiotic regimes should be encouraged to move children to a low-order diet incorporating meat and dairy products. Unfortunately, it is also part of the Zen macrobiotic philosophy to avoid medical consultation and recourse has been made to court orders in the treatment of such children. Anthropometric studies of preschool children in the USA and Holland have shown that the height and weight of children raised on macrobiotic diets can be significantly less than omnivores and other vegetarian children (Dwyer *et al.*, 1983; van Staveren *et al.*, 1985).

### The Fruitarian diet

This represents a highly restricted vegan diet with only fruit, nuts and seeds being acceptable and normally eaten uncooked. Extremely careful planning is needed to ensure that nutrient requirements are met. Vitamin $B_{12}$, riboflavin and vitamin D supplementation should be advised. It has been suggested that vitamin A might be deficient in such a diet as the better fruit sources of the provitamin, e.g. melons, apricots and mangoes, are expensive in the UK (Dickerson and Fehily, 1979).

Children weaned on to such a diet should be regarded as being at risk and severe malnutrition has been reported in such cases.

## Vitamin abuse

Diets or dietary supplementation regimes designed to increase the intake of vitamins to levels 20–600 times the RDA (Recommended Daily Allowance) have been reported. The misguided rationale behind such a scheme is usually 'if a little is good – then a lot must be even better' and by achieving a 'mega dose' level of a vitamin in the diet the metabolic process in which the vitamin is involved will be maximized. This is assumed to enhance the health of the individual either generally or in respect of a specific disorder. Often the established therapeutic value of a vitamin is wrongly seen as conferring preventative properties.

The toxic nature of vitamins A and D has long been recognized and because of the limited excretion of these vitamins their potential toxicity to man has been acknowledged by health care professionals. However, for some time it was considered that the toxic potential of the water soluble vitamins was negligible as ingested excess would be excreted in the urine. This, however, is not the case. Six vitamins, three water soluble and three fat soluble, can be considered to be hazardous to health if abused. These are as follows:

1. *Vitamin A* The harmful effects of vitamin A have been reported to occur at daily intakes of 5–10 mg retinol equivalents (RE) (Dubick and Rucker, 1983). The UK RDA for adults is 750 $\mu$g RE (DHSS, 1979). There are two possible reasons why the intake of retinol might be high. Parents may be over enthusiastic in giving vitamin drops and cod liver oil to children; secondly there has been an increase in the media interest in vitamin A due to the successful use of retinoids, vitamin A and substances with vitamin A-like activity in skin diseases and cancer. Retinoids are of value in the treatment of severe acne and psoriasis; they have also been used in the

treatment of some epithelial cancers although their use is limited by their toxicity. Because vitamin A is seen as having a preventative role in these disorders the abuse of the vitamin and vitamin rich foods is being encouraged. One of the classic symptoms of retinol toxicity is an increased intracranial pressure which mimics the effects of a brain tumour. In a recent American survey of 50 individuals with pseudo tumour of the brain, five were found to have a bizarre attitude to the place of liver in the diet, two routinely purchasing more than 6 lbs/week for consumption (Brooke *et al.*, 1980). Some carotenes are included in the generic description 'vitamin A'. Excessive intake of carotenes can produce a symptom referred to as xanthosis cutis which can represent a 'cosmetic' hazard rather than a health hazard. Although carotenes are non-toxic and as such do not represent a health hazard this condition is indicative of a bizarre attitude to vitamin A. Indeed a fatal case of retinol toxicity was reported in the UK in 1975 in a male whose intake of carrot juice was phenomenal (Leitner *et al.*, 1975).

2. *Vitamin D* Daily intakes of 1–8 mg have been reported to be harmful to man (10 μg is the RDA for elderly housebound adults (DHSS, 1979). Excessive intakes can result in high blood calcium levels, irreversible renal failure and calcification of soft tissues (Baker and Bender, 1982).
3. *Vitamin E* Harmful effects have been noted on intakes of 900 mg/day. There is no RDA in the UK but 8–10 mg/day is the RDA published by the National Academy of Sciences (1980). Excessive intakes of vitamin E result in an interference with vitamin A and K metabolism; depression, fatigue, cramps and blurred vision are frequently reported (Dubick and Rucker, 1983).
4. *Pyridoxine* Pyridoxine, or vitamin $B_6$ has gained wide public acceptance as a remedy for pre-menstrual syndrome (PMS), especially for the relief of oedema. Also it is frequently used as part of body building schemes. The American adult RDA for pyridoxine is 1.8–2.2 mg. In a recent study of 58 women self-administering pyridoxine at levels of 50–300 mg/day for relief from symptoms of PMS nearly 40 per cent had abnormally elevated serum pyridoxine levels and symptoms of sensory neuropathy. After 2 months without a supplement, all reported an overall improvement (Dalton, 1985). It seems that the potential toxicity of pyridoxine might have been underestimated because previous reports of toxic effects had been at much higher levels of intake (Rudman and Williams, 1983).
5. *Niacin* Harmful effects have been reported at intakes of 6 g/day. The maximum RDA for adults is 18 mg/day (DHSS, 1979). Niacin can have a transient vasodilatory effect in man; it is also hepatotoxic if administered at high levels for long periods (Baker and Bender, 1982).
6. *Vitamin C* Vitamin C is often discussed as being potentially harmful at megadose levels – however, there is very little evidence to support this (Couleham, 1979; Basu and Schorah, 1982) especially in view of the popularity of the vitamin. Rebound scurvy has, however, been reported to develop in individuals who abruptly stop taking large doses and there is evidence of possible interference with drug metabolism (see also p. 426).

## Conclusion

There is no single 'ideal' diet and it is possible to derive all the nutrients needed to sustain health from a wide range of dietary practices. However, if the range of foods consumed is restricted because of cultural practices, religious beliefs or philosophical views a greater knowledge of food composition is needed to ensure nutritional adequacy. Knowledge of the effects of these various influences is very important to health care professionals, particularly in a multi racial society.

## References


Aslam, M. (1979). Interaction between curry ingredient (Karela) and drug (Chlorpropamide). *Lancet*, i, 607.

Barker, B.M. and Bender, D.A. (1982). *Vitamins in Medicine* Vol. 1. 4th ed. Heinemann: London.

Basu, T.K. and Schorah, C.J. (1982). *Vitamin C in Health and Disease*. Croom Helm: London.

Bender, A.E. and Readi, G.B. (1982). Toxicity of kidney beans (phaseolus vulgaris) with particular reference to lectins. *J. Plant Foods*, **4**, 15–22.

Brooke, O.G., Brown, I.R.F., Bone, C.D.M., Carter, N.D., Cleeve, H.J.W., Maxwell, J.D., Robinson, V.P. and Winder, S.M. (1980). Vitamin D supplements in pregnant Asian women: effects on calcium status and fetal growth. *Br. Med. J.*, **280**, 751–4.

Burr, M.L. and Sweetnam, P.M. (1982). Vegetarianism, dietary fiber and mortality. *Am. J. Clin. Nutr.*, **36**, 873–7.

Campbell, M., Loffes, W.S., Gibbs, W.N. (1982). Rastafarianism and the vegan syndrome. *Br. Med. J.*, **285**, 1617–18.

Carlson, E., Kipps, M., Lockie, A. and Thomson, J.A. (1985). Comparative evaluation of vegan, vegetarian and omnivore diets. *J. Plant Foods*, **6**, 89–100.

Chanarin, I., Malkowska, V., O'Hea, A.M., Rinsier, M.G., Price, A.B. (1985). Megaloblastic anaemia in a vegetarian Hindu community. *Lancet*, **ii**, 1168–72.

Couleham, J.L. (1979). Ascorbic acid and the common cold. *Postgrad. Med.*, **66**, 153–60.

Dalton, K. (1985). Pyridoxine overdose in premenstrual syndrome. *Lancet*, **i**, 1168–9.

Davidson, S., Passmore, R., Brock, J.F. and Truswell, A.S. (1979). *Human Nutrition and Dietetics*. 6th ed. Churchill Livingstone: Edinburgh.

Davies, G.J., Crowder, M., Reid, B. and Dickerson, J.W.T. (1986). Bowel function measurements of individuals with different eating patterns. *Gut*, **27**, 164–9.

DHSS. (1979). *Report on health and social subjects 15. Recommended daily amounts of food energy and nutrients for groups of people in the United Kingdom*. HMSO: London.

Dickerson, J.W.T. and Fehily, A.M. (1979). Bizarre and unusual diets. *Practitioner*, **222**, 643–7.

Dubick, M.A. and Rucker, R.B. (1983). Dietary supplements and health aids – a critical evaluation. Part I – Vitamins and minerals. *J. Nut. Educ.*, **15**, 47–53.

Dunnigan, M.G., McIntosh, W.B., Sutherland, G.R. *et al.*, (1981). Policy of prevention of Asian rickets in Britain: a preliminary assessment of the Glasgow rickets campaign. *Br. Med. J.*, **282**, 357–60.

Dwyer, J.T., Andrew, E.M., Berkey, C., Valadin, I. and Reed, R.B. (1983) Growth in 'new' vegetarian preschool children using the Jenss-Bayley curve fitting technique. *Am. J. Clin. Nutr.*, **37**, 815–27.

Editorial. (1980). Heart disease in different ethnic groups. *Br.Med. J.*, **281**, 469–70.

Gear, J.S.S., Ware, A., Fursdon, P., Mann, J.I., Nolan, D.J., Brodribb, A.J.M. and Vessey, M.P. (1975). Symptomless diverticular disease and intake of dietary fibre. *Lancet*, **i**, 511–14.

Goodwin, G., (1980). The problems of Vietnamese childen in Britain. *J. Maternal Child Health*, **August**, 307–12.

Immerman, A.M. (1981). Vitamin $B_{12}$ status on a vegetarian diet. A critical review. *World Rev. Nutr. Diet.*, **37**, 38–54.

James, J.A., Clark, C. and Ward, P.S. (1985). Screening Rastafarian children for nutritional rickets. *Br. Med. J.*, **290**, 899–900.

Jivani, S.K. (1984). Dietary problems in Asian children. *The Physician*, **2**, 572–6.

Kenny, R.A. (1980). Chinese restaurant syndrome. *Lancet*, **i**, 311–12.

Leitner, Z.A., Moore, T. and Sharman, I.M. (1975). Fatal self medication with retinol and carrot juice. *Proc. Nutr. Soc.*, **34**, 44A.

MacLean, W.C. and Graham, G.G. (1980). Vegetarianism in children. *Am. J. Dis. Child.*, **34**, 513–19.

Mann, G.V. (1980). Food intake and resistance to disease. *Lancet*, **i**, 1238–9.

Marmot, M.G., Adelstein, A.M., Bulusu, L. (1984). Lessons from the study of immigrant mortality. *Lancet*, **i**, 1455–8.

McKeigue, P.M., Marmot, M.G., Adelstein, A.M., Hunt, S.P., Shipley, M.J., Butler, S.M., Riemersma, R.A. and Turner, P.R. (1985). Diet and risk factors for coronary heart disease in Asians in Northwest London. *Lancet*, **ii**, 1086–90.

Miller, D.S. and Mumford, P. (1972). The nutritive value of western vegan and vegetarian diets. *Plant foods in Hum. Nutr.*, **2**, 201–13.

National Academy of Sciences National Research Council Food and Nutrition Board. (1980). *Recommended Dietary Allowances*, 9th Ed. Washington DC.

Nnakwe and Kies C. (1985). Calcium and phosphorus utilization by omnivores and lacto-ovo-vegetarians fed laboratory controlled lacto-vegetarian diets. *Nut. Reps. Int.*, **31**, 1009–14.

O'Riordan, J.L.H. (1974). Bone. In *Clinical Physiology*, 4th Ed., pp. 383–415. Eds. Campbell, E.J.M., Dickinson, C.J. and Slater, J.D.H. Blackwell Scientific Publn: Oxford.

Paul, A.A. and Southgate, D.A.T. (1978). *McCance and Widdowson's The Composition of Foods*. 4th ed. HMSO: London.

Qureshi, B.A. (1986). Management of Ethnic Asian Patients in General Practice. *The Medical Annual*, pp. 155–65. John Wright: Bristol.

Roberts, I.F., West, R.J., Ogilvie, D. *et al.*, (1979). Malnutrition in infants receiving cult diets. A form of child abuse. *Br. Med. J.*, **1**, 296–8.

Rudman, D. and Williams, P.J. (1983). Megadose vitamins. *N.E.J.M.*, **309**, 488–90.

Sanders, T.A.B., (1983). Vegetarianism: dietetic and medical aspects. *J. of Plant Foods*, **5**, 3–14.

Sanders, T.A.B., Ellis, F.R. and Dickerson, J.W.T. (1977). Haematological studies on vegans. *Br. J. Nutr.*, **40**, 9–15.

Sanders, T.A.B., Ellis, F.R. and Dickerson, J.W.T. (1978). Studies of vegans: the fatty acid composition of plasma choline phosphoglycerides, erythrocytes, adipose tissue and breast milk and some indicators of susceptibility to ischaemic heart disease in vegans and omnivore controls. *Am. J. Clin. Nutr.*, **31**, 805–13.

Sanders, T.A.B. and Purves, R. (1981). An anthropometric and dietary assessment of the nutritional status of vegan pre-school children. *J. Hum. Nutr.*, **35**, 349–57.

Selhorst, J.B., Jennings, S., Corbett, J.J. (1984). Liver lovers headache: Pseudomotor cerebri and vitamin A intoxication. *JAMA*, **252**, 3365.

Springer, L. and Thomas, J. (1983). Rastafarians in Britain: a preliminary study of their food habits and beliefs. *Hum. Nutr.: Appl. Nutr.*, **37A**, 120–27.

van Staveren, W.A., Dhuyvetter, J.H.M., Bons, A., Zeelan, M. and Hautvast, J.G.A.

(1985). Food consumption and height/weight status of Dutch pre-school children on alternative diets. *J. Am. Diet. Assoc.*, **85**, 1579–84.
Swales, J.D. (1980). Dietary salt and hypertension. *Lancet*, **i**, 1177–9.
Tunstall-Pedoe, H., Clayton, D., Morris, J.N., Brigden, W. and McDonald, L. (1975). Coronary attacks in East London. *Lancet*, **ii**, 833–8.

# 20 Nutrition and alcohol

John Wright



## Introduction

The recreational use of alcohol[1] is a world-wide phenomenon which dates back to antiquity. In the United Kingdom alcohol consumption which, based on excise records, was at its highest during the 18th century, has been increasing steadily over recent years. About three quarters of a million people in England and Wales – around 2 per cent of the adult population – can be classified as alcoholics (Paton *et al.*, 1981) and in some regions, particularly North-East England and Scotland, the prevalence is much higher (Chick, 1982). Alcohol abuse is now a factor in up to one quarter of admissions to hospital in the United Kingdom (Jariwalla *et al.*, 1979; Jarman and Kellett, 1979) and the incidence of alcohol-related conditions, especially cirrhosis, is steadily increasing, particularly in women and younger people.

In man, alcohol in the body is derived almost exclusively from exogenous sources (Lester, 1961). Only trace amounts are formed by bacterial fermentation in the gut; much higher amounts are produced in herbivorous animals, particularly ruminants, in which alcohol generation is a significant means by which energy is derived from otherwise indigestible carbohydrate.

[1]Alcohol in this chapter refers exclusively to ethanol or ethyl alcohol. These terms are used interchangeably.

There is some confusion about the way in which the alcohol content of drinks is expressed because of the variety of units used. 'Pure' distilled alcohol contains 95 per cent ethanol and 5 per cent water; further purification steps are needed to produce absolute, 100 per cent ethanol. Ethanol has a density relative to water of approximately 0.8 and 1 gramme of alcohol, therefore, occupies a volume of either 1.25 ml (absolute alcohol) or 1.32 ml (pure, distilled alcohol). The alcohol content of a solution can be expressed either as 'g/100 ml' or 'per cent by volume' (% vol. or v/v); a solution containing 10 g/100 ml contains 12.5 per cent by volume.

The range of alcohol content in beverages is shown in Table 20.1.

The content of most drinks is expressed as '% by volume' but the situation is further confused by the use of 'proof' scales and the fact that the UK proof differs from US proof. For UK and Canadian proof, 100 per cent is defined as 57.15 per cent vol. (45.5 g/100 ml); 100 per cent US proof is equal to 50 per cent vol. (40 g/100 ml). In the UK, spirits are usually 70 per cent proof (40 per cent vol., 32 g/100 ml); one standard bottle of spirits in the UK (700 ml), therefore contains 224 g alcohol. In the USA most spirits are 90 per cent proof (45 per cent vol, 36 g/100 ml). A single standard measure of most drinks (half pint of beer or lager, one glass of wine, one single measure of spirits) all contain about the same amount of alcohol (approximately 8–10 g) as shown in Table 20.1. Alcoholic beverages also contain a vast number of other compounds (so-called 'congeners') including higher alcohols, aldehydes, ketones, acids and esters as well as aliphatic and aromatic compounds which appear as by-products of the fermentation process. Over 200 such substances have been

Table 20.1 Average alcohol, carbohydrate and energy content of selected alcoholic drinks

| | Alcohol content | | Contents of a typical measure or drink | | | |
|---|---|---|---|---|---|---|
| | g/100 ml | % vol. | Volume (ml) | Alcohol (g) | Sugar (g) | Energy (kcals) |
| *Beverage* | | | | | | |
| Beer, lager, cider | 2.2–4.00 | 2.8–5.00 | 280 | 6.2–11.2 | 4.2–11.8 | 60–120 |
| Strong beers* | 4.00–6.6 | 5.00–8.3 | 280 | 11–18.5 | 12–18.5 | 100–200 |
| Wines | 8–11 | 10–14 | 120 | 9.6–13.2 | 0.4–7 | 70–90 |
| Fortified wines** | 13–16 | 16.3–20 | 45–60 | 7.8–9.6 | 1–9.5 | 40–50 |
| Spirits | 32 | 40 | 24 | 7.7 | 0 | 55 |
| *Mixers* | | | | | | |
| Regular | 0 | 0 | 120 | 0 | 10 | 40 |
| Sugar free | 0 | 0 | 120 | 0 | 0 | 0 |

* e.g. 'Extra' stout, strong ales, barley wines
These beers may be served in smaller measures than ½ pint.
** Sherry, Vermouths, Port
Sources – Paul and Southgate (1981), Marks (1978), Wallgren and Barry, (1970)

identified in distilled spirits, for example, most in trace amounts only (Smuckler, 1979). The metabolic effects of most of these congeners are unknown although they may play a role in the symptoms of hangover.

By convention, the concentration of alcohol in body fluids is usually expressed in mass rather than molar terms. The molecular weight of alcohol is 46 and a concentration of 1 mmol/litre is therefore equivalent to 4.6 mg/dl.

The pharmacological effects of alcohol which form the basis for its social use are exerted predominantly on the central nervous system. Like other general anaesthetics, alcohol is a CNS depressant, its stimulatory effect probably being due to depression of inhibitory control mechanisms (Goodman and Gilman, 1985). The higher cerebral centres involved in functions such as judgement, discrimination, concentration, memory and insight are the earliest affected, resulting in the characteristic features of drunkenness. Ultimately, lower cerebral centres are affected with potentially fatal depression of the respiratory centre occurring when blood alcohol concentration rises above 400 mg/dl and possibly with levels as low as 200 mg/dl (Odesanmi, 1983).

In addition to its importance as a drug of abuse and a cause of organic disease, alcohol deserves consideration from a nutritional standpoint both as a nutrient in its own right and because of the effects of alcohol consumption on the intake, absorption and metabolism of the other dietary constituents.

## Metabolism of alcohol

Alcohol is readily absorbed from the upper small intestine and, to a lesser extent, the stomach. It is rapidly distributed throughout total body water and has been used to measure the volume of this compartment.

Less than 10 per cent of ingested alcohol is excreted unchanged in the urine, sweat or breath, the remainder being metabolized in the liver by one of three pathways. The most important of these, accounting for at least 80 per cent of alcohol metabolism, is catalyzed by the enzyme alcohol dehydrogenase (ADH):

$$C_2H_5OH + NAD^+ \rightarrow CH_3CHO + NADH + H^+$$

The generation of hydrogen ions and NADH in this reaction causes a shift in the redox state in the cytosol of the hepatocyte which has important consequences for a number of biochemical processes including fat and carbohydrate metabolism (Lieber and Davidson, 1962; Lieber, 1980).

The second pathway involves the microsomal ethanol oxidizing system (MEOS), a mixed function cytochrome P-450 oxygenase system which is also responsible for the metabolism of numerous drugs and xenobiotics (Lieber and De Carli, 1968). The MEOS catalyses the reaction:

$$C_2H_5OH + NADPH + H^+ + O_2 \rightarrow CH_3CHO + NADP^+ + 2H_2O$$

The precise contribution of this pathway to ethanol metabolism is unclear but since (a) it is an inducible system and (b) it has a much higher $K_m$ for ethanol than ADH (7–9 vs 0.5–1.0 mmol/litre), it may be important in chronic alcohol abuse or in the face of high ethanol concentrations.

The third pathway involves the enzyme catalase:

$$C_2H_5OH + H_2O_2 \rightarrow CH_3CHO + 2H_2O$$

This system makes only a minimal contribution to the metabolism of ethanol.

Almost all of the acetaldehyde generated in these reactions is metabolized to acetate within the liver by the enzyme aldehyde dehydrogenase (AlDH) with further generation of NADH and $H^+$. Such is the efficiency of this system that acetaldehyde does not normally enter the general circulation during alcohol metabolism (Eriksson, 1983) and it is, therefore, unlikely that acetaldehyde is responsible for any of the extrahepatic effects of alcohol. However, dysfunction of the AlDH enzyme complex can result in symptoms of systematic acetaldehyde toxicity consisting of flushing, nausea, vomiting and, when severe, prostration. Such a reaction occurs in a high proportion of Chinese and Japanese who lack the mitochondrial isoenzyme of AlDH (Goedde *et al.*, 1983), and during treatment with drugs such as disulfiram ('Antabuse'); an AlDH inhibitor used in the treatment of alcoholism, and in some diabetics taking sulphonylureas, particularly chlorpropamide (so-called 'chlorpropamide-alcohol flushing' or CPAF) (Leslie and Pyke, 1978).

The acetate produced from ethanol metabolism is either converted to acetyl CoA which enters the TCA cycle (which provides most of the ATP from ethanol oxidation), or acts as a precursor for the synthesis of fatty acids and triglycerides.

The rate of alcohol metabolism is probably determined by the activity of the enzyme alcohol dehydrogenase rather than the rate of reoxidation of NADH although fructose, by regenerating $NAD^+$, can produce a small increase in the rate of alcohol metabolism (see Marks, 1978). The rate of metabolism is most commonly expressed in terms of its disappearance from blood; normal values are in the range 15–20 mg/dl/hr but values more than twice this may be seen in chronic alcoholics (Winek and Murphy, 1984). There is considerable debate as to whether this is due to an increase in activity of ADH or MEOS (see Crow, 1985).

## Alcohol as food

Alcohol consumption in the United Kingdom per head of the adult population averages approximately 20 g per day (Levi and Chalmers, 1978). Based on an energy value for alcohol of 7.1 kcal/g, this represents about 7 per cent of mean dietary energy intake for the whole population while in some individuals the calculated contribution of alcohol is clearly much greater than this. (A standard 0.7 litre bottle of spirits, containing 224 g of alcohol, is theoretically equivalent to 1590 kcals.) However, it is clear that man does not act as a simple bomb calorimeter and, in terms of its effect on body weight at least, the actual contribution of alcohol to energy intake is less than the theoretical value. The addition of between 650 and 1800 kcal as alcohol to an otherwise adequate diet has been shown to produce either no weight gain (Mezey and Faillace, 1971) or even a slight weight loss (McDonald and Margen, 1976). In another study, the addition of as much as 2000 kcal as alcohol resulted in a weight gain of only 6 g/day compared with 198 g/day when the same number of calories were given as chocolate (Pirola and Lieber, 1976). This study also showed that alcohol cannot be considered equivalent to carbohydrate since isocaloric substitution of alcohol for carbohydrate accounting for 50 per cent of total energy intake resulted in significant weight loss. These experimental data support clinical observations in alcoholics who frequently lose weight despite a high ethanol-calorie intake (Morgan, 1982).

The reasons for these findings are unclear. Thyroid function is not affected by alcohol and although catecholamine secretion may be stimulated by both high dose and prolonged drinking, no consistent effect of alcohol on metabolic rate has been described. Similarly, the thermic effect of alcohol feeding has not been found to be higher than the effect of isocaloric carbohydrate, although alcohol metabolism is associated with increased hepatic oxygen uptake along with depressed activity of the Krebs cycle (Videla *et al.*, 1973). A number of factors may be involved including an increase in the production of lactate rather than pyruvate due to alteration in cytosolic redox state when alcohol is metabolized by ADH or, when metabolism by MEOS predominates, the wasteful production of NAPDH which cannot be coupled to oxidative phosphorylation (Pirola and Lieber, 1976). Whatever the cause, it has even been suggested that alcohol-derived calories should be disregarded completely when predicting dietary-induced changes in body weight (World *et al.*, 1984); this is particularly true in the presence of high alcohol consumption when MEOS probably play a more important role.

There is also good evidence that alcohol impairs the absorption of a number of nutrients from the gut and interferes with a number of metabolic processes, although none which obviously results in energy wastage. These aspects are considered below.

Ethanol has been used in the past as a constituent of intravenous feeding solutions. In view of the ready availability of either glucose or lipid emulsion as an energy source, there is no longer any justification for using ethanol in this way; its use is associated with a number of potential dangers (particularly lactic acidosis and hypoglycaemia), and no advantages other than inducing mild intoxication.

## Malnutrition in alcoholics

Malnutrition is a frequent but not invariable concomitant of alcohol abuse (Halsted, 1980; Morgan, 1982). However, a distinction must be made between the under-nourished, skid-row, down-and-out alcoholic on the one hand and the adequately nourished (frequently over-nourished), affluent alcoholic on the other. The differences between the two are obviously due more to social and economic facts than metabolic effects. Many of the most widely quoted reports, particularly those from the USA, are based upon studies in poorer, socially deprived subjects (Leevy *et al.*, 1965; Patek *et al.*, 1975). However, in these groups other factors are clearly important. In one study of unselected patients in a large city hospital, for example, the nutritional status of alcoholic patients was no worse than that of non-alcoholic patients admitted to hospital for other medical reasons. In the United Kingdom, it is estimated that down-and-out alcoholics represent less than 10 per cent of the total and, while the nutritional problems of this minority may have been well described, the situation in the larger group of more affluent alcoholics has been less well documented.

A number of factors may predispose to malnutrition in alcoholics:

1. *Inadequate nutrient intake due to*:
   Preference for alcohol
   Anorexia
   Vomiting
2. *Impaired digestion and absorption of nutrients due to*:
   Changes in gastrointestinal motility
   Alcohol-induced malabsorption
   Pancreatic and biliary insufficiency

## Inadequate nutrient intake

Dietary deficiencies may be determined in some groups by economic factors with the choice of alcohol in preference to food decided by limited financial resources. In view of the very poor nutritional value of nearly all alcoholic beverages this will inevitably lead to a reduced intake of other essential nutrients. In chronic alcoholics, food intake may be further reduced by the anorexia and vomiting which accompany the development of gastritis.

Increasingly, however, studies from more affluent communities report excessive alcohol consumption in addition to an otherwise adequate diet (for example Neville *et al.*, 1968; Hurt *et al.*, 1981). Care is needed in the interpretation of such studies if, when assessing total energy intake, those calories derived from alcohol are included; as mentioned above, alcohol calories may be 'wasted' and calculations based upon a contribution of 7.1 kcal/g alcohol are probably invalid. In addition, although the absolute intake of nutrients other than alcohol may appear adequate, the proportion of calories supplied by protein, fat and carbohydrate will clearly be lower if the energy from alcohol is included (Morgan, 1982).

Clinical estimates of nutritional status of individual alcoholics frequently correlate poorly with nutrient intake and it is clear that a number of other factors are involved, particularly the effects of alcohol on gastrointestinal function.

## Impaired digestion and absorption

Of all tissues, the gut and the liver are exposed to the highest concentrations of alcohol and bear the brunt of tissue damage. Gastrointestinal symptoms (anorexia, nausea, abdominal discomfort or pain, diarrhoea) are common and are the presenting feature in over one-third of alcoholics admitted to hospital. Structural lesions in the gastrointestinal tract which may be caused by alcohol include oesophagitis and oesophageal cancer, acute and chronic gastritis, and acute haemorrhagic duodenitis and jejunitis; the incidence of peptic ulceration is probably not increased in alcoholics. In addition to structural injury, alcohol has a number of important effects on gastrointestinal function.

### Altered gastric emptying and gastrointestinal motility

Alcohol has long been used socially to accelerate gastric emptying – a glass of Schnapps or Calvados between courses, for example. Although moderate doses may produce this effect, high concentrations within the stomach (above

10 g/dl) may delay gastric emptying due to either a direct irritant or hyperosmolar effect.

Alcohol also causes an increase in small intestinal motility. This may be due to a direct, irritant effect; following an oral dose as low as 1 g/kg body weight, the concentration within the jejunum will be around 5 g/100 ml which has been shown to produce haemorrhagic lesions in the mucosa (Gottfried *et al.*, 1976). However, since an increase in motility may also occur following intravenous ethanol, central mechanisms may also be involved. The resulting changes in motility may contribute to both the diarrhoea and the malabsorption which are associated with alcohol abuse.

**Small intestinal malabsorption**

Steatorrhoea along with malabsorption of xylose, vitamin $B_{12}$, folate and thiamine has been well documented in up to 50 per cent of recently drinking alcoholics, and in volunteer subjects fed alcohol for several weeks malabsorption of $B_{12}$ but not xylose, fat and folate develops (Lindenbaum and Lieber, 1975). The effects of alcohol are more marked on those nutrients for which there is an active intestinal transport mechanism, probably due to direct epithelial damage with consequent loss of membrane-bound enzymes such as disaccharidases and Na-K ATPase (Wilson and Hoyumpa, 1978; Halsted, 1980), while the absorption of substances which cross the intestinal mucosa by passive diffusion is relatively unaffected. Iron absorption, also, is unaffected and may in fact be enhanced by alcohol. Certainly, liver iron stores are frequently raised in chronic alcoholics, occasionally making it difficult to distinguish between alcohol abuse and iron overload (haemochromatosis) as a cause of cirrhosis.

Malnutrition *per se* and folate deficiency in particular can cause or exacerbate malabsorption, and maintenance of adequate nutrient intake in addition to alcohol appears to protect against its development; with a poor intake, there is the risk of a vicious cycle of increasingly severe malabsorption and malnutrition (Halsted, 1980).

Although steatorrhoea is common in alcoholics, the precise effect of alcohol on fat absorption is complex. In moderate doses, alcohol enhances the lipaemic response to fat ingestion (alimentary hyperlipaemia) due in part to an increase in the rate of fatty acid incorporation into triglycerides during re-esterification in the small intestinal mucosa. More prolonged exposure to high doses, however, appears to reduce intestinal triglyceride synthesis which may contribute to the steatorrhoea in alcoholics (Lieber and Savolainen, 1984).

**Pancreatic and biliary insufficiency**

The development of either cirrhosis or pancreatitis, both of which are common complications of chronic alcoholism will, by reducing the production of either bile salts or pancreatic exocrine secretion, further reduce fat absorption and exacerbate steatorrhoea.

## Interaction with other nutrients

### Carbohydrates

Alcohol has a number of major effects on carbohydrate metabolism which have been reviewed recently (Wright and Marks, 1984). Alcohol is an important cause of hypoglycaemia (see Marks and Rose, 1984) which can be reliably induced by intravenous or oral ethanol in normal subjects who have fasted for at least 36 hours; maintenance of blood glucose concentration in this situation, when liver glycogen stores are exhausted, depends upon gluconeogenesis which is inhibited by alcohol, probably as a result of the change in intracellular redox status (Krebs, 1968). Similarly, the action of insulin is enhanced by alcohol and this may precipitate severe and occasionally fatal hypoglycaemia in insulin-treated diabetics (Arky *et al.*, 1968).

Although ethanol does not stimulate insulin secretion directly, the insulin response to carbohydrate feeding is enhanced in the presence of alcohol and in susceptible individuals this may result in reproducible hypoglycaemia developing about 3 hours after a meal (O'Keefe and Marks, 1977); since the neurological effects of alcohol and hypoglycaemia are additive, this may result in marked impairment of cerebral function at such times. In about one quarter of chronic alcoholics, the counter-regulatory hormone (cortisol, growth hormone and catecholamine) response to induced hypoglycaemia is blunted which increases the susceptibility to hypoglycaemia and delays recovery (Wright, 1978).

Paradoxically, alcohol may occasionally cause acute hyperglycaemia probably due to a combination of stress and liver damage, which may be subclinical. Occasionally, alcohol abuse may precipitate frank diabetes (Philips and Safrit, 1971) which improves when alcohol is withdrawn but does not always resolve completely, suggesting an underlying diabetic tendency in such subjects. However, in the treatment of diabetes, there is ordinarily no reason to exclude alcohol completely from the diet. The fact that alcohol can enhance the insulin response to carbohydrate feeding suggests that it might even have a role in the treatment of non insulin-dependent diabetes although this has yet to be demonstrated.

### Lipids

An abnormality of lipid metabolism is perhaps the commonest metabolic derangement seen in association with alcohol abuse, with triglyceride levels being particularly affected as alcohol influences both the exogenous and endogenous pathways of triglyceride metabolism (see Janus and Lewis, 1978; Lieber and Savolainen, 1984). The degree of alimentary lipaemia is enhanced by alcohol, partly due to increased VLDL production in the small intestine. The lipaemia is further increased by the metabolism of alcohol in the liver in preference to fat particularly (Cramp, 1984). In addition, there is an increase in hepatic triglyceride synthesis because of the increased cytosolic NADH:NAD ratio, and an increase in the rate of VLDL release from the liver. Together, these factors can result in an increase in both intra hepatic and circulating triglyceride levels. Occasionally extremely high plasma triglyceride levels are found which may not return completely to normal during abstinence indicating a concomitant genetic predisposition.

The effect of alcohol on cardiovascular mortality is the subject of a continuing debate. In recent years a number of reports have indicated that moderate alcohol intake exerts a protective effect on the development of ischaemic heart disease, with cardiovascular mortality higher in teetotallers than in moderate drinkers consuming around 20–40 g alcohol per day (Barboriak *et al.*, 1977; Blackwelder *et al.*, 1980; Klatsky *et al.*, 1981). At higher doses, mortality increases due to factors other than atherosclerosis. One possible explanation for these observations is provided by the fact that HDL cholesterol levels are increased by alcohol although possibly not the more protective, HDL2 fraction (Haskell *et al.*, 1984; see also Barboriak, 1974). These data are inconclusive and certainly insufficient to recommend alcohol as a cardioprotective agent, not least because of the narrow margin between safe and potentially dangerous drinking.

## Protein and amino acids

The effects of alcohol on protein and amino acid metabolism are less well documented. Amino acid transport systems are inhibited by ethanol and the consequent impairment of amino acid absorption from the small intestine may contribute to the malnutrition of alcoholism (Israel *et al.*, 1969). However, the abnormalities in plasma amino acid seen in alcoholics with raised levels of glutamic acid and reduced levels of methionine and branched chain amino acids (Siegel *et al.*, 1964) and the changes following alcohol loading suggest that other factors are also involved. Studies of the effect of alcohol on hepatic protein synthesis have produced conflicting results with some suggesting an acute inhibitory effect which improves with chronic alcohol administration (e.g. Lieber, 1980) and other suggesting just the reverse (e.g. Morland *et al.*, 1983).

In chronic alcoholics, a low plasma albumin concentration is a common finding. In most cases this will be the result of liver damage rather than undernutrition and care must therefore be taken in assessing nutritional status in the alcoholic if the level of serum albumin is a major factor in any calculation. The clinical consequences of hypo-albuminaemia include peripheral oedema, ascites, hypovolaemia and secondary hyperaldosteronism. In addition, the levels of other proteins synthesized in the liver, particularly vitamin K dependent clotting factors, may be reduced.

## Vitamins and minerals

With the exception of beer which contains nicotinic acid at a concentration of 3–5 mg/litre (Paul and Southgate, 1978), the vitamin content of alcohol beverages is uniformly low. Vitamin deficiencies may therefore develop in alcoholics because of inadequate dietary intake, impaired absorption or altered metabolism of vitamins, reduced hepatic storage, or an increased physiological requirement (Ryle and Thomson, 1984).

A number of studies, particularly those carried out in large American city hospitals, have demonstrated a high incidence of vitamin deficiencies in chronic alcoholics, with low levels of folate, vitamin $B_6$ and thiamine in over half the subjects studied, and of nicotinic acid, vitamin $B_{12}$, vitamin C and pantothenic acid in a further quarter. In a high proportion of these patients, reduced dietary intake was almost certainly a major factor.

Malabsorption of vitamins may occur either as a result of impairment of carrier-mediated transport (e.g. $B_{12}$, folate, thiamine), gastro-intestinal damage, or pancreatico-biliary insufficiency which reduces the absorption of fat-soluble vitamins.

The development of alcoholic liver damage may accelerate the development of vitamin-deficiency syndromes. The liver is the major site of activation of many vitamins (e.g. thiamine, pyridoxine and folic acid), of storage (e.g. vitamins A, $B_{12}$) and of synthesis of vitamin-K dependent clotting factors. The failure of these processes may account for the increased requirements of many vitamins in alcoholics (Ryle and Thomson, 1984).

Of the vitamin-deficiency syndromes which occur in alcoholics, the most important is the Wernicke–Korsakoff syndrome which combines the features of Wernicke's encephalopathy (mental confusion, ataxia and opthalmoplegia) and Korsakoff's psychosis with loss of short-term memory. This condition is associated with chronic thiamine deficiency but although the encephalopathy responds well to high-dose thiamine treatment, the psychotic element responds poorly and 50 per cent of patients show no improvement. The precise role of vitamin deficiencies in the pathogenesis of the delirium tremens (DTs) of alcohol withdrawal is unknown. Multiple vitamin deficiencies may be demonstrable and high-dose multivitamin therapy is used in treatment but a firm causative link has not been established.

The effects of alcohol on mineral metabolism are rather confused but obviously variable with no regular pattern (see McIntyre, 1984). Low levels of both zinc and calcium have been observed in alcoholics but have not been related to any specific clinical effect. A more definite and consistent effect of alcohol on magnesium has been described. Hypomagnesaemia is common in alcoholics, mainly due to an increase in urinary magnesium excretion, vomiting and diarrhoea. It has been suggested that low magnesium levels may cause the fits and tremulousness associated with alcohol withdrawal. However, the correlation between magnesium levels and individual clinical symptoms is poor (Heaton *et al.*, 1962), and treatment with magnesium fails to affect the course of delirium tremens (Brooks and Adams, 1975).

## Alcohol, nutrition and liver disease

Liver disease is the major complication and cause of death in alcoholics (Scheuer, 1982; Sherlock, 1982; Lieber, 1984). Four distinct but interrelated patterns of liver disease can be identified histopathologically:

### Acute fatty liver (steatosis)

Acute fatty liver is characterized by the presence of triglyceride-filled vacuoles in hepatocytes throughout the liver and can be induced in normal subjects given moderate doses of alcohol (equivalent to 68–130 g per day) for only one or two weeks (Rubin and Lieber, 1968). This is a non-progressive lesion which resolves completely within a few weeks of stopping drinking.

## Alcoholic hepatitis

Alcoholic hepatitis follows heavier and more prolonged alcohol abuse. It is often accompanied by an acute febrile illness with jaundice and abdominal pain. Microscopically, the liver shows hepato-cellular necrosis with infiltration by polymorphonuclear leucocytes. Complete resolution which may take several weeks or even months occurs in most cases if drinking is stopped but a proportion of patients go on to develop cirrhosis.

## Cirrhosis

Cirrhosis represents end-stage irreversible hepatic disease with general loss of liver architecture, fibrosis and nodular regeneration. It may not be preceded by clinical evidence of fatty liver or hepatitis. The complications of cirrhosis, which may prove fatal, include heptato-cellular failure with hepatic coma (encephalopathy), portal hypertension resulting in ascites and, occasionally, massive haemorrhage from oesophageal varices, hypoalbuminaemia with oedema, and a bleeding tendency due to deficiency of clotting factors.

## Hepatocellular carcinoma (hepatoma)

Hepatocellular carcinoma develops in up to 30 per cent of patients with cirrhosis and is associated with rapidly declining health and deterioration of liver function.

Until fairly recently, nutritional deficiencies rather than alcohol itself were thought to be responsible for the development of liver damage. Deficiencies of methionine and particularly choline can produce fatty liver in rodents in the absence of alcohol (Best *et al.*, 1949) but in man and primates neither an adequate diet nor choline supplementation can prevent the development of fatty liver or cirrhosis in response to alcohol feeding (Rubin and Lieber, 1968 and 1974). Nevertheless, the recent finding that reduced hepatic vitamin A levels may predispose to the development of liver disease suggests that nutritional factors may, after all, play a role (Leo *et al.*, 1983). The major factor, however, is clearly alcohol itself and, more specifically, the metabolism of alcohol in the liver. This causes:

1. An alteration in the intracellular redox state (increased NADH:NAD ratio) which results in increased synthesis and reduced oxidation of triglyceride.
2. Increased oxygen consumption which results in centrilobular hypoxia and necrosis.
3. Production of acetaldehyde, a highly reactive compound which may bind with phospholipids and proteins (Lieber, 1980).

In addition, genetic factors may influence susceptibility to alcohol although some studies have failed to confirm this (see Eddleston and Davis, 1982).

Hepatic cirrhosis develops only after prolonged and heavy alcohol abuse and most cirrhotics will have consumed over 150 g daily. (However, one study has shown that as little as 40 g daily in men and only 20 g daily in women for just five years is associated with a significantly increased risk of cirrhosis (Pequignot, 1974).

## Nutritional anaemia in alcoholism

Alcohol abuse may give rise to a variety of haematological abnormalities which may or may not be associated with anaemia.

1. Macrocytosis of alcoholism
2. Megaloblastic anaemia
3. Iron deficiency anaemia
4. Sideroblastic aneamia

Macrocytosis is seen in up to 90 per cent of alcoholics consuming more than 80 g alcohol per day (Wu *et al.*, 1974). In the majority of cases the macrocytosis is moderate (MCV usually between 100 and 110 fl), haemoglobin is normal and there are no other features of megaloblastic anaemia in either the peripheral blood or bone marrow. The macrocytosis is not associated with either vitamin $B_{12}$ or folate deficiency and is unresponsive to treatment with either. The cause of the macrocytosis of alcoholism is unclear; alcohol appears to exert a direct action on the developing red cell, possibly producing changes in the phospholipid and cholesterol content of the membrane.

True megaloblastic anaemia due to nutritional folate deficiency also occurs in alcoholism but much less commonly than simple macrocytosis. Other characteristic features of megaloblastic anaemia are also present including a raised mean cell haemoglobin concentration (MCHC), anaemia, multi-segmented neutrophils and megaloblastic changes in the bone marrow; serum or red-cell folate concentration is usually low. The folate deficiency may be due either to inadequate intake or malabsorption (which, itself, may be exacerbated by folate deficiency).

Severe megaloblastic anaemia in alcoholics is occasionally associated with sideroblastic features. Such patients are usually ill, poorly nourished and may have an associated deficiency of pyridoxine. Iron-deficiency anaemia is an uncommon feature of alcohol abuse; indeed, alcohol enhances absorption of iron from the small intestine and alcoholic cirrhosis is sometimes associated with features of iron overload (haemochromatosis). The presence of iron deficiency suggests the possibility of gastrointestinal bleeding.

## Fetal alcohol syndrome

Alcohol abuse during pregnancy can result in fetal and neonatal death as well as congenital abnormalities. The fetal alcohol syndrome (Jones and Smith, 1973) is a characteristic pattern of abnormalities which include prenatal and postnatal growth deficiency, developmental delay, microcephaly, short palpebral fissures, maxillary hypoplasia, joint anomalies, abnormal palmar creases and cardiac abnormalities. Long-term follow-up of affected children reveals persistent growth deficiency and intellectual handicap, the severity of which is related to the extent of the craniofacial abnormalities (Streissguth *et al.*, 1985). The syndrome is clearly related to excessive maternal alcohol consumption, particularly in early pregnancy, but the precise way in which alcohol causes the damage is not known. It is most probably due to a direct teratogenic effect of alcohol, the severity of the syndrome being related to the level of alcohol consumption. The contribution of other factors such as disturbance in amino acid supply to the fetus, and maternal malnutrition and smoking is unknown but the susceptibility of the developing fetus, especially in the first weeks of pregnancy, highlights the importance of preconception counselling. Alcohol should be avoided completely during the first trimester and this should be instituted prior to conception whenever possible. For the remainder of the pregnancy, alcohol consumption should be kept to a minimum and should not exceed two drinks (15 g ethanol) per day at any time. In women with a history of alcohol abuse, vitamin supplementation should be given at the same time.

## Detection of alcohol abuse

Despite the fact that many, if not all, alcoholics will attempt to conceal or minimize the extent of their drinking, a carefully taken history, with or without the use of a specially designed questionnaire, remains the surest way of detecting alcohol abuse. Of the laboratory methods available for confirming the diagnosis, measurement of alcohol itself should not be overlooked. The detection of significant amounts in either blood or urine outside normal social drinking hours, particularly in individuals who deny drinking, or the finding of high levels without signs of inebriation are highly suspicious. The standard reference technique for the measurement of alcohol, and the standard method for medico-legal purposes, is by gas liquid chromatography, but spectrophotometric methods using alcohol dehydrogenase, although less specific, are adequate for clinical use (Denney, 1984).

A variety of biochemical and haematological parameters may be affected by alcohol abuse. Of these, the most useful are measurements of mean red cell volume (MCV) and the enzyme gamma glutamyl transferase (gamma-GT). The sensitivity of either alone is between about 50 per cent (for MCV) and 75 per cent (for gamma-GT). Using both tests, at least one abnormal parameter will be found in up to 85 per cent of alcoholics (Rosalki, 1984). Other tests which have been used include the enzyme glutamate dehydrogenase (which is less sensitive in chronic alcoholics than a gamma-GT but may be more useful in binge drinkers), and measurement of plasma urate and triglycerides which are non-specifically elevated in a proportion of heavy drinkers.

## References


Arky, RA, Veverbrants, E and Abramson, EA (1968). Irreversible hypoglycaemia: a complication of alcohol and insulin. *JAMA*, **206**, 575–8.

Barboriak, J.J. (1984). Alcohol, lipids and heart disease. *Alcohol*, **1**, 341–5.

Barboriak, J.J., Rimm, A.A., Anderson, A.J., Schmidhoffer, M. and Tristani, F.E. (1977). Coronary artery occlusion and alcohol intake. *Br. Heart J.*, **39**, 289–93.

Best, C.H., Hartroft, W.S., Lucas, C.C. and Ridout, J.H. (1949). Liver damage produced by feeding alcohol or sugar and its prevention by choline. *Br. Med. J.*, **2**, 1001.

Blackwelder, W.C., Yano, K., Rhoads, G.G., Kagan, A., Gordon, T. and Palesch, Y. (1980). Alcohol and mortality: the Honolulu heart study. *Am. J. Med.*, **68**, 164–9.

Brooks, B.R. and Adams, R.D. (1975). Cerebral spinal fluid acid-base and lactate changes after seizures in unanesthetized man II. Alcohol withdrawal seizures. *Neurology (Minneap)*, **25**, 935–42.

Chanarin, I. (1982). Haemopoiesis and alcohol *Br. Med. Bull.*, **38**, 81–6.

Chick, J. (1982). Epidemiology of alcohol use and its hazards. *Br. Med. Bull.*, **38**, 3–8.

Cramp, D.G. (1984). Lipid abnormalities in alcoholism. In *Clinical Biochemistry of Alcoholism*, Ed. Rosalki. Churchill Livingstone: Edinburgh.

Crow, K.E. (1985). Ethanol metabolism by the liver. *Reviews on Drug Metabolism and Drug Interactions*, **5**, 113–58.

Denney, R.C. (1984). Measuring alcohol. In *Clinical Biochemistry of Alcoholism*, Ed. Rosalki. Churchill Livingstone: Edinburgh.

Eddleston, A.L.W.F. and Davis, M. (1982). Histocompatibility antigens in alcoholic liver disease. *Br. Med. Bull.*, **38**, 13–16.

Eriksson, C.J.P. (1983). Human blood acetaldehyde concentration during ethanol oxidation (Update 1982). *Pharmacol. Biochem. Behav.*, **18** (Suppl.) **1**, 141–50.

Goedde, H.W., Agarwal, D.P. and Harada, S. (1983). Pharmacogenetics of alcohol sensitivity. *Pharmacol. Biochem. Behav.*, **18**, (Suppl). **1**, 161–6.

Goodman, L.S. and Gilman, A. (1985) *The Pharmacological Basis of Therapeutics*. Macmillan: New York.

Gottfried, E.B., Korsten, M.A. and Lieber, C.S. (1976). Gastritis and duodenitis induced by alcohol: an endoscopic and histologic assessment. *Gastroenterology*, **70**, 890.

Halsted, (1980). Alcoholism and malnutrition. *Am. J. Clin. Nutr.*, **33**, 2705–8.

Halsted, (1980). Folate deficiency in alcoholism *Am. J. Clin. Nutr.*, **33**, 2736–40.

Haskell, W.L., Camargo, C., Williams, P.T., Vranizan, K.M., Krauss, R.M., Lindgren, F.T. and Wood, P.D. (1984). The effect of cessation and resumption of moderate alcohol intake on serum high density lipoprotein subfractions *N. Eng. J. Med.*, **310**, 805–10.

Heaton, F.W. Pyrah, L.N., Beresford, C.C., Bryson, R.W. and Martin, D.F. (1962). Hypomagnesaemia in chronic alcoholism. *Lancet*, **2**, 802–805.

Hurt, R.D., Higgins, J.A., Nelson, R.A., Morse, R.M. and Dickson, E.R. (1981) Nutritional status of a group of alcoholics before and after admission to an alcoholism treatment unit. *Am. J. Clin. Nutr.*, **34**, 386–92.

Israel, Y., Valenzuela, J.E., Salazar, I. and Ugaste, G. (1969). Alcohol and amino acid transport in the human small intestine. *J. Nutr.*, **98**, 222–4.

Janus, E.D. and Lewis, B. (1978). Alcohol and abnormalities of lipid metabolism. *Clin. Endocrinol. Metabol.*, **7**, 32–332.

Jariwalla, A.G., Adams, P.H. and Hore, B.D. (1979). Alcohol and acute general admissions. *Health Trends*, **11**, 95–7.

Jarman, C.M.B. and Kellett, J.M. (1979). Alcoholism in the general hospital. *Br. Med. J.*, **2**, 469–72.

Jones, K.L. and Smith, D.W. (1973). Recognition of the fetal alcohol syndrome in early infancy. *Lancet*, **2**, 999–1001.

Klatsky, A.L., Friedman, G.D. and Siegelaub, A.B. (1981). Alcohol and mortality; a ten-year Kaiser-Permanente experience. *Ann. Int. Med.*, **95**, 139–45.

Krebbs, H.A. (1968). The effects of alcohol on the metabolic activities of the liver. *Adv. in Enz. Reg.*, **6**, 467–80.

Leo, M.A., Sato, M. and Lieber, C.S. (1983). Effect of hepatic vitamin A depletion on the liver in humans and rats. *Gastroenterology*, **84**, 562–72.

Leslie, R.D.G. and Pyke, D.A. (1978). Chlorpropamide-alcohol flushing: a dominantly inherited trait associated with diabetes. *Br. Med. J.*, **2**, 1519–21.

Lester, D. (1961). Endogenous alcohol: a review. *Q. J. Stud. Alc.*, **22**, 554–74.

Levi, A.J. and Chalmers, D.M. (1978). Recognition of alcoholic liver disease in a district general hospital. *Gut*, **19**, 521–5.

Leevy, C.M., Baker, H., Hove, W., Frank, O. and Cherrick, G.R. (1965). B-complex vitamins in liver disease of the alcoholic. *Am. J. Clin. Nutr.*, **16**, 339–46.

Lieber, C.S. and Savolainen, M. (1984). Ethanol and lipids. *Alcoholism Clin. Exp. Res.*, **8**, 409–23.
Lieber, C.S. and Davidson, C.S. (1962). Some metabolic effects of ethyl alcohol. *Am. J. Med.*, **33**, 319–27.
Lieber, C.S. (1980). Alcohol, protein metabolism and liver injury. *Gastroenterology*, **79**, 373–90.
Lieber, C.S. and De Carli, L.M. (1968). Ethanol oxidation by hepatic microsomes. *Science*, **162**, 917.
Lieber, C.S. (1984). Alcohol and the liver: 1984 update. *Hepatology*, **4**, 1243–60.
Lindenbaum, J. and Lieber, C.S. (1975). Effect of chronic ethanol administration on intestinal absorption in man in the absence of nutritional deficiency. *Ann. N.Y. Acad. Sci.*, **252**, 228–34.
Lindenbaum, J. and Roman, M.J. (1980). Nutritional anaemia in alcoholism. *Am. J. Clin. Nutr.*, **33**, 2727–35.
Marks, V. (1978). Alcohol and carbohydrate metabolism. *Clin. Endocrinol. Metabol.*, **7**, 333–50.
Marks, V. (1981). Alcohol and the diabetic. *Balance* (December).
Marks, V. and Rose, F.C. (1984). *Hypoglycaemia*, 2nd ed. Blackwell Scientific Publications: Oxford and London.
McIntyre, N. (1984). The effects of alcohol on water, electrolytes and minerals. In *Clinical Biochemistry of Alcoholism*. Ed. Rosalki. Churchill Livingstone: Edinburgh.
McDonald, J.T. and Margen, S. (1976). Wine versus ethanol in human nutrition 1. Nitrogen and calorie balance. *Am. J. Clin. Nutr.*, **29**, 1093–103.
Mezey, E. and Faillace, L.A. (1971). Metabolic impairment and recovery time in acute ethanol intoxication. *J. Nerv. Ment. Dis.*, **153**, 445–52.
Morgan, M.Y. (1982). Alcohol and Nutrition. *Br. Med. Bull.*, **38**, 21–9.
Morland, J., Bessesen, A., Smith-Kielland, A., and Wallin, B. (1983). Ethanol and protein metabolism in the liver. *Pharmacol. Biochem. Behav.*, **18**, (Suppl.) **1**, 251–6.
Neville, J.N., Eagles, J.A., Samson, G. and Olson, R.E. (1968). Nutritional status of alcoholics. *Am. J. Clin. Nut.*, **21**, 1329–40.
Odesanmi, W.O. (1983). The fatal blood alcohol level in acute alcohol poisoning. *Med. Sci. Law.*, **23**, 25–30.
O'Keefe, S.J.D. and Marks, V. (1977). Lunchtime gin and tonic: a cause of reactive hypoglycaemia. *Lancet*, **1**, 1286–8.
Patek, A.J., Toth, I.G., Saunders, M.G., Castro, G.A.M. and Engel, J.J. (1975). Alcohol and dietary factors in cirrhosis. *Arch. Internal Med.*, **135**, 1053–7.
Paton, A., Potter, J.F. and Saunders, J.B. (1981). ABC of Alcohol: Nature of the problem. *Br. Med. J.*, **283**, 1318–19.
Paul, A.A. and Southgate, D.A.T. (1978). In *The Composition of Foods*. Eds. McCance and Widdowson. HMSO: London.
Pequignot, G. (1974). Augmentation du risque du cirrhose en fonction de la ration d'alcool. *Revue de l'acoolisme*, **20**, 191–202.
Philips, G.B. and Safrit, M.F. (1971). Alcoholic diabetes: induction of glucose intolerance with alcohol. *J.A.M.A.*, **217**, 1513–19.
Pirola, R.C. and Lieber, C.S. (1976). Hypothesis: energy wastage in alcoholism and drug abuse: possible role of hepatic microsomal enzymes. *Am. J. Clin. Nutr.*, **29**, 90–93.
Pratt, O.E. (1982). Alcohol and the developing fetus *Br. Med. Bull.*, **38**, 43–52.
Rosalki, S.B. (1984). In *Clinical Biochemistry of Alcoholism*, Ed. Rosalki. Churchill Livingstone: Edinburgh.
Rubin, E. and Lieber, C.S. (1968). Alcohol-induced hepatic injury in non alcoholic volunteers. *N. Engl. J. Med.*, **278**, 869–76.
Rubin, E. and Lieber, C.S. (1974). Fatty liver, alcoholic hepatitis and cirrhosis

produced by alcohol in primates. *N. Engl. J. Med.*, **290**, 128–35.
Ryle, P.R. and Thomson, A.D. Nutrition and vitamins in alcoholism. In *Clinical Biochemistry of Alcoholism*, Ed. Rosalki. Churchill Livingstone: Edinburgh.
Sherlock, S. (1982). Alcohol-related liver disease. *Br. Med. Bull.*, **38**, 67–70.
Siegel, F.L., Roach, M.K. and Pomeroy, L.R. (1964). Plasma amino acid patterns in alcoholism: the effects of ethanol loading. *Proc. Natl. Acad. Sci.*, **51**, 605–11.
Scheuer, P.J. (1982). Morphology of alcoholic liver disease. *Br. Med. Bull.*, **38**, 63–8.
Smuckler, E.A. (1979). The composition of alcoholic beverages, the absorption, distribution and excretion of their components. In *Metabolic Effects of Alcohol*, pp. 27–38. Eds. Avogaro, Sirtori and Tremoli. Elsevier: Holland.
Streissguth, A.P., Clarren, S.K. and Jones, K.L. (1985). Natural history of the fetal alcohol syndrome: a ten-year follow-up of eleven patients. *Lancet*, i, 85–91.
Videla, L., Bernstein, J. and Israel, Y. (1973). Metabolic alteration produced in the liver by chronic ethanol administration: Increased oxidative capacity *Biochem. J.*, **134**, 507–14.
Wallgren, H. and Barry, H. (1970). *Action of Alcohol*. Elsevier: Amsterdam.
Wilson, F.A. and Hoyumpa, A.M. (1978). Ethanol and small intestinal transport. *Gastroenterology*, **76**, 388–403.
Winek, C.L. and Murphy, K.L. (1984). The rate and kinetic order of alcohol elimination. *Forensic Sci. Int.*, **25**, 159–66.
World, M.J., Ryle, P.R., Pratt, O.E. and Thomson, A.D. (1984). Editorial: Alcohol and body weight. *Alcohol and Alcoholism*, **19**, 1–6.
Wright, J. (1978). Endocrine effect of alcohol. *Clin. Endocrinol. Metabol.*, **7**, 351–68.
Wright, J. and Marks, V. (1984). The effects of alcohol on carbohydrate metabolism. In *Clinical Biochemistry of Alcoholism*. Ed. Rosalki. Churchill Livingstone: Edinburgh.
Wu, A., Chanarin, I. and Levi, A.J. (1974). Macrocytosis of chronic alcoholism. *Lancet*, **i**, 829–31.

# 21 Assessment of nutritional status

Susan M. Goodinson and
John W.T. Dickerson



## Introduction

Recent surveys have suggested a substantial and alarming prevalence of protein-energy malnutrition (PEM) in hospital patients. Independent studies (Bistrian *et al.*, 1976; Hill *et al.*, 1977; Weinsier *et al.*, 1979), have shown that 30–50 per cent of general medical and surgical patients are malnourished on admission, others may undergo progressive deterioration of nutritional status during hospitalization, due to the effects of disease, the side-effects of therapy and to neglected aspects of nutritional care. PEM results in poor wound healing, depressed immunocompetence, decreased enzyme synthesis, alterations in drug metabolism, a lowered tolerance to radiotherapy and chemotherapy, decreased psychological well-being and increased mortality (Grant, 1981; Seltzer *et al.*, 1982).

These findings underline the need for early identification of individuals at risk, so that optimal nutritional support can be offered in the hope of improving the patient's outcome. An essential first step in achieving this is to adopt a policy of routine nutritional assessment on admission and during subsequent progress, as part of the overall evaluation of care. High risk categories of patients who are either already malnourished or likely to become so include the elderly, unconscious, those in the perioperative period, and individuals suffering from burns, trauma, sepsis, acute or chronic renal failure, gastrointestinal disease, liver failure and those admitted with cancer or receiving therapy for it (see also 'dietary history').

For purposes of the present discussion, nutritional assessment is considered under the following headings: general consideration and methods; assessment of energy protein, vitamin and mineral nutriture.

## General consideration and methods

### Aims of nutritional assessment

A nutritional assessment aims to:

1. Define nutritional status at a particular time and evaluate the adequacy of recent nutrient intake.
2. Detect overt and subclinical malnutrition and identification of individuals requiring support.
3. Provide guidelines on relative amounts of nutrients required.
4. Evaluate, by repeated assessment, the effectiveness of nutritional support.

Apart from physical examination and dietary history, an imposing array of biochemical, anthropometric, immunological and morphological investigations can be used to define nutritional status. However, confusion exists as to which positive findings are necessary to make a diagnosis and some of the methods used are controversial. Indeed, do we have any 'ideal' markers of nutritional status? Buzby and Mullen (1985) have defined the criteria for such a marker as follows:

1. consistent abnormality in patients with PEM demonstrating a high sensitivity and low incidence of false negative results;
2. consistent normality in patients without PEM demonstrating a high specificity and low incidence of false positive results;
3. unaffected by non-nutritional factors (i.e. nutrition-specific);
4. normalized by nutritional support, demonstrating a high sensitivity to nutritional repletion.

These criteria pose a challenge because no single currently available measure meets them all. Thus, several investigations must be carried out in parallel to overcome the deficiencies of any single measure. Furthermore, serial measurements must be made over a period of time; 'one-off' estimates are of little value. Ideally, the investigations which are selected must be simple to perform, inexpensive, readily available and non-invasive. A suggested protocol for nutritional assessment is summarized in Table 21.1. This chapter reviews some of the methods currently used to assess nutritional status with particular reference to patients.

### Methods of assessment

#### Dietary history

The first clues to the aetiology and presence of malnutrition are often provided by the patient's history. Nurses and medical staff should elicit dietary

Table 21.1 Protocol for nutritional assessment

| Investigation | On admission | Weekly | Other |
|---|---|---|---|
| Clinical examination | + | | Repeated as necessary |
| Dietary history | + | | |
| Weight | + | + | |
| Arm muscle circumference | + | + | |
| Triceps skinfold thickness | + | + | |
| Serum albumin | + | + | |
| Serum transferrin | + | + | |
| Serum retinol binding protein | + | + | |
| Serum thyroxine<br>Serum prealbumin | + | + | |
| Delayed hypersensitivity tests | + | + | |
| Blood urea and electrolytes | + | | Daily or twice weekly |
| Nitrogen balance | + | | Four consecutive collections each week (24-hour urine) |
| Creatinine height/index | + | | As above |

information when patients are interviewed on admission; this could be easily incorporated as part of the nursing history.

Relevant information includes patterns of food intake prior to current illness and any alterations in the types and quantities of foods consumed since its onset. Of particular importance are the presence of symptoms affecting food intake or absorption of nutrients (e.g. anorexia, nausea, taste changes, dysphagia, dysgeusia, vomiting, diarrhoea and constipation). The presence of chronic diseases which require long term dietary modification, such as diabetes mellitus, renal, hepatic and cardiac disease, should be noted together with any difficulties in complying with prescribed therapeutic diets. Questions should be included on those social factors which may affect diet such as resources for purchasing, storing and preparing food. Of particular importance in the elderly are living circumstances and whether any care and assistance is required with activities of living and physical and psychological conditions.

The possible impact of drug therapy on nutritional status should also be considered. Chronic administration of steroids can lead to fluid retention, enhanced protein catabolism and insulin resistance. Common side-effects of drugs used in the chemotherapy of malignant disease include nausea, vomiting, diarrhoea, folate deficiency (methotrexate) and thiamine deficiency (5-fluorouracil).

The history of any weight change should be noted. Blackburn (1979) suggests that a non-intentional weight loss of 10 per cent usual body weight is clinically significant over a 6 month period, as is a loss of 5 per cent body weight over one month. Greater losses in shorter periods are regarded as severe and are associated with an increased risk of postoperative morbidity and mortality.

**Clinical examination**
To the trained observer a number of physical signs may indicate nutritional deficiency; they can, however, also be manifestations of underlying disease. Attention should be directed to the patient's general and physical appearance; i.e. a patient's excessive over or underweight appearance may be suggestive of obesity or starvation whilst muscle wasting or tenderness may indicate thiamine deficiency or a lack of protein. Skeletal deformities can suggest vitamin D deficiency and bruised or dry, rough, inflamed skin depletion of vitamin C, K or A. Classic oral signs associated with vitamin deficiency states are the swollen red tongue with papillary atrophy characteristic of vitamin B complex deficiency and spongy, bleeding, receding gums typical of a lack of vitamin C. Examination of the central nervous system may reveal sensory loss associated with thiamin depletion or the listlessness, apathy and depression associated with deficiency of the vitamin B complex.

**Surveys of dietary intake**
In some circumstances more detailed information regarding dietary intake may be needed to identify nutrient deficiency states in hospitalized patients or in the community. A variety of methods can be used to provide such information, including weighed food intakes usually measured for 7 days, and dietary recall over periods ranging from 24 hours to 1 month. The advantages and disadvantages of these approaches have been extensively reviewed (Marr, 1971; MacLeod, 1974; Burke and Bryson, 1980). If a recall method is selected, the subject is asked to give details of all foods and drink consumed during the relevant period. Each day is reviewed slowly and systematically, bearing in mind that recall can be difficult, particularly in the elderly. Marr (1971) stresses the need for the investigator to elicit information in an unbiased way, avoiding leading questions whilst maintaining the subject's interest, confidence and co-operation. Using a structured questionnaire this can be simply and rapidly carried out, especially if the data is subsequently computerized for analysis. However, recall methods covering short periods may miss day-to-day variations or seasonal changes in the diet and can be subject to memory errors. Another problem, that of difficulties in estimating portion sizes, can be overcome by using food models and household measures to quantify the foods consumed. Precise descriptions of each food item consumed are also required. Day-to-day variations may be less of a problem in estimating the nutrient intake of elderly individuals because they often consume a monotonous diet (MacLeod, 1974). A good correlation has been obtained between 24-hour and 7-day dietary recall in such individuals.

Weighing methods, in which food is weighed before meals and any remaining is reweighed at the end, can provide a greater degree of accuracy in estimating nutrient intakes, but they are relatively expensive to undertake. This method is time consuming, it may miss week-to-week and seasonal variations and can involve a delay in serving food which alters its aesthetic appeal, thus adversely affecting consumption (Marr, 1971). If the patient undertakes the weighing of food before and after each meal a great deal of co-operation, motivation and initial supervision are required to ensure accuracy. A disadvantage is the possibility of introducing behavioural bias. Furthermore, poor eyesight and physical disability can limit participation by elderly subjects and compliance may be decreased if the survey is extended beyond 7 days.

Whatever method is selected, once the type and quantity of foods consumed are obtained, daily energy and nutrient intake can be calculated using computerized standard tables of food composition (Paul and Southgate, 1978). Tropical food tables are also available for use in immigrant groups (Platt, 1962). The composition of proprietary enteral feeds and supplements can be obtained from the manufacturers' literature, as may details of newly marketed processed foods not presently included in standard tables. Within the confines of a metabolic laboratory where balance studies are undertaken, food composition can be estimated with a high degree of accuracy by chemically analysing duplicate aliquots for their nutrient content.

Once daily energy and nutrient intakes are obtained these can be compared with recommended intakes (DHSS, 1979) and any gross deficiencies identified. In making comparisons and drawing conclusions, care is needed as the data provided by these tables is drawn from population studies. Individuals whose intakes fall marginally below recommended values may not therefore be nutritionally 'at risk', but intakes which are consistently less than 60 per cent of that recommended are cause for concern and should be further investigated. It is also important to bear in mind that the energy and nutrient requirements of hospitalized patients may be altered by the metabolic response to injury, trauma and other factors, including bed-rest, related to disease. Guidelines for providing nutrient intakes which meet the requirements of these individuals are discussed at length by Jensen (1983), Silk (1983) and Long (1985).

## Protein energy malnutrition

### Anthropometry

#### Body weight

This is the sum of fat, protein, water and bone mineral mass. Total body energy (kcal) equals the sum of that contained in fat stores, protein reserve and glycogen store. It is important to distinguish between the terms 'store' and 'reserve' when applied here to fat and protein respectively. Almost all the fat store is available for utilization as a metabolic fuel during periods of negative energy balance. In contrast, while the protein reserve has the *potential* for use as a 'back-up' metabolic fuel, its primary utilization is in the maintenance of a complex array of cell functions. Depletion of the reserve can then lead to serious functional impairment.

Assuming constancy of bone mineral mass and the absence of serious derangements in fluid balance, serial measurements of weight provide an approximation of changes in body energy stores. A negative energy balance causes weight loss and vice-versa (Heymsfield *et al.*, 1985). Weight loss is an important easily obtained indicator of impaired nutritional status which correlates with PEM and an increased risk of postoperative morbidity and mortality. Currently there are no standardized methods of expressing either weight or weight loss. Reference values that can be used for body weight include 'average' values obtained from surveys of healthy populations, e.g. the Health and Nutrition Examination Survey (HANES) carried out in the USA (National Centre for Health Statistics, 1979), and the DHSS, UK, Survey

(Knight, 1984). Alternatively, the ideal body weight derived from actuarial data based on mortality statistics, e.g. Metropolitan Life Insurance tables (1959; 1979) can be used. It cannot be assumed that 'average' and 'ideal' weights are synonymous.

If the Metropolitan Life Insurance tables (1959; 1979) are used, actual body weight can be compared with ideal body weight for height, sex and frame size and the percentage ideal body weight calculated as follows:

$$\text{Percentage Ideal Body Weight (IBW)} = \frac{\text{Current Weight}}{\text{Ideal Body Weight}} \times 100$$

Interpretations vary, but a current weight of 60–80 per cent IBW suggests moderate, and less than 60 per cent, severe malnutrition (Blackburn, 1979). However, Grant (1981) suggests that the use of percentage IBW may incorrectly detect malnutrition in a normal ectomorph and overlook possible depletion in the obese. Further limitations inherent in using the Metropolitan Life Insurance tables are that the 1959 data is now nearly thirty years out of date, and did not incorporate a rigorous assessment of frame size which is known to exert a significant impact on IBW. However, the 1979 tables incorporate a correction for frame size derived from elbow breadth; other researchers have modified the data to incorporate frame size derived from a height:wrist circumference ratio (Grant, 1982).

Percentage weight loss, and the time-scale over which this occurs, may be more important than the percentage of ideal weight.

$$\text{Percentage Weight Change} = \frac{\text{Usual Weight} - \text{Current Weight}}{\text{Usual Weight}} \times 100$$

A constraint here is that the patient's usual weight is obtained from memory, which can be associated with an error as great as 3.6 kg (Morgan *et al.*, 1980). Blackburn *et al.*, (1977) suggest that losses of 10 per cent body weight (or more) over any time period are significant, whilst losses in excess of 30 per cent body weight greatly increase postoperative morbidity and mortality regardless of initial nutritional status (Cruse and Foord, 1973; Steffee, 1980).

*Accuracy and limitations*

To obtain accurate body weights, patients should be weighed at the same time each day, preferably before breakfast, to avoid diurnal variation, and wearing the same clothing. If comparison with reference tables is to be made, the clothing to be worn is usually also specified. The scales used should be accurate to ± 0.1 kg and calibrated frequently using standard weights.

Height is measured using a stadiometer observing the guidelines for design, stance and head position (Frankfurt plane) advocated by Knight (1984) in the DHSS survey.

Although serial measurements of body weight evaluated over a period of several weeks can provide a useful guide to depletion of energy stores, they are unreliable in the presence of dehydration, expansion of the extracellular volume, oedema and ascites. It is therefore important to monitor weight changes in conjunction with fluid balance records and other indices of hydration. The possible impact of drug therapy on fluid balance should also be borne in mind particularly with regard to diuretics which promote renal sodium and water loss, and corticosteroids which cause their retention.

Other factors which affect the interpretation of weight changes are massive tumour growth and organomegaly, while weight change *per se* does not indicate the nature of tissue loss.

Lipschitz and Mitchell (1985) have reviewed the problems involved in evaluating weight changes in the elderly. Changes in height, weight and body composition all occur with advancing years. Height declines due to degenerative changes in the vertebral column, weight increases up to the fifth decade then plateaus and may decline, while the proportion of body weight as fat increases. Current standards of reference are not suitable for use in the elderly. The HANES data (1974) can only be applied to subjects up to 74 years and the DHSS Survey (Knight, 1984) up to 64 years of age. Total arm length may provide a more accurate alternative to height in nutritional assessment of the elderly, since long bone measurements are less affected by ageing (Mitchell and Lipschitz, 1982; Roche, 1982).

Other points to note with regard to the use of reference tables on body weight are that the values published in the HANES, 1974, study (National Centre for Health Statistics, 1979) relate body weight for age to population percentile for men and women and are *not* analysed for frame size or height. The DHSS survey (Knight, 1984) gives percentage distributions of weight at each height and average weights for adult men and women in the age range 16–64 years, analysed by social and demographic variables. Other indices of weight for height are examined and Body Mass Index (BMI) values for the survey population are included and also analysed by demographic variables, which is particularly useful.

The data incorporated in all the reference tables currently available refer solely to the population and age ranges surveyed; they may not be applicable to other ethnic groups.

### Measurements of body fat

As approximately 50 per cent of the body fat is located subcutaneously, measurement of one or more skinfolds, or limb fat areas, can give an approximation of changes in total body fat. Rapid decrements in fat indices suggest a marked negative energy balance.

Skinfolds can be most reliaby measured using Harpenden or Lange calipers which possess a high resolution scale reading to ± 0.1 mm and apply a standard pressure of 10 g/mm$^2$. Skinfolds can be measured at six sites: the biceps, triceps, subscapular, surprailiac, thigh and calf. An estimate of total body fat can be obtained from the sum of the skinfold thicknesses at the first four sites (Durnin and Womersley, 1974). The most commonly measured skinfold thickness is the triceps (TSF), midway between the acromium process of the scapula and olecranon process of the ulna, on the posterior aspect of the arm. Traditionally the non-dominant arm is held vertical and relaxed at the side during measurement. Whatever site is used, the skinfold is grasped firmly with the thumb and forefinger and lifted clear of the underlying tissues. The calipers are applied midway between the apex and the base of the skinfold and a reading taken after 3 seconds. The average of three measurements is taken which can be compared to the standard values given by Jelliffe (1966) and Blackburn (1979) (Table 21.2) or reference percentiles (Frisancho, 1981). If

Table 21.2 Triceps skinfold thickness in adults (Blackburn, 1979)

| | Standard (mm) | 90 % | 80 % | 70 % | 60 % |
|---|---|---|---|---|---|
| Male | 12.5 | 11.3 | 10.0 | 8.8 | 7.5 |
| Female | 16.5 | 14.9 | 13.2 | 11.0 | 9.9 |
| | | Not depleted | Mildly depleted | Moderately depleted | Severely depleted |

the latter are used moderate depletion of fat depots is assumed if values fall between the 25–35 percentiles and severe if the value is below the 25 percentile.

**Mid arm muscle circumference**

Measurement of mid arm muscle circumference provides an indirect assessment of skeletal muscle protein reserves. This is obtained by measuring the mid upper arm with a non-stretchable tape measure at the same site as the triceps skinfold thickness. Care must be taken to maintain the tape horizontal and to avoid compressing the skin. Measurements must be made in triplicate to the nearest mm and an average taken. Arm muscle circumference is then obtained from the following formula:

Mid Arm Muscle circumference (MAMC)
= Mid Arm circumference − (0.314 × TSF)
All measurements in centimetres

Comparison can then be made with reference standards as before (Table 21.3). Values less than 70 per cent or 60 per cent of the standard are suggestive of moderate and severe malnutrition respectively.

**Sources of error**

Care must be taken to eliminate possible inter and intra observer error when making any anthropometric measurement. Specifically trained personnel should be used; the same observer should record the measurement for each patient and the site should be marked with indelible ink.

**Accuracy and limitations**

Although anthropometric techniques are useful, inexpensive and non-invasive, their accuracy when applied to individuals can be limited by a number of variables. Useful points to bear in mind when interpreting data are listed below.

1. Skinfold compressibility varies with age, sex, anatomical site and hydration status.
2. Distribution of body fat varies with sex, ethnic group and age.
3. Changes in muscle mass can occur independently of changes in muscle composition.
4. Limb oedema and subcutaneous surgical emphysema render the measurements invalid.
5. Assumptions are made in the calculations described earlier, that in cross-section the arm is circular when it is elliptical; bone area is also neglected.

**Table 21.3** Mid arm muscle circumference in adults (Blackburn, 1979)

| | Standard (mm) | 90 % | 80 % | 70 % | 60 % |
|---|---|---|---|---|---|
| Male | 25.3 | 22.8 | 20.2 | 17.7 | 15.2 |
| Female | 23.2 | 20.9 | 18.6 | 16.2 | 13.9 |
| | | Not depleted | Mildly depleted | Moderately depleted | Severely depleted |

6. Skinfold measurements at multiple sites provide the most accurate representations of changes in body fat.

Heymsfield *et al.*, (1982; 1985), describe advanced equations for calculating limb fat and muscle areas; some of these include corrections for bone area and the neuro-vascular bundle. More sophisticated, but expensive, techniques can also be used to provide highly accurate measurements, for example ultrasound for measuring the thickness of the fat layer and either computerized tomography or nuclear magnetic resonance (NMR) to estimate limb muscle cross sectional area.

A number of reference standards can be used to interpret anthropometric data, some of which are controversial. Those collated by Jelliffe (1966) have been widely used in clinical practice (Blackburn, 1979, see Tables 21.2 and 21.3). However, they have attracted criticism (Harries *et al.*, 1983) with regard to the population sample surveyed and the different sites at which arm measurements were taken in males and females. A further difficulty is that where results are presented as an average measurement with no standard deviation, there is no clue as to whether a patient fits into a 'normal' range. More recently, age- and sex-specific percentiles for triceps skinfolds and upper arm fat and muscle area have been published (Frisancho, 1981; Bishop *et al.*, 1981) based on data obtained in the HANES (1981) survey in the USA. The latter was based on a cross-sectional sample of 19 097 white subjects aged 1–74 years, of whom 8204 were males and 10 093 were females. The advantage of presenting data in percentiles is that the reference population need not show a Gaussian distribution and, in fact, many anthropometric surveys produce a skewed distribution of the population. Harries *et al.*, (1983) have compared the reference standards of Jelliffe (1966) and Frisancho (1981) in assessing the nutritional status of 318 subjects. They found no consistent agreement between the two standards of reference both in and between sexes, but of the subjects included in the survey only 106 were 'healthy'; 212 were suffering from inflammatory bowel disease.

The applicability of current reference standards to the elderly population poses a further problem. A community study by Sherman *et al.*, (1983) assessed the nutritional status of elderly patients of both sexes in the age range 64–95 years. Data was compared with that obtained by HANES (1974) and a statistically significant difference in all parameters, both anthropometric and biochemical, was found. This is not surprising, since lean body mass decreases and the proportion of body weight constituted by fat increases with age. A redistribution of body fat, with increased deposition around internal organs, accompanies these changes. Mitchell and Lipschitz (1982) have also found

MAMC to be of limited value in the assessment of elderly patients, while Vir and Love (1980) suggest that abdominal girth may prove to be the most valuable anthropometric parameter to measure in this group.

In summary, given the current state of the art with regard to reference standards, it would seem timely to adopt the suggestion of Heymsfield *et al.*, (1985), that patients followed over a period of time can act as their own controls and that the *relative* changes which are observed are as important as comparisons with reference populations. Current standards may well not be valid for the aged and different ethnic groups hence further surveys are urgently needed. Ideally, anthropometric measurements should be used to predict functional outcome, but we do not know if this is possible using the reference data presently available. Finally, it is important to note that in evaluating the response to nutritional therapy, small increments in body fat over short periods of time are impossible to measure accurately using anthropometry.

## Functional tests on skeletal muscle

Since visible muscle wasting is one of the most obvious effects of prolonged malnutrition, changes in contractility, relaxation and endurance rate which may precede the overt signs are currently under investigation for their potential use as indicators of nutritional status.

Lopes *et al.*, (1982) performed these tests on 22 healthy and 10 malnourished individuals by measuring the response of the adductor pollicis muscle to stimulation of the ulnar nerve. A slower maximum relaxation rate and an increased force loss during endurance tests was demonstrated in malnourished individuals when compared with healthy subjects. Maximal contractile force obtained by stimulation at high frequencies was also reduced in the malnourished. A significant improvement in these functional parameters was subsequently observed in four patients who received total parenteral nutrition (TPN) for one month. Russell *et al.*, (1985) have corroborated these findings in obese individuals subjected to short term hypocaloric fasting and in malnourished individuals suffering from anorexia nervosa. In the former group, muscle biopsy data obtained during fasting showed atrophy of type II fibres, 2-band degeneration, an increase in the intracellular muscle calcium concentration and diminished activity of key regulatory enzymes such as phosphofructokinase. The authors hypothesize that malnutrition may result in increased muscle breakdown by activation of an intracellular calcium-dependent proteinase.

Further research is needed to extend these preliminary findings before muscle function tests can be assimilated into the battery of those routinely used to assess nutritional status. How reliable an indicator is this likely to be? Possible limitations on its use are suggested by the other factors which can lead to functional changes in muscle. These include neurological disorders, muscle myopathies and drugs acting on the central nervous system which may cause muscle weakness as a side-effect. In critically ill patients, serious disturbances in the extracellular potassium, hydrogen and calcium ion concentrations can occur, resulting in profound changes in muscle excitability. Further problems in this group are the effects on muscle metabolism and function of respiratory and circulatory failure.

Although in its early stages of development, dynamometry may provide another useful rapid, non-invasive and inexpensive method of assessing skeletal muscle reserves, specifically those of arm muscle protein. Grip strength (in kg) is measured using a simple hand grip dynamometer. Three readings are taken, allowing a suitable period of relaxation between each, and a mean value recorded. A study by Klidjian *et al.*, (1980) suggested that hand grip strength was a highly sensitive indicator in predicting complications in patients admitted for major abdominal surgery. 'Appreciable' protein depletion was defined by this study as a hand grip strength below 85 per cent of control values (Males 48.8 $\pm$ 7.0 kg; Females 34.4 $\pm$ 4.7 kg). Grip strength was significantly decreased in 87 per cent of patients who developed postoperative complication. Further work is urgently needed to corroborate these findings and develop age related standards for grip strength. This method of assessment is unsuitable for use where grip strength is impaired by paralysis, arthritis, trauma, muscle myopathies, or any of the other factors described earlier which adversely affect muscle contraction, relaxation and endurance. Martin *et al.*, (1985) investigated the effects of non-nutritional factors (age, posture, circadian rhythm, drugs and certain pathological processes) on the relationship of grip strength to creatinine excretion, and forearm muscle area to lean body mass.

## Biochemical indices of PEM

### The 'creatinine-height index'

Phosphocreatine and creatine in muscle are non-enzymatically dehydrated to form creatinine, which is quantitatively excreted in the urine. If the proportion of phosphocreatine and creatine in muscle is constant then the excretion of creatinine per 24 hours should provide a measure of muscle mass. The excretion of less than 60 per cent of the amount of creatinine predicted for height at the ideal weight is said to indicate 'severe muscle mass deficit' (Taylor and Anthony, 1983). The use of creatinine as a measure of muscle mass in this 'creatinine-height index' depends on the constancy of its excretion. There is now considerable evidence that creatinine excretion is, in fact, so variable (Webster and Garrow, 1985) that its measurement in a single 24-hour urine sample gives an unreliable estimate of muscle mass. Webster and Garrow found a coefficient of variation of 8.7 to 34.4 per cent and a poor correlation with measures of lean body mass such as density, body water or body potassium.

Standards for the urinary creatinine per cm height in men and women of ideal weight for their height are given by Dickerson (1983).

### 3-Methylhistidine excretion

The 24-hour urinary excretion of 3-methylhistidine is another marker of skeletal muscle mass. This compound is released during the breakdown of actin and myosin and is not re-utilized. However, studies in the rat showed that only about half the excreted 3-methylhistidine could be accounted for by skeletal muscle (Millward *et al.*, 1982). Rennie and Millward (1983) have questioned the value of 3-methylhistidine as an indicator of change in skeletal muscle mass, pointing out that approximately 25 per cent of that excreted is derived from non-skeletal muscle pools, which are in rapid turnover.

However, Fürst (1982) concluded that 3-methylhistidine provides a useful tool in the study of muscle protein metabolic responses under a variety of nutritional, pathological and physiological circumstances. However, this worker commented that there are many factors which make blind acceptance of results dangerous and advised caution in their interpretation.

Long (1985) has suggested that in stable, chronically ill patients on a constant diet, 3-methylhistidine excretion provides a reliable index of skeletal muscle mass. In such malnourished individuals a significant reduction in excretion occurs with time, as the skeletal muscle mass is progressively reduced in size during starvation.

The excretion of 3-methylhistidine can be used to calculate myofibrillar protein catabolic rate (MPCR), the percentage turnover of myofibrillar protein (TMP%) and the rate of muscle protein breakdown (MPB). Fürst (1982) summarized values in the literature in various clinical conditions.

**Measurement of nitrogen balance**

Estimates of nitrogen balance can be used to determine whether or not an individual is gaining or losing tissue protein. If protein is being catabolized due to an inadequate intake, then negative balances can be corrected by readjusting the dietary intake of energy and protein.

Nitrogen intake is readily calculated from the daily protein intake, on the basis that 6.25 g protein contain 1 g nitrogen. For accurate balances it is essential to analyse the diet to determine the nitrogen intake. Hartley and Lee (1975) have devised a formula for the calculation of nitrogen balance over a 24 hour period:

$$\text{Nitrogen Balance} = \frac{\text{Protein Intake (g)}}{6.25} - \begin{matrix}\text{Urinary urea}\\ \text{nitrogen} + 4\text{ g}\end{matrix}$$

In the calculation of losses, correction factors can be used to allow for changes in the blood urea and proteinuria (if any) and to take account of the fact that urinary urea nitrogen constitutes only 80 per cent of the total urinary nitrogen; 20 per cent is in the form of creatinine, small peptides, uric acid and amino acids. A value of 4 g is added to allow for extrarenal losses of nitrogen in hair, sweat, skin and faeces. Individuals with leaking fistulas and diarrhoea may lose considerably more, so these fluids must be collected and their nitrogen content determined to provide an accurate estimate of total losses. Nitrogen balance studies are usually carried out over three consecutive 24-hour periods, necessitating three 24-hour urine collections, to provide a reliable estimate of balance. In non-catabolic patients, Silk (1983) advocates that nitrogen requirements are calculated to exceed losses by 3–5 g/day. Nitrogen requirements are drastically increased during the peak catabolic response to injury, trauma or infection. Guidelines for the provision of nutritional support, including maintenance of nitrogen balance during this period, are discussed by Silk (1983) and Long (1985).

**Visceral transport proteins as indicators of PEM**

Attempts have been made to measure changes in the visceral protein mass by estimating serum concentrations of the transport proteins synthesized by the liver, i.e. albumin, transferrin, retinol binding protein (RBP) and thyroxine binding prealbumin. It is assumed that a decrease in their serum concentrations reflects decreased liver protein synthesis due to malnutrition. However, this is an over-simplification, since serum concentrations are dependent on the rate of metabolic utilization, excretion, transfer between the intra- and extravascular compartments and hydration status. The intravenous administration of protein products including blood, plasma and albumin solutions can also alter serum concentrations (Grant, 1981).

*Albumin*

Albumin has been used extensively to assess visceral protein depletion. However, it is a poor indicator of acute changes in nutritional status due to its long half-life (19 days) and large body pool size (5 g) per kg body weight. Mobilization of albumin from the extravascular pool during periods of protein depletion also ensures that the serum concentration does not decline immediately. The normal range is 40–50 g/litre. Generally values of 28–35 g/litre are indicative of mild depletion, 21–27 g/litre of moderate depletion and $< 21$ g/litre of severe depletion.

A number of studies have shown a significant correlation between a low serum albumin and an increased risk of morbidity and mortality in hospitalized patients (Seltzer *et al.*, 1979; Mullen *et al.*, 1980; Harvey *et al.*, 1978). The outcome of surgical treatment as related to the response of the serum albumin level to nutritional support was investigated by Ching and Grossi (1980). Only survivors demonstrated an increase in the serum albumin level to 35 g/litre with intensive nutritional support.

As a nutritional marker, albumin is easy to measure and provides a useful index of long-term changes in nutritional status. In situations where the serum level declines, as, for example, the result of severe injury, liver disease, neuropathy and enteropathy, its use as a nutritional marker is unreliable.

Serum albumin estimations have been incorporated, together with other weighed parameters of nutritional status, into a single prognostic nutritional index (Mullen and Buzby 1979; Buzby *et al.*, 1980) (see later).

*Transferrin*

Transferrin is the $\beta$ globulin which transports iron in plasma. It has a smaller body pool size (100 mg/kg/body weight) and a shorter half-life (9 days) than albumin; these characteristics render it far more sensitive to acute changes in nutritional status. It can be measured directly by radial immunodiffusion or by extrapolation from the total iron binding capacity (TIBC) using the following formula proposed by Blackburn *et al.*, (1977).

$$\underset{\text{(mg/dl)}}{\text{Serum Transferrin}} = 0.8\ \underset{\text{(mg/dl)}}{\text{TIBC}} - 43$$

Other laboratories have noted that the relationship between TIBC and transferrin is not quite as predicted by this equation and have produced modified formulae based on their assay method for TIBC (Dennis *et al.*, 1981; Miller *et al.*, 1981).

Normal ranges for serum concentrations of transferrin are 250–300 mg/dl. Values between 100–150 mg/dl are indicative of moderate, and < 100 mg/dl of severe visceral protein depletion. In considering the usefulness of transferrin as an indicator of PEM, it is important to bear in mind the other conditions which can affect the serum concentration. It rises in pregnancy, iron deficiency and hypoxia due to enhanced synthesis and declines in liver disease, the acute phase of trauma, chronic infection, pernicious anaemia and any protein-losing enteropathy or nephropathy.

*Thyroxine binding prealbumin*

The very short half-life of this protein (2 days) renders it extremely sensitive to a decreased protein and energy intake of a few days duration. Fischer (1982) has suggested that it declines in 3 days in response to a lowered energy intake, even when protein intake is adequate. It is encouraging to note that the independent studies of Douville (1982), Carpentier *et al.*, (1982) and Bourry (1982) have demonstrated that while prealbumin declines drastically in PEM, the response towards normal values resulting from the administration of nutritional support (TPN) is equally prompt.

Serum concentrations of prealbumin are rapidly depressed in liver disease, infection, stress and also in trauma, hence it is of limited value immediately after surgery. As measured by radial immunodiffusion normal ranges are reported to lie between 160–360 mg/litre (Bourry *et al.*, 1982; Grant, 1981). Values of 50–100 mg/litre are indicative of moderate and < 50 mg/litre of severe protein depletion.

*Retinol binding protein (RBP)*

A rapid decline in response to decreased protein and energy intakes has been reported for this transport protein with a half-life of only 12 hours (Shetty *et al.*, 1979; Ingenbleek *et al.*, 1975) showed that low serum RBP levels associated with malnutrition in Senegalese children returned to normal following nutritional support. In protein-depleted patients, RBP levels returned to normal after 5 days of TPN (Carpentier, *et al.*, 1982).

Unfortunately, a number of other factors influence serum RBP concentrations, notably liver disease, trauma, zinc deficiency and hyperthyroidism, which all decrease it. Serum levels may be raised in renal failure due to impaired glomerular filtration and decreased renal metabolism.

Low RBP levels are a cause of low retinol (vitamin A) levels (Atukorala *et al.*, 1979). The normal range for RBP has been reported to be 30–65 mg/litre (Shetty *et al.*, 1979) and 26–76 mg/litre (Grant, 1982).

*Fibronectin*

Recently, attention has been focused on the potential use of fibronectin, a plasma glycoprotein and opsonin of the reticulo-endothelial system, as a nutritional marker. Scott *et al.*, (1979) and Chadwick *et al.*, (1985) have demonstrated the exquisite sensitivity of plasma fibronectin to starvation and repletion in healthy subjects. Its short half-life (4 hours) and the fact that it is not synthesized by the liver and subject to many of the variables affecting the visceral transport proteins, are advantageous.

Further investigation is necessary to identify other factors which may affect its concentration in plasma. A fall follows burns (Grossman *et al.*, 1980); sepsis (Scovill *et al.*, 1978) and surgery or shock (Saba, 1975). More recently, Jung (1986) has described changes in the fibronectin concentration in patients suffering from neoplasms of the digestive system, breast, reproductive tract and lung.

**Immunocompetence and PEM**

Depressed immunocompetence and increased incidence and severity of infection are associated with PEM (Chandra and Newberne, 1977). Although malnutrition appears to exert a particularly important influence on cell mediated immunity, the humoral response, phagocytosis and the complement system are also adversely affected (Gross and Newberne, 1980). Specific effects of PEM on immune function include the following:

1. A decreased total lymphocyte count.
2. Depressed neutrophil chemotaxis.
3. Absence of a delayed hypersensitivity response.
4. A decrease in all complement components especially C3.
5. A decrease in secretory 1gA.

The most widely available tests are the total lymphocyte count, and delayed cutaneous hypersensitivity testing.

Moderate and severe PEM have been associated with lymphocyte counts of 800–1000 and $< 800$ per $mm^3$ respectively (Grant, 1982). As yet, no conclusive evidence has emerged to correlate changes in the peripheral lymphocyte count with an increased risk of morbidity and mortality (Mullen *et al.*, 1980).

PEM can also be evaluated by delayed hypersensitivity skin testing using at least three antigens to which most individuals have received prior sensitization, e.g. mumps, candida albicans, tuberculin, streptokinase-streptodornase. The antigens are injected intradermally and the site inspected after 24–48 hours. A normal, positive response in a healthy subject is demonstrated by an area of inflammatory induration $> 5$ mm in diameter at the site of infection. Anergy, a complete lack of response, is seen in PEM. Interpretation must, however, be cautious since anergy may also occur as a result of stress, uraemia, cancer, sepsis, and treatment with immunosuppressive drugs, cytotoxic agents, $H_2$ blockers and some anaesthetics. Anergy is also a concomitant of ageing.

Studies by Meakins *et al.*, (1977) and Mullen and co-workers (1979) reported a positive correlation between anergy, postoperative sepsis and mortality. In Meakin's study, reversal of anergy followed the institution of TPN and was associated with an improved prognosis, corroborating earlier findings (Law *et al.*, 1974).

To date, neither total lymphocyte counts nor delayed hypersensitivity testing have been widely used in routine nutritional assessment. Evidence is lacking on the sensitivity of total lymphocyte counts in PEM and so many other factors which may co-exist with malnutrition can impede the interpretation of skin tests. Recent research concerning the interrelationships between PEM, infection and immunocompetence is, in some instances, inconclusive and occasionally controversial. More substantive evidence is urgently required regarding the complex effects of PEM on immunocompetence and its reversal with nutritional support. Mullen *et al.*, (1979) have used delayed hypersensitivity tests in the development of a prognostic nutritional index.

## Prognostic nutritional indices (PNIs)

The correction or prevention of nutritional deficiencies which could exert a negative impact on a patient's progress, in terms of morbid complications and mortality, is the prime objective of nutritional support. Identification of the patient at risk is one of the most crucial objectives of a nutritional assessment yet, as described earlier in this chapter, many of the measures which may be of use in identifying high risk populations can present difficulties when made as single observations or when applied to individuals.

A clinician who carried out a range of tests using a protocol such as that in Table 21.1 may be presented with a conflicting array of normal and abnormal data. How then should these be interpreted in terms of risk to the patient of suffering nutrition-related complications? Can the risk be quantified and allow identification of those individuals who require nutritional support?

In an attempt to answer these questions, Mullen *et al.*, (1979) developed a PNI which utilized several assessment parameters to quantify risk. One hundred and sixty one patients admitted for major intrathoracic or abdominal surgery were given a full nutritional assessment prior to surgery. This included measurement of biochemical, anthropometric and immunological parameters. Their subsequent postoperative progress was monitored and baseline nutritional status correlated with outcome in terms of morbidity and mortality. Computer regression analysis identified the most sensitive predictive variables to be serum albumin and transferrin concentrations, triceps skinfold thickness and delayed cutaneous hypersensitivity testing. Discriminant analysis was used to develop a linear predictive model; this provided a (PNI) relating morbid complications to the four predictive variables of nutritional status (Buzby and Mullen, 1985).

$$\text{PNI}\ \% = 158 - 16.6\,\underset{\text{g/dl}}{(\text{serum albumin})} - 0.78\,\underset{\text{mm}}{(\text{Triceps skinfold thickness})}$$

$$- 0.2\,\underset{\text{mg/dl}}{(\text{Serum transferrin})} - 5.8\ {}^{+a}(\text{Hypersensitivity test})$$

[a] Maximal skin test reactivity to any of three recall antigens

+Graded 0 if non-reactive
1 if 5 mm reactive
2 if > 5 mm reactive

Mullen *et al.*, (1980) evaluated the validity of the PNI in a group of patients admitted for gastrointestinal surgery, comparing predicted risk with outcome. The model correctly classified as high (PNI 40–49 per cent) risk 89 per cent of the patients who developed complications, 92 per cent of those who developed sepsis and 95 per cent of those who died. Other prospective studies (Smale *et al.*, 1979; Simms and Smith, 1981) have also used this PNI in the successful identification of at risk patients. The PNI does not, however, appear to be as useful as a predictor of outcome if the assessment is carried out in the immediate postoperative period on critically ill patients (Eisenberg *et al.*, 1981).

Since Mullen's early work on PNIs others have developed their own indices. Broden *et al.*, (1984) found serum albumin and transferrin concentrations to be most useful in predicting postoperative morbidity but noted that diagnosis and age of the patients also exerted a significant impact. Rainey-McDonald *et al.*, (1983) also found that a two-variable index using the serum albumin and transferrin gave the best prediction of outcome.

Mullen *et al.*, (1980) have used their PNI to identify candidates for preoperative nutritional support. In a non-randomized study, pre-operative TPN was found to reduce the incidence of morbidity and mortality in patients identified as high risk (PNI > 50 per cent) when compared with high risk patients not receiving TPN.

A pilot study by Detsky *et al.*, (1984) evaluated the accuracy of seven nutritional assessment techniques in predicting a single nutrition-associated complication (infection) in a group of 59 high and low risk surgical patients. The techniques evaluated were serum albumin, transferrin, creatinine-height index, delayed cutaneous hypersensitivity, anthropometry, a PNI (Mullen *et al.*, 1979) and 'subjective global assessment' (SGA) which comprised a very thorough dietary history, physical examination and functional assessment of performance related to activities of daily living. The best combination of sensitivity and specificity was found to be the SGA, and the second best was either the PNI or creatinine-height index. These preliminary findings should be confirmed in a larger group of patients. The inclusion of questions related to performance of activities of daily living in the SGA is apposite, since malnutrition can exert a significant impact on quality of life.

## Future directions

Nutritional assessment is in an early stage of development and the search for new indicators which are unaffected by non-nutritional factors continues. It is encouraging to note that a number of sophisticated research techniques can now provide accurate assessments of changes in body cell mass, e.g. measurements of total body potassium ($^{40}$K a radio-isotope present in small amounts in the body) and exchangeable potassium (using $^{42}$K in an isotope dilution method). Total body neutron activation analysis can provide accurate estimates of total body nitrogen and hence, of lean body mass. However, it is difficult to see such complex, sophisticated and expensive techniques becoming widely available.

Recently, attention has been focused on the potential for functional indices to provide a reliable assessment of nutritional status; these include cognitive ability, disease response, reproductive competence, physical activity, work performance and social/behavioural performance (Solomons and Allen, 1983).

## Assessment of vitamin status

Vitamins are organic substances that are essential to health. They cannot be made in the body, at least not in amounts sufficient to meet metabolic requirements, and must therefore be supplied in the diet. With one notable exception (vitamin D, or cholecalciferol), vitamins function as co-factors for enzyme systems. Vitamins are divided into two groups depending on whether they are water- or fat-soluble. Large amounts of some vitamins are taken by persons susceptible to the publicity given to largely unfounded claims of beneficial effects. The 'mega' doses of vitamins taken in this way may produce ill-effects. Deficiency results in specific clinical conditions. The effects of deficiencies and excesses are more serious in the rapidly growing fetus and child than in the adult. However, deficiencies of some vitamins are a public health problem in certain ethnic minorities, particularly Asians, and in the elderly.

It is important to recognize that the absence of a deficiency disease is not reliable evidence of satisfactory vitamin status. Deficiency diseases are the end result of a series of changes and take time to develop (Fig. 21.1). A carefully taken history is of considerable value in identifying risk factors and early warning signs. Social conditions, medical history, drug consumption and a carefully taken qualitative dietary history may give valuable clues about possible deficiencies (Table 21.4). It is generally cheaper to provide vitamin supplements on the basis of information gained in this way than to undertake biochemical assessment of vitamin status. Moreover, with few exceptions, such as folate and vitamin $B_{12}$, biochemical assessment of vitamin status is not readily available in hospital biochemical laboratories.

### Clinical examination

Persons recognized as vulnerable to vitamin deficiency should always be examined for clinical evidence of deficiency. In the developed nations overt vitamin deficiency diseases are rare but may occur amongst the vulnerable groups already mentioned, the elderly and ethnic minorities, and also amongst food faddists. Symptoms associated with developing, or less severe, deficiencies have only been established as the result of studies in which previously healthy individuals have been deprived of a single vitamin and physical and psychological symptoms noted. Studies of this kind are difficult to perform due to the length of time needed to deplete the tissues. Moreover, the symptoms are often vague and their description necessarily subjective. The diet consumed in

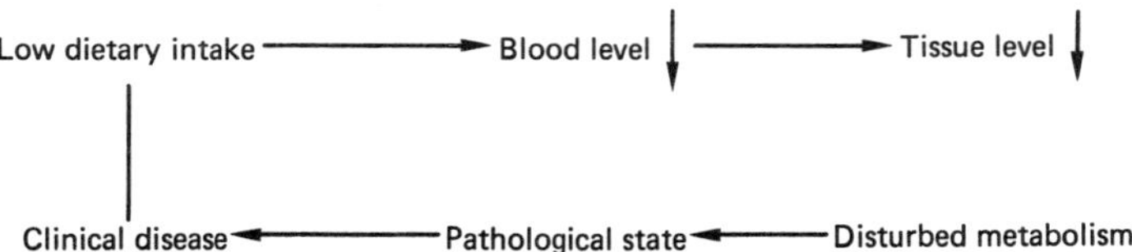


**Fig. 21.1** Sequence of changes leading to the development of a deficiency disease (From Dickerson, 1983).

Table 21.4 Findings in the medical history suggesting increased risk of vitamin deficiency (Adapted from Selhub and Rosenberg, 1985)

| |
|---|
| Recent weight loss |
| Restricted dietary intake |
| Drastic weight reducing diet |
| Fad diets |
| Liquid or soft diets |
| Anorexia, bulimia |
| Excessive alcohol use |
| Chronic disease |
| Increased losses due to gastrointestinal disorders such as malabsorption and diarrhoea |
| Drugs that interfere with vitamin utilization or increase requirements for vitamins |
| In the elderly – poor health, mental or physical disability, social isolation, dependence on meals-on-wheels |

studies of this sort must be adequate in respect of all nutrients other than the vitamin under investigation.

The diseases due to vitamin deficiencies and the symptoms associated with deficiency are shown in Table 21.5 (from Dickerson and Booth, 1985).

## Recommended allowances

The amounts of folic acid, vitamin $B_{12}$ and ascorbic acid shown in Table 21.5 as the level at which symptoms begin to appear are the minimum amounts required to relieve deficiency symptoms. It is likely that there are differences between individuals in the amounts of the various vitamins required for health. Allowance is made for this variability in arriving at the recommended daily intakes (DHSS, 1979). The intakes of the various vitamins recommended by different governments vary considerably and the reason for the different values is not always clear. The recommended intakes of ascorbic acid vary between 30 mg per day in the UK to 75 mg per day in the USSR. There may well be a case for considering that the UK figure is too low (Dickerson, 1979) for it is based on the amount of ascorbic acid required to cure scurvy and is thus related to only one function of the vitamin. Also, it is to be noted that there are some vitamins for which the British Authorities felt unable to make a recommendation. The absence of a value for folic acid is attributed to uncertainty about the folic acid content of foods. This vitamin is very difficult to determine accurately with currently available methods because the different forms in which the vitamin is present in food are assayed to a varying extent. No value is given for pyridoxine, a vitamin which is present in small amounts in a wide variety of foods. The US recommended value of 1.5–2.0 mg per day is often used. This is the amount present in the average US diet. The clinical biochemistry of vitamin $B_6$ has been discussed by Rosalki (1979). The requirement for vitamin E varies with the amount of polyunsaturated fatty acids in the diet (Witting, 1974). Vitamin E is an antioxidant and prevents peroxidation of lipids. However, most foods that contain large amounts of polyunsaturated fats also contain large amounts of vitamin E.

Table 21.5 Diseases and clinical evidences of deficiency of certain vitamins (modified from Pike and Brown, 1975), (from Dickerson and Booth, 1985) Dietary intake below which symptoms appear is shown in brackets

| Vitamin | Deficiency disease | Clinical symptoms associated with deficiency |
|---|---|---|
| Thiamin (<0.2–0.3 mg/ 1000 kcal) | Beri-beri | Anorexia; nausea with vomiting; constipation; calf muscle tenderness; weakness; irritability; depression; confusion; lowered blood pressure |
| Riboflavin (<0.6 mg/day) | | Cheilosis; angular stomatitis; seborrheic dermatitis (particularly nasolabial) |
| Nicotinic acid (<4.4 mg/ 1000 kcal) | Pellagra | Dermatitis; glossitis; stomatitis; diarrhoea; proctitis and vaginitis; mental depression, anxiety |
| Vitamin $B_6$ (<1.25 mg/day) | | Seborrheic dermatitis; glossitis; stomatitis, cheilosis; depression; confusion; abnormal electro-encephalogram |
| Folic acid (< 50 μg/day) | Macrocytic anaemia | Weakness; tiredness; dyspnoea; sore tongue; irritability and forgetfulness; diarrhoea; headache; palpitation |
| Vitamin $B_{12}$ (<0.5 μg/day | Pernicious anaemia | Weakness; tiredness; sore tongue; paraesthesia; constipation; headache; palpitation; macrocytic anaemia; neurological damage |
| Ascorbic acid (<10 mg/day) | Scurvy | Hyperkeratotic papules; petechiae; perifolliculosis; swollen, spongy gums; poor wound healing; fatigue; coiled hair; muscular aches; swollen joints; oedema |
| Vitamin A (<23–40 IU/kg) | Xerophthalmia<br>Keratomalacia<br>Blindness | Poor dark adaptation; white papules; abnormal electroretinogram; acne; follicular hyperkeratosis; abnormalities of balance, taste, and smell |
| Vitamin D | Rickets<br>Osteomalacia | Swollen wrists, knees and ends of ribs (rachitic rosary); bowing of legs; open fontanelle; osteomalacia marked by bone pain and muscle weakness giving rise to 'waddling' gait |
| Vitamin E (<3 mg/day) | Haemolytic anaemia in babies | Oedema (infants); anaemia; increased erythrocyte haemolysis |

Other factors known to affect the requirement for vitamin E at least in animals include the dietary content of selenium, sulphur-containing amino acids and vitamin A. Little clinical information is available about the relevance of these observations to man. A complicating factor that is relevant to man is the considerable variation in the vitamin E contents of raw materials, such as vegetables, foods and diets (Bunnell *et al.*, 1965; Smith *et al.*, 1971).

Assessments of dietary intakes of vitamin E from food tables are unreliable. Measurements of vitamin E intake of whole diets in the UK have given low values (Smith *et al.*, 1971). The range is of the order of 1–8 mg $\alpha$-tocopherol. In the US intakes tend to be higher averaging 3–18 international units per day (Bieri and Evarts, 1973) (1 international unit in the activity of 1 mg DL-$\alpha$-tocopherol); $\alpha$-tocopherol, in fact, probably is the major form of vitamin E in the diet.

In the UK about 10 mg per day is the usual dietary intake (DHSS, 1979) but it must be remembered that no single figure is applicable to all circumstances (Losowsky, 1979).

## Biochemical assessment

Biochemical methods available for the assessment of vitamin status are shown in Table 21.6 (from Dickerson, 1983). For some vitamins plasma or serum

Table 21.6 Biochemical methods for the determination of vitamin status (From Dickerson, 1983)

| Vitamin | Methods | Comments |
|---|---|---|
| A | Plasma retinol and $\beta$ carotene | Normal levels of vitamin A taken as 50–100 $\mu$g/100 ml. |
| | Plasma retinol-binding protein | Low levels alone do not indicate deficiency. Deficiency should be confirmed by assessment of dietary intake and measurement of dark adaptation. |
| D | Plasma alkaline phosphatase | Raised levels of alkaline phosphatase occur in rickets and osteomalacia but are non-specific for vitamin D deficiency. |
| | Plasma 25-hydroxy-cholecalciferol | Normal values for 25-hydroxycholecalciferol vary with the method used |
| E | Plasma tocopherol | Plasma level varies with total plasma lipids. Representative lower limits of normal taken as 5 $\mu$g/ml or 0.8 mg/g lipid. |
| | Erythrocyte haemolysis | High peroxide haemolysis not specific to vitamin E deficiency. |
| Thiamine | Blood pyruvate and lactate | Raised levels non-specific for thiamin deficiency |
| | Red cell (or whole blood) transketolase and stimulation (TPP % value) | Red cell transketolase and particularly raised TPP % value is most reliable index. Values > 15 probably indicate deficiency. |
| | Urinary excretion of thiamin | |
| Riboflavin | Red cell glutathione reductase (GR) and GR stimulation ratio | Stimulation or activation ratios >1.30 indicative of riboflavin deficiency. |
| | Urinary excretion of riboflavin | |

Table 21.6 *Continued*

| Vitamin | Methods | Comments |
|---|---|---|
| Nicotinic acid | Urinary excretion of N′-methyl nicotinamide (NMN) | Excretion of <0.6 mg/6 h is subnormal; excretion of 0.2 mg or less/6 h indicative of deficiency.<br>Ratio of NMN to creatinine in 2 h urine collected between 10 AM and 12 AM similar to values obtained on 24 h urine. |
| | Urinary excretion of NMN after an oral dose of nicotinamide | For load test, 50–200 mg nicotinamide given. Normally nourished subjects excrete 20 % of dose as NMN in 24 h. |
| Pyridoxine | Red cell aspartate transaminase (AST) and red cell AST stimulation | The red cell AST stimulation test is a convenient method of determining pyridoxine status. |
| | Enzymological assay of pyridoxal phosphate with tyrosine decarboxylase | After a tryptophan load, deficient individuals excrete an increased amount of xanthurenic acid and an increased ratio of hydroxykynurenine:hydroxyanthranilate. |
| | Tryptophan load test | |
| Folate | Serum folate | Normal range 3–25 $\mu$g/l. Concentrations reduced by loss of appetite. Low value not sufficient to diagnose deficiency. Indicates negative folate balance at the time. |
| | Red cell folate | Normal range 150–600 $\mu$g/l packed cells.<br>Normal range varies considerably in different laboratories.<br>Low levels always indicative of folate deficiency.<br>Diagnosis confirmed by satisfactory treatment with 200 $\mu$g/d. |
| | Histidine load test | 15 g L-histidine given. Folate deficiency indicated by excretion of >18 mg formimino-glutamic acid (FIGLU) in first 8 h. |
| $B_{12}$ | Serum concentration | Normal range quoted as 170–1000 $\mu$g/ml but varies with the method used. |
| | Methylmalonic acid (MMA( excretion | Normal range 0.2–15.3 mg MMA/24 h.<br>Level of excretion increased in $B_{12}$ deficiency particularly if urine is collected after giving valine or isoleucine.<br>Less sensitive and less convenient than measurement of $B_{12}$. |
| Ascorbic acid | Plasma and leucocyte ('buffy coat') concentrations | Plasma levels reflect recent intake but repeated values <0.2 mg/100 ml probably indicate deficiency.<br>Leucocyte concentrations reflect tissue concentrations.<br>Values <25 $\mu$g/$10^8$ cells indicate deficiency. |
| | Saturation test | Adequately nourished individuals excrete most of the load. Depleted individuals retain a proportionately greater amount. |

levels can be measured. A single observation of a low level is of no value as an indication of low status, but repeated low values of, for instance, plasma ascorbic acid are more reliable. For other vitamins, for example niacin or nicotinic acid, the urinary excretion of a metabolite provides a more reliable indication of status than blood levels. Due to the difficulty of obtaining reliable 24-hour urine collections, urinary metabolites are often related to creatinine excretion but this varies with the muscle mass, is affected also by renal function and changes with age so that different 'normal' or reference values must be used for subjects of different ages.

Because vitamins function as coenzymes at various stages of metabolic pathways, deficiency of a vitamin will lead to a reduction in the activity of a particular enzyme and may lead to the increased excretion of a metabolite formed prior to that point in the metabolic pathway. This forms the basis for the load tests used for the investigation of, for example, folic acid (histidine load test) and pyridoxine (tryptophan load test) status.

Determination of status with respect to a number of vitamins in the B group (thiamine, riboflavin and pyridoxine) can be made by measuring the activities of enzymes in the red cell for which they act as co-factors. A more reliable index of status is given by the 'activation coefficient' which is the rise in enzyme activity when the vitamin is added to deficient red cells. This can be expressed as a ratio or as a percentage.

More information about the assessment of vitamin status is given in the review by Selhub and Rosenberg (1985).

## Assessment of essential inorganic micronutrient (trace element) status

The first edition of a standard textbook of nutrition published in 1967 stated that 'Trace elements are required in extremely small amounts in the diet and are so widely distributed in foodstuffs that even diets inadequate in other respects usually contain sufficient quantities of these nutrients' (Pike and Brown, 1975).

Improved methods of determination of trace minerals have shown that deficiencies of some of them are associated with specific clinical conditions and deficiencies of others occur in a variety of diseases (see Stamp, Chapter 14). Interest in the inorganic micronutrients has further been stimulated by the occurrence of clinical evidence of deficiency in patients maintained on total parenteral nutrition (see Lee, Chapter 23), and the need to provide adequate amounts in intravenous solutions (Fell and Burns, 1978; Fell, 1985). Assessment of mineral status is complex because these micronutrients are bound to carrier proteins and changes in the synthesis and catabolism of these proteins may occur in disease states. It follows that changes in serum, or plasma, concentrations may occur without any change in cellular concentrations. Haemodilution may also lower serum values.

At least fourteen trace elements (Cr, Co, Cu, F, I, Fe, Mn, Mo, Ni, Se, Si, Sn, V, Zn) are known to be required for the normal growth and development of one or more animal species and some of these are discussed elsewhere in this book (Chapter 4). It seems likely that all of these are involved in some way in the regulation of biochemical pathways. Some are present in metalloenzymes whilst others activate or inhibit many intracellular processes. It seems likely that with increasing knowledge of these biochemical pathways it will be possible to select for each mineral an appropriate laboratory test to confirm suspected deficiency. Thus, selenium deficiency can be assessed by measuring the Se–containing enzyme glutathione peroxidase and chromium status can be assessed by studies of glucose or cholesterol metabolism.

Though plasma or serum levels are commonly measured (Table 21.7), there is interest in the possibility that other body fluids such as saliva and urine can be used. As already mentioned, however, it is likely that body fluid concentrations may be a poor index of cellular levels. The most accessible cells are the leucocytes and these have been used for the assessment of zinc status (see below).

Hair has certain advantages as a biopsy material, not least the fact that obtaining the sample is virtually non-invasive. Considerable popular interest in hair analysis and the commercial availability of a service has tended to encourage health fanatics and virtually unqualified health 'consultants' to attach considerable importance to the mineral content and to use it as a means of diagnosing all kinds of ailments. Clearly, hair is much more liable to contamination than body fluids or leucocytes and high values for any mineral should probably be viewed with some suspicion. However, providing that the preparation and analysis of the sample is done with appropriate care, low values may well indicate low status, as has been found to be the case for chromium (Hambidge, 1974). There is a tendency to look for a correlation between hair and serum levels, but hair grows slowly and the levels therefore represent mineral status over time – a chronic picture, whereas serum concentrations are subject to acute variations and are subject to the other influences mentioned above. On this basis, any correlations might be surprising rather than expected.

Much of the developing interest in the possible role of trace elements in clinical conditions, such as psychiatric disorders, centres not so much on

Table 21.7 Dietary content, intestinal absorption, recommended dietary intake and serum concentrations of some essential trace minerals

| | Daily dietary content | Intestinal absorption (%) | Recommended dietary intake[3] | Serum concentration ($\mu$g/100 ml) |
|---|---|---|---|---|
| Zinc | 7–17[1] | 10–40 | 15[1] | 80–165 |
| Copper | 1–3[1] | 30 | 2–3[1] | 75–150 |
| Manganese | 1–8[1] | 50 | 2.5–5.0 | 2–3 |
| Chromium | 5–100[2] | 10–25 | 0.05–0.2[1] | – |
| Selenium | 60 (average)[2*] | – | 0.05–0.2[1] | 10–34 |
| Vanadium | 25 (average)[2*] | – | – | 35–48 |
| Iodine | – | – | 50–300† | – |

[1,2] Values are shown [1] in mg, and [2] in $\mu$g
[3] From Recommended Dietary Allowances, Revised 1980. Food and Nutrition Board, National Academy of Sciences – National Research Council
* United States values
† From various sources

deficiency or excess of a single mineral but on relationships between minerals. Changes in ratios of related minerals, such as zinc and copper, may be more important than the absolute concentration of either independently. Such considerations mean that there is a need to determine the concentrations of a number of minerals in the same sample. This adds further to the attraction of hair as a biopsy material.

## Recommended allowances

Requirements for minerals can be determined by carrying out balance studies – measuring the intake in the diet and the output in urine and faeces. In normal adults the difference between input and output should be zero and the person 'in balance'. The requirement would then be the amount required in the diet to equal the amounts lost in urine and faeces. However, other components of the diet, as well as the form in which the mineral is present in food, affect intestinal absorption (Table 21.7). It is therefore not surprising that only recently have attempts been made to provide 'recommended dietary intakes' (Table 21.7). Considering the many factors that affect the intestinal absorption of minerals it is clear that individuals may be 'in balance' on greatly different intakes.

## Assessment of zinc status

The laboratory criteria for the assessment of zinc status are not clearly established. Red blood cells contain approximately 75 per cent of whole blood zinc with plasma containing about 22 per cent (Lindeman, 1985). Thus, only slight haemolysis may be sufficient to significantly raise serum or plasma levels. Levels in these fluids are also raised in conditions in which there is leakage of zinc from tissues that are rich in zinc. This is particularly serious in conditions such as trauma, including burns. In these conditions large amounts of zinc may be excreted in the urine at a time when serum levels are within the normal range. Thus, in conditions in which there is leakage of zinc from cells serial measurements of serum or plasma concentrations should be combined with measurements of the 24-hour urinary excretion of zinc. The plasma zinc concentration in healthy subjects is $112 \pm 12$ μg/dl.

Leucocyte zinc concentrations have been considered to reflect tissue concentrations (Meadows *et al.*, 1981). However, there is evidence that the zinc concentration differs in the different leucocytes so that the leucocyte concentration will be changed in conditions in which there are changes in the leucocyte population.

Zinc is present in parotid saliva but its concentration may be a poor indicator of zinc status (Mathur *et al.*, 1977). Normal levels for hair zinc concentrations are quoted on $193 \pm 18$ μg/g.

Because of uncertainties about the laboratory diagnosis of zinc status it may be that clinical response to zinc supplementation is the most reliable index for diagnosing deficiency (Prasad *et al.*, 1975).

## Conclusions

Many methods have been used to assess nutritional status. The methods to be used in a given situation depend on the nature and severity of the suspected deficiencies. For some nutrients it is only by combining different methods that a reliable assessment can be obtained.

## Acknowledgements

We thank Mrs. S. Holmes for permission to reproduce material from the Proceedings of the 'Nutrition in Nursing Practice' Conference held at the University of Surrey, April, 1986. We are also grateful to Baillière Tindall for permission to reproduce material from 'Nursing'.

## References

Atukorala, S., Basu, T.K., Dickerson, J.W.T. *et al.*, (1979). Vitamin A, zinc and lung cancer. *Br. J. Cancer*, **40**, 927–31.

Bieri, J.G. and Evarts, R.P. (1973). Tocopherols and fatty acids in American diets. *J. Am. Diet. Ass.*, **62**, 147–51.

Bishop, C.W., Bowen, P.E. and Ritchey, S.J. (1981). Norms for nutritional assessment of American adults by upper arm anthropometry. *Am. J. Clin. Nutr.*, **34**, 2530–9.

Bistrian, B.R., Blackburn, G.L., Vitale, J. *et al.*, (1976). Prevalence of malnutrition in general medical patients. *J.A.M.A.*, **235**, 1567–70.

Blackburn, G. (1979). Nutritional assessment and treatment of hospital malnutrition. *Infusiontherapie*, **6**, 238–50.

Blackburn, G.L., Bistrian, B.R., Maini, B.S. *et al.*, (1977). Nutritional and metabolic assessment of the hospitalised patient. *J. Parenteral. Enteral. Nutr.*, **1**, 11–22.

Bourry, J., Milano, G., Caldani, C. and Schneider, M. (1982). Assessment of nutritional proteins during the parenteral nutrition of cancer patients. *Ann. Clin. Lab. Sci.*, **12**, 158–62.

Broden, G., Bark, S., Nordenvall, B. and Backman, L. (1984). Nutritional assessment and post-operative morbidity. A prospective study in 286 consecutive surgical patients. *Acta Chir. Scand.*, (Suppl.), **502**, 27–32.

Bunnell, R.H., Keating, J., Quaresimo, A. and Parman, G.K. (1965). Alpha-tocopherol content of foods. *Am. J. Clin, Nutr.*, **17**, 1–10.

Burke, M. and Bryson, E. (1980). Dietary intakes, resting metabolic rates and body composition in benign and malignant gastrointestinal disease. *Br. Med. J.*, **1**, 211–15.

Buzby, G.P. and Mullen, J.L. (1985). Analysis of nutritional assessment indices: prognostic equations and cluster analysis. In *Nutritional Assessment*, pp. 141–55. Eds. Heymsfield, S. and Wright, R. Blackwell Scientific Publications: Oxford.

Buzby, G.P., Mulen, J.L., Matthews, D.C. *et al.*, (1980). Prognostic nutritional index in gastrointestinal surgery. *Am. J. Surg.*, **139**, 160–67.

Carpentier, Y.A., Barthel, J. and Bruyns, J. (1982). Plasma protein concentration in nutritional assessment. *Proc. Nutr. Soc.*, **41**, 405–17.

Chadwick, S.J.D., Sim, A.J.W. and Dudley, H.A.F. (1986). Changes in plasma fibronectin during acute nutritional deprivation in healthy human subjects. *Br. J. Nutr.*, **55**, 7–12.

Chandra, R.K. and Newberne, P.M. (1977). *Nutrition, Immunity and Infection. Mechanisms of Interaction*. Plenum Press: New York.

Ching, N. and Grossi, C. (1980). The outcome of surgical treatment as related to the response of the serum albumin level to nutritional support. *Surg. Gynec. Obstet.*, **151**, 199–202.

Cruse, P.J. and Foord, R. (1973). A five year prospective study of 23,649 surgical wounds. *Arch. Surg.*, **107**, 206–10.

Dennis, R.S., Long, C.L. and Slickers, K. (1981). A correlation of total iron binding capacity and serum transferrin in a clinical setting. *Fed. Proc.*, **40**, 933 (Abstract).

Department of Health and Social Security (1979). *Recommended daily amounts of energy and nutrients*. Report No. 15. HMSO: London.

Detsky, A.S., Baker, J.P., Mendelson, R.A. *et al.*, (1984). Evaluating the accuracy of nutritional assessment techniques applied to hospitalized patients: methodology and comparisons. *J. Parenteral Enteral. Nutr.*, **8**, 153–9.

Dickerson, J.W.T. (1979). Man's need for vitamins – a need for review? In *The Importance of Vitamins to Human Health*, pp. 1–7. Ed. Taylor, T.G. MTP Press: Lancaster.

Dickerson, J.W.T. (1983). Malnutrition and vitamin and mineral deficiencies and excesses. In *Biochemistry in Clinical Practice*, pp. 113–38. Eds. Williams, D.L. and Marks, V. William Heinemann Medical Books: London.

Dickerson, J.W.T. and Booth, E.M. (1985). Recommended allowances. In *Clinical Nutrition for Nurses, Dietitians and other Health Care Professionals*, pp. 52–64. Faber and Faber: London.

Douville, P., Talbot, J., LaPointe, R. and Balanger, L. (1982). Potential usefulness of serum prealbumin in total parenteral nutrition. (Letter) *Clin. Chem.*, **28**, 1706–1707.

Durnin, J.V.G.A. and Womersley, J. (1974). Body fat assessed from total body density and its estimation from skinfold thickness measurements. *Br. J. Nutr.*, **32**, 77–97.

Eisenberg, D., Silberman, H. and Marynulk, J. (1981). Inapplicability of the prognostic nutritional index in critically ill patients. *Surg. Forum*, **32**, 109–11.

Fell, G.S. (1985). Essential inorganic micronutrients. In *Advances in Diet and Nutrition*, pp. 221–226. Ed. Horwitz, C. John Libbey: London.

Fell, G.S. and Burns, R.R. (1978). Zinc and other trace elements. In *Advances in Parenteral Nutrition*, pp. 241–61. Ed. Johnson, I.D.A. MTP Press: Lancaster.

Fischer, J.E. (1982). Plasma proteins as indicators of nutritional status. In *Nutritional Assessment: Present Status and Future Directions and Prospects*, pp. 25–6. Ed. Levenson, S.M. Report of Second Ross Conference on Medical Research. Ross Laboratories: Columbus, Ohio.

Frisancho, A.R. (1981). New norms of upper limb fat and muscle areas for assessment of nutritional status. *Am. J. Clin. Nutr.*, **34**, 2540–5.

Fürst, P., Bergstrom, J. and Liljedahl, S.O. (1982). Nutritional assessment in severe trauma. In *Nutritional Assessment: Present Status and Future Directions and Prospects*, pp. 26–9. Ed. Levenson, S.M. Report of the Second Ross Conference on Medical Research. Ross Laboratories: Columbus, Ohio.

Grant, J. (1981). Current techniques of nutritional assessment. *Surg. Clin. N. Amer.*, **61**, 437–63.

Gross, R.L. and Newberne, P.M. (1980). Role of nutrition in immunologic function. *Physiol. Rev.*, **60**, 188–302.

Grossman, J.E., Demling, R.H., Duy, N.D. and Mosher, D.F. (1980). Response of plasma fibronectin to major body burns. *J. Trauma*, **20**, 967–70.

Hambidge, K.M. (1974). Chromium nutrition in man. *Am. J. Clin. Nutr.*, **27**, 505–14.

Harries, A.D., Jones, L.A., Heatley, R.V. and Rhodes, J. (1983). Assessment of nutritional status by anthropometry: a comparison of different standards of reference. *Hum. Nutr.: Clin. Nutr.*, **37C**, 227–31.

Hartley, T.F. and Lee, H.A. (1975). A method of determining daily nitrogen requirements. *Postgrad. Med. J.*, **51**, 441–5.

Harvey, K.B., Ruggiero, C.S. and Regan, C.S. (1978). Hospital morbidity – mortality risk factors using nutritional assessment. *Clin. Res.*, **26**, 581A (Abstract).

Heymsfield, S.B., McManus, C.B., Seitz, S.B. *et al.*, (1985). Anthropometric assessment of adult protein-energy malnutrition. In *Nutritional Assessment*, pp. 27–82. Eds. Wright, R.A., and Heymsfield, S.B. Blackwell Scientific Publications: Oxford.

Heymsfield, S.B., McManus, C., Smith, J. *et al.*, (1982). Anthropometric measurement of muscle mass: equations for calculating bone-free muscle mass. *Am. J. Clin. Nutr.*, **36**, 680–90.

Hill, G.L., Blackett, R.L., Pickford, I. *et al.*, (1977). Malnutrition in surgical patients: an unrecognised problem. *Lancet*, **i**, 689–92.

Ingenbleek, Y., Can den Shriek, H.G., De Nayer, P. *et al.*, (1975). Albumin, transferrin and thyroxine binding prealbumin/retinol binding protein (TBA/RBP) complex in assessment of malnutrition. *Clin. Chim. Acta.*, **63**, 61–7.

Jelliffe, D.B. (1966). *The assessment of nutritional status of the community. WHO Monograph No. 53.* WHO: Geneva.

Jensen, T.G. (1983). *Nutritional assessment: a manual for practitioners.* Appleton Century Crofts: Hartford CT.

Jung, S. (1986). Blood fibronectin changes in various neoplasms. *Presse Med.*, **15**, 197–8: 203–204 (English Abstract).

Klidjian, A.M., Foster, K.J., Kammerling, R.M. *et al.*, (1980). Relation of anthropometric and dynamometric variables to serious post-operative complications. *Br. Med. J.*, **281**, 899–901.

Knight, I. (1984). *The heights and weights of adults in Great Britain.* Office of Population Censuses and Surveys. HMSO: London.

Law, D.K., Dudrick, S.J. and Abdou, N.I. (1974). The effects of protein-calorie malnutrition on immune competence of the surgical patient. *Surg. Gynaecol. Obstet.*, **139**, 257–66.

Lindeman, R.D. (1985). Assessment of trace element depletion. In *Nutritional Assessment*, pp. 239–61. Eds. Wright, R.A., and Heymsfield, S.B. Blackwell Scientific Publications: Oxford.

Lipschitz, D.A. and Mitchell, C.O. (1985). Nutritional assessment of the elderly: special considerations. In: *Nutritional Assessment*, pp. 131–9. Eds. Wright, R.A. and Heymsfield, S.B. Blackwell Scientific Publications: Oxford.

Long, C. (1985). The energy and protein requirements of the critically ill. In *Nutritional Assessment*, pp. 157–81. Eds. Wright, R.A. and Heymsfield, S.B. Blackwell Scientific Publications: London.

Lopes, J., Russell, D. McR., Whitwell, J. and JeeJeeBhoy, K.N. (1980). Skeletal muscle function in malnutrition. *Am. J. Clin. Nutr.*, **36**, 602–609.

Losowsky, M.S. (1979). Vitamin E in human nutrition. In *The Importance of Vitamins to Human Health*, pp. 101–10. Ed. Taylor, T.G. MTP Press: Lancaster.

Macleod, C.C. (1974). *Methods of Dietary Assessment.* Gerontological Research Unit Publication. Department of Geriatric Medicine, University of Glasgow.

Marr, J.W. (1971). Individual dietary surveys: purposes and methods. *World Rev. Nutr. Diet.*, **13**, 105–64.

Martin, S., Neale, G. and Elia, M. (1985). Factors affecting maximal momentary grip strength. *Hum. Nutr.: Clin. Nutr.*, **39C**, 137–47.

Mathur, A., Wallenius, K. and Abdulla, M. (1977). Relation between zinc content in saliva and blood in healthy human adults. *Scand. J. Clin. Lab. Invest.*, **37**, 469–72.

Meadows, N.J., Ruse, W., Smith, M.F. *et al.*, (1981). Zinc and small babies. *Lancet*, **ii**, 1135–6.

Meakins, J.L., Pietsch, J.B., Bubenick, O., *et al.*, (1977). Delayed hypersensitivity: indicator of acquired failure of host defences in sepsis and trauma. *Ann. Surg.*, **186**, 241–9.

Metropolitan Life Insurance Company. *Statistical Bulletin (1959). 40*, Nov–Dec. and

(1979) *Build Study*: Society of Actuaries and Association of Life Insurance Medical Directors of America, Courtesy of Metropolitan Life.

Miller, S.F., Morath, M.A. and Finley, R.K. (1981). Comparison of derived and actual transferrin: A potential source of error in clinical assessment. *J. Trauma*, **21**, 548–50.

Millward, D.J., Bates, P.C., Broadbent, P. and Rennie, M.J. (1982). Sources of 3-methylhistidine in the body. In *Clinical Nutrition '81*. Proceedings of IIIrd. European Congress on Parenteral and Enteral Nutrition, pp. 190–203. Ed. Wesdorp, R.I.C. Churchill–Livingstone: Edinburgh.

Mitchell, C.O. and Lipschitz, D.A. (1982). Arm length measurement as an alternative to height in nutritional assessment of the elderly. *J. Parenteral Enterol. Nutr.*, **6**, 226–9.

Morgan, D.B., Hill, G.L. and Burkinshaw, L. (1980). The assessment of weight loss from a single measurement of body weight: The problems and limitations. *Am. J. Clin. Nutr.*, **33**, 2101–5.

Mullen, J.L. and Buzby, G.P. (1979). Prediction of operative morbidity and mortality by preoperative nutritional assessment. *Surg. Forum*, **30**, 80–82.

Mullen, J.L., Buzby, G.P. and Matthews, D.C. (1980). Reduction of operative morbidity and mortality by combined preoperative and post-operative nutritional support. *Ann. Surg.*, **192**, 604–13.

National Center for Health Statistics (1979). *Weight by height and age for adults 18–74 years: United States 1971–74* Rockville, M.D.: (Vital and Health Statistics. Series 11: Data from the National Health Survey, No. 208). (DHEW publication No. (PHS) 79–1656).

Paul, A. and Southgate, D.A.T. (1978). *McCance and Widdowson's 'The composition of foods'* (4th. ed.) MRC Special Report No. 297. HMSO: London.

Pike, R.L. and Brown, M.L. (1975). *Nutrition: An integrated approach*. 2nd ed. p. 195. John Wiley and Sons: Chichester.

Platt, B.S. (1962). *Tables of representative values of foods commonly used in tropical countries*. MRC Special Representative Service. No. 302. HMSO: London.

Prasad, A.S., Schoomaker, E.B., Ortega, J. *et al.*, (1975). Zinc deficiency in sickle cell disease. *Clin. Chem.*, **21**, 582–7.

Rainey-MacDonald, C.G., Holliday, R.L., Wells, G.A. and Donner, A.P. (1983). Validity of a two variable nutritional index for use in selecting candidates for nutritional support. *J. Parenteral Enteral. Nutr.*, **7**, 15–20.

Rennie, M.J. and Millward, D.J. (1983). 3-Methylhistidine excretion and the urinary 3-methylhistidine creatinine ratio are poor indicators of skeletal muscle breakdown. *Clin. Sci.*, **65**, 217–25.

Roche, A.F. (1982). Anthropometric variables effectiveness and limitations. In *Assessing Nutritional Status of the Elderly: State of the Art*. p. 22. Ross Laboratories: Columbus, Ohio.

Rosalki, S.B. (1979). Clinical biochemistry of vitamin $B_6$. In *The Importance of Vitamins to Human Health*. pp. 53–60. Ed. Taylor, T.G. MTP Press: Lancaster.

Russell, D.M., Atwood, H.L. and JeeJeeBhoy, K.N. (1985). Nitrogen versus muscle calcium in the genesis of abnormal muscle function in malnutrition. *J. Parenteral Enteral. Nutr.*, **9**, 415–21.

Saba, T.M. (1975). Reticulo-endothelial system host defence after surgery and traumatic shock. *Circ. Shock*, **2**, 91–108.

Scott, R.L., Sohmer, P.R. and MacDonald, M.G. (1982). The effect of starvation and repletion on plasma fibronectin in man. *J.A.M.A.*, **248**, 2025–7.

Scovill, W.A., Saba, T.M. Blumenstock, F.A., *et al.*, (1978). Opsonic alpha - 2 surface binding glycoprotein therapy during sepsis. *Ann. Surg.*, **188**, 521–9.

Selhub, J. and Rosenberg, I.H. (1985). Assessment of vitamin depletion. In *Nutritional Assessment*. pp. 209–38. Eds. Wright, R.A., and Heymsfield, S.B. Blackwell Scientific Publications: Oxford.

Seltzer, M.H., Bastidas, J.A., Cooper, D.M., *et al.*, (1979). Instant nutritional assessment. *J. Parenteral Enteral. Nutr.*, **3**, 157–9.
Seltzer, M.H., Slocum, B.A., Cataldi-Betcher, E.L. *et al.*, (1982). Instant nutritional assessment: Absolute weight loss and surgical mortality. *J. Parenteral Enteral. Nutr.*, **6**, 218–21.
Sherman, M., Brickner, P.W., Greenbaum, D. *et al.*, (1983). Nutritional parameters in homebound persons of greatly advanced age. *J. Parenteral Enteral. Nutr.*, **7**, 378–80.
Shetty, P.S., Watrasiewicz, K.E., Jung, R.T. and James, W.P.T. (1979). Rapid-turnover transport proteins: an index of subclinical protein-energy malnutrition. *Lancet*, **ii**, 230–32.
Silk, D.B.A. (1983). *Nutritional Support in Hospital Practice*. Blackwell Scientific Publications: Oxford.
Simms, J.M. and Smith, J.A.R. (1981). A prognostic index for surgical patients. *J. Parenteral. Enteral. Nutr.*, **5**, 353.
Smale, B.F., Mullen, J.L. and Buzby, G.P. (1979). Prognostic nutritional index in cancer surgery. *Proc. Amer. Soc. Clin. Oncol.*, **20**, 336. (Abstract).
Smith, C.L., Kelleher, J., Losowsky, M.S. and Morrish, N. (1971). The content of vitamin E in British diets. *Br. J. Nutr.*, **26**, 89–96.
Solomons, N.W. and Allen, L.H. (1983). The functional assessment of nutritional status: principles, practice and potential. *Nutr. Rev.*, **41**, 33–50.
Steffee, W. (1980). Malnutrition in hospital patients. *J.A.M.A.*, **244**, 2630–35.
Taylor, K.B. and Anthony, L.E. (1983). *Clinical Nutrition*. p. 31. McGraw-Hill: New York.
Vir, S.C. and Love, A.H. (1980). Anthropometric measurements in the elderly. *Gerontology*, **26**, 1–8.
Webster, J. and Garrow, J.S. (1985). Creatinine excretion over 24 hours as a measure of body composition or of completeness of urine collection. *Hum. Nutr.: Clin. Nutr.*, **39**, 101–106.
Weinsier, R.L., Hunker, E.M., Krumdieck, C.L. and Butterworth, C.E. (1979). Hospital malnutrition: a prospective evaluation of general medical patients during the course of hospitalization. *Am. J. Clin. Nutr.*, **32**, 418–26.
Witting, L.A. (1974). Vitamin E – polyunsaturated lipid relationship in diet and tissues. *Am. J. Clin. Nutr.*, **27**, 952–9.

# 22 Enteral feeding

Harry A. Lee



## Introduction

Malnourishment occurs, or soon develops, in many patients after an acute illness or operation. It is also seen in patients who have been in an Intensive Care Unit or in the elderly entering a geriatric ward. There has been a tendency in the past to think of nutritional support for such patients only in terms of total parenteral nutrition (TPN). However, over the past 10 years there have been considerable advances with tube feeding, otherwise known as nasogastric or naso-enteral feeding. The commercial preparations are very acceptable nutritionally, their efficacy undoubted and the delivery systems used much easier to manipulate by the nursing staff. All too often, when there is perfectly normal gut function TPN is inappropriately used which is much more costly and difficult to administer. Enteral nutrition has been the 'Cinderella' of metabolic/nutritional support yet should occupy a place of paramount importance. The majority of patients who require aggressive comprehensive nutritional support can have this by the enteral route. Enteral feeding should not be seen simply as the cheap and ready way of providing nutritional support but it, too, like TPN, requires careful consideration, careful patient assessment, choosing the best preparation, making sure the right prescription is written with respect to all macro and micro nutrient requirements. It needs collaboration between nutritional support staff and nursing staff to make sure that the whole feed is given over a given period. No longer are commercial preparations seen as convenience feeds but as scientifically prepared diets which completely meet a patient's needs and which, in fact, do not prove more costly than using the former blenderized hospital food approach which is often suspect from bacteriological contamination.

Many ill patients are simply too weak or lack motivation to want to eat of their own accord. This relative anorexia does not mean the gastrointestinal tract is not functional and, therefore, one must proceed immediately to TPN. Furthermore, there is still far too much laxity in noticing what a patient does not eat rather than what he does eat. It is therefore the responsibility of nursing staff to carefully document rejects so that the attendant clinicians really do have an idea what the patients are actually taking, not only to meet their basic requirements, but also to meet previous losses or excess losses as a result of their catabolic status. There can be no excuse for delay in instituting enteral nutrition which is a very economic and safe way of providing nutritional support with modest facilities.

## Physiology of starvation

Many studies have shown the adaptive response of the body to cachexia and starvation. Thus, protein breakdown is minimized and the body draws upon its fat reserve for the major energy contribution. Thus, the starving individual becomes keto adapted, the ketones providing an important energy source. However, one should not confuse the adaptive physiological mechanisms of starvation with that of acute malnutrition that complicates many critically ill patients. Unfortunately, when physicians do ward rounds they rarely state 'this patient is starving' or has gone into negative nitrogen balance. Nevertheless, careful consideration of the total patient profile will often show they have features of negative nitrogen balance (see Table 22.1). It is important, therefore, that enteric sources of nutrition supply energy that approximates to a normal dietary intake (i.e., 50 per cent carbohydrate, 50 per cent fat) and that whole protein together with full electrolyte, vitamin, essential biological elements requirements are given. It is well understood that in the postoperative phase there is a tendency for salt and water retention due to ADH activity which often results in hyponatraemia, often the prime occupation of many clinicians. Again, there can be no excuse for delaying the commencement of enteral nutrition, for the longer the delay, the more rapid the depletion of intestinal mucosal enzyme content therefore making later absorption of enteric nutrients more difficult.

Therefore, the question asked of the clinician when a patient requires nutritional support is, which route should be used? There is only one real answer to this and that is whether or not the gastrointestinal tract is functional. If it is, then use it, by naso-gastric route, by naso-enteric route, or by feeding jejunostomy. The practical approach to this question is shown in Fig. 22.1. The advantages of sip feeding should not be underestimated in the debilitated patient. Commercially prepared sip feeds given over a 24-hour period can provide 60 g of protein and 2000 kcals quite readily, whilst still allowing the patient to 'pick at' other hospital food. It is important whenever one considers nutritional support in hospital that this (sip feed) is distributed over the normal

Table 22.1 Clinical associations with negative nitrogen balance

| |
|---|
| Loss of body weight |
| Diminished muscle mass |
| Hypoproteinaemic oedema |
| Impaired immunocompetence – humoral and cellular |
| Increased susceptibility to infection |
| Poor wound healing; dehiscence |
| Apathy |
| Increased morbidity and mortality |

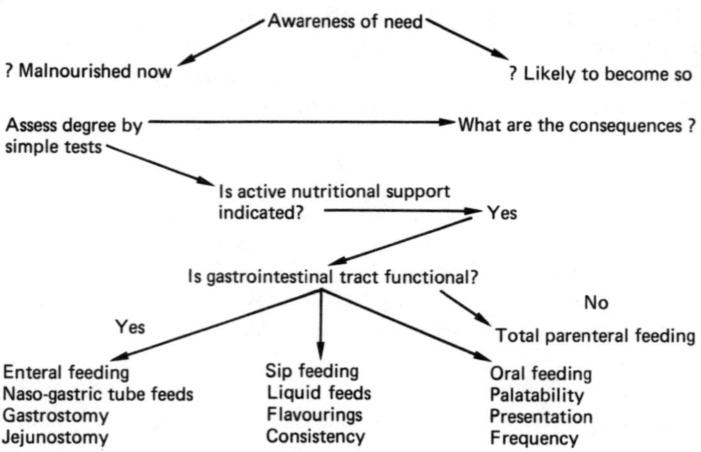


Fig. 22.1 Which nutritional treatment?

feedings hours of daytime and not condensed simply into some 8 hours or less to suit nursing and other administrative practices.

Having decided what route to use, the next question is what is available? Nowadays, there are a number of ACBS approved nutrient preparations (List A and B, BNF) which really cover the whole range of clinical demands. In my view there is no need for specific preparations orientated towards specific end-organ failure. The whole protein feeds containing energy sources (both carbohydrate and fat) or simply protein sources to which carbohydrate and fat sources can be added (Table 22.2) fully meet nutritional requirements of all patients. When considering enteral nutrition nitrogen sources the choice is between protein containing diets, predigested chemically defined elemental diets and only rarely special formulations (also predigested) for such conditions as liver failure. However, if the gut is normal use whole protein preparations. Questions arise as to whether peptide preparations are required. Further studies are required but in general it is safe to use whole protein preparations in all patients with normal gut function but where there is uncertainty about gut function the newer peptide preparations such as 'Nutranel' and 'Reabilan' may have a useful role. These remarks, of course, relate to adult nutrition only. It must be emphasized that many of the commercially available enteric feeds are not suitable as a source of sole nutrition for the infant or very young adult. It is now common practice for many hospitals to hold a limited 'pantry' of commercially available nutritional products which makes life much easier for the prescribing physician (Table 22.3). Having decided what he requires for his patient, this is then interpreted by the dietitian using commercial preparations and making them up to an appropriate volume. Another important factor is that the commercial preparations are not only being very cost effective but are absolutely sterile and free from bacterial contamination. This has certainly been far from the case with respect to hospital kitchen prepared blenderized tube feeds. On the other hand, it must be made clear that the whole question of enteral feed contamination causing septicaemia in adult patients has been grossly overstated.

Table 22.2 Nutritional support for adults (from Advisory Committee on Borderline Substances (ACBS) – List B)

A. a. *Nutritionally complete feeds* (chemically defined diets – whole protein based) – for oral, sip or tube feeding.
  1. *Gluten free*
   Clinifeed
   Fortisip Energy-Plus
   Fortisip Standard
   Fortison Energy-Plus
   Fortison Standard
   Triosorbon

'There is a cross index listing clinical conditions and the products which the ACBS has approved for the management of those conditions. It is essential to consult List A for more precise guidance.'

  2. *Lactose and gluten free*
   Ensure
   Ensure Plus
   Ensure Powder
   Isocal
   MCT (1) Powder (with appropriate vitamin and mineral supplements)
   Nutrauxil Liquid and Sip
   Portagen

 b. *Elemental and low lactose*
  Flexical
  Nutranel
  Vivonex

B. *Nutritional source supplements*
 See synthetic diets
  malabsorption states
 a. *Carbohydrates* – lactose free and gluten free
  Calonutrin
  Caloreen*
  Fortical*
  Hycal*
  Maxijul
  Maxijul LE*
  Polycal
  * Have low electrolyte content
 b. *Fat*
  Calogen
  Prosparol
  Medium chain triglycerides
  Alembicol D
  MCT oil
  Liquigen

C. *Nitrogen sources*
 Albumaid complete (hydrolysed protein based)
 Casilan (whole protein based, low sodium)
 Forceval protein (whole protein based, low sodium)
 Maxipro HBV (whole protein based, low sodium)

D. *Minerals*
 Aminogran mineral mixture
 Metabolic mineral mixture

Table 22.3 (a) Request for nutritional support. (b) Commonly used standard regimens

Request for nutritional support.
(St. Mary's Hospital, Portsmouth)

Patient's Name:.................... D.O.B. .................... Hosp. No ....................
Ward .................... Consultant ....................
Clinical Details

Prescription:

| | | | |
|---|---|---|---|
| Protein | g/day | Energy | Kcal/day |
| Electrolyte: e.g. | Na | K | mmol/day |

Enteral

Nasogastric – Preferably one of the standard regimens overleaf A.B.C.D.
Oral/sip Feeds Will be supplied by the Dietition from a range of products

| Standard Regimen IV or Enteral | Composition | Start time and Duration | Signature | Date |
|---|---|---|---|---|
| | | | | |
| | | | | |
| | | | | |
| | | | | |
| | | | | |

In case of doubt or technical difficulty please contact the Nutrition Support Team through the Dietition or the Clinical Nutrition Nurse or Pharmacy

(b)

| Enteral | Volume (ml) | Protein (Nitrogen g) | Energy kcal (Non protein) | Na mmol | K mmol | Ca mmol | Cl mmol | $PO_4$ mmol |
|---|---|---|---|---|---|---|---|---|
| A. Clinifeed ISO 6 units × 375 ml | 2250 | 63 (10) | 2250 (2000) | 34 | 86 | 34 | 66 | 30 |
| B. Clinifeed Favour 6 units × 375 ml | 2250 | 85 (14) | 2250 (1900) | 68 | 64 | 26 | 73 | 29 |
| C. Nutrauxil (also Fresubin) 6 units × 500 ml | 3000 | 114 (18) | 3000 (2545) | 99 | 96 | 37 | 99 | 58 |
| D. Fortison Standard 6 units × 500 ml | 3000 | 120 (19) | 3000 (2520) | 105 | 115 | 37 | 67 | 48 |

1. Fine bore tube (1 mm = Gauge 6; 1.5 mm = Gauge 8) is preferable; (up to Gauge 10 acceptable) – gravity feed will normally suffice. Enteral pump may be available on request.
2. Ensure continuous flow and not bolus feeding.
3. Label the reservoir/bottle clearly.
4. For patients who have not been fed for 4–5 days begin with ½ strength, but full volume of feed.
5. If cartons of feed supplied from diet kitchen these must be completely stored in the fridge.

Some idea of external secretions from the body is important in compiling the electrolyte constituents required in any enteral feed (Table 22.4).

Although there has been a tendency to over-prescribe energy and nitrogen for patients receiving TPN this has been less so with enteral approaches. The requirements for patients are still of the same order of 30–35 kcals/kg body weight energy divided preferably on an equi-energetic basis between carbohydrate and fat and 0.2 g of nitrogen/kg body weight. The preparations must contain sufficient amounts of sodium, potassium, calcium, magnesium and, of course, vitamins and essential biological elements, particularly copper and zinc. Most whole protein feeds nowadays contain adequate amounts of essential fatty acids.

In addition to these essential principles of enteric feeding, other points need careful consideration (see Table 22.4). It is generally accepted that the placement of a fine-bore nasogastric or naso-enteric tube is a basic prerequisite for good enteric feeding. Such tubes have an internal diameter of either 1.0 or 1.5 mm and these tubes are easy to place and can be maintained long-term, be that in hospital or at home. The frequency of changing such tubes can now be as infrequent as once per month. In certain situations a nasogastric or naso-enteric tube can be placed at the time of operation. For example, it is well known that in gastric surgery, gastric atony may persist for some days even though small intestinal function returns rapidly after operation. Elsewhere, for example, in head and neck surgery, it is sensible to place a fine-bore tube at the end of operation so that this route is available for nutritional support whereas it might be difficult or impossible to place such a tube postoperative. Another myth that has pervaded modern tube feeding is that after placement of a fine-bore tube a chest X-ray must be taken. There are simple tests such as blowing air down the feeding tube and listening to bubbling over the stomach

Table 22.4 Composition of some body external secretions (after Lee, 1974)

| Secretion | Sodium mmol/litre | Potassium mmol/litre | Chloride mmol/litre | Bicarbonate mmol/litre | Volume litre/24 h |
|---|---|---|---|---|---|
| Parotid saliva | 112 | 19 | 40 | – | 1.5 |
| Gastric juice | 50 (10–110) | 15 (5–40) | 140 (125–150) | 0–15 | 2–3 |
| Pancreatic juice | 130 (110–160) | 5 (2–10) | 55 (40–95) | 110 | 0.5–1 |
| Bile | 145 (130–160) | 5 (2–10) | 100 (90–120) | 38 | 0.5–1 |
| Jejunal juice | 140 | – | 130 | Variable | – |
| Ileal juice | 140 | 11 | 70 | Variable | – |
| Succus entericus | 80–150 | 2–8 | 40–135 | 20–40 | 3 |
| Ileostomy (adapted) | 50 | 4 | 25 | – | 0.5 |
| Colostomy | 60 | 15 | 40 | – | 0.1–0.2 |
| Diarrhoea | 30–140 | 30–70 | – | 20–80 | Variable |
| Normal stool | 20–40 | 30–60 | 20 | – | 0.1 |
| Insensible sweat | 12 | 10 | 12 | – | 0.5 |
| Visible sweat/°C | 58 | 10 | 45 | – | 0.5 |

or simply aspirating a millilitre or two (which can be done from such tubes) and testing against litmus paper. It is completely illogical that tubes are sometimes placed and that there is another 24-hour delay before patients receive any feeding because of the insistence that a chest X-ray is mandatory.

There is also the important question of osmolar loading with tube feeding and the inducement of diarrhoea. All too often tube feeding is blamed as a cause of diarrhoea when, in fact, it is bad practice that causes this. The overriding principle to remember is that it is osmolar loading per unit time and not per unit volume that often causes profound diarrhoea. Again, a common problem is failure to adequately dilute feed in the mistaken belief that too much fluid is likely to precipitate the elderly patient into congestive cardiac failure. Thus, the principle of continuous flow feeding as opposed to bolus feeding is mandatory.

It must be appreciated with enteral feeding, as opposed to parenteral feeding, that one usually has to gradually build up the full dosage of nutritional support over a 2–3 day period dependent upon the length of pre-existing period of malnutrition. Before assuming that the enteral feed is the cause of diarrhoea, one should carefully check a patient's therapeutic chart as to whether he is receiving drugs, e.g., antibiotics, in particular, which are notorious for producing diarrhoea. By and large, provided that adequately diluted feeds are used in a continuous feeding system, then diarrhoea is a particularly rare occurrence. If it does occur, then it is reasonable to give codeine phosphate syrup (30–60 mg b.d.) to control it. At the other end of the scale when regurgitation occurs, metaclopramide may be used to overcome delayed gastric emptying.

The whole question of osmolar loading can best be illustrated by the effect of enteral feeding on the immature kidney in the infant. If too much nitrogen is given without any water a solute diuresis (urea induced) will occur leading to hyperosmolar dehydration. One gram of urea equals approximately 0.5 g of nitrogen which equals 3 g of protein, and 1 g of urea equals 17 mmol. Thus, if a patient receives a diet containing 60 g of protein with 60 mmol of sodium and say 60 mmol of potassium, he would have an osmolar load to excrete of 460 mmol. If then his urine concentration ability was only 300 mmol/litre he would require a minimal urine volume of 1.5 litres daily to excrete this solute load. Then allowing for 1 litre daily for essential losses his tube feed will have to be diluted to a minimum of 2.5 litres in order to maintain normal water balance. The glucose contribution, assuming that it is non-excessive, from the diet does not need to be considered provided that hyperglycaemia does not occur as glucose is metabolized to water, $CO_2$ and energy production. Thus, tube feeding in infants, as well as in the elderly needs to be tailored within reason to the limits of renal function. The question of dilution needs to be further tempered against the known fact that if a patient is pyrexial, then water losses are accentuated and for every degree centrigrade elevation an extra 500–750 ml of water must be given.

## Patient assessment and monitoring

The parameters for patient assessment are exactly the same as given in the following chapter concerning TPN (see Table 23.3). As with any other therapeutic modality it is important to measure the initial state of malnutrition

Table 22.5 Potential complications of enteral feeding

1. Unpalatability (orally taken feeds)
2. Nasopharyngeal ulceration if large, inflexible NG tubes used
3. Gastric erosions (dependent upon type of NG tube)
4. Aspiration (particularly in elderly and debilitated or comatose patients)
5. Gastric retention
6. Nausea, vomiting, cramps
7. Diarrhoea
8. Disturbances of water balance
   a Hypertonic dehydration
   b Hyperosmolar non-ketonic coma
   c Osmotic diuresis (e.g. hyperglycaemia)
9. Skin rashes e.g. Zn or EFAD
10. Hypoprothrombinaemia
11. Essential biological element deficiency
12. Essential fatty acid deficiency (EFAD)

Table 22.6 Monitoring enteral feeding

1. Daily weight (in kg)
2. Urine volume; fluid balance
3. Stool frequency, consistency and volume
4. Serum and urine osmolarities
5. Blood glucose
6. PCV and haemoglobin
7. Serum electrolytes, urea and creatinine
8. Urine electrolytes and urea
9. Serum albumin, transferrin and complement C3
10. Weekly skin fold thickness and mid arm muscle circumference

and then to ensure that the therapeutic modality used is actually effective in combating or improving the situation under treatment. There can be no excuse for simply giving enteral nutrition and hoping for the best.

It is well recognized that metabolic complications of enteral nutrition are very limited. One could give an exhaustive list of potential complications but really these are minimal and the most frequent are as indicated in Table 22.5. Indeed, the infrequency of complications of enteral nutrition ranks amongst the other advantages, which include wide application, ease of administration, cost effectiveness, minimal personnel involvement, availability, simplicity and flexibility. The amount of monitoring required in such patents is minimal as indicated in Table 22.6. It is important to realize, as with parenteral nutrition, enteral feeding can induce liver enzymes and thus it is not unusual to see elevations of serum alkaline phosphatase, serum $\gamma$ GT and 5NT soon after starting enteral nutrition.

## Delivery system

It is now well established that when using commercial feeds these are best diluted in the diet kitchen and delivered as a total volume in two or three aliquots to the ward. However, it is important to brief the ward staff that such aliquots should not be stored on radiators, on top of cookers or elsewhere, but within the refrigerator. Otherwise, there is the real risk of secondary bacterial contamination. All commercial feeds, even though many are presented as isotonic preparations, can still be diluted at the preliminary introduction of enteral feeding. All too often at ward level there is far too much emphasis on provision of fluid allowance only and not taking into account nutritional requirements. Therefore, it is better if enteral feeds are diluted to a degree that takes into account the full fluid requirements of patients, thus preventing further manipulation of these feeds at ward level.

All commercially available preparations are capable of delivery by the fine-bore nasogastric/enteric tube. As for the containers to deliver the enteral feed, these vary from bottles and bags to cannisters, which in turn may be delivered by gravity feed or enteral feed pumps of which there are a growing number available on the market, all of which are reasonably priced. In the critically ill patient, as with parenteral nutrition, it is often advisable that enteral feeds are delivered via pump systems to ensure a continuous even delivery thus avoiding a major complication, e.g. diarrhoea, whilst at the same time ensuring proper delivery over a 24-hour period of the nutritional requirements. In the home setting, where enteral feeding is practised by community nurses and, indeed, relatives of the ill patient, it is sufficient to rely upon gravity feeding.

## Application

As initially stated, whenever a patient requires nutritional support and has a functional gastrointestinal tract, then enteral feeding is the normal approach. This applies to oral feeding, sip feeding, nasogastric, naso-enteral and, to a much lesser degree in this country, feeding via gastrostomies or jejunostomies. It must be emphasized that there is no diagnostic index of indications for enteral feeding. When a patient is unable to take adequate nutritional support voluntarily, but has a normal gastrointestinal tract, then nasogastric/enteric feeding becomes mandatory. There are now commercially available preparations which need very little tailoring for individual patient requirements (see Table 22.2). Thus, any acutely ill patient can be fed in this manner, not to mention those who have equally dramatic onset of their illnesses, but are not hypercatabolic by definition. I refer to such patients who have had strokes or elderly patients coming into geriatric wards with a previous history of poor nutritional intake. All of these patients can benefit dramatically by prompt application of nasogastric feeding and provided the rules are observed, respond very quickly and without complications to this approach.

It must not be forgotten that when patients are being weaned from TPN there often is a period of up to 1 week when an equivalent amount of nasogastric feeding is given to compensate for the equal withdrawal of TPN. There can be little doubt that many elderly patients are admitted to hospital in a malnourished state and are also confused and can benefit dramatically by nasogastric feeding. As mentioned in an earlier chapter, fine-bore tube nasogastric feeding can have a dramatic impact upon the anorexia nervosa patient. Finally, many elderly patients who hitherto have been kept in hospital simply for nutritional support can now be managed in the community as a result of fine-bore nasogastric feeding practices. It has now become the norm for community nurses to attend many day release courses on nutritional support of critically ill and chronically ill patients.

## Further reading


Bothe, A., Wade, J.E. and Blackburn, G. (1981). *Enteral Nutrition – an Overview in Nutrition and the Surgical Patient*, pp. 76–103 Ed. Hill, G.L. Churchill Livingstone: Edinburgh.

Grant, A. and Todd, E. (Eds.) (1982). *Enteral and Parenteral Nutrition: A Clinical Handbook*. Blackwell Scientific Publications: Oxford.

Johnston, I.D.A. and Lee, H.A. (eds). (1979). *Developments in Clinical Nutrition. Research and Clinical Forums* 1. No. 1 MCS Consultants: Tunbridge Wells.

Karran, S.J. and Alberti, K.G.M.M. (eds). (1980). *Practical Nutritional Support*. Pitman Medical: Tunbridge Wells.

Lee, H.A. (1981). Choice of methods: enteral or parenteral nutrition. In *Parenteral and Enteral Nutrition*. Eds. Wright, P.D. and Elliott, M. *Acta Chir. Scand.* (Suppl.) **507**, 181–90. W.B. Bett Ltd.: Tillicoultry.

Russell, R.I. (1986). Enteral feeding. In *Clinical Nutrition in Gastroenterology*, pp. 97–115. Eds. Heatley, R.V. Losowsky, M.S. and Kelleher, J. Churchill Livingstone: Edinburgh.

# 23 Parenteral nutrition

Harry A. Lee



## Introduction

Many surveys have shown that the incidence of clinical malnutrition amongst all acute hospital admissions may be as high as 45–50 per cent although only some 15 per cent at most will require energetic nutritional support. Nevertheless, it is important to emphasize that it has been shown that malnourished hospital patients continue to lose weight whilst in hospital and therefore hospitalization stay is prolonged and morbidity is increased. Probably of the 15 per cent requiring careful nutritional support, about one-third will require parenteral nutrition. The absolute indication for parenteral nutrition is gastro-intestinal failure, though on occasion there will be patients who require simultaneously both forms of nutritional support. Previously there has been too much parenteral nutrition practised when enteral nutrition would suffice. It is important to remember that anorexia ends at the mouth and that many such patients have perfectly normal gastrointestinal tracts.

For a long while many clinicians have considered that parenteral nutrition should be handled by specialists, and therefore many patients in outlying hospitals have not benefited from this therapeutic procedure. The prescription and provision of parenteral nutrition has been simplified with advances over the past 10 years. Many hospitals have Nutritional Support teams whose members include physicians, surgeons, pharmacists, dietitians and nurses able to help a clinician with any parenteral nutritional regimen.

Much is now understood about the metabolic response to trauma and stress and how best this can be contained by appropriate therapeutic manoeuvres. It is known that the carbohydrate (glycogen) reserves are rapidly utilized and that in the majority of patients fat energy reserves are then called upon which together with gluconeogenetic processes maintain a supply of fuel for vital tissue processes. However, it has been shown that 10 per cent of all patients are not able to immediately draw upon their fat reserves for reasons which are not yet clear and, therefore, such patients do not become immediately 'keto adapted'. These patients tend to go into a greater degree of negative nitrogen imbalance and have a higher morbidity and mortality rate.

In addition to the dissolution of energy reserves in the body, the body muscle mass is also reduced as part of the process of gluconeogenesis induced by adrenal cortical hormones. Thus, muscle protein reserves are rapidly broken down and the nitrogen and carbon residues from amino acid and glucose metabolism respectively combine to form alanine which is then taken to the liver (alanine shuttle) and incorporated via gluconeogenic process into production of more glucose, the nitrogen residue appearing as urinary urea which is a useful marker of the catabolic response. Over the years many studies have been undertaken to see whether drugs might modify or reduce the catabolic response to trauma but in reality no useful drug has been found which has practical or clinical significance. Although it has been shown that nursing patients with burns in a high environmental temperature can reduce the catabolic response, this is a rather isolated example of environmental or therapeutic manipulation to modify the metabolic response.

Thus, any individual who has severe trauma complicated by multiple operations and infection is bound to waste with the attendant consequences if he cannot maintain an adequate oral intake, be that voluntarily or by nasogastric or naso-enteric route. It is in just this sort of patient that 'starvation in the midst of plenty' may continue with disastrous results. For the patient who cannot, must not or will not take adequate oral nutrition, then parenteral nutrition is the answer.

There is still too often the tendency to delay far too long before instituting complete parenteral nutrition. In my view there is no place for partial parenteral nutrition (protein sparing therapy); a patient either requires full enteral support or parenteral support and half way measures only cloud the issues and complicate matters.

Previously, there has been far too much discussion about which energy substrates to use, which type of amino acid preparations were required and whether or not certain nutrients could be mixed in a 3 litre bag. Nowadays, the whole issue is simplified as many pharmacies can now provide a 3 litre bag in which *all* ingredients are mixed and can be delivered by one line (usually a central venous one) to a patient. Therefore, the clinician, having decided that he wants parenteral nutrition, can write a prescription out indicating how much energy and nitrogen he requires and his pharmacy colleagues will mix appropriate solutions in the 3 litre bag, the pharmacists having all the knowledge about miscibility, stability and the precipitation of particulate matter (Table 23.1). Again, there is often confusion about the concept of a central venous line and the need to give hypertonic solutions only via this route. For those clinicians with less manual dexterity, it is a simple matter to insert a peripheral drum catheter with its tip ending centrally and thereby still delivering hypertonic solutions, i.e., a 3 litre bag via this route. Where a pharmacy service is not available, then it is still possible to give amino acids and glucose together giving the fat emulsion sequentially over a 24-hour period. The unavailability of a 3 litre bag should not be seen as a reason for not undertaking parenteral nutrition.

Table 23.1 (a) Request for nutritional support. (b) Commonly used standard regimens

(a) Request for nutritional support

Patient's Name:.................... D.O.B. .................... Hosp. No ....................

Ward .................... Consultant ....................

Clinical details

Prescription: Protein g/day Energy Kcal/day

Electrolyte: Na K mmol/day

Mode of feeding: Parenteral

Preferably one of the standard regimens overleaf

Pharmacy must receive the day's prescription by 10.00 a.m. (based on the previous day's electrolyte results). If new requests for I.V. feeding arise over the weekend, it is recommended that bottles and Travenol W-sets be used.

Is a central venous line in place? YES/NO

| Date | Standard Regimen No. IV or Enteral | Electrolyte requirement if different from Standard | Start time and Duration | Signature |
|---|---|---|---|---|
| | | | | |
| | | | | |
| | | | | |
| | | | | |
| | | | | |

For standard IV regimens up to a maximum of 100 mmols of additional monovalent ions e.g. $Na^+$, $K^+$ may be requested.

In case of doubt or technical difficulty please contact the Nutrition Support Team through the Dietition or the Clinical Nutrition Nurse or Pharmacy

| | | Volume (ml) | Nitrogen (G) | Energy (non protein) kcals | Na | K | Ca mmol | Cl | $PO_4$ |
|---|---|---|---|---|---|---|---|---|---|
| E. | Vamin N | 1000 | | | | | | | |
| | Glucoplex 1000 | 1000 | 9.4 | 2000 | 100 | 50 | 7.5 | 135 | 25.5 |
| | Intralipid 20 % | 500 | | | | | | | |
| F. | Aminoplex 12 | 1000 | | | | | | | |
| | Glucoplex 1000 | 1000 | 12.4 | 2000 | 85 | 60 | 5.0 | 147 | 18.0 |
| | Intralipid 20 % | 500 | | | | | | | |
| $G_1$. | Vamin N | 1500 | | | | | | | |
| | Glucoplex 1000 | 1000 | 14.1 | 2000 | 125 | 60 | 8.75 | 163 | 25.5 |
| | Intralipid 20 % | 500 | | | | | | | |

| | | Volume (ml) | Nitrogen (G) | Energy (non protein) kcals | Na | K | Ca mmol | Cl | $PO_4$ |
|---|---|---|---|---|---|---|---|---|---|
| $G_2$. | Vamin N | 1500 | | | | | | | |
| | Glucoplex 1600 | 1000 | 14.1 | 2600 | 125 | 60 | 8.75 | 163 | 25.5 |
| | Intralipid 20 % | 500 | | | | | | | |
| H. | Vamin 18 Stability | 1000 | | | | | | | |
| | Glucoplex 1600 under test | 1000 | 18.0 | 2600 | 50 | 30 | 5.0 | 80 | 25.5 |
| | Intralipid 20 % Available shortly | 500 | | | | | | | |

(All with standard additives: Addamel, Solivito and Vitlipid)

1. Central venous line essential.
2. 1 g N = 6.25 g protein; requirement may be established by the following formula:
   24 hour urinary urea (mmol) × 0.035 = g N.
3. Best mixed in a 3 litre bag in the pharmacy.
4. Infuse preferably by volumetric pump over 12–24 hours.

## Energy substrates

There is now general agreement that only two non-protein energy sources need be considered when preparing a TPN regimen, i.e., glucose and a fat emulsion – normally a soybean derived emulsion. There is no longer any need to consider xylitol, sorbitol, fructose, maltose and various combinations of these in TPN. Whilst for many years there was a vogue to practise the 'American hyperalimentation approach' this, too, has now been overcome by more modern considerations showing that the provision of fat and carbohydrate on equi-energetic basis or 40 per cent fat with 60 per cent carbohydrate yields the best physiological and metabolic result. The advantages of a combined glucose fat energy regimen for TPN are shown in Table 23.2. In the past, there was the overall tendency to provide far too much energy. It still remains true that the severe burns case may require 3500–4500 kcal/day but for the vast majority of other patients 2000–2500 kcal is now the accepted norm. Initially, fat emulsions were made the scapegoat for many complications attendant upon TPN. However, considerable evidence has accrued to show that glucose energy only regimens have far more complications. In the past it was considered inappropriate to give fat emulsions to many intensive care patients, particularly those on ventilators and who had concurrent sepsis. There is now overwhelming evidence to show that acutely ill septic patients tolerate fat emulsions extremely well and, indeed, in some instances, metabolize these preferentially to carbohydrate only. It has been claimed that fat emulsions were the cause of the 'white lung syndrome' though there is no good evidence to support this.

There is general acceptance that to give more than about 600 g of glucose daily to any patient will overload that individual's intermediary metabolic

Table 23.2 Advantages of combined glucose/fat (Intralipid) energy regimen for total parenteral nutrition

| |
|---|
| Smaller energy osmolar load |
| Less chance of hyperosmolar dehydration syndrome |
| Less possible wastage of energy into urine (glycosuria) |
| Need to add soluble insulin rare |
| Metabolically remain within individual energy substrate tolerance limits |
| Less water gain component in total weight gain compared to glucose only |
| Greater positive effect upon protein anabolism |
| Less risk of hypercarbia and respiratory compromise compared to glucose only |
| Less demand upon myocardium to meet increased oxygen requirements by increasing cardiac output in glucose only regimens |
| Stress state of catabolic patients not exacerbated by excess noradrenalin secretion (cf. glucose only) |
| Less risk of fatty liver |
| Overall requirements for monitoring decreased |

pathways with attendant problems. Studies have shown that increasing the rate of glucose infusion up to 5 mg/kg body weight/minute is associated with a stepwise increase in oxidation of glucose. Thus, for a 70 kg man this would represent an infusion of 504 g of glucose/day equivalent to some 2066 kcal. However, to proceed beyond that point leads to such metabolic problems as hypertriglyceridaemia, fat deposition in the liver resulting in a less cost effective and nutritional situation. Another misunderstanding in the past has been to infuse more and more glucose at higher rates in an attempt to induce greater protein synthesis. There have been attempts to induce these mechanisms by using large amounts of soluble insulin but studies have now shown that this is not physiologically effective and simply maintains normo-glycaemia. However, this does not imply that insulin is inappropriate in the diabetic patient or those with severe 'stress diabetes'. Whilst it is not doubted that insulin is a valuable anabolic hormone, its role in TPN is minimal. It is no longer my practice to use glucose-insulin regimens. If both glucose and fat energy substrates are given simultaneously, then the individual's tolerance limits for each substrate will not be exceeded, again reducing the need for concomitant insulin infusion.

Many studies have shown that to give glucose only may constitute a severe physiopathological insult to the patient. Thus, in high dose glucose regimens in the catabolic patient, increased carbon dioxide production occurs, leading to an increased ventilatory effort to eliminate the $CO_2$, the increased ventilatory drive of itself requiring a higher energy ($O_2$) input. Furthermore, if such patients are already on ventilators, high glucose TPN may delay their weaning from a ventilator because of the increased respiratory load. Conversely, if any individual has a degree of respiratory compromise, e.g., the elderly chronic bronchitic, then he may actually be forced on to a ventilator by this nutritional approach. Again, in the elderly patients with compromised myocardial function, cardiac failure may be precipitated because of increased oxygen requirement and therefore increased cardiac output needed to metabolize excess glucose. Finally, high glucose load infusions have been shown to stimulate the secretion of catecholamines (particularly noradrenalin) which may, in turn, cause cardiac arrhythmias, further compromising the unstable myocardium.

Precise metabolic studies have clearly shown that when glucose only regimens have been used, patients showed a greater weight gain as a result of water retention compared to when glucose and fat were used together, this resulting in greater protein acquisition and less fat deposition and water retention. Therefore, glucose only regimens are more likely to cause a fatty liver as opposed to the infusion of a fat emulsion which used to be thought the cause. It is established that infused triglycerides (fat emulsions) are not metabolized by the liver. In single pass studies it has been shown that the liver is the least important organ in the metabolism of an infused fat emulsion. The role of the liver is to produce ketone bodies (acetoacetic acid and betahydroxybutyric acid) from fatty acids released from peripheral fat stores or after the breakdown of infused fat emulsions by tissue lipoprotein lipases. The muscle mass utilizes by far the greatest amount of any infused fat.

From the practical standpoint, glucose solutions and fat emulsions can be mixed with certain amino acid solutions in a 3 litre bag and stability studies have shown such preparations can be stored for up to 1 week without fear of destabilization. Formerly it was customary to think about 200 kcal/1 g of nitrogen but, in fact, a ratio nearer to 150:1 is now more generally accepted as physiologically appropriate.

Studies have been undertaken to see whether adding acylcarnitine to fat emulsions or a simultaneous infusion might improve the utilization of infused fat. Although some experimental work has proved promising the general application to patient care is not yet possible. In summary, therefore, glucose and fat should be used on nearly an equi-energetic basis, rarely more than 2500 kcal/day is required and the need for insulin infusions has been almost eradicated.

## Nitrogen sources

Over the last decade there has been a proliferation of nitrogen source solutions, i.e., amino acid preparations, to meet the needs of TPN. There has been a tendency to try and develop specific solutions for those acutely ill patients who have primary cardiac disease, liver disease, renal disease or gastrointestinal disease and possibly lung disease. However, in the final analysis, there is very little evidence indeed to show that organ specific solutions for the acutely ill patient have any major advantage over a carefully constructed 'general' TPN regimen. Indeed, in my view, far too many amino acid solutions are currently available. Many solutions are equipotent in terms of their efficacy, i.e., protein anabolism, and it is their compatibility with energy substrates and cost which need to be considered when formulating a TPN regimen. Most districts with their 'Nutritional Support Teams' have decided upon a high nitrogen source amino acid solution, a maintenance nitrogen source and, of course, specific requirements for paediatric practice. In my view there is absolutely no need for any specific amino acid profile, provided the amino acid solution contains all the essential amino acids and a full profile of the non-essential. It is preferable that the essential amino acid nitrogen content should be in the range of 30–40 per cent of the total nitrogen content. Some clinicians prefer amino acid solutions only without electrolytes, others are happy to use electrolyte containing amino acid solutions.

In recent years there has been much attention given to the branched chain amino acid content of amino acid solutions but the evidence does not support that increasing the percentage of isoleucine, leucine and valine in any solution results in a net better anabolic effect, even in the liver compromised patient.

Whilst it is true that the branched chain amino acids may be of benefit pharmacologically for the cirrhotic patient in the pre-coma stage, there is no evidence to show that in the long-term they have increased patient survival. Indeed, the early studies were hindered by lack of controlled investigations. Certainly, there is no need to have specially defined amino acid solutions for acute renal failure patients as the readily available solutions may be used and the patient dialysed or haemofiltered as often as necessary. The earlier work suggesting the specificity of acute renal failure solutions was based on the *misconception* that the urea nitrogen recycling was nutritionally beneficial to the patient.

In the past there has been a tendency to provide too much energy, now there is a tendency to provide far too much nitrogen. Thus, very concentrated amino acid solutions providing up to 25 g/litre have been made but which have little other value than reducing the volume of infusion to achieve optimal nitrogen infusion in those patients with severe fluid intake restriction. However, in my view, and based on available evidence, there is rarely ever a case to be made for exceeding 20–22 g of nitrogen daily for efficient metabolic care and achieving nitrogen equilibrium in catabolic patients. If more nitrogen is given, then the liver's ability to cope with such a nitrogen load is exceeded and more deamination occurs with a greater urea production and appearance of urinary nitrogen. It must be emphasized that although some patients may excrete 30–40 g nitrogen/day (assuming none of this derives from absorption of trauma haematomata or blood in the gastrointestinal tract) one is not aiming to catch up with actual measured losses. As already mentioned the liver's inability to cope with a greater load prevents this and the aim of TPN here is to contain what otherwise might be disastrous effects of the metabolic response to trauma.

Whether amino acid solutions should be made pure or may have added energy is a moot point. Clearly, if an amino acid solution already contains some energy, then this is taken into consideration when making up a total prescription for a 3 litre bag. As mentioned above, there may be a case for having some amino acid solutions without any electrolyte content.

It is not the intention here to go through the relative merits of all the many amino acid solutions made, for each pharmacy will stock a selected number of solutions which will always be able to meet the clinical requirements. This, of course, makes the ease of overall prescription that much greater for the clinician who simply decides how much he wants to give.

In the past much has been written about protein sparing therapy and the use of peripheral amino acid solutions. The main attraction of isotonic amino acid solutions was that they could be given through peripheral veins and therefore 'some nitrogen' was better than none. However, amino acid solutions alone are not the basis of TPN in the critically ill patient. The concept behind isotonic amino acid solutions was that they would not stimulate insulin activity and therefore lipolysis could proceed uninhibited with production of ketone bodies, an important fuel substrate for all patients. In my view, isotonic amino acids have little to recommend them and many studies have shown their inefficiency. Indeed, to give peripheral isotonic amino acids is probably one of the most expensive ways of giving sterile water to a patient.

## Other nutrients

There are now a number of commercial preparations that provide a full profile of vitamins which cover the basic daily recommended allowances. Serum concentrations of vitamins are extremely difficult to measure and, indeed, with the use of the currently available vitamin solutions, vitamin deficiency syndromes in the critically ill patient on TPN are very rarely encountered. Even in patients on home TPN such preparations still suffice. The requirements for zinc, copper, manganese, are now well understood and for short-term TPN, i.e., under 6 weeks, there is no real evidence to suggest that chromium and selenium additions are required. Of course, just as in the past a drop of water with a dash of salt was thought to be parenteral nutrition, nowadays one must be wary of the concept that a little nitrogen with some sweetener is equally beneficial. It is important to carefully construct the overall regimen and to ensure that all nutrients are given to obtain optimal metabolic/nutritional benefit.

## Delivery systems

As indicated earlier, the advent of the 3 litre bag has revolutionized the delivery of TPN to patients. Having the single bag approach with all the nutrients contained therein, needs only one line for delivery which is normally a central venous access point. However, alternatively a long flexible drum catheter inserted peripherally can equally well be used, requiring an equally meticulous aseptic approach. Where a 3 litre bag facility is not available, then 1 litre bottles may be used and all nutrients can be given simultaneously through 'Travenol' W sets or Y sets giving amino acids and glucose together followed by a fat emulsion. With the use of 3 litre TPN bags, it is customary and probably preferable to use some form of infusion pump to ensure a steady delivery to the patient. Clearly, this is mandatory in patients on home TPN where they are infused for say, 10 or 12 hour periods overnight only. Again, pump controlled parenteral nutrition is vital in paediatric practice. There are many catheters now available for TPN and individual clinicians get to know their type of catheter best and in their hands obtain the best results irrespective of what others may advise them.

## Patient assessment

As with any other therapeutic manoeuvre, so with TPN, it is important to assess the effectiveness of treatment or if treatment is not succeeding to have parameters whereby adjustments may be made. Unfortunately, there is a tendency with TPN to simply give it and 'hope for the best'. There is no one single marker of malnutrition any more than there is for infection.

Table 23.3 Profile of measurements for monitoring malnutrition

| Tests for malnutrition | Equipment required | Result in malnutrition |
|---|---|---|
| 1. *Body weight in kg and recent loss | Various scales | >10 % |
| 2. *Triceps skin fold thickness (TST) Fat energy reserves | Holtain skin fold calipers | <10 mm in males <13 mm in females |
| 3. *Mid-arm muscle circumference (MAMC) Muscle protein reserves (MAMC = arm circumf. − $\pi$(TST)) | Tape measure in cm | <23 cm in males <22 cm in females |
| 4. *Serum albumin (visceral protein) | Routine lab. test | <35 g/litre |
| 5. Serum transferrin, Complement $C_3$ } short half-life proteins | Routine lab. test | <2 g/litre (not reliable) |
| 6. *Retinol binding protein Thyroxine binding pre-albumin | Special tests | |
| 7. Urinary hydroxyproline | Special test | ↑ Collagen turnover |
| 8. Lymphopaenia | Routine lab. test | <1.2 × $10^9$/litre |
| 9. Plasma amino acid profile | Specialized tests | Changing valine/glycine ratio |
| 10. Urine 3 methylhistidine | Specialized tests | Increased muscle breakdown |
| 11. Hair root morphology | Tweezers and microscopy | More telogens and dysplastic hairs |
| 12. Finger dynamometry | Dynamometer and interested clinician | Diminished power |
| 13. Skin responses to intradermal injections of antigenic material | e.g. DNCB, candida | Skin anergy (time consuming and little value) |
| 14. *Visual assessment of patient | Eyes! and clinical acumen | |

* The most useful tests. Do no. 1 and 14 daily; no. 2, 3 and 6 twice weekly (e.g. Mon. and Thurs. as a routine). No. 4 alternate days.

Nevertheless, it is useful to have a fairly simple practical profile of measurements that can give not only useful information about the existence of malnutrition, but about deterioration or improvement according to treatment or lack of. Such measurements are shown in Table 23.3, all of which are simple, do not require expensive or complicated equipment and can be equally practised by nurses, medical staff and nutritionists. It is unfortunate that in the last decade there have been times when the nursing role has been so modified that the nutritional care of patients has not been one of their responsibilities but rather delegated to 'ward maids'. Fortunately, with the introduction of such specialized groups as BITA, (British Intravenous Therapists Association) and the advent of 'Nutrition Clinical Nurse Specialist', it is hoped once again that this aspect of patient care will merit the emphasis it deserves. There are now increasing numbers of day release courses organized by the RCN devoted to nutritional care and incorporating these in EBS Courses. Equally, however, it is deplorable that many physicians and surgeons are guilty of not calling in other expert nutritionist personnel to help with patient care when nutritional support is of paramount importance. Hopefully, with the growing recognition that nutrition is important for a patient's survival, even in hospital, and with the currently available Nutritional Support Teams, more and more integrated co-ordinated approaches will be made when prescribing nutritional support for critically ill patients. It is fortunate that with nutrition there are a number of biometric assessments which are meaningful and reproducible at ward level.

## Application

Who really requires parenteral nutrition? As previously stated, the absolute indication is gastrointestinal failure. Alternatively, there will be occasions when a combination of parenteral and enteral nutrition provides the best metabolic-nutritional management of a critically ill patient. It must be emphasized that the application of TPN is not dependent upon a 'diagnostic index' disease approach. Parenteral nutrition is essentially designed to improve the nutritional status of any patient who cannot take adequate oral, naso-gastric or enteral nutrition. Again, because nowadays we have the simplified approaches not only for prescribing TPN but for its delivery, there can be no excuse for dilatoriness, which all too frequently still occurs. The guidelines for optimal TPN support are given in Table 23.4. The advent of parenteral nutri-

Table 23.4 Guidelines for efficient, safe total parenteral nutrition

1. Scrupulous, aseptic technique for insertion and aftercare of catheter (central or peripheral).
2. Immediate chest x-ray to check catheter correctly located.
3. Correct patient assessment using anthropometric, biochemical and physiological measurements.
4. Nitrogen (full profile amino acid solution) 0.2–0.25 g/kg body weight.
5. Energy 30–35 kcal/kg body weight.
6. Energy (kcal):nitrogen (g) ratio 140:1 (catabolic patients); up to 180:1 less catabolic
7. Derive energy equally from glucose and fat. Do not exceed 700 g glucose per day.
8. Give energy and nitrogen simultaneously – gives best anabolic effect.
9. Nitrogen (g): potassium (mmol); magnesium (mmol), phosphorus (mmol) ratios of 1:5–7; 1:1; 1:0.5.
10. Water-soluble vitamins from onset (protect from light); after 2 weeks fat soluble vitamins.
11. Essential biological elements Zn, Cu, Mn; essential fatty acids.
12. HPPF, plasma or blood for immediate restoration of serum oncotic pressure or haemoglobin concentration.
13. Folinic acid 5 mg daily.
14. Use IV feeding line for nutritional purposes only.
15. Mobilize patient as soon as possible – promotes anabolism.
16. Reassess and recalculate requirements (do *not* speculate).
17. Monitor appropriately and frequently.

tion has made a significant advance in the management of upper gastrointestinal fistulae. Whereas both morbidity and mortality used to be high, i.e., approximately 40 per cent, with TPN this figure has been reduced to 10 per cent or less, particularly with high intestinal fistulae. Furthermore, in the management of patients with gastrointestinal fistulae not only has the success rate improved, but the hospital duration of treatment has been reduced by half.

Many intensive care patients with multiple problems of:

1. ventilation;
2. associated acute renal failure;
3. liver compromise and;
4. gastrointestinal failure

can be successfully managed by routine TPN *not* requiring specialized solutions. Again, I must re-emphasize that if a patient requires TPN then currently available solutions should be used and with the help of pharmacy colleagues, a 3 litre bag can be prepared that can materially alter the prognosis of a patient. For example, it has been shown with acute renal failure patients that, given the dialysis/haemofiltration techniques are fairly standard, then the addition of TPN can improve the prognosis in some groups by as much as 20 per cent. This has to be borne in mind against the overall appalling survival prognosis of 50 per cent for such patients.

The value of TPN in cancer patients has to be put into perspective. Clearly, if a patient has an inoperable carcinoma which is not amenable to chemotherapy and/or radiotherapy, there can be little justification for starting TPN. On the other hand, in certain types of cancer, particularly head and neck surgery, and of the small bowel, a case can be made for giving TPN so that effective chemotherapy and/or radiotherapy can be delivered and the patient simultaneously kept in an acceptable nutritional state so he can benefit from the effects of specific anti-cancer treatment. Conversely, TPN is not the answer to cancer cachexia when no other therapy is available for the primary lesion. It has long since been recognized that negative nitrogen balance and cancer cachexia have many common metabolic and immunological sequelae. In cancer patients with a poor nutritional intake yet continuing normal or accelerated metabolic losses, the host amino acid pool decreases (catabolism) whilst the tumour amino acid pool increases (anabolism). Investigations have shown that 50 per cent of cancer patients have anergy to a number of skin antigens. It has been clearly shown that patients can gain weight on TPN. Does the weight gain *per se* matter? Yes, for it has been shown that increased weight gain correlates with:

1. positive nitrogen balance;
2. improved physical and psychological well being;
3. widening of the surgical interventions that can be attempted;
4. few interruptions of specific anti-cancer therapy be that chemo- or radiotherapy.

This seems in turn to relate to the improved immunocompetence that follows improved nitrogen balance as reflected in the fact that conversion of skin anergy results in better anti-cancer therapy response.

It has been previously debated whether or not critically ill patients with associated sepsis (a very common accompaniment) can benefit from TPN. The answer must be an unreserved yes, and as indicated above, comprehensive TPN with standard nutrients is able to effect the best results. Regrettably, in many Intensive Care Units, there is still some reluctance to practise conventional (as by modern day standards) TPN and they still rely on the old glucose (with insulin infusions) and amino acid regimens only.

Parenteral nutrition has made a considerable contribution to the management of patients who have extensive loss of the gastrointestinal tract (GIT), particularly those with Crohn's disease. Results with malignant disease of the GIT are less impressive. Nevertheless, in the UK alone, over 200 patients have benefitted from home TPN with remarkably good results. It is likely that 2–3 patients per million will benefit from this therapeutic modality. The gut, unlike many other organs, has a remarkable power of adaptation. Therefore, many patients who embark upon home TPN treatment therapy, in contrast to home haemodialysis (or CAPD) can benefit from weaning of treatment. In other words, often the gut will hypertrophy and will physiologically adapt so that oral nutrition can be restarted.

In summary, it is clear that many patients can benefit by 'life itself' by the early application of comprehensive TPN and nowadays complications are minimal. The approach has been simplified, delivery systems made simple and patient acceptability is good.

## Monitoring

Careful monitoring of TPN is essential if complications are to be avoided not only from the regimens administered but by virtue of excess or deficiencies of nutrient elements supplied or metabolic complications arising from end organ failure. All too often in the past clinicians have blamed the TPN regimen for metabolic complications occurring. This is a somewhat naive approach and it must be realized that in critically ill patients the 'milieu interieure' will change because of different end-organ function. The optimal observations (Table 23.5) to prevent complications of TPN (Table 23.6) are shown in the accompanying tables.

Often for example, nutritional substrates are blamed for, say, the occurrence of lactic acidosis. Again, from a clinical standpoint, lactic acidosis is not differentiated from lactic acidaemia. However, if the liver or kidney are involved in disease processes then inevitably, since both are responsible for the elimination of lactate from the blood, a metabolic acidosis may occur irrespective of the nutritional regimen given. This is particularly true nowadays when energy substrates are, or indeed should be, derived only from glucose and fat emulsion substrates.

Clearly, the amount of monitoring will differ from patient to patient, dependent upon their own particular illness and the chief end-organs involved. An indication of the tests required, and their frequency, is given in Table 23.5.

The complications of TPN, though now minimal, are nevertheless illustrated in Table 23.6. Fortunately, with the modern day rationalization of TPN most of the basic metabolic complications are totally avoidable.

There is general agreement that the major complication of TPN is that of

Table 23.5 Optimal observations during intravenous nutrition

*Biochemical*

1. Routine:
   - Blood urea, serum creatinine and electrolytes (daily)
   - SMA 12/60 profile* (every 2nd or 3rd day)
   - Serum lactate, pyruvate (in unexplained anion gap)
   - Blood glucose (frequently with glucose meter according to IV regimen used)
   - Liver function tests (at least weekly)
   - Serum magnesium (weekly)
   - Serum transferrin, complement $C_3$ (weekly)
   - Serum and urine osmolality
   - Observation of spun plasma each morning when using fat emulsion
   - 24-hour urine urea, sodium (daily)
   - Acid-base balance; blood gases
2. Special:
   - Serum amino acid profile
   - Serum and urine, zinc and copper (especially in hypercatabolic patients)
   - Any specific test determined by illness

*Haematological*

- Hb, WBC, platelets, PCV (daily or less frequently depending on circumstances)
- BPR (prothrombin index)
- Serum folate (rarely)

*Physiological*

- Vital signs – pulse, respiration, BP, temperature, colour
- CVP (line not mandatory)
- Weight (weigh bed invaluable)
- Fluid balance (urine volume, etc.)

*Mechanical*

- Line inspection (filter changes, care with connections)
- Flow rates
- Catheter insertion point
- Pump checks
- Meniscus levels in bubble traps
- Back-flow up 'piggy-back' lines
  (particularly with solutions of low density, e.g. fat emulsion)

*Bacteriological*

- Blood cultures (once a week at least)
- Viral agglutination titres (e.g. cytomegalovirus)
- Watch carefully for Candida or other fungus infections

*Radiological*

Chest x-ray
1. Must have initial one immediately after catheter insertion
2. Subsequently one a week depending on clinical condition

* Includes albumin, calcium, phosphorus, bilirubin, urate, alkaline phosphatase, LDH, aspartate transaminase, creatinine

infection, and this comes back to intravenous angio access technique and subsequent nurse management. It cannot be over-emphasized how important it is to insist upon obsessional care of the access site which, after all, is the lifeline for such patients.

Table 23.6 Potential complications of total parenteral nutrition

| Problem | Possible cause |
|---|---|
| *Metabolic* | |
| Metabolic acidosis; lactic acidosis | Fructose*, sorbitol*, ethanol*, carbohydrate combinations; infection; liver or renal insufficiency |
| Metabolic alkalosis | Gastric aspiration; inadequate potassium supplements |
| Hyperosmolar dehydration syndrome | Hypertonic glucose; sorbitol |
| Hyperuricaemia | Fructose, sorbitol, xylitol* |
| Oxalaemia and oxaluria | ? Xylitol |
| Hypertriglyceridaemia | Excess glucose; sorbitol; fat emulsion |
| Hyperlipidaemia | Excess fat emulsion; bacterial infection or toxaemia |
| Hypophosphataemia | Phosphorus free glucose regimens |
| Essential fatty acid deficiency | Fat free regimen |
| Hyperammonaemia | Protein hydrolysate solution |
| Folate metabolism disturbance | Ethanol; methionine |
| Hypercarbia | Excess glucose provision |
| Fatty liver | Excess glucose provision |
| Eczematous rash (acrodermatitis enteropathica) | Zn deficiency |
| Bone marrow hypoactivity (red and white cell series) | Cu deficiency |
| Altered cerebration | Poorly designed amino acid solutions |
| Hyponatraemia | Water overload, rarely inadequate sodium provision |
| Hypercalcaemia | Amino acid solution ? mechanism |
| Bleeding diathesis | Vitamin K deficiency |
| *Vascular access* | |
| Thrombosis | Hypertonic solution via short peripheral catheter |
| Infection, septicaemia, endocarditis | Poor technique |
| Catheter embolus | Avoid catheters with sharp needle casings |
| Drainage to structures during central venous catheterization (e.g. nerve injury, haematoma haemorrhage, pneumothorax) | Poor technique; inexperience |

N.B. *Glucose and a fat emulsion (e.g. Intralipid) should nowadays be the only energy sources used.

## Value of parenteral nutrition

Regrettably, in my view, there are still those who would ask whether TPN can do anything for the critically ill patient. Clearly, as is manifestly evident from the literature, this therapeutic modality when correctly practised has enormous benefits on patient survival. However, TPN is no short cut to metabolic and/or nutritional success. It needs to be carefully planned, carefully applied and monitored with care. Those who still argue that the risks of TPN outweigh any advantages are clearly not well informed. The ultimate proof, perhaps, of TPN is with HTPN patients. Here we find patients can be managed for years at a time without any adverse metabolic and/or nutritional sequelae. At the same time, it has to be admitted that many of the advances made in TPN have accrued as a result of prolonged observations on HTPN patients. Over the past decade, many of the myths surrounding TPN have been removed. There is first of all a simplified approach with respect to nutritional ingredients and secondly re the delivery approach. Furthermore, there is a growing awareness that one does not need end-organ failure dependent nutritional regimens. Although TPN, if practised inappropriately is expensive, when practised properly, it is extremely cost effective.

The fact must not be lost sight of that if any critically ill patient loses more than 30 per cent of his initial body weight in any acute metabolic illness then he has only a remote chance of survival. When it is considered that many such patients will lose between 10 and 20 g of nitrogen/day, i.e., 0.3–0.6 kg of muscle mass per day, then it is readily appreciated how quickly the net loss of body weight can occur. It is worth re-emphasizing that the consequences of negative nitrogen balance are not only loss of body weight but increased susceptibility to infection, increased incidence of wound dehiscence, hypoproteinaemic oedema, all leading ultimately to increased morbidity and mortality. The provision in time of correctly prescribed parenteral nutrition can only but decrease the morbidity and mortality rate. It is imperative that all District General Hospitals have a Nutritional Support Team which can offer advice on any nutritional problems thereby removing the embarrassment or, indeed, arrogance of clinicians who, whilst not knowing what are the prerequisites of TPN, can derive support from such teams. No longer can the excuse be offered that TPN is the prerogative of Teaching Hospitals or that it is too difficult to implement or there are too many controversies surrounding its application. Nowadays, there are not any contraindications to TPN in those patients who require this particular therapeutic approach. Once a patient is recognized as being in need of TPN then all the clinician need do is to write a prescription and the pharmacy or other members of the Nutritional Support Team can advise how best to supply the basic requirements for a given patient. In conclusion, TPN is a therapeutic modality that can be given to any patient, in any hospital, at any time, by any clinician who considers any patient requires this treatment.

## Further reading

Askanazi, J. Nordenstrom, J., Rosenbaum, S.H., Elwyn, D.H., Hyman, A.I., Carpentier, Y.A. and Kinney, J.M. (1981). Nutrition for the patient with respiratory failure: glucose vs. fat. 1 *Anaesthesiology*, **54**, 373–7.

Baker, J.P., Detsky, A.S., Stewart, S., Whitwell, J., Marliss, E.B. and Jeejeebhoy, K.N. (1984). Randomized trial of total parenteral nutrition in critically ill patients: metabolic effects of varying glucose-lipid ratios as the energy source. *Gastroenterology*, **87**, Part I. pp. 53–9.

Clark, R.G. (1981). Parenteral nutrition. In *Recent Advances In Clinical Nutrition*. **1**. pp. 107–12. Eds. Howard, A. and McLean Baird, I. John Libbey: London.

Grant, A. and Todd, E. (Eds). (1982). *Enteral and Parenteral Nutrition: A Clinical Handbook*. Blackwell Scientific Publications: Oxford.

Heatley, R.V. and Tredree, R. (1986). Intravenous feeding. In *Clinical Nutrition in Gastroenterology*, pp. 116–29. Eds. Heatley, R.V., Losowsky, M.S. and Kelleher, J. Churchill Livingstone: Edinburgh.

Jeejeebhoy, K.N. (1981). *Intravenous Nutrition – an overview in Nutrition and the surgical Patient*, pp. 118–32. Ed. Hill, G.L. Churchill Livingstone: Edinburgh.

Jeejeebhoy, K.N. (Ed.) (1983). *Total Parenteral Nutrition in the Hospital and at Home*. CRC Press: Florida.

Johnston, I.D.A. (ed). (1983). *Advances in Clinical Nutrition*. MTP Press: Lancaster.

Karran, S.J. and Alberti, K.G.M.M. (eds). (1980). *Practical Nutritional Support*. Pitman Medical: London.

Lee, H.A. (1982). *Intravenous Feeding in Intensive Care*, pp. 1–30. Ed. Sherwood Jones, E. MTP Press Ltd: Lancaster.

Lee, H.A. (1983). *Parenteral Nutrition in Current Medical Treatment*, 5th ed., pp. 525–34. Ed. Havard, C.W.H. Ballière Tindall: Eastbourne.

Lee, H.A., (1986). Parenteral aspects of intravenous feeding. In *Clinical Nutrition in Gastroenterology*, pp. 86–96. Eds. Heatley, R.V., Losowsky M.S. and Kelleher, J. Churchill Livingstone: Edinburgh.

McEntee, G.P., Moran, K., Duinan, J.P. and O'Malley, E. (1986). Monitoring nitrogen losses in parenteral therapy. *J. Parenteral Therapy*, 7, 124–6.

MacFie, J., Smith, R.C., Hill, G.L. (1981). Glucose or fat as a non-protein energy source? *Gastroenterology*, **80**, 103–107.

Nanni, G., Sitegel, J.H., Coleman, B., Fader, P., and Castiglione, R., (1984). Increased lipid fuel dependence in the critically ill septic patient. *J. Trauma*, **24**, 14–29.

Roulet, M., Detsky, A.S., Marliss, E.B., Todd, T.R.J., Mahon, W.A., Anderson, G.H., Stewart, S. and Jeejeebhoy, K.N. (1983). A controlled trial of the effect of parenteral nutritional support on patients with respiratory failure and sepsis. *Clin. Nutrit.*, **2**, 97–105.

Wright, P.D., and Elliott, M., (Eds). (1981). Parenteral and enteral nutrition. *Acta. Chir. Scand., (Suppl.)*, **507**, W.M. Bett Ltd.: Tillicoultry.

# Appendix

Table 1 Gluten-free diet (from Davidson *et al.*, 1975). Reproduced by permission of Churchill Livingstone, Edinburgh

| | |
|---|---|
| *Indications* | For patients with coeliac disease or gluten-induced enteropathy |
| *Nutrients* | Energy and protein intake adjusted according to age and activity. All cereals containing gluten (gliadin), i.e. wheat, oats, rye, barley and buckwheat must be omitted |
| | *Sample daily menu* |
| *Breakfast* | Fruit *or* fruit juice<br>Cornflakes or puffed rice with milk and sugar<br>Egg and bacon<br>Gluten-free bread (toasted) with butter and marmalade or jelly<br>Coffee or tea with milk and sugar |
| *Midday meal* | Soup made with meat or vegetable stock and thickened with gluten-free flour; rice, barley, peas or lentils may be added<br>Meat *or* fish; any gravy is thickened with cornflour or other gluten-free flour<br>Potato *or* rice<br>Vegetables, avoiding those prepared with mayonnaise or sauce (e.g. canned baked beans)<br>Salad with dressing made without flour<br>Fruit or permitted dessert/pudding; special brands of ice cream<br>Coffee or tea, with milk and sugar |
| *Evening meal* | Fruit *or* fruit juice<br>Main dish with an egg, cheese, fish or meat<br>Potato *or* rice<br>Vegetables<br>Gluten-free bread or roll with butter<br>Fruit *or* permitted dessert<br>Tea with milk and sugar |

*Management*

*Forbidden foods*: Bread, biscuits, cakes, cookies, crackers, crispbreads, doughnuts, flour (white or wholemeal), muffins, pancakes, pastry, pies, pretzels, rolls, rusks, scones, toast and waffles. Breakfast cereals made with wheat or oatmeal, e.g. All Bran, Wheat Flakes, Puffed Wheat, Shredded Wheat, Weetabix, Shreddies, Sugar Smacks, Grapenuts, oatmeal, wheat germ. Macaroni, noodles, spaghetti, semolina, vermicelli and other pasta. Meat pie, luncheon meat, canned meat, meat loaf, commercial hamburgers, sausages, bologna and frankfurters. Canned soups and soup mixes. Vegetables with cream sauces or crumbs, e.g. baked beans. Proprietary sauces and ketchups, gravies, commercial salad dressings. Packet and pudding mixtures, pastry mixtures, patent infant foods. Malted milk, ovaltine, postum and beer, commercial milk flavourings. Baking powder. Cheese spreads. Most ice creams (except those listed below). Commercial chocolates and liquorice sweets.

*Foods that may be used freely*: Milk (all kinds) and yogurt; may be flavoured with home-made syrup or unprocessed cocoa. Fresh meats and poultry and bacon, fish (fresh or canned), shellfish, organ meats. Gravies made with cornstarch or rice flour. Cheese and egg (boiled, poached, scrambled, omelet and in mixed dishes). Vegetables (fresh, frozen, canned), raw or cooked. Potatoes and rice. Nuts. All fruits and fruit juices. Bread and flour made from wheatstarch, arrowroot, cornmeal, soyabean, rice or potato flour. Breakfast cereals made from rice and maize. Cream, butter, margarine, peanut butter, cooking fats and oils. Sugar, jam, jelly, marmalade, honey syrup, boiled sweets, hard candies, home-made candy, plain chocolate. Desserts and puddings made with gelatine, tapioca, sago, rice and cornstarch. Cakes and cookies made with gluten-free flour. Coffee, tea and carbonated beverages. Salt, pepper, mustard, spices, garlic and vinegar. Ice cream (in UK made by Walls, Lyons, Eldorado or Hoods).

Successful treatment depends on complete elimination of all foods containing even traces of gluten. Many mixed and manufactured foods contain small amounts of wheat flour, and lists of forbidden and permissible foods should be continuously checked and brought up to date. A current list of gluten-free foods and recipes can be obtained from the Coeliac Society, P.O. Box No. 181, London, NW2 2QY.

Table 2 Low protein dietary regimens for treatment of hepatic encephalopathy

In order to provide a diet which will be acceptable to the individual patient's taste an exchange system can be used, as follows:

*Meat exchanges* (= 6 g protein)
1 exchange is one of the following:
- 25 g cooked meat (40 g raw meat)
- 25 g cooked fish (40 g raw rish)
- 50 g cooked sausage
- 1 egg (size 5, 50 g)
- 200 g milk or yogurt
- 25 g cheese
- 100 g cooked lentils, haricot, red or butter beans (3 tablespoons)
- 25 g shelled almonds or peanuts
- 50 g shelled chestnuts or walnuts

*Bread exchanges* (= 2 g protein)
1 exchange is one of the following:
- 25 g bread (1 large thin slice)
- 25 g plain cake, pastry or flour
- 4 plain biscuits (e.g. cream crackers)
- 25 g Cornflakes, Rice Krispies (= 5 tablespoons)
- 125 g (5 tablespoons) cooked porridge
- 50 g peas, broadbeans
- 150 g boiled potato (= 3 small)
- 100 g boiled rice (= 4 tablespoons)
- 50 g icecream (1 brickette)
- 25 g baked beans (= 1 tablespoon)
- 100 g cooked dhall (= 3 tablespoons)

*Minimal protein diet*

*Foods forbidden*
Milk, meat, eggs, fish, cheese, bread, flour, pulses, spinach, mushrooms, nuts, jelly

*Foods allowed*
Glucose, sugar, honey, jam
Potatoes, rice, low-protein pasta protein-free bread, protein-free crispbread, tapioca, sago, fruit, low protein vegetables, butter, oil, double cream (50 % fat)

Energy intake should be kept as high as possible by the use of glucose or sugar in fruit drinks etc., a minimum of 1600 kcal (6.7 MJ) being given daily in this form. The use of a glucose polymer* can be helpful as these products are less sweet than glucose and therefore less nauseating to the patient.
*suitable glucose polymers include:
Maxijul and Maxijul L.E. (Scientific Hospital Supplies)
Caloreen (Roussel) Polycal (Cow and Gate)
Calonutrin (Geistlich) Polycose (Abbotts)

---

*20 g protein diet*
1 meat exchange as milk, for tea etc.
1 meat exchange, divided between two meals
4 bread exchanges
Fruit, low protein vegetables, sugar, jam, honey, butter, oil, double cream

---

*40 g protein diet*
1 meat exchange as milk for tea etc.
4 meat exchanges divided between three meals
5 bread exchanges
Fruit, low protein vegetables, sugar, jam, honey, butter, oil, double cream

---

*60 g protein diet*
1 meat exchange as milk, for tea etc.
5 meat exchanges, divided between three meals
9 bread exchanges
Fruit etc. as above

---

Table 3 Example low sodium diet

No salt to be used in cooking or added at table

| | |
|---|---|
| *Breakfast* | Fruit or fruit juice if desired |
| | Shredded Wheat, Puffed Wheat or porridge made without salt |
| | 1 egg, tomatoes or mushrooms |
| | Salt-free bread, matzos or salt-free crispbread |
| | Salt-free butter |
| | Jam, marmalade or honey |
| | Milk from allowance on cereal and in tea |
| *Mid-morning* | Tea or coffee, milk from allowance |
| *Lunch* | 50 g (2 oz) meat or fish |
| | Potatoes, rice or pasta, or salt-free bread |
| | Vegetables or salad |
| | Fruit, jelly, unsalted pastry |
| | 'Milk' pudding made from double cream (50 % fat) |
| *Tea* | Tea with milk from allowance |
| | Salt-free cake or biscuit |
| *Supper* | As lunch |
| *Bed-time* | Remainder of milk in tea or coffee |
| | Salt-free bread with salt-free butter and jam, or |
| | Salt-free cake or biscuit |
| *Daily* | 250 ml (½ pint) for tea, cereal etc. |
| | (natural yogurt may be exchanged for milk if desired) |

This regimen provides approximately 20 mmol sodium daily. The diet can be increased to 40 mmol daily by the addition of 4 slices of ordinary bread, instead of salt-free bread. 1 slice (25 g approx) ordinary bread contains about 5 mmol sodium.

Salt should not be used in cooking or added at table in either diet and foods forbidden and allowed are the same for both regimens, apart from bread:

| *Foods allowed freely* | *Foods not allowed* |
|---|---|
| Fruit, fresh, canned or frozen | Ordinary bread, biscuits, cakes |
| Fresh or frozen vegetables, except spinach, celery, beetroot | Spinach, celery, beetroot |
| Salt-free bread, matzos | Self-raising flour, baking powder |
| Salt-free crispbread | Cornflakes, Rice Krispies, All-Bran |
| Puffed Wheat, Shredded Wheat | Ham, bacon, tinned meats, meat paste |
| Sugar Puffs, unsalted porridge | Tinned fish, smoked fish, fish paste |
| Meat, fish, eggs, milk, in limited quantities only | Cheese, yogurt, icecream<br>Meat extract, yeast extract |
| Double cream (50 % fat) | Tinned vegetables |
| Sugar, glucose, honey, marmalade, jam | Tinned or packet soups |
| Pepper, herbs, spices, vinegar | Sauces, pickles, ready-made mustard |
| Powdered mustard | Chocolates, toffees, fudge, golden syrup, fruit gums, fruit pastilles |
| Salt substitutes (based on potassium chloride) may be used if serum potassium is normal or low | Tomato juice<br>Sultanas, raisins |
| Boiled sweets, peppermints, chewing-gum | |

Table 4 Low fat diet, with added MCT – suitable for child*

Long-chain fat should be restricted, to reduce steatorrhoea, and medium-chain triglycerides should be added to the diet to increase the energy content. The sample diet below is suitable for a child of 3- to 6-years old, and provides 50 g protein, 1500 kcal (6.3 MJ), 10 g LCT, and 50 g MCT.

| | |
|---|---|
| *Daily* | 500 ml (1 pint) MCT milk (see below) |
| *Breakfast* | Cereal, plus MCT milk and sugar<br>1 slice bread, toasted, no butter, with 2 tablespoons baked beans<br>1 cup MCT milk, with flavouring if desired |
| *Mid-morning* | Orange or blackcurrant fruit drink |
| *Dinner* | 25 g (1 oz) lean meat, or white fish<br>Potatoes, mashed or fried with 1 teaspoon MCT<br>Vegetables, no added fat<br>Custard or milk pudding, made with separated milk and 1 teaspoon MCT<br>Tinned fruit or jam |
| *Tea* | 25 g (1 oz) lean meat<br>Tomato or lettuce<br>1 slice bread, with MCT margarine (see below)<br>Fresh fruit<br>Cake or biscuit, made with MCT |
| *Bed-time* | MCT milk and flavouring |

Medium chain triglyceride oil (MCT) should be introduced slowly into the diet over several days, as it may cause gastrointestinal disturbance in the early stages, if administered rapidly. The oil should never be given undiluted, as a medicine, but always mixed with at least an equal quantity of fluid or food.

*MCT milk*
60 g skimmed milk powder
30 ml MCT oil
Water to 500 ml
Whisk together well
Commercially prepared milk powders containing MCT may be used if preferred.

*MCT margarine*
30 ml water
30 g (2 tablespoons) skimmed milk powder
15 ml (1 tablespoon) MCT
1–2 drops yellow colouring
Salt to taste
Mix the water and milk powder well, to a smooth cream. Whisk in the oil gradually, preferably with an electric mixer or rotary whisk. Add colouring and salt. Allow to thicken in the refrigerator for a few hours before use as a spread on bread.

*Vitamins* supplementation with 3 Ketovite tablets plus 5 ml Ketovite liquid (Paines & Byrne) is recommended.

---

* Dorothy E.M. Francis, *Diets for Sick Children*, Oxford: Blackwell

# Index